NICE SHOULDER COURSE

2010

Dépôt légal : mai 2010

I.S.B.N. : 978-2-84023-676-4
E.A.N. : 9782840236764

Imprimé en France

SHOULDER CONCEPTS 2010

THE GLENOID

under the direction of

G. WALCH, P. BOILEAU,D. MOLÉ,

L. FAVARD, C. LÉVIGNE, F. SIRVEAUX

sauramps medical

Montpellier - Paris

11, boulevard Henri IV - 34000 Montpellier
E-mail : sauramps.medical@wanadoo.fr

CONTRIBUTORS

Ghassan ALAMI, MD
Department of Orthopeadics
L'Archet 2 Hospital - University of Nice-Sophia-Antopilis
151 route de St Antoine de Ginestière
06200 Nice - France

Pascal BOILEAU, MD
Department of Orthopaedics
L'Archet 2 Hospital - University of Nice-Sophia-Antipolis
151, route de St Antoine de Ginestière
06200 Nice - France

Nicolas BONNEVIALLE, MD
Department of Orthopaedics
L'Archet 2 Hospital - University of Nice-Sophia-Antipolis
151 route de St Antoine de Ginestière
06200 Nice - France

Timothy BUNKER, MD
Nuffield Health Exeter Hospital
Wonford Road
Exeter Devon EX2 4UG
United Kingdom

W. Z. BURKHEAD, Jr, MD
WB Carrell Memorial Clinic
2909 Lemmon Ave
Dallas, TX 75204 2311
USA

Robert S. CHURCHILL, MD
Aurora Advanced Healthcare
12203 N. Corporate Pkwy,
Mequon, WI 53092
USA

Philippe CLAVERT, MD
Shoulder and Elbow Service
CCOM-CHU Strasbourg
10, avenue Baumann
67400 Illkirch - France

Robert H. COFIELD, MD
Orthopedic Surgery
Mayo Clinic in Rochester
200 First St. S.W.
Rochester, MN 55905
USA

Philippe COLLIN, MD
Service d'Orthopédie
Centre Hospitalier Privé
6 rue de la Boutière
35768 St Grégoire Cedex
France

Joe De BEER, MB, ChB, M Med
Cape Shoulder Institute
Cape Town
South Africa

Lieven De WILDE, MD
Dept. of Orthopaedic Surgery
Ghant University Hospital
De Pintelsan 185
9000 Gent
Belgium

T. Bradley EDWARDS, MD
Fondren Orthopedic Group, LLC
740 South Main Street
Houston, Texas 77030-4509
USA

Roger EMERY, MBBS, FRCS
Shoulder Unit
Hospital of St John and St Elizabeth
60 Grove End Road
London NW8 9NH
United Kingdom

Giuseppe FAMA, MD
Ortopedia e Traumatologia
Azienda Ospedaliera-University of Padua
Via Giustiniani, 2
35128 Padova
Italy

Alain FARRON, MD
Orthopédie et traumatologie
University of Lausanne
Avenue Pierre-Decker 4
CH-1011 Lausanne
Switzerland

Luc FAVARD, MD
Department of Orthopaedics-Traumatology I
CHU Trousseau
37044 Tours Cedex 1
France

Marc FRANKLE, MD
13020 Telecom Pkwy N
Temple Terrace, FL 33637
USA

François GADÉA, MD
44 rue Losserand
37000 Tours
France

Arnaud GODENÈCHE, MD
Centre Médical Santy
24 Avenue Paul Santy
69008 Lyon
France

Frank GOHLKE, MD
Orthopädische Klinik
König Ludwig Haus
Brettreistrasse, 11
97074 Wurzburg
Germany

Peter HABERMEYER, MD
ATOS Praxisklinik
Bismarckstr 9-15
Heidelberg, 69115
Germany

Heinz R. HOENECKE, MD
Sport Clinic
Sports Medicine, MS-116
10666 N Torrey Pines Rd
La Jolla, CA 92037
USA

Joseph IANNOTI, MD,PhD
Orthopaedic and Rheumatologic Institute
Cleveland Clinic Main Campus
Mail Code A41
9500 Euclid Avenue
Cleveland, OH 44195
USA

Bernhard JOST, MD
Uniklinik - Balgrist Forchstr.
340 CH-8008 Zürich
Switzerland

Simon LAMBERT, MD
The Shoulder and Elbow Service
Royal National Orthopaedic Hospital
Stanmore UK, HA7 4LP
United Kingdom

Christophe LÉVIGNE, MD
Clinique du Parc
86 Boulevard des Belges
69006 Lyon
France

William N. LEVINE, MD
Columbia Orthopaedics
622 West 168 Street, PH11-Center
New York, NY 10032
USA

Markus LOEW, MD
Department of Shoulder and Elbow Surgery
Orthopaedic University Clinic
Schlierbacher Landstr. 200a
69118 Heidelberg
Germany

Pierre MANSAT, MD, PhD
Department of Orthopaedics
CHU Purpan
Place du Dr Baylac
31059 Toulouse Cedex
France

Barbara MELIS, MD
Department of Orthopaedics
L'Archet 2 Hospital - University of Nice-Sophia-Antipolis
151 route de St Antoine de Ginestière
06200 Nice
France

Grégory MOINEAU, MD
Department of Orthopaedics
L'Archet 2 University Hospital
151 route de St Antoine de Ginestière
06200 Nice
France

Daniel MOLÉ, MD
Clinique Traumatologique et Orthopédique CS 5211
49, rue Hermite
54052 Nancy Cedex
France

Lionel NEYTON, MD
Centre Médical Santy
24 Avenue Paul Santy
69008 LYON
France

Tom NORRIS, MD
Orthopaedics
California Pacific Medical Center
2351 Clay St, #510
San Francisco, CA 94115 1931
USA

Dominique ROULEAU
Orthopedics
Sacré-Cœur Hospital
5400 Gouin Blvd W
Montréal QC H4J 1C5
Canada

François SIRVEAUX, MD, PhD
Clinique de Traumatologie et d'Orthopédie
49 rue Hermite
54000 Nancy
France

Alexandre TERRIER, MD
EPFL STI CBT LBO
Ecole Polytechnique Fédérale de Lausanne
AI 1137 (Bâtiment AI) Station 15
CH-1015 Lausanne
Switzerland

Philippe VALENTI, MD
Institut de la Main
6 Square Jouvenet
75016 Paris
France

Gilles WALCH, MD
Centre Médical Santy
24 Avenue Paul Santy
69008 Lyon
France

W. Angus WALLACE, MD
Division of Orthopaedic & Accident Surgery
Queen's Medical Centre
Nottingham NG7 2UH
United Kingdom

Allan YOUNG
Centre Médical Santy
24 Avenue Paul Santy
69008 Lyon
France

TABLE OF CONTENTS

Preface
P. BOILEAU

ANATOMY & BIOMECHANICS OF THE GLENOID

Genetic and Biomechanical Determinants of Glenoid Version: Implications for Glenoid Implant Placement in Shoulder Arthroplasty
J.P. LANDAU, H.R. HOENECKE 13

Anatomy of the Glenoid Revisited - Morphobiometry of the Scapula
P. CLAVERT, J. BOUCHAÏB, J.-F. KEMPF 23

Glenoid Implants: History, Design, & Rationale-PE/MB, Flat/Curved, Peg/Keel, Screws, Reverse
A. GODENÈCHE 29

Biomechanics of anatomical & resurfaced glenoid
A. FARRON, A. TERRIER 33

Does implant design influence glenoid constraints: A finite element analysis
P. MANSAT, J. BRIOT, M. MANSAT, P. SWIDER 37

THE MULTICENTER STUDY: PRESENTATION & METHODOLOGY

The Glenoid in the Horizontal Plane : Walch Classification - Revisited Humeral Subluxation and Glenoid Retroversion
D.M ROULEAU, J.F. KIDDER, J. PONS-VILLANUEVA, S. DYNAMIDIS, M.J DEFRANCO, G. WALCH 45

The Glenoid in the frontal plane: the Favard and the Hamada radiographic classifications of cuff tear osteoarthritis
L. FAVARD, G. ALAMI 53

THE GLENOID IN HEMIARTHROPLASTY

Results of Hemiarthroplasty in Primary Osteoarthritis
W.N. LEVINE 59

Biological Resurfacing for Glenohumeral Arthritis Then and Now
W.Z. BURKHEAD J[R], S.G. KRISHNAN 67

Arthroscopic Biological Resurfacing of the Glenoid in Glenohumeral Arthritis: Two to five year outcomes of a pilot study
J.F. DE BEER, D.N. BHATIA 71

Hemiarthroplasty: Long-Term Survorship and Outcomes
F. GADEA, G.B. ALAMI, J. KIDDER, M. PFAHLER, C. LÉVIGNE, L. FAVARD 75

Predictive Factors of Glenoid Erosion
G. FAMA, F. SIRVEAUX, G. PAPE, F. GADEA, L. FAVARD 85

What is the ideal etiology and preoperative glenoid status for shoulder hemiarthroplasty?
L. FAVARD, D. MOLÉ, J.C. BALESTRO, C. TROJANI, G. ALAMI, F. GADEA 93

THE GLENOID IN ANATOMICAL TOTAL SHOULDER ARTHROPLASTY

Long-term results of a flat-back polyethylene glenoid component in primary osteoarthritis - a multi-center study
G. WALCH, A. YOUNG, F. GOHLKE, R. PHILIPPE, L. FAVARD, P. BOILEAU 103

Results of the convex back cemented keeled glenoid component in primary osteoarthritis - Multicentric study with a follow-up > 5 years
G. WALCH, A. YOUNG, B. MÉLIS, D. GAZIELLY, M. LOEW, P. BOILEAU 117

A 10 Year Radiological Comparison of Two All-Polyethylene Glenoid Component Designs - A Prospective Trial
P. COLLIN, A. TAY, B. MELIS, P. BOILEAU, G. WALCH 131

Results of Uncemented, Metal-Backed Glenoid Implants: A North American Experience
R.H. COFIELD, M.J. TAUNTON 141

Results of Uncemented, Metal-back Glenoid Implants: The UK Experience
W.A. WALLACE 145

Long-term Results and Survival of Uncemented Metal-Back Glenoid Implants in Primary Glenohumeral Osteoarthritis
G. MOINEAU, A. GODENÈCHE, N. MORIN SALVO, B. MÉLIS, C. LÉVIGNE, L. FAVARD, D. MOLÉ, M. CARLES, G. WALCH, P. BOILEAU 149

Factors for proper exposure, preparation and cementing technique of the glenoid implant
M. LOEW, D. GAZIELLY, P. RAISS, G. PAPE 163

Radiographic comparison of pegged and keeled glenoid components using modern cementing techniques: A prospective randomized study
T.B. EDWARDS, J.E. LABRIOLA, R.J. STANLEY, D.P. O'CONNOR, H.A. ELKOUSY, G.M. GARTSMAN 167

Pegged Versus Keeled Glenoids: A Retrospective Study
R.H. COFIELD, T.W. THROCKMORTON 179

Clinical and Radiographic Analysis of a Partially Cemented Glenoid Implant - 5 Year Minimum Follow-Up
R.S. CHURCHILL, C. ZELLMER, H.J. ZIMMERS, R. RUGGERO 185

HOW TO DEAL WITH GLENOID DEFICIENCY

Hybrid glenoid resurfacing: experience and results
S.M. LAMBERT 195

Clinical and radiological follow-up of the Aequalis third-generation cemented total shoulder replacement - A minimum ten-year study
A. KHAN, T.D. BUNKER, J.B. KITSON 203

Glenoid failure: Material or Surgical Failure. Assessment of polyethylene-wear patterns in relation to glenoid component positioning in Total Shoulder Replacement: A three-dimensional CT study
R. EMERY, T. GREGORY 215

Recentering the Humeral Head in the Horizontal Plane in TSA
P. HABERMEYER 221

New Methods of Pre Operative Planning for Management of Glenoid Bone Loss
J.P. IANNOTTI 233

Horizontal glenoid deficiency (B2 & C) results of glenoid bone graft in primary TSA
C. LÉVIGNE, J. GARRET, P. BOILEAU, C. MORAGA, G. WALCH 243

Augmented Glenoid Component for Bone Deficiency
R.H. COFIELD, R.S. RICE 251

THE ERODED GLENOID & THE LOOSE GLENOID - GLENOID RECONSTRUCTION & REVISION

Revision of humeral head replacement to total shoulder arthroplasty for glenoid erosion: outcomes of the anatomic versus the reverse glenoid
F. SIRVEAUX, F. WEIN, J. ARMENGOL, J. PORCELLINI 255

Lessons Learned from the Hylamer Experience & Technical Salvage for Glenoid Reconstruction
T.R. NORRIS, S. ABDUS-SALAAM 265

Glenoid removal or glenoid bone grafting?
L. NEYTON, B. MELIS, N. BONNEVIALLE, P. BOILEAU 279

Aseptic Glenoid Loosening or Failure in Total Shoulder Arthroplasty: Results of Revision with Glenoid Reimplantation
N. BONNEVIALLE, B. MELIS, L. NEYTON, C. TROJANI, P. BOILEAU 287

Aseptic Glenoid Loosening or Failure in Total Shoulder Arthroplasty: Results of Revision with Reverse Shoulder Arthroplasty
B. MELIS, N. BONNEVIALLE, L. NEYTON, G. WALCH, P. BOILEAU 299

Revision of failed hemi-arthroplasty to reverse total shoulder arthroplasty through a transhumeral approach
F. GOHLKE, J. STEHLE, B. WERNER 313

THE GLENOID IN REVERSE SHOULDER ARTHROPLASTY

Reverse total shoulder arthroplasty and glenoid notching
B. JOST, C. GERBER 323

Biomechanics of Reverse Shoulder Arthroplasty
M. WALKER, M. WILLIS, J. BROOKS, M. FRANKLE 329

Lateralization in the design of the reverse shoulder arthroplasty. Is it dangerous? Is it useful?
P. VALENTI, D. KATZ, P. SAUZIERES, A. KILINC 353

Biomechanical Rationale for BIO-RSA & Metallic Lateralization
A. TERRIER, A. FARRON 365

Bony Increased-Offset Reversed Shoulder Arthroplasty (BIO-RSA): The Benefits of Bony Lateralization
P. BOILEAU, G. MOINEAU, Y. ROUSSANNE, K. O'SHEA 371

Polyethylene Wear in Anatomic and Reversed Shoulder Prostheses
A. FARRON, A. TERRIER 389

Influence of Sphere Diameter on Radiographic and Clinical Results of RSA
L. DE WILDE 393

Results of glenoid bone graft in primary reverse shoulder arthroplasty
C. LÉVIGNE, J. GARRET, S. GROSCLAUDE 403

Revision of glenoid component in Reverse Shoulder Arthroplasty
D. MOLÉ, C. DEZALY, F. SIRVEAUX 411

Long-term outcomes with the reverse shoulder prosthesis: 10 to 15 years of follow-up
L. FAVARD, G. ALAMI, A. YOUNG, C. DEZALY, V. FALAISE 421

Pattern of loosening of polyethylene keeled glenoid components in primary osteo-arthritis - A multicenter study with follow-up >5 years
G. WALCH, A. YOUNG, P. BOILEAU 427

PREFACE

Both hemiarthroplasty and total shoulder arthroplasty have proven to be effective in pain relief and improvement of function in patients with an arthritic shoulder. This procedure has changed the life of thousands of people over the world who had a painful, stiff shoulder. However, the glenoid remains the weak link of shoulder replacement, whether it has been resurfaced or not. There are concerns regarding the occurrence of glenoid component loosening and glenoid erosion.

To date, too many questions regarding the glenoid remain unanswered. What is the biomechanics of the glenoid? Where does glenoid wear take place in anatomical total shoulder arthroplasty? What is the real benefit of glenoid resurfacing for the patient with osteoarthritis? In primary glenohumeral osteoarthritis, should the surgeon do a hemiarthroplasty or total shoulder arthroplasty? Is glenoid resurfacing always necessary? What are the long-term results of hemiarthroplasty in the different diagnoses? What is the place of humeral resurfacing? Are they alternatives to prosthetic glenoid resurfacing? What is the place of biologic resurfacing? In case of glenoid resurfacing, should the surgeon use an all-polyethylene cemented or a metal-back uncemented glenoid component? A flat-back or a keeled convex glenoid implant? A pegged or a keeled glenoid implant? Where are we today with new implants and new technologies? What is the exact survival rate of glenoid cemented and uncemented glenoid resurfacing? Which are the factors that contribute or are associated with glenoid loosening or failures: prosthesis malpositioning, secondary rotator cuff tears, prosthetic instability, polyethylene wear, low-grade infection? In case of glenoid loosening or failure, how to evaluate and quantify the glenoid bone defect? How to reconstruct the glenoid? What are the complications associated with glenoid loosening or failure? What are the results of glenoid reconstruction and revision surgery? Is it logical to reimplant a glenoid implant or should we just remove and/or bone graft the glenoid? If a glenoid implant is needed, should the surgeon re-implant a non-constrained glenoid component or a reverse glenoid component? Which approach to expose the glenoid in RSA? What are the limits of prosthetic reimplantation? What are results of reverse reimplantation with and without Bone Graft? What is the influence of lateralization on radiological and clinical results of the RSA?

A glenoid data base of more than 1600 patients operated on for a shoulder replacement, with or without glenoid resurfacing, has been created to answer some of these questions. Eight multicenter studies have been performed and are the basis of this 'Glenoid Day' and of this book.

This extensive experience will be reported in Nice, France on May 22, 2010 during the Nice Shoulder Course. We hope that the material presented here will help shoulder surgeons to provide the best care for their patients and will serve as a basis for future studies and research.

Pascal Boileau, Gilles Walch, Daniel Molé,
Luc Favard, Christophe Lévigne, François Sirveaux
Nice, May 7, 2010

GENETIC AND BIOMECHANICAL DETERMINANTS OF GLENOID VERSION: IMPLICATIONS FOR GLENOID IMPLANT PLACEMENT IN SHOULDER ARTHROPLASTY

J.P. LANDAU, H.R. HOENECKE

INTRODUCTION

Glenoid version (defined as the angle between the glenoid face and the scapular body) changes significantly with arthritis. In shoulder arthroplasty, restoration of glenoid version to normal values is recommended. The relationship of the glenoid cavity to the scapular body, however, is extremely variable. This raises the question of the relevance of the relationship of the glenoid face to the scapular body.

The current understanding of the relationship between scapular osseous anatomy and function is limited. There are some currently accepted definitions of "normal" relationships that theoretically carry some implications on biomechanics, function, and the development of pathologic states.

Clinicians have made assumptions about the relationships between pathologic conditions of the glenohumeral joint and abnormalities in glenoid version. The mature adult glenoid neck and face may be considered the final target or end result of scapular development. From a simplified point of view, the ultimate goal in the development of the scapula is to create a stable articular platform to allow force transmission across the glenohumeral joint. Keeping this target in mind, an analysis of the embryologic and genetic determinants of osseous anatomy will help to understand the anatomic and biomechanical pathologic changes seen in glenohumeral disease states.

The goal of this paper is to advance our conceptual understanding of scapular morphology in health and diseased states through an exploration of the existing literature regarding scapular anatomy, genetics, and embryology. The relationship between osseous and soft-tissue developmental factors will be analyzed by evaluating specific disease states such as brachial plexus birth palsy, glenoid retroversion with posterior glenohumeral subluxation, glenoid hypoplasia, and Sprengel's Deformity. Through analysis of these disease states, we hope to elucidate the genetic and biomechanical determinants of glenoid version.

GLENOID VERSION

Our current conceptual model of scapular biomechanics and function is based on a range of accepted "normal" relationships between the glenoid and the scapular body. Before CT scans, the technique for measuring glenoid version was based on axial radiographs. The technique described by Saha in 1971 is to draw a line from the center point of the glenoid to the junction between the medial border of the scapula and the scapular spine [14]. The glenoid version is defined as the angle between this line and the line between the most anterior and the most posterior margin of bone of the glenoid. Friedman *et al.* [5] adapted this technique to provide a measurement technique for glenoid version based on CT scans (fig. 1). They found a mean of 2 degrees ± 5 degrees of glenoid anteversion in 63 normal control subjects. They found 11 degrees ± 8 degrees of retroversion in patients with osteoarthritis or inflammatory arthritis. The conclusion based on this data was that reconstructive surgical techniques should aim to restore glenoid version to approximately 2 degrees of anteversion utilizing eccentric reaming or posterior bone grafting.

We have used 3-D CT technology to study the variability in the relationship between the glenoid and the scapular body (fig. 2). The axial images can be processed to produce a slice outline of the bony anatomy of the scapular body, neck, and glenoid at the level of the glenoid center (fig. 3). The osseous relationship appears to be extremely variable. This broad range of variability is not characteristic of most other bones. The variability seems to be organized into three categories: body shape (curved vs. flat), glenoid translation (anterior, centered, posterior), and glenoid version (anteversion, neutral, retroversion). Figure 4 depicts these categories conceptually. The scapular morphology appears to be somewhat modular, with the body being one component and the glenoid being a second component. These two components are situated separately in space, and then joined by a bridge of tissue forming the glenoid vault.

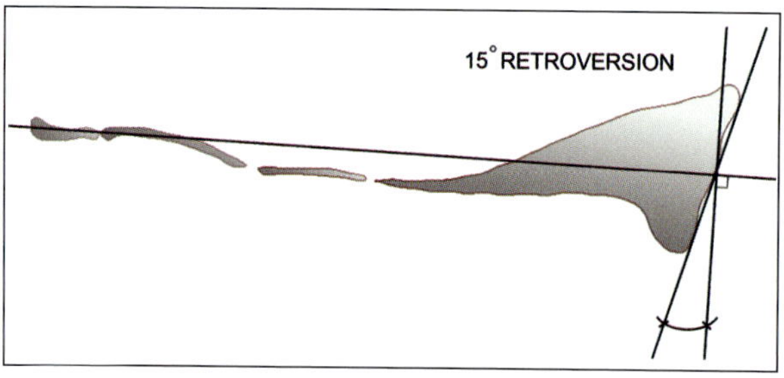

Fig. 1: Measurement of Glenoid Version

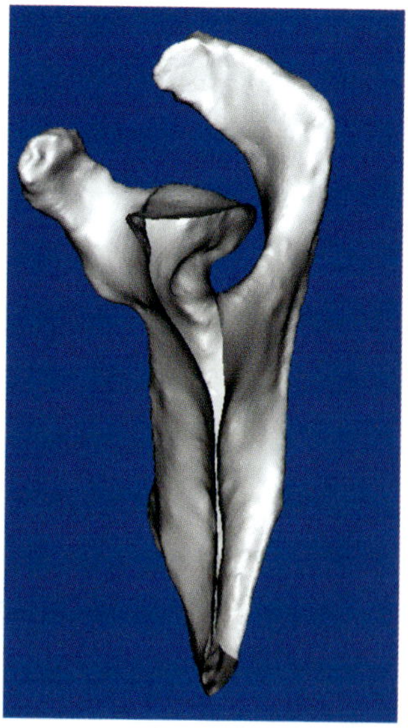

Fig. 2: Example of a 3-D CT reconstruction used to identify the center of the glenoid and to create a slice outline to analyze the relationship between the scapular body, the neck, and the glenoid in normal subjects.

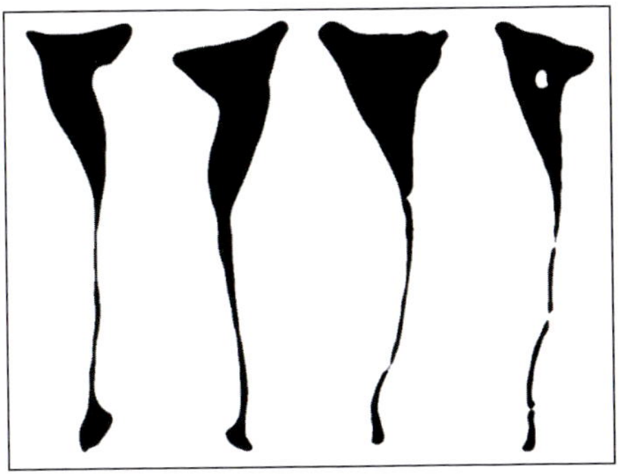

Fig. 3: CT scan slice outlines of the right scapulae from four different normal cadaveric subjects.

The osseous development of the scapula is mostly formed by intramembranous ossification by at least eight ossification centers (fig. 5) [6]. There are multiple growth centers that ossify to form the acromion, one for the body of the scapula, one for the medial border, one for the inferior angle, two for the coracoid, and two for the glenoid. The glenoid has one superior growth center that is at the base of the coracoid, and one horseshoe shaped growth center inferiorly. The inferior center is thin at its center and thicker peripherally to form the concavity and shape of the glenoid.

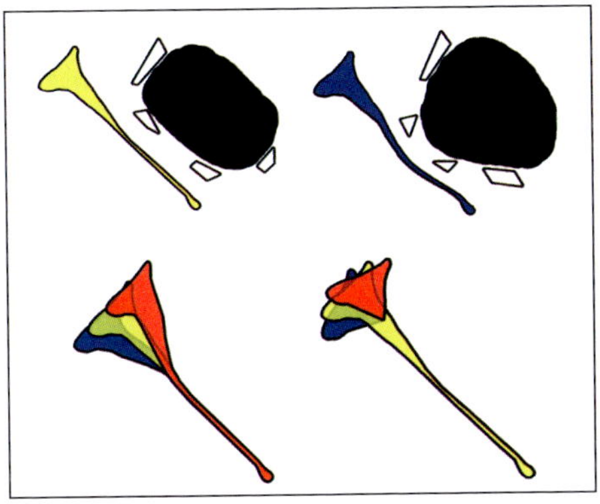

Fig. 4: The modular scapula: variations in normal scapular morphology can be expressed in terms of the shape of the scapular body, the glenoid translation, and the glenoid version.

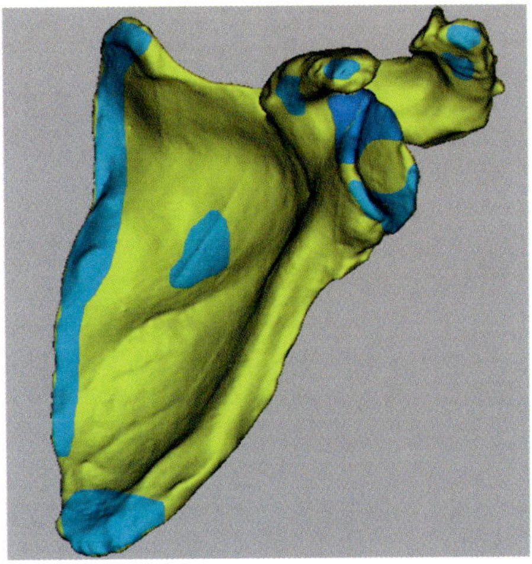

Fig. 5: Ossification Centers of the Scapula

SCAPULAR EMBRYOLOGY AND GENETICS

Why is there so much variability in scapular morphology? How is the scapula formed and are malformations the result of intrinsic genetic developmental mishaps, or the result of pathological influences from extrinsic sources?

The scapula differentiates at fetal week five and is located at the level of the fourth, fifth, and sixth cervical vertebrae [7]. By eight weeks of development, all limb structures are present. Early on, the scapula is wider than it is tall, as is the case in quadrupeds. As the human fetus develops, the scapular body elongates until the length is greater than the width. This allows for increased motion of the upper extremity for a bipedal human.

Additionally, there is a caudal migration of the scapula as there is differential growth within the spine resulting in the final position of the scapula to be at the level of the second through seventh thoracic ribs. In Sprengel's Deformity, the scapula remains undescended and develops in a different muscular and bony milieu. The normal elongation does not occur, and the surrounding musculature becomes infiltrated with fibrofatty tissue [2]. Additionally, the scapular body is curved over the superior aspect of the chest wall, as if accommodating to the shape of the thoracic cage. This will interfere with normal scapulothoracic motion if this deformity is not addressed at the time of corrective surgery. Although the position of the scapula can be surgically lowered with respect to the thorax, the shape of the scapular body still matches the curvature of the upper part of the thorax, thereby resulting in scapulothroacic incongruency. Even in patients without Sprengel's Deformity, it appears that the bodies of some scapulae are curved, and some are flat and this appears to be dependent upon the shape of the adjacent rib cage (fig. 4). From the undescended scapula, it appears as if the shape of the body is at least heavily influenced if not determined by the surrounding muscular and bony envelope, rather than a predetermined genetic design.

Where does the tissue that forms the scapula come from? Shoulder girdle development is commonly grouped together with the limb formation, however this is probably not an accurate conceptual grouping. There are three embryologic structures that appear to play a significant role in limb development: the apical ectodermal ridge (AER), the Wingless-type (Wnt) pathway, and the Zone of Polarizing Activity (ZPA). Multiple studies have shown, however, that interfering with these pathways interferes with limb development but does not affect the scapula or shoulder girdle [15, 16].

There are, however, a number of genes that have been found to govern specific portions of scapular development. These include the Pax1 gene, the Emx2 gene, and the Hoxc6 gene. Figure 6 summarizes these genes and their location of primary influence.

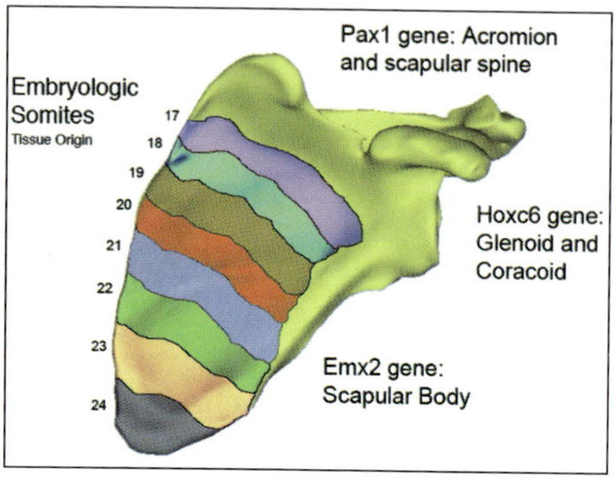

Fig. 6: Regions of genetic influence governing scapular development.

The Pax1 gene controls development of the acromion and scapular spine. Genetic knockout analysis has found that if the Pax1 gene is lacking, then the acromion and part of the scapular spine is missing [19].

The Emx2 gene controls development of the scapular body, as well as the ilium. Knockout mice lacking Emx2 results in a complete absence of the body of the scapula, while the distal end of the acromion is present and articulates with the clavicle. The coracoid and the glenoid cavity develop normally, and glenoid articulates with the humeral head normally [13]. Interestingly, these mice also lacked the majority of the ilium. This implies that the iliac wing may be a homolog to the scapular body. This pattern of pathology has been noted clinically in humans by Cousin *et al.* [4] who described pelviscapular dysplasia with bilateral agenesis of the wing of the scapula and hypoplasia of the ilium. It appears that scapular body development is not governed by the same genetic mechanism that governs the development of the acromion, coracoid, and glenoid.

Emx2 is also intensely expressed in the mesonephros, the tissue that forms the urogenital system is being formed [13]. Some have hypothesized that spine, cardiac, scapular, and urogenital pathological congenital conditions are often associated because these structures are all being formed at the same embryological time period. This genetic link, however, may implicate a genetic etiology, rather than an environmental insult to the fetus at a vulnerable time period.

The Hoxc6 gene controls the development of the coracoid and glenoid. Isolated abnormalities of the coracoid and glenoid have been seen with Hoxc6 defects. Expanding expression of Hoxc6 genes results in duplicate shoulder coracoid and acromion formation in chick embryos [11]. This has been seen clinically in humans (fig. 7) as reported by McClure *et al.* [10]

Additional information on the origin of the scapular tissue has been further elucidated through an avian model. Huang *et al.* [8] found that the scapula has a dual origin. The glenoid and acromion is formed from the somatopleura. In contrast, the body of the scapula is derived from a compartment called the dermomyotome that also serves as the precursor for all the musculature of the trunk. Why does the scapular body have so many different muscular attachments? Huang *et al.* found that the scapular body was divided into segments, formed by the coalescence of tissue derived from multiple embryologic somites. Interestingly, each somite is responsible for creating a portion of the bone, as well as the respective muscle and connective tissue that is attached to that specific segment (fig. 6). This implies that the scapular body is not a skeletal element proper, but rather an ossifying muscle attachment [3].

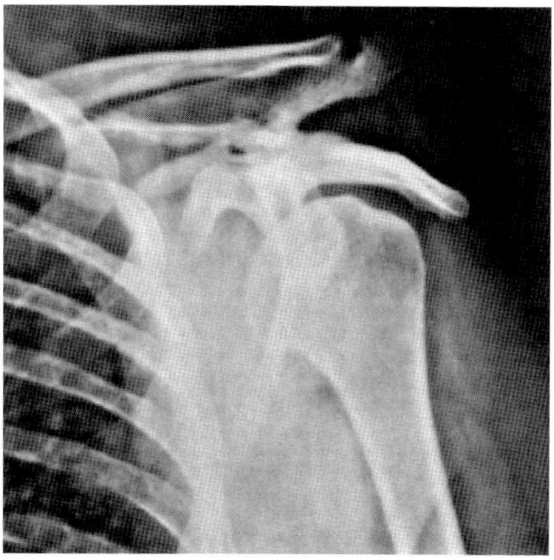

Fig. 7: Double acromion and coracoid process. *(Reprinted with permission from McClure et al. [10])*

Kieny *et al.* [9] found that transplanted cervical presomites into the thorax did not form ribs, but did form normal scapula. This implies that the scapula is formed based on local environmental cues. Alternatively, transplanting thoracic somites into the cervical region causes cervical ribs to form, but does not form scapula, further supporting that the scapula only forms according to the correct environmental cues. From this information combined with the information we learned by analyzing the scapular deformity seen with Sprengel's Deformity, it appears that the scapular body and the surrounding ligaments and musculature are formed within a soft-tissue sleeve that depends on signals and structure from the local environment. This development is governed by separate genes and is from distinctly separate tissue than those controlling the acromion, coracoid, and glenoid development.

By analyzing the embryology and genetics governing scapular development, it appears that the scapular body and the glenoid develop from two completely separate tissues, and are governed by independent forces. The body seems to be more of an ossified muscular attachment whose development depends on the surrounding muscular sleeve, while the glenoid has separate ossification centers and develops according to genetic composition.

POSTERIOR GLENOHUMERAL SUBLUXATION

How do these embryological findings help us understand glenoid retroversion and posterior subluxation? Are these manifestations of an isolated developmental bony deformity? How much does soft-tissue balance play a role?

Historically, orthopaedic surgeons have approached understanding the glenohumeral relationship from primarily a bony standpoint. In the case of glenoid retroversion and posterior subluxation, the solution intuitively would be to fix the retroversion, which should theoretically center the humeral head, resulting in less pain, and less progression of arthritis. Brewer *et al.* [1] reported a small series of five patients who underwent corrective glenoid osteotomy with posterior capsular imbrication for the treatment of non-traumatic adolescent patients with posterior instability. All shoulders became stable and functional (one required revision due to loss of correction), but with only one to two years follow-up, and glenoid version analysis was performed with axillary radiographs, rather than computed tomography.

In contrast, Walch *et al.* [17] studied a small select population of patients under forty years old who presented with retroversion of the glenoid and posterior subluxation and performed glenoid neck corrective osteotomies. In their first two patients, they performed corrective glenoid osteotomies with capsular imbrication. They abandoned this procedure because it did not successfully center the humeral head. The posterior subluxation continued despite changing the angle between the glenoid face and the scapular body. The cause-and-effect relationship between glenoid version and humeral subluxation is not as straightforward as it seems. Glenohumeral subluxation is likely governed by a complex interaction between bony architecture and soft-tissue balance.

Brewer *et al.* [1] implicate faulty ossification centers of the glenoid as the cause for the excessive glenoid retroversion, stating that abnormalities of the ossification center at the base of the coracoid explain posterior rotation of the glenoid (fig. 5). Similarly, abnormalities of the horseshoe shaped ossification in the mid-glenoid area results in flattening of the glenoid fossa. Interestingly, these ossification centers appear at 10 and 15 years old respectively. It may be that there is a combination of osseous developmental abnormalities and soft-tissue imbalances that both contribute to posterior subluxation and an incongruous joint.

BRACHIAL PLEXUS BIRTH PALSY

The relationship between osseous deformity and soft-tissue balance becomes more clearly elucidated by studying the glenoid changes seen in Brachial Plexus Birth Palsy (BPBP). Pearl and Edgerton [12] studied 25 children with internal rotation contractures from BPBP with arthrograms to define glenoid deformities due to chronic shoulder abduction and external rotation palsy. Seven had normal glenoids, there were 17 abnormal posterior glenoids. Five of these had flattening, seven biconcave, six had pseudoglenoid with a concavity separate and posterior from the original articular surface. The severity of glenoid abnormality was directly associated with the severity of the internal rotation contracture. Although all types of deformity were seen at all ages, there was a significant correlation between age and severity of glenoid deformity.

In a similar study, Waters *et al.* [18] prospectively followed ninety-four patients with BPBP to determine the relationship of age and severity of muscular weakness on glenohumeral joint deformity. Only forty-two patients had persistent weakness. These patients were evaluated with CT and MRI. They found mean retroversion of 25 degrees compared to 5 degrees on the contralateral normal side. They also found that the more glenoid deformity, the more posterior subluxation of the humeral head. They also found an association between retroversion and age. Interestingly, the osseous anatomy of scapular body and the glenoid vault was typically normal as seen on a plain x-ray with the changes in the scapula confined to the cartilage covering the glenoid face. This implies that the growth disturbance was not an intrinsic problem with the bone, but rather an impairment of the cartilaginous development of the posterior glenoid. Given that the contralateral shoulder was normal in these children, extrinsic muscle imbalance must play a significant role in the symmetric growth of the glenoid. Genetic influences do not appear to be significant. The severe glenohumeral osseous deformities were not seen until patients were past their adolescent growth spurt. One of their conclusions was that severe muscle imbalance leads to early dislocation, rather than an osseous abnormality. It is noted that infantile shoulder dislocation leads to rapid severe osseous deformity. It appears that if bony abnormalities do not cause posterior subluxation then correcting the bony deformity may not correct the subluxation.

From examining patients with Brachial Plexus Birth Palsy, it is clear that the development of osseous deformity of the glenoid is governed or at least strongly influenced by extrinsic muscular balance across the glenohumeral joint.

GLENOID HYPOPLASIA

Now that we have an understanding of the different tissue sources and genetic variables involved in creating a normal scapular body and glenoid, we can look clinically at cases where this developmental process goes astray.

Wirth, Lyons, and Rockwood [20] reported on sixteen patients who were found to have what they termed "hypoplasia of the glenoid". Thirteen were bilateral, and the presenting complaint was pain. Severe hypoplasia was defined as having extensive hypoplasia of the inferior part of the glenoid, marked dysplasia of the humeral head, varus angulation of the humeral head, apparent joint incongruity, and associated scapular abnormalities, including an enlarged and inferiorly directed acromion, a prominent coracoid process, and hooking of the distal part of the clavicle. In this study, the patients did well with conservative physiotherapy treatment. They did not find a familial pattern. All patients had pain, six lost range of motion, and five had symptomatic instability. The severity of hypoplasia correlated with the loss of range of motion. Interestingly, one patient with ten years of symptoms with moderate hypoplasia had an arthroscopic examination, which revealed a congruent joint space and normal-appearing cartilage. They noted that only two patients in the study developed osteoarthrosis and during the course of the study they performed more than 600 reconstructive shoulder procedures, and not one of these operations was for the treatment of problems associated with glenoid hypoplasia.

SUMMARY

Understanding the embryology and genetics of scapular development can help us understand the pathomechanics and pathoanatomy found in various forms of glenohumeral disease states. The glenoid is formed from two ossification centers: a subcoracoid superior center, which may be implicated in the determination of physiologic glenoid version and an inferior horseshoe-shaped center that may be implicated in glenoid hypoplasia and the development of a shallow socket. The shapes of the glenoid and the scapular body are governed by separate forces. The body is dependent upon the surrounding thoracic shape and the surrounding muscular sleeve. The glenoid face and vault seem to connect to the scapular body in a modular-type fashion, with resultant normal variations in glenoid translation and version. The Emx2 gene appears to be integral to the body formation. In contrast, the Hoxc6 gene is integral for glenoid development. The Pax1 gene governs development of the acromion. Patients with brachial plexus birth palsy teach us that the glenoid development is an ongoing process through the course of childhood development and is highly dependent on the balance of muscular forces across the glenohumeral joint. In the adult patient with static posterior glenohumeral subluxation, corrective glenoid osteotomy does not necessarily correct posterior humeral subluxation, suggesting that abnormalities of glenoid version may not be the primary cause of the subluxation. The osseous glenoid and scapular body should be considered independently. The angle formed between the glenoid face and the scapular body may be less important in understanding glenohumeral biomechanics than we previously have thought. The traditional definition of glenoid version therefore may be less relevant when making decisions regarding the position of glenoid prosthesis placement during shoulder arthroplasty. Understanding soft-tissue and muscular balance and their interaction with the developing anatomy of the scapula may assist in the proper treatment of glenohumeral disorders.

ACKNOWLEDGEMENTS

Cesar Flores and David Avi Gordon for contributions in graphic development.

REFERENCES

[1] BREWER BJ, WUBBEN RC, and CARRERA GF. Excessive retroversion of the glenoid cavity. A cause of non-traumatic posterior instability of the shoulder. *J Bone Joint Surg Am 1986; 68: 724-31.*

[2] CAVENDISH ME. Congenital elevation of the scapula. *J Bone Joint Surg (Br) 1972; 54-B:395-408.*

[3] CHRIST B, and WILTING J. From somites to vertebral column. *Ann Anat 1992; 174: 23-32.*

[4] COUSIN J, WALBAUM R, CEGARRA P, HUGUET J, LOUIS J, PAULI A, *et al* Familial pelvi-scapulary dysplasia with anomalies of the epiphyses, dwarfism and dysmorphy: a new syndrome? *Arch Fr Pediatr 1982; 39: 173-75.*

[5] FRIEDMAN RJ, HAWTHORNE KB, and GENEZ BM. The use of computerized tomography in the measurement of glenoid version. *J Bone Joint Surg Am 1992; 74: 1032-37.*

[6] GARDNER E, and GRAY DJ. Prenatal development of the human shoulder and acromioclavicular joints. *Am J Anat 1953; 92: 219-76.*

[7] GROGAN DP, STANLEY EA, BOBECHKO WP. The congenital undescended scapula. *J Bone Joint Surg (Br) 1983; 65-B, N° 5: 598-605.*

[8] HUANG R, ZHI Q, PATEL K, WILTING J, CHRIST B. Dual origin and segmental organisation of the avian scapula. *Development 2000; 127(17): 3789-94.*

[9] KIENY M, MAUGER A, and SENGEL P. Early regionalization of the somite mesoderm as studied by the development of the axial skeleton of the chick embryo. *Dev Biol 1972; 28: 142-61.*

[10] McCLURE JG, RANEY RB. Double acromion and coracoid process: Case report of an anomaly of the scapula. *J Bone and Joint Surg Am 1974; 56: 830-32.*

[11] OLIVER G, DE ROBERTIS EM, WOLPERT L, TICKLE C. Expression of a homeobox gene in the chick wing bud following application of retinoic acid and grafts of polarizing region tissue. *EMBO J 1990; 9: 3093-99.*

[12] PEARL ML, EDGERTON BW. Glenoid Deformity Secondary to Brachial Plexus Birth Palsy. *J Bone Joint Surg Am 1998; 80: 659-67.*

[13] PELLEGRINI M, PANTOANO S, FUMI MP, LUCCHINI F, FORABOSCO A. Agenesis of the scapula in Emx2 Homozygous Mutants. *Dev Biology 2001; 232: 149-56.*

[14] SAHA AK. Dynamic stability of the glenohumeral joint. *Aeta Orthop. Scandinavica 1971. 42: 491-505.*

[15] SAUNDERS JW. The proximo-distal sequence of origin of the parts of the chick wing and the role of the ectoderm. *J Exp Zool 1948; 108: 363-403.*

[16] SPATER D, HILL TP, GRUBER M, HARTMANN C. Role of canonical wnt-signaling in joint formation. *European Cells and Materials 2006; 12: 71-80.*

[17] WALCH G, ASCANI C, BOULAHIA A, NOVE-JOSSERAND L, EDWARDS TB. Static posterior subluxation of the humeral head: an unrecognized entity responsible for glenohumeral osteoarthritis in the young adult. *J Shoulder Elbow Surg 2002; 11(4): 309-14.*

[18] WATERS PM, SMITH GR, and JARAMILLO D. Glenohumeral Deformity Secondary to Brachial Plexus Birth Palsy. *J Bone Joint Surg Am 1998; 80: 668-77.*

[19] WILM B, DAHL E, PETERS H, BALLING R, and IMAI K. Targeted disruption of Pax1 defines its null phenotype and proves haploinsufficiency. *Proc Natl Acad Sci 1998; 95: 8692-97.*

[20] WIRTH MA, LYONS FR, ROCKWOOD CA. Hypoplasia of the glenoid. A review of sixteen patients. *J. Bone Joint Surg. Am. 1993; 75: 1175-84.*

ANATOMY OF THE GLENOID REVISITED - MORPHOBIOMETRY OF THE SCAPULA

P. CLAVERT, J. BOUCHAÏB, J.-F. KEMPF

INTRODUCTION

The mobility of the upper limb involves the glenohumeral joint and also the scapulothoracic joint. The glenoid is the articular surface of the scapula in contact with the humeral head. Its complex anatomy reflects all the functions of the upper limb and obeys a paradox: it has to have a strong fulcrum to allow the prehension and the technical movements executed by the upper limb; but it also has to respect imperatives of stability and adaptation to the mechanical constraints to maintain a functional joint. The scapulo-humeral joint is a compromise between mobility and stability. The restoration of the biomechanics of the shoulder is an essential pre-requisite for a prosthetic replacement.

A CONFIGURATION FAVORABLE TO MOBILITY

The osseous development of the scapula is mostly formed by intramembranous ossification of 8 ossification centers. It differentiates at fetal week 5. As the human fetus develops, the scapular body elongates until the length is greater than the width [1]. This allows for increased motion of the upper extremity. Additionally, there is a caudal migration resulting in the final position of the scapula to be at the level of the 2nd through 7th thoracic ribs [2].

Descriptive Anatomy [3]

The scapula is a flat, triangular bone. It suspends the upper limb to the thorax. It allows the mobility through its articular surface, the glenoid, and through the scapulothoracic bursae. The scapula is oriented anteriorly at an angle of 30° to the thorax. in the resting position, the scapula is oriented 3° upward and medial in the frontal plan; and 20° upward and anteriorly in the sagittal plan [4-6].

Most standard anatomical textbooks describe the glenoid cavity as pear-shaped or having a inverted comma-shape. It is globally ovoid, flared downward. It faces the humeral head and is directed forward, upward and laterally. On average it measures 35 mm of carnio-caudal diameter and 25 mm of antero-posterior diameter [7]. The anterior edge of the glenoid is disrupted by a more or less marked notch around the upper one-third (located slightly below the junction between 2 ossification centers), allowing one to disting with several shapes of glenoids. At least it divides the glenoid into 2 parts with regard to the tilting angle and radius of curvature (the lower part, directed slightly anteriorly with a small radius of curvature, and the upper part, directed posteriorly with a large radius of curvature), conducive to glenohumeral motion and stability [7].

The orientation of the scapula and of the glenoid can be easily analyzed by CT-scan. With regard to the axis of the scapula, the glenoid is retroversed, from -10 to 10°; the relationship of the glenoid cavity to the scapular body is extremely variable. Moreover, this angle varies according to the level of axial cut of the glenoid, with a retroversion that decreases for the most inferior part of the articular surface.

The glenoid is slightly concave and centered by a small osseous projection, the glenoidal tubercle (Assaki's tubercle), below which the concavity of the glenoid slightly increases. The radius of curvature of the glenoid is about 25 mm (larger in the cranio-caudal axis than in the antero-posterior axis). It exceeds the radius of curvature of the humeral head by 8 to 9 mm; the surface area ratio of the humeral head to glenoid fossa is about 3:1 [8]. The cancellous bone has a conic shape in the axial and frontal plane. The osseous density of the subchondral bone varies; the problem of the bone tissue lies in its anisotropy as well as in its inhomogeneity. The thickness of the subchondral plate is on average 1.9 mm. The trabeculae of cancellous bone are denser in the postero-superior part of the glenoid. The cancellous Young's modulus was found to vary from 183 to 3500 Mpa [9, 10]. The articular surface is covered with hyalin cartilage, the thickness of which is not uniform and becomes thicker in the central zone of the bottom part of the glenoid. The "bare spot" of the glenoid cavity has been described as a consistent reference point to identify the center of the glenoid, nevertheless its absence has been observed in half of the cases. In vivo glenohumeral contact locations are variable among subjects, but the centroid of contact on the glenoid surface is more than 5 mm away from the geometric center of the glenoid articular surface. On the humeral head surface, the centroids of contact are located at the superomedial quarter [8, 11]. This means that "ball-and-socket" kinematics do not govern normal shoulder function [11].

At its rim, the glenoid is completed by the labrum, a triangular fibro-cartilage [12]. It decreases the radius of curvature of the articular surface to improve the congruence of 2 articular surfaces and to increase their contact area. It enhances glenoid fossa depth by about 50%.

Adaptation of anatomy and function

The shoulder is a complex structure, consisting of 3 bones and 4 joints. Muscles mainly ensure its stability. Through the interplay of these elements, the shoulder provides for the hand a wide reachable workspace, but it also provides a stable support for fine manipulation tasks. This freedom is allowed by the arrangement of the articular surfaces and their low congruence, as well as the muscular and neurologic conditions. This balanced compromise between mobility and stability, however, can be easily disturbed if one of the shoulder elements fails. Indeed, the anatomy of the scapula and the glenohumeral joint adapts itself to the position at hand, i.e. they interact among each other, or with prosthesis, to move.

The acquisition of the vertical position came along with important morphological modifications. The anteroposterior diameter of the thorax decreased, and the scapula moved towards the back on the rib cage. This translation directed the glenoid laterally, freeing the upper limb of the carrying function, and increasing the amplitude of articular mobility. We observed an increase of size in the infraspinatus fossa associated with an increase in the length of the scapular spine. This change of proportions lowers the scapulothoracic index (width of the scapula with regard to the length) and testifies to the greater role of the posterior muscles of the rotator cuff with the sagittal orientation of the glenoid.

The development of the scapulabody is dependent upon the surrounding thoracic shape and the surrounding muscular sleeve. The glenoid face and vault seem to connect to the scapular body in a modular-type fashion, with resultant normal variations in glenoid translation and version. Its development is highly dependent on the balance of muscular forces across the glenohumeral joint. From a finalist point of view, the goal in the development of the scapula is to create a stable articular platform to allow force transmission across the glenohumeral joint [13].

BIOMECHANICS [14]

The liberation of the glenohumeral joint of its weight bearing function does not however relieve it of important biomechanical constraints. The glenoid is subjected to the forces exerted by muscles on the joint, to the forces applied by the upper limb across the articular surface of the humerus, and to the reaction force of the articular surface [13]. Moments applied by these forces to the glenoid vary with the position of the arm. So, during a movement, compression forces on the glenoid are maximal when the arm is in 90° of abduction and in external rotation, with an intensity that can achieve up to half of the weight of the body. The value of the moment of the compression forces also varies according to the speed of the movement: the more the angular speed increases, the less the moment of the forces applied to the glenoid. The orientation of the muscle fibers of the supraspinatus is such that during the movement of abduction it exerts on the glenoid compression in the axis of the movement [15-17]. On the other hand, the deltoid fibers, which are not quite directed in the same plans associate with the compression forces an effect of translation of the head on the glenoid during abduction [18]. Because of this balance of the muscular forces and the anatomy of the articular surfaces, the point of application of the forces on the glenoid slides during abduction of the upper limb from anterior to posterior and from caudal to cranial. On the other hand, if compression of the humeral head into the glenoid fossa is lessened (rotator cuff tears), there is an increase in anterior directed forces that may, over time, result in instability. Infraspinatus muscle tears result in increased IGHL strain, and decrease in the force required to dislocate the joint [17].

According to Wolf's Law, the trabecular architecture of bone may be altered by variation in the loading conditions [19]. The magnitude of the principal stress plays an important role in the bone strength or apparent density of the trabeculae of the cortical and cancellous bone.

The glenoid is usually considered to be a low-density cancellous structure. The density of the trabecular bone varies from approximately 45% in the posterior glenoid to approximately 11% in the deep anterior glenoid [9, 20]. The results of our 3-dimensional study have proved that most parts of the glenoid trabecular bone have a preferred horizontal orientation. Nevertheless the juxtaarticular cancellous region also revealed supero-inferiorly connected trabeculae secondary to the primary trabecular orientation, suitable for the absorption of shear stresses generated during the physiologic translational movement of the humeral head on the glenoid joint surface [9].

CONCLUSION

The anatomy of the glenoid is variable according to individuals, but always obeys this paradox: it has to guarantee sufficient articular motion with the conservation of a stable and painless joint. This configuration exposes it to pathologies ensuing directly from these properties: the glenoid wear that arises in glenohumeral degenerative osteoarthritis and glenohumeral instability. The consideration of the anatomical characteristics of the glenoid and the understanding of its functional role allow the explanation of the limits of early treatments and to elaborate therapeutic techniques more and more adapted to these pathologies.

REFERENCES

[1] FEALY S, RODEO S, DICARLO E, O'BRIEN S. The developmental anatomy of the neonatal glenohumeral joint. *J Shoulder Elbow Surg 2000: 9: 217-22.*

[2] O'BRIEN S, ALLEN A, FEALY S, RODEO S, ARNOCZKY S. Developmental anatomy of the shoulder and anatomy of the glenohumeral joint. In: Rockwood CJ, Matsen F, eds. The Shoulder 2nd edition. *Philadelphia: WB Saunders, 1998: 1-33.*

[3] CODMAN E. The anatomy of the human shoulder. In: Codman E, eds. The shoulder. *Malabar FLA: Krieger Publishing, 1984: 1-31.*

[4] CHURCHILL R, BREMS J, KOTOSCHI H. Glenoid size, inclination, and version: an anatomic study. *J Shoulder Elbow Surg 2001: 10: 327-32.*

[5] LANDAU J, HOENECKE H. Genetic and biomechanical determinants of glenoid version: implications for glenoid implant placement in shoulder arthroplasty. *J Shoulder Elbow Surg 2009: 18: 661-7.*

[6] HERNIGOU P, DUPARC F, HERNIGOU A. Determining humeral retroversion with computed tomography. *J Bone Joint Surg 2002: 84(A): 1753-62.*

[7] SOSLOWSKY L, FLATOW E, BIGLIANI L, MOW V. Articular geometry of the glenohumeral joint. *Clin Orthop 1992: 285: 181-90.*

[8] WARNER J, BOWEN M, DENG X *et al.* Articular contact patterns of the normal glenohumeral joint. J Shoulder Elbow Surg 1998: 7: 381-8.

[9] FRICH L. Bone strength and materials properties of the glenoid. *J Shoulder Elbow Surg 1997: 6: 97-104.*

[10] ANGLIN C, TOLHURST P, WYSS U, PICHORA D. Glenoid cancellous bone strength and modulus. *J Biomech 1999: 32: 1091-7.*

[11] SOSLOWSKY L, FLATOW E, BIGLIANI L, *et al.* Quantitation of in situ contact areas at the glenohumeral joint: a biomechanical study. *J Orthop Res 1992: 10: 524-34.*

[12] CLAVERT P, KEMPF J, WOLFRAM-GABEL R, KAHN J. Are there induced morphologic variations of the superior glenoid labrum? About 100 shoulder arthroscopies. *Surg Radiol Anat 2005: 27: 385-8.*

[13] MATSEN F, FU F, HAWKINS R. The shoulder: A balance of mobility and stability. In: Matsen F, Fu F, Hawkins R, eds. The shoulder: A balance of mobility and stability. *Rosemont, IL: American Academy of Orthopaedic Surgeons, 1993: 279-304.*

[14] PERRY J. Biomechanics of the shoulder. In: Rowe C, eds. The shoulder. *New York: Churchill Livingstone, 1988: 1-35.*

[15] DEBSKI R, SAKONE M, WOO S *et al.* Contribution of the passive properties of the rotator cuff to glenohumeral stability during anterior-posterior loading. *J Shoulder Elbow Surg 1999: 8: 324-9.*

[16] McMAHON P, DEBSKI R, THOMPSON W *et al.* Shoulder muscle forces and tendon excursions during glenohumeral abduction in the scapular plane. *J Shoulder Elbow Surg 1995: 4: 199-208.*

[17] PARSONS I, APRELEVA M, FU F, WOO S. The effect of rotator cuff tears on reaction forces at the glenohumeral joint. *J Orthop Res 2002: 20: 439-46.*

[18] BILUART F, GAGEY O, SKALLI W, MITTON D. Biomechanics of the deltoideus. *Surg Radiol Anat 2006: 28: 76-81.*

[19] HOBATHO M, RHO J, ASHMAN R Atlas of mechanical properties of human cortical and cancellous bone. In vivo assessment of bone quality by vibration and wave propagation techniques. Part II Editors: Van der Perre G LG. Atlas of mechanical properties of human cortical and cancellous bone. In vivo assessment of bone quality by vibration and wave propagation techniques. *Leuven: ACCO; 1992.*

[20] LEHTINEN T, TINGART M, APRELEVA M, WARNER J. Total, trabecular, and cortical bone mineral density in different regions of the glenoid. *J Shoulder Elbow Surg 2004: 13: 344-48.*

GLENOID IMPLANTS: HISTORY, DESIGN, & RATIONALE-PE/MB, FLAT/CURVED, PEG/KEEL, SCREWS, REVERSE

A. GODENÈCHE

Despite the improved longevity and performance of newer shoulder prostheses, the fixation of the glenoid component remains the greatest challenge in total shoulder arthroplasty.

Glenoid loosening represents one third of all reported complications and is the most common indication for revision [1-7].

Anatomic or oval-shaped glenoid components are available. The anatomic glenoid may provide the advantage of avoiding internal impingement of nonarticular structures with overhanging polyethylene. However, having a smaller upper portion of the component decreases the surface area available for contact. This decrease in wall height in the superior portion of the component theoretically decreases the force required for dislocation or subluxation. No matter which component – anatomic (pear-shaped) or oval – is used, the key is to size the glenoid appropriately to allow for minimum overhang.

A curved-back design has superior loosening characteristics to a flat-backed component [8, 9].

Polyethylene is much stiffer than the cartilage and labrum; therefore, shock absorption and humeral translations are not present in a conforming prothetic glenoid. Nonconformity of the prosthetic articular surfaces, with a glenoid surface radius larger than the humerus, allows physiologic translations without rim loading [10, 11]. Increasing the glenoid radius with respect to the humeral radius, so long as the wall height is the same, has no clinically significant effect on glenohumeral stability [12]. In a large clinical series by Walch *et al.* [13] articular mismatch was directly correlated with improved loosening scores. The best clinical results occurred with 5 to 7 mm of radial mismatch. Although glenohumeral-radial mismatch may have advantages, one of the disadvantages is potentially increased levels of stress transmitted to the glenoid and cement [10, 14]. As the degree of mismatch increases, there is a decrease in contact area and an increase in the contact pressures with the potential risk of polyethylene failure. No one has ever shown the effects of mismatch on the wear characteristics of polyethylene or the effect of *in vivo* use on initial glenoid component radius.

Prosthetic glenoid components can be anchored by use of cemented, cementless, or hybrid techniques.

Several component design variations of cemented glenoid implants exist and can be divided into 2 main groups: keeled and peg-shaped glenoid components [15].

The peg-shaped anchorage systems provide greater theoretical stability against shear forces. Angling *et al.* [8] and Lazarus *et al.* [16] concluded that radiolucencies at the cement-bone interface and incomplete component seating occurred more frequently with keeled components versus pegged components. Anterior offset of the keel with respect to the surface of the component demonstrates better resistance to bending compared with a centered keel [17].

Cementless glenoid components consist of multiple designs, including 2-piece metal-backed components with a polyethylene inlay, 1-piece metal-backed polyethylene components, and hybrid components with metal sleeves for all-polyethylene pegged components. Most of the metal-backed components contain a surface treatment to encourage biologic ingrowth. All-polyethylene components generate lower stress concentrations and are more compliant and conforming than metal-backed components [18]. The theoretical advantages of metal-backed components are great because of the potential for permanent ingrowth and immediate initial fixation. There are several reports of polyethylene dissociation and screw breakage before bony ingrowth in 2-piece metal-backed components [19]. The survival rate of cementless metal-backed glenoid components has been shown to be inferior to that of cemented all-polyethylene components in most series [20, 21].

The possibility of permanent biologic fixation continues to drive research into metal-backed glenoid components [22, 23].

Constrained shoulder systems were born to address the problem of rotator cuff deficiency in shoulder arthroplasty. These implants were generally non-anatomic, and very few constrained options remain today. Paul Grammont took a different approach. His prosthesis placed the center of rotation more medial at the bony glenoid by placing a hemisphere directly mounted on its surface. The first version of this implant, designed in 1985, was upgraded to the Delta III implant. This system employs a medialized rotation center, reducing torque moments on the glenoid and allowing for better deltoid recruitment in elevation and abduction [24, 25].

Persistent challenges included problems with instability, inability to restore external rotation motion and strength, and notching of the scapula by the prosthesis [25].

Short-term results with this reverse system have been encouraging as well [26]. However, challenging issues such as glenoid fixation, rotator cuff deficiency, and prosthesis revision still demand more of the same from our community.

REFERENCES

[1] FENLIN JM, RAMSEY ML, ALLARDYCE TJ, FRIEMAN BG Modular total shoulder replacement. *Clin Orthop 1994; 307: 37-46.*

[2] FRANKLIN JL, BARRETT WP, JACKINS SE, MATSEN FA. Glenoid loosening in total shoulder arthroplasty. *J Arthrolplasty 1988; 3: 39-46.*

[3] HAWKINS RJ, GREIS PE, BONUTTI PM. Treatment of symptomatic glenoid loosening following unconstrained shoulder arthroplasty. *Orthopedics 1999; 22: 229-34.*

[4] NEER CS II, KIRBY RM. Revision of humeral head and total shoulder arthroplasties. *Clin Orthop 1982; 170: 189-95.*

[5] SPERLING JW, COFIELD RH, ROWLAND CM Neer hemiarthroplasty and Neer total shoulder arthroplasty in patients fifty years old or less. *J Bone Joint Surg Am 1998; 80: 464-73.*

[6] TORCHIA ME, COFIELD RH, SETTERGREN CR. Total shoulder arthroplasty with the Neer prosthesis: long-term results. *J Shoulder Elbow Surg 1997; 6: 495-505.*

[7] WIRTH MA, ROCKWOOD CA. complications of shoulder arthroplasty. *Clin Orthop 1994; 307: 47-69.*

[8] ANGLIN C, WYSS UP, NYFFELER RW, GERBER C. Loosening performance of cemented glenoid prosthesis design pairs. *Clin Biomech (Bristol, Avon) 2001; 16: 144-50.*

[9] COLLINS D, TENCER A, SIDLES J, MATSEN F III. Edge displacement and deformation of glenoid components in response to eccentric loading. The effect of preparation of the glenoid bone. *J Bone Joint Surg Am 1992; 74: 501-7.*

[10] KARDUNA AR, WILLIAMS GR, WILLIAMS JL, LANNOTTI JP. Kinematics of the glenohumeral joint: influences of muscle forces, ligamentous constraints, and articular geometry. *J Orthop Res 1996; 14: 986-93.*

[11] MATSEN FA, ROCKWOOD CA, WIRTH MA, LIPPITT SB. Glenohumeral arthritis and its management. In: Rockwood CA, Matsen FA, editors. The shoulder. *Philadelphia: Saunders; 1999. p. 233-76.*

[12] KARDUNA AR, WILLIAMS GR, WILLIAMS JL, LANNOTTI JP. Joint stability after total shoulder arthroplasty in a cadaver model. *J Shoulder Elbow Surg 1997; 6: 506-11.*

[13] WALCH G, EDWARDS TB, BOULAHIA A *et al.* The influence of glenohumeral prosthetic mismatch on glenoid radiolucent lines: results of a multicenter study. *J Bone Joint Surg Am 2002; 84: 2186-91.*

[14] COUTEAU B, MANSAT P, ESTIVALEZES E *et al.* Finite element analysis of the mechanical behaviour of a scapula implanted with a glenoid prosthesis. *Clin Biomech (Bristol, Avon) 2001; 16: 566-75.*

[15] HABERMEYER P, EBERT T. Current status and perspectives of shoulder replacement (in German). *Unfallchirurg 1999; 102: 668-83.*

[16] LAZARUS MD, JENSEN KL, SOUTHWORTH C, MATSEN FA III. The radiographic evaluation of keeled and pegged glenoid component insertion. *J Bone Joint Surg Am 2002; 84: 1174-82.*

[17] ORR TE, CARTER DR, SCHURMAN DJ. Stress analyses of glenoid component designs. *Clin Orthop 1988; 232: 217-24.*

[18] STONE KD, GRABOWSKI JJ, COFIELD RH, MORREY BF, AN KN. Stress analyses of glenoid components in total shoulder arthroplasty. *J Shoulder Elbow Surg 1999; 8: 151-8.*

[19] LEVY O, CAPELAND SA. Rotational dissociation of glenoid components in a total shoulder prosthesis: an indication that sagittal torque forces may be important in glenoid component design (letter). *J Shoulder Elbow Surg 2001; 10: 197.*

[20] BOILEAU P, AVIDOR C, KRISHAN SG *et al.* Cemented polyethylene versus uncemented metal-backed glenoid components in total shoulder arthroplasty: a prospective, double-blind, randomized study. *J Shoulder Elbow Surg 2002; 11: 351-9.*

[21] RODOSKY MW, WEINSTEIN D, POLLOCK R. On the rarity of glenoid component failure. *J Shoulder Elbow Surg 1995; 4S:13.*

[22] COFIELD RH, DALY PJ. Total shoulder arthroplasty with a tissue ingrowth glenoid component. *J Shoulder Elbow Surg 1992;1: 77-85.*

[23] WALLACE AL, PHILLIPS RL, MACDOUGAL GA, WALSH WR, SONNABEND DH. Resurfacing of the glenoid in total shoulder arthroplasty. A comparison, at a mean of five years, of prostheses inserted with and without cement. *J Bone Joint Surg Am 1999; 81: 510-8.*

[24] GRAMMONT PM, BAULOT E. Delta shoulder prosthesis for rotator cuff rupture. *Orthopedics 1993; 16-65-68.*

[25] BOILEAU P, WATKINSON DJ, HATZIDAKIS AM, BALG F. Grammont reverse prosthesis: Design, rationale, and biomechanics. *J Shoulder Elbow Surg 2005; 14: S147-61.*

[26] FRANKLE M, SIEGAL S, PUPELLO D, SALEEM A, MIGHELL M, VASEY M. associated with severe rotator cuff deficiency: A minimum two-year follow-up study of sixty patients. *J Bone Joint Surg 2005; 87A: 1967-1705.*

BIOMECHANICS OF ANATOMICAL & RESURFACED GLENOID

A. FARRON, A. TERRIER

BACKGROUND

The gleno-humeral joint is not congruent. Therefore the stability is mainly provided by static (bone and cartilage; labrum; capsule and ligaments) and dynamic (rotator cuff; stabilizers of the scapula) factors.

These properties allow for natural sliding and gliding movements of the humeral head on the glenoid. For example, during abduction, the contact point is located at the lower part of the glenoid at the beginning of the movement, moves at the superior part of the glenoid at 90° and then moves down again at 120°, inducing a physiological "rocking horse" phenomenon.

After anatomical TSA, these biomechanical principles are preserved. Consequently, an eccentric loading of the glenoid is also observed during movements, leading to significant stress within cement and bone. Even if subjective and functional midterm results after anatomical TSA are good, the risks of glenoid loosening and the high rate of radiolucencies are still a matter of concern. The role of the eccentric loading in these situations is not yet well known.

Many factors are involved in joint stability and biomechanics of the resurfaced glenoid:
- Anatomy and geometry of the humeral head and the glenoid;
- Rotator cuff and stabilizers of the scapula;
- Design of the glenoid implant.

Our goal was to specifically analyze the influence of these factors on biomechanics of the prosthetic glenoid, in order to improve our knowledge of the mechanisms of glenoid loosening.

METHOD

A numerical musculoskeletal model of the shoulder was used for this comparative study. The model included the scapula, the humerus and 6 scapulo-humeral muscles: middle, anterior, and posterior deltoid, supraspinatus, subscapularis and infraspinatus combined with teres minor.

Arm motion and joint stability was achieved by muscles, allowing for natural translation of the humeral head. The muscle activation patterns were derived from EMG data and controlled by a synchronization algorithm. The movements of abduction were simulated, with 1 kg in the hand. Aequalis prosthesis was positioned in the numerical model according to manufacturer recommendations.

6 pathologic situations were tested and then compared to the standard (normal) resurfaced glenoid:

- 15° of glenoid retroversion,
- Humeral head placed 5mm to high,
- Humeral head placed 5 mm to low,
- Complete deficiency of the supraspinatus muscle,
- Partial deficiency (50%) of the subscapularis muscle,
- Inversion of the scapulothoracic rhythm (2:1).

The location of the humeral contact point on the glenoid, the glenoid pressure and the stress within the cement were measured.

The design of the glenoid implant was than modified (custom made glenoid) for optimizing the loading of the glenoid in order to decrease the stress within the cement.

RESULTS

For the 6 pathologic situations tested, we observed an aggravation of the eccentric loading of the glenoid during abduction, leading to significant increase of the glenoid pressure (except for the supraspinatus deficiency).

Consequently, the stress measured in the cement rose also dramatically (fig. 1).

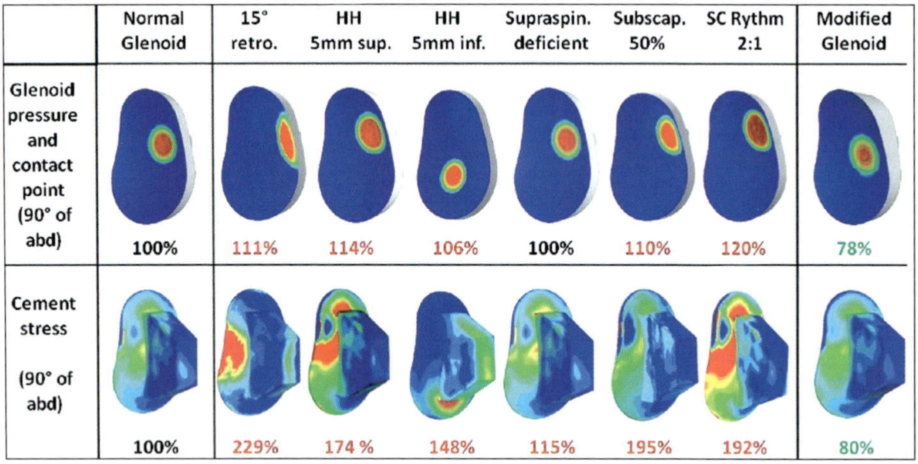

Fig. 1 : Contact point and glenoid pressure (top), and cement stress (bottom) at 90° of abduction, measured in different pathologic situations (glenoid retroversion, humeral head malposition, rotator cuff deficiency, inversion of scapula-thoracic rhythm), compared to standard (normal) and modified glenoids.

The custom made modification of the glenoid design allowed decreasing either the eccentric loading of the glenoid and the glenoid stress.

CONCLUSIONS

After anatomical TSA, as for the natural gleno-humeral joint, the shoulder is still not congruent, allowing for sliding and gliding of the humeral head on the glenoid.

Therefore, the stability of the prosthetic joint is provided either by the implants, the bone support and the dynamic stabilizers. Any deficiency in these stabilizing structures may lead to an aggravation of the eccentric loading of the glenoid, inducing a consecutive significant increase of cement stress, and could be implicated in the mechanisms of glenoid loosening.

To restore a "physiological" shoulder biomechanics after anatomical TSA, anatomical reconstruction of the humeral head, optimal orientation of the glenoid, and integrity of the rotator cuff seems to be essential.

The development of "anatomical" custom made glenoid implants, in order to decrease joint stress and limit the risks of loosening, could probably be a way of study in the near future.

ACKNOWLEDGEMENT

This study was partly supported by Tornier Inc., Edina, MN.

DOES IMPLANT DESIGN INFLUENCE GLENOID CONSTRAINTS: A FINITE ELEMENT ANALYSIS

P. MANSAT, J. BRIOT, M. MANSAT, P. SWIDER

ABSTRACT

Total shoulder arthroplasty has become a successful surgical procedure through design improvements. However, lucent lines around the glenoid component are of major concern leading to component loosening. To better understand the mechanism causing loosening, a finite element biomechanical model of an *in-vivo* scapula was implemented. The effect of eccentric loading was analyzed on a keel glenoid implant and a peg glenoid implant. Results indicated that eccentric loading increases greatly stresses in the cement mantle at the bone-cement interface and no significant difference was predicted between keel and peg implants. The results suggested that eccentric loading is a likely cause for initiation of cracks in the cement layer especially at the posterior side. Moreover, these results along with other studies indicate that geometric and bone properties of the scapula may be more important factors in the success of shoulder arthroplasty than implant design.

INTRODUCTION

Total shoulder arthroplasty is a difficult surgery because of the little available space for implant fixation. Even though shoulder replacement has been performed for the last thirty years, long term follow-up clinical studies are scarce in the literature [22, 24]. Most of the clinical studies report an average follow-up of three to four years [16, 17, 25]. The main complication is glenoid component loosening and it is likely to become more important as long-term follow-up studies are available. Glenoid component loosening is mainly associated with radiolucencies in the bone-cement layer used to fix glenoid component. These radiolucencies may be created by high stresses in the cement layer [3, 7].

To better understand the failure scenario of glenoid components, 2D finite element (FE) analyses were first performed to quantify stresses within the glenoid component, the cement layer, and the surrounding bone [9, 13, 20]. So far, 3D studies have been designed to address the importance of minimizing stresses within the cement layer and to study the effect of different types of design. Peg components are superior to keel components for normal bone but worse for low bone-density glenoids [12]. Offset keel components perform better than centered keel components [19] and metal-backed component does not perform better than total polyethylene designs [10, 12]. A thick cement layer can result in higher cement stresses [7].

All FE studies have been performed on cadaveric scapulae or non-pathologic patients [4, 7, 23]. However, patients with osteoarthritis or rheumatoid arthritis have different bone properties and geometries than normal scapulae [8]. This is expected to change the way the load is transferred. In this study, a 3D FE analysis was performed on an *in-vivo* patient with primary osteoarthritis. It was hypothesized that the effect of *in-vivo* bone properties and geometries will be more important factors than glenoid component design. The results of the study have already been published [15].

METHODS

A female patient of 76 years diagnosed retrospectively with primary osteoarthritis was CT-scanned on a Siemens Somaton Plus 4. Two millimeters thick contiguous CT-images were taken with a resolution of 0.22 mm. Bone contours of the CT-images were outlined using a custom-written software, and exported into Patran v7.5 (MSC Software®). Two glenoid components were investigated: a Cofield® keel component (Smith & Nephew) and its peg counterpart. The same FE mesh grid was used to model these two implants. Thus, the two different types of implants were simulated by changing the mechanical properties assigned to the elements. The implant was then inserted into the bone model so that the faces of the keel or the pegs were aligned with the scapular faces. A cement layer of one-millimeter thickness was modeled between the keel or pegs and the surrounding bone. Fully bonded interfaces were modeled. The mesh involved 33393 8-node cubic elements. Models were solved using MSC Marc® with all materials being modeled as linear elastic isotropic.

The implants were made of polyethylene with a Young's modulus of 965 MPa and a Poisson's ratio of 0.34. PMMA bone cement had a Young's modulus of 2000 MPa and Poisson's ratio of 0.23. Inhomogeneous bone properties were assigned to the elements to account for the true non-homogeneous distribution of bone density within the patient's scapula [14]. The material properties were assigned by using relationship between CT number and mechanical parameters. As this relationship has not been defined for the glenoid, an average of relationships found in the literature [2, 6, 11, 21] for other bones was used. The following relationship was obtained:

$$E = 2.696 X CT + 163.95 \qquad (1)$$

where E was the Young's modulus of cancellous bone. For CT numbers between 900 and 1300, a Young's modulus of 11800 MPa was used and for CT numbers greater than 1300 a Young's modulus of 16000 MPa was used [5]. A Poisson's ratio of 0.3 was assigned to all bone elements.

Load cases have been chosen in order to simulate balance and imbalance of soft tissues. Proximal migration in total shoulder arthroplasty is frequently observed. Moreover, the shoulder can be anteriorly or posteriorly unstable [3, 18, 25]. In this study, three loading cases were simulated. The first one was represented by a centered load to simulate a stable shoulder; the second and third ones were applied in the superior-anterior and superior-posterior locations to represent migration of the humeral head in the anterior and posterior directions respectively. A constant load of 1.8 BW (1300 N) was used to represent daily activities of elderly people like standing from a chair or walking with a cane [1]. The scapula was restrained from any movement along the blade.

RESULTS

The Von-Mises stress distribution within the glenoid component indicated that eccentric loading could create very high stresses on the rim of the glenoid (Fig. 1). With central loading, stresses remained low with a value of 7 MPa at the junction between the keel and the glenoid. On the other hand with superior-anterior or superior-posterior loading, stresses up to 20 MPa were found under the area of loading.

Glenoid component loosening is generally believed to occur through high stresses in the cement at the bone-cement interface. When a central load was applied, low maximum principal stress was found at this interface in the order of 2 to 3 MPa (Fig. 2). However, when the glenoid component was loaded in the superior-anterior direction, very high maximum principal stresses were predicted at the tip of the keel and at the edge of the base of the keel with the component. Stresses of up to 8 MPa were predicted in the posterior side, due to a bending of the component in the anterior-posterior plane. When the component was loaded in the superior-posterior direction, a mainly compressive

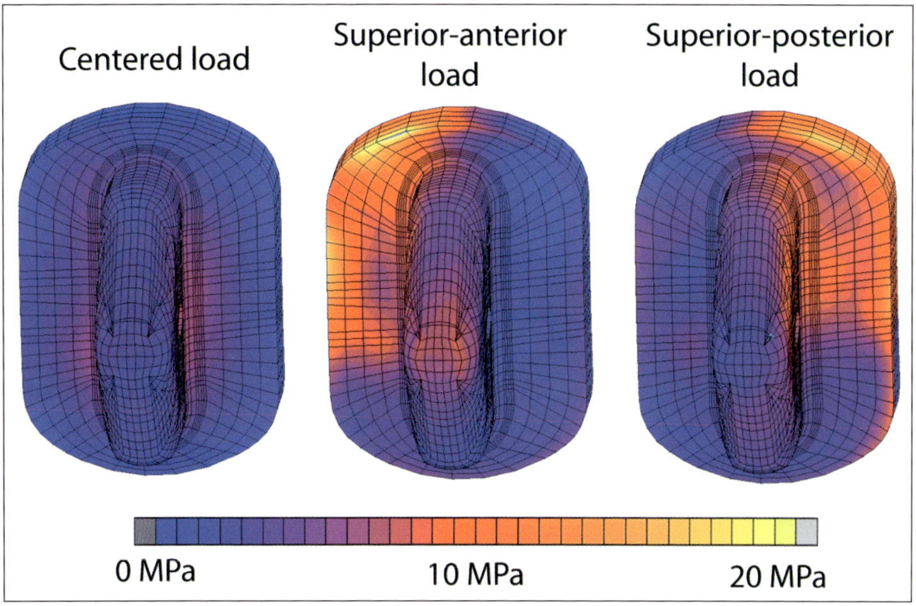

Fig. 1: Von-Mises stress in the keel glenoid component for the three load cases investigated

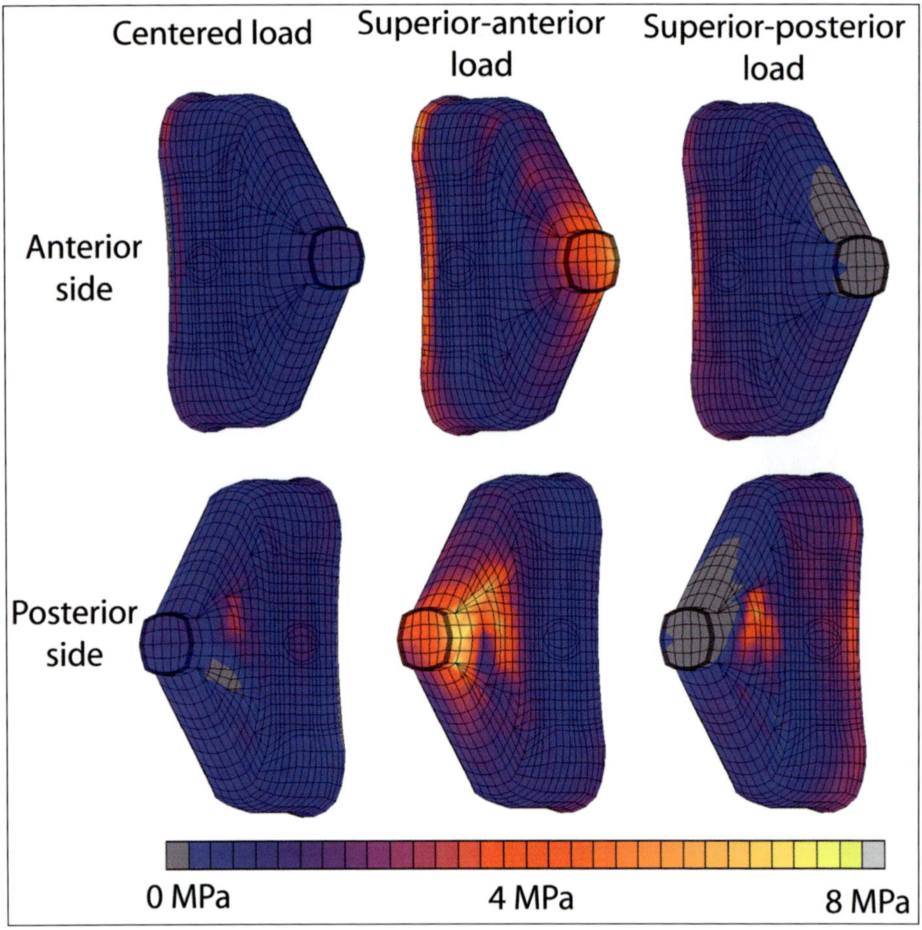

Fig. 2: Maximum principal stress in the cement layer at the bone-cement interface

stress was predicted at the tip of the keel. Some peak tensile stresses were found in the posterior side and on the rim of the cement layer.

The maximum shear stresses at the bone-cement interface in the anterior-posterior and superior-inferior directions indicated higher shear stress in the posterior side (Fig. 3). The component was more prone to bending in the anterior-posterior direction than in the superior-inferior direction. Micro-movement at the bone-cement interface due to high shear stress might be responsible for glenoid component loosening.

No significant differences were predicted between keel and peg implants (Fig. 4). The same stress distribution was predicted for the maximum and minimum principal stress at the bone-cement interface.

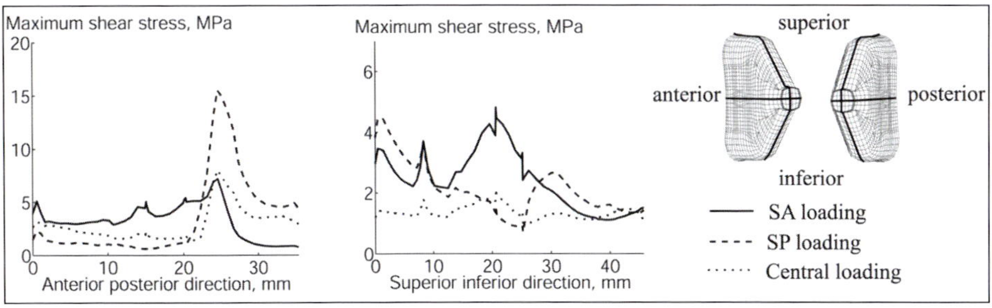

Fig. 3: Maximum shear stress at the bone-cement interface along the anterior-posterior and superior-inferior paths of the cement layer

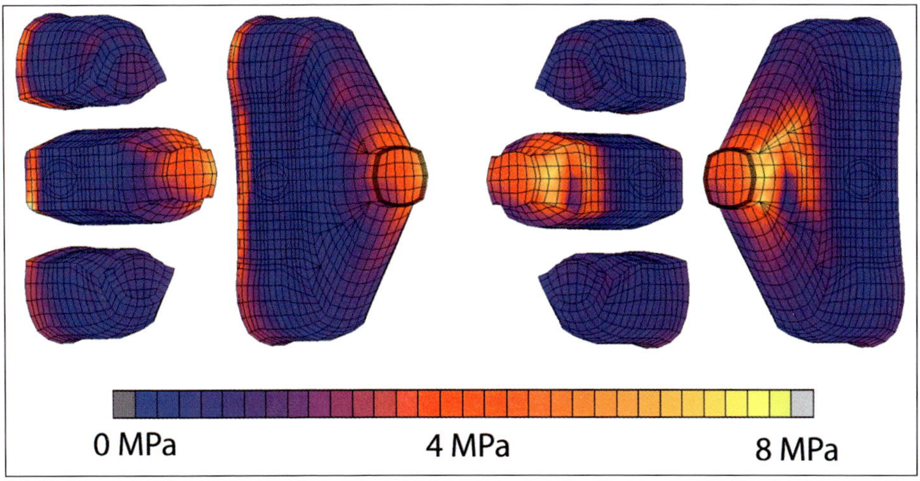

Fig. 4: Maximum principal stress in the cement layer at the bone-cement interface for a load in the superior-anterior direction. Comparison between keel and peg components

DISCUSSION

This study showed that the effect of eccentric loading after total shoulder arthroplasty was of prime importance for the survival of glenoid component. Reasonably low stresses were predicted with a central loading, whereas stresses largely above fatigue failure of bone cement were predicted for a loading in the superior-anterior or superior-posterior directions. Stresses predicted in the cement layer were believed to explain the high rate of glenoid component loosening. Several limitations exist in this study. The effect of eccentric loading was investigated by changing the location and direction of the gleno-humeral force. However, no other muscle forces were included. The stresses were calculated for perfectly bonded interfaces between the implant, the cement and the bone. These conditions were assumed to represent reasonably well the interface situation immediately post-operatively. As crack initiation occurs and debonding at the bone-cement interface proceeds, it is expected that the stress distribution within the cement layer will change.

Very similar stress distributions were found between keel and peg glenoid components. Our results suggest that the design of the glenoid component did not alter the surrounding cement mantle. This result was different than the results found by Lacroix *et al.* [12] who found that a keel implant was better than a peg implant for normal bone and worse for a bone with low bone density. However, in our study the bone was not normal but pathologic and thus an inner remodeling of the posterior side was observed resulting in a higher bone density in the glenoid than normal (379 ± 179 CT) [8]. This might explain the small effect of component design on the load transfer in this specific scapula.

Our results indicated high stresses in the posterior side of the cement when the loading was in the superior-anterior position. This was explained by the very small space available between the implant and the bone cortex on the posterior side. Moreover, due to the inner remodeling in that region, high stresses are produced in the cement mantle in contact with this

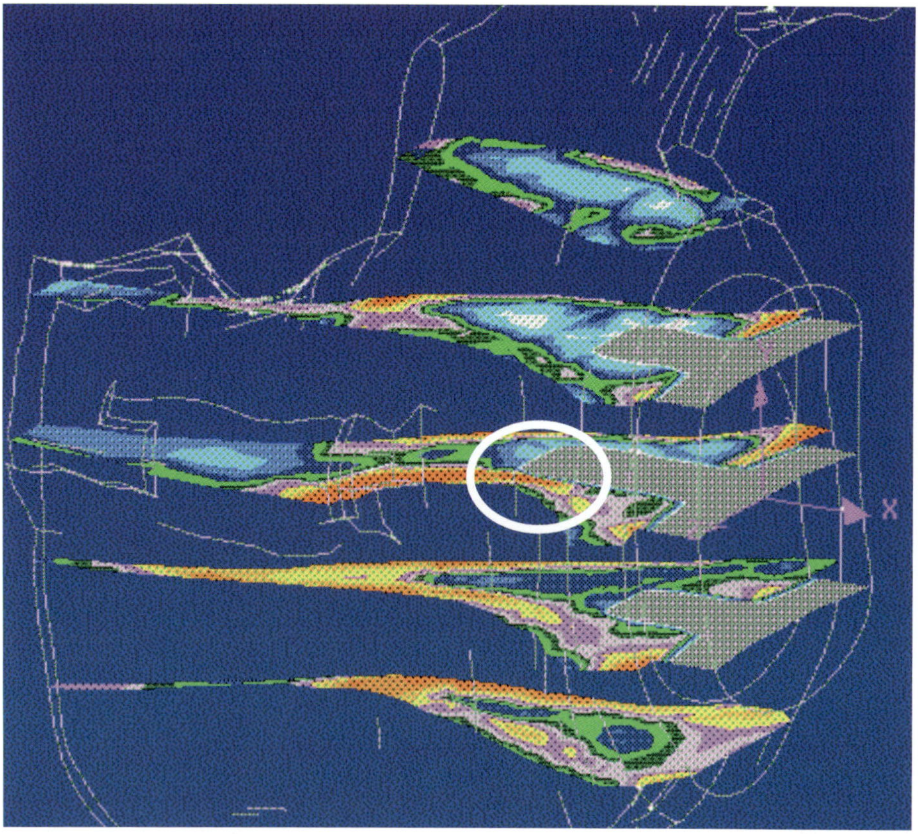

Fig. 5: Position of the implant on the osteoarthritic scapula. Note the contact of the implant with the bone cortex on the posterior side leading to high stresses in the cement mantle

region (Fig. 5). This result suggested that implant position was critical in the values of stresses within the cement. Different angles of the keel would result in various cement stresses. It is possible that for each patient, an optimum position exists where stresses are the lowest.

This fundamental result may indicate that for total shoulder arthroplasty it is more important to take account of the geometry and bone properties of the patient than the actual design of the prosthesis. It is thus recommended in the future to perform specific pre-operative planning that would account for both patient specifications and manufacturer implant design. The progress of imaging techniques with the use of automatic meshing and structural FE modeling could result in a biomechanical analysis that would be useful for surgical pre-operative planning.

ACKNOWLEDGEMENT

We would like to thank B. Couteau and D. Lacroix who initiated this study, and Smith & Nephews Company, which funded this study.

REFERENCES

[1] ANGLIN C, WYSS UP, PICHORA DR. Glenohumeral contact forces. *Proc. Inst. Mech. Eng. [H] 2000; 214: 637-644.*

[2] CIARELLI MJ, GOLDSTEIN SA, KUHN JL, CODY DD, BROWN MB. Evaluation of orthrogonal mechanical properties and density of human trabecular bone from the major metaphyseal regions with materials testing and computed tomography. *J Orthop Res 1991; 9: 674-682.*

[3] COFIELD RH, EDGERTON BC. Total shoulder arthroplasty: complications and revision surgery. *Instructional course lectures 1990; 39: 449-462.*

[4] COUTEAU B, MANSAT P, DARMANA R, MANSAT M, EGAN J. Morphological and mechanical analysis of the glenoid by 3D geometric reconstruction using computed tomography. *Clinical Biomechanics 2000; 15 Suppl 1: S8-12.*

[5] COUTEAU B. Modélisation par la méthode des éléments finis du fémur humain. Application à l'étude des prothèses sur-mesure. *Thèse d'Université, Paul Sabatier, Toulouse, 1997; 2677.*

[6] COUTEAU B, HOBATHO MC, DARMANA R, BRIGNOLA JC, ARLAUD JY. Finite element modelling of the vibrational behaviour of the human femur using CT-based indivisualized geometrical and material properties. *J Biomech 1998; 31: 383-386.*

[7] COUTEAU B, MANSAT P, ESTIVALEZES E, DARMANA R, MANSAT M, EGAN J. Finite element analysis of the mechanical behavior of a scapula implanted with a glenoid prosthesis. *Clin Biomech 2001; 16: 566-575.*

[8] COUTEAU B, MANSAT P, MANSAT M, DARMANA R, EGAN J. In vivo characterisation of glenoid using computed tomography. *J. Shoulder Elbow Surg 2001; 10: 116-122*

[9] FRIEDMAN RJ, LABERGE M, DOOLEY RC, O'HARA AL. Finite element modelling of the glenoid component: effect of design parameters on stress distribution. *J Shoulder Elbow Surg 1992; 1: 261-270.*

[10] GUPTA S, VAN DER HELM FCT, VAN KEULEN A. Stress analysis of cemented and uncemented glenoid prostheses. *Proc Europ Soc Biomech Dublin 2000; 161.*

[11] HVID I, HANSEN SL. Trabecular bone strength patterns at the proximal tibial epiphysis. *J Orthop Res 1985; 3: 464-472.*

[12] LACROIX D, MURPHY LA, PRENDERGAST PJ. Three-dimensional finite element analysis of glenoid replacement prostheses: a comparison of keeled and pegged anchorage systems. *J Biomech Eng 2000; 122: 430-436.*

[13] LACROIX D, PRENDERGAST PJ. Stress analysis of glenoid component designs for shoulder arthroplasty. *Proc Instn Mech Engrs Part H 1997; 211: 467-474.*

[14] MANSAT P, BAREA C, HOBATHO MC, DARMANA R, MANSAT M. Anatomical variation of the mechanical properties of the glenoid. *J Shoulder Elbow Surg 1998; 7: 109-115.*

[15] MANSAT P, BRIOT J, MANSAT M, SWIDER P. Evaluation of the glenoid implant survival using a biomechanical finite element analysis: influence of the implant design, bone properties, and loading location. *J Shoulder Elbow Surg 2007; 16: 79S-83S.*

[16] MANSAT P, GUITY MR, BELLUMORE Y, MANSAT M. Shoulder arthroplasty for late sequelae of proximal humeral head fractures. *J Shoulder and Elbow Surg 2004; 13: 305-12.*

[17] MANSAT P, MANSAT M, BELLUMORE Y, RONGIÈRES M, BONNEVIALLE P. Résultats à moyen terme de la prothèse d'épaule dans l'omarthrose primitive. *Rev Chir Orthop 2002; 88 : 544-552.*

[18] MOECKEL BH, ALTCHEK DW, WARREN RF, WICKIEWICZ TL, DINES DM. Instability of the shoulder after arthroplasty. *J Bone Joint Surg (Am) 1993; 75: 492-497*

[19] MURPHY LA, PRENDERGAST PJ, CHRISTIE R, RESCH H. Finite element analysis predicts lower stress for an offset-keel glenoid component compared to a center-keel design. *Trans ORS San Francisco, 2000; 787.*

[20] ORR TE, CARTER DR, SCHURMAN DJ. Stress analysis of glenoid component designs. *Clin Orthop 1988; 232: 217-224.*

[21] RHO JY, HOBATHO MC, ASHMAN RB. Relation of mechanical properties to density and Ct numbers in human bone. *Med Eng Phys 1995; 17: 347-355.*

[22] SPERLING JW, COFIELD RH, ROWLAND CM. Neer hemiarthroplasty and Neer total shoulder arthroplasty in patients fifty years old or less: long-term results. *J Bone Joint Surg (Am) 1998; 80: 464-473.*

[23] STONE KD, GRABOWSKI JJ, COFIELD RH, MORREY BF, AN KA. Stress analysis of glenoid component in total shoulder arthroplasty. *J Shoulder Elbow Surg 1999; 8/2: 151-158.*

[24] TORCHIA ME, COFIELD RH, SETTERGREN CR. Total shoulder arthroplasty with the Neer prosthesis: long-term results. *J Shoulder Elbow Surg 1997; 6: 495-505.*

[25] WIRTH MA, ROCKWOOD CA. Currents concept review: complications of total shoulder replacement arthroplasty. *J Bone Joint Surg (Am) 1996; 78: 603-616.*

THE GLENOID IN THE HORIZONTAL PLANE:
WALCH CLASSIFICATION REVISITED HUMERAL SUBLUXATION AND GLENOID RETROVERSION

D.M ROULEAU, J.F. KIDDER, J. PONS-VILLANUEVA, S. DYNAMIDIS, M.J DEFRANCO, G. WALCH

INTRODUCTION

Glenohumeral osteoarthritis is a common diagnosis encountered by orthopedic surgeons. Given the rising incidence of primary and revision shoulder replacements, more and more attention has been placed on the knowledge of shoulder disorders. Walch *et al.* in 1999 published one study on the glenoid in glenohumeral osteoarthritis (fig. 1). The classification has come under closer scrutiny in the literature in recent years, and, with the advent of more sophisticated imaging modalities (3D CT), its future use by orthopedic surgeons in describing glenohumeral osteoarthritis has been questioned. These authors (Scalise *et al.* 2008, Nowak *et al.* 2010) obtained low reliability when using the classification in small group of patients (n<30). They recommend that a modification of the classification could help. We revisited the classification to establish its validity in a larger number of patients and we tried a different reorganisation of its subgroups to obtain better reliability. Results on this topic will be presented in ***Section I***.

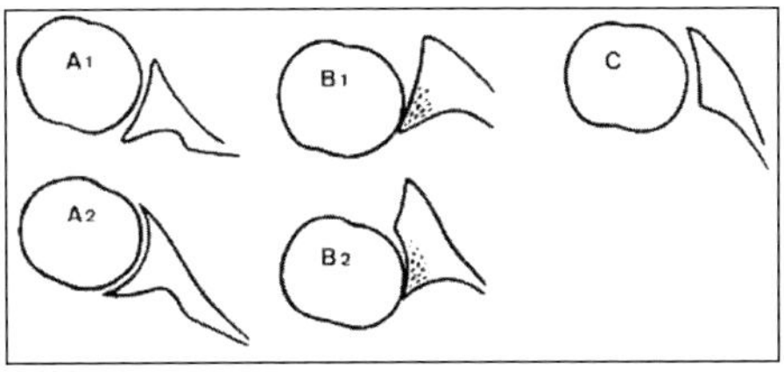

Fig. 1 : Glenoid Classification, Walch et al., 1999.

Section II of this chapter concerns the measurement of glenoid version. Recognition of the glenoid version is important for evaluation of different pathologies. Surgical strategies in shoulder reconstruction can change significantly in the presence of major retroversion. Despite acknowledgment of the importance of this crucial morphologic particularity in the pathological shoulder, there is no consensus on the method to use to evaluate version on a regular CT scan. An overview of the literature showed two main techniques for the assessment of glenoid version on a CT scan. Friedman (1992) described a measuring method using a

Some Data and images included in this chapter are from Authors' previous scientific publication or articles in press. All figures are published with the author's permission

line between the tip of the medial border of the scapula to the center of the glenoid joint as a reference line for the scapula axis. Also, we can use the general axis of the scapula body on a CT-scan. These two techniques are shown in Figure 2. In this specific example, the scapula body is curved and each reference technique gives a different line.

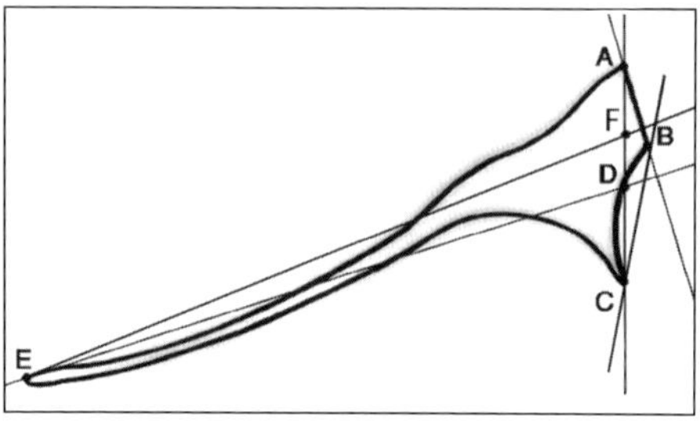

Fig. 2 : Measurement of retroversion according to Friedman line (ED) and Scapula body (EF)
AB = Paleoglenoid
AC = Intermediate glenoid
BC = Neoglenoid

Section III is dedicated to quantification of posterior humeral subluxation. Humeral head static posterior subluxation is important information in the evaluation of osteoarthritis. Subluxation of the humeral head can lead to posterior wear or erosion of the glenoid and after surgery can lead to prosthetic instability, increased glenoid polyethylene wear, and early loosening of a glenoid component, often resulting in revision and worse outcomes for patients.

Recent articles have shed some light onto this perplexing entity of posterior subluxation; however, more research is needed to understand and improve our treatment of shoulder arthritis in its presence. Proposals for standardization of subluxation measurements have been advocated for decades, but no universal standard exists. Different techniques exist to measure subluxation, but none have ever been validated and we currently do not know which is most predictable regarding the complication rates of shoulder arthroplasty in patients with glenohumeral osteoarthritis. Subluxation can be assessed according to a perpendicular line to the joint surface, the mediatrice (fig. 3). It can also be measured following a scapular axis reference line as utilized in other research groups (fig. 4). The purpose of this section is to investigate different methods to measure subluxation of the glenohumeral joint and to compare them in terms of absolute difference and reliability.

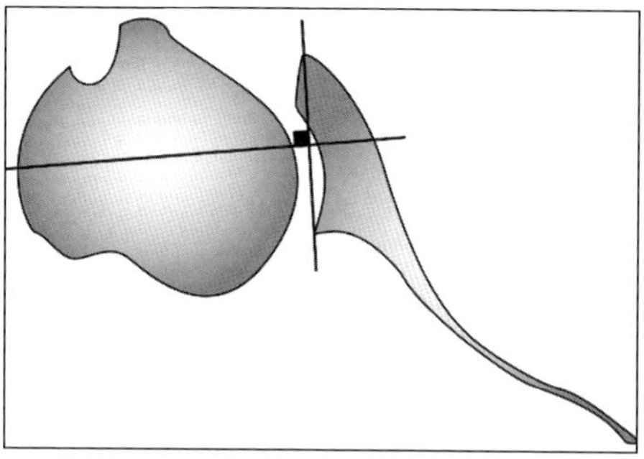

Fig. 3 : Assessment of glenohumeral subluxation according to the mediatrice line.

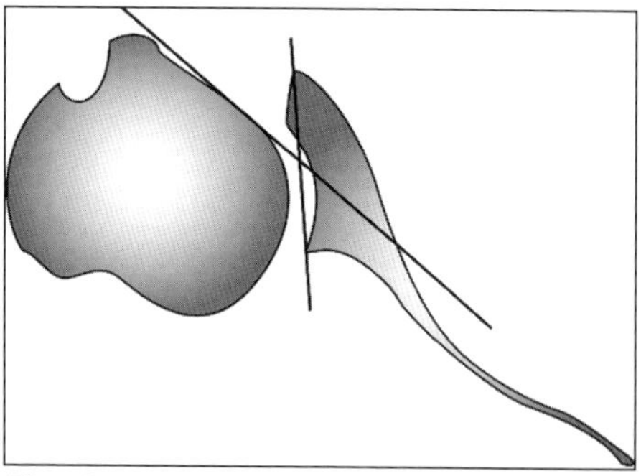

Fig. 4 : Assessment of glenohumeral subluxation using the Friedman line.

MATERIALS AND METHODS

One hundred sixteen consecutive shoulder CT scans of patients with primary glenohumeral arthritis were selected by an independent evaluator. The axial cut inferior to the coracoid process was selected. The patient demographics on the images were made anonymous and presented randomly to three independents evaluators. The evaluators were of different levels of experience (one general orthopaedic surgeon with two years' experience, one shoulder fellow, and one mid-level orthopaedic resident) and from different countries (Spain, United States of America, and Italy) reflecting different training backgrounds. The evaluators were asked to classify glenoid wear according to the Walch classification two separate times at a one-week interval. Each surgeon received and reviewed the original paper to understand the classification as described by Walch *et al.* Also, evaluators were asked to measure glenoid version and glenohumeral subluxation following the different methods mentioned earlier. Validity of these methods was then established.

Section I: Walch classification revisited

The agreement between different evaluators in classifying fracture type or other radiological element using categorical classification is calculated with the Kappa statistic. The Kappa statistic is an evaluation of agreement between two sets of observations. It is important to underline the fact that some agreement between two observers can be due only to chance. The Kappa statistics was developed to express the amount of agreement not due to chance. A Kappa of 1 means full agreement. A Kappa of 0 means that present agreement is only due to chance. For example, if the shoulder image in this study were classified randomly by two monkeys, we would probably find some agreement due to chance but it will still give a Kappa close to 0. It is generally accepted that a Kappa < 0.4 is poor; Kappa =0.4-0.59 is fair; Kappa =0.6-0.74 is good; Kappa >0.74 is excellent. The validation study was done for three sets of data:

- **Set A:** The complete classification with categories and sub categories: A1, A2, B1, B2, C.
- **Set B:** Regrouping data with main categories: A, B, C
- **Set C:** Regrouping with categories according to glenoid facet morphology (fig. 5):
  - Normal concavity: A1, A2, B1
  - Biconcave glenoid: B2
  - Retroverted glenoid: C

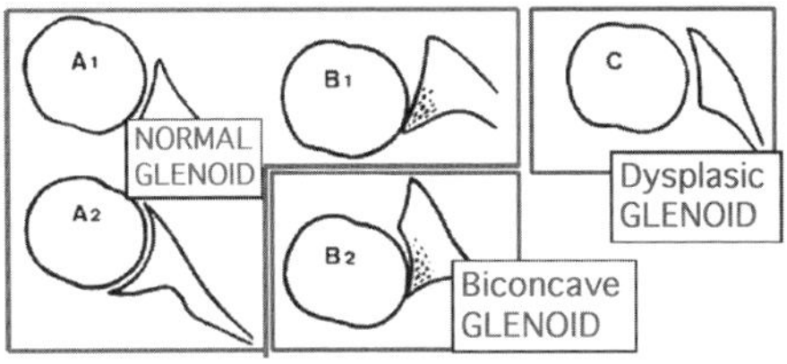

Fig. 5: Regroupment of Walch Classification (original figure from Walch et al. 1999).

The CT-scans of 116 shoulders were evaluated by the three independent observers in a blinded and randomized method as described above. The intra-observer Kappa values for Observer 1, 2, and 3 were 0.899, 0.927, and 0.773 with an average of 0.866 for set A (the complete classification including sub categories); all indicating excellent intra-observer reliability. For Set B (major categories, no sub-categories), the kappa values for observer 1, 2, and 3 were 0.955, 0.975, and 0.814, with an average of 0.915; all excellent values. For set C (normal concavity, biconcave B2, and C), the values were 0.897, 0.948, and 0.777, with an average of 0.874; all excellent values.

The Kappa values for inter-observer reliability for Set A (complete classification) were 0.776, 0.512, and 0.574, with an average of 0.621; indicating good values. For Set B (major categories, no sub-categories), the values averaged 0.759 (0.880, 0.713, 0.685), indicating excellent inter-observer agreement. For Set C, the average was 0.642 (0.825, 0.519, 0.581), indicating good inter-observer agreement.

According to these results, this most recent study of the Walch classification demonstrates excellent reproducibility and good to excellent agreement among observers. The strengths of the classification described by Walch *et al.* include high levels of reliability when used properly, even in the hands of less experienced orthopedic surgeons. The repeat study was performed with three independent observers: one practicing general orthopedic surgeon, one shoulder fellow, and one mid-level orthopedic resident. Each observer was from a different country, with differences in training and experience; however, the good to excellent intra- and inter-observer values noted in this study are evidence for a classification that is reproducible for all orthopedic surgeons, regardless of training or experience. Another strength is the large number of patients used for validation in this study and the original paper by Walch *et al.*, each over 100 (116 and 113, respectively). Cohen, in his original paper in 1960 on Kappa statistics, points out that the Kappa distribution will become normal when N is greater than 100. Results obtained with too small a sample have a greater chance to be non-representative of the population.

Strength of the classification is that 2D axial CT slices are easily available and very familiar to most practicing orthopedic surgeons. CT analysis of glenoid morphology and the definition of different types of glenoid have shown a wide range of polymorphism and evolution.

Like other classifications (e.g., AO classification), inter-observer reliability increased when only three types of glenoid categories were used (A, B, C). *Set C of data did not improve reliability; therefore this restructuring of the classification is not advocated.* Therefore, the classification proposed by Walch *et al.* is valid, simple, and continues to be a reliable and valuable method to assess the glenoid in osteoarthritic glenoids.

Section II: Glenoid version measurement

Two different reference lines were compared to evaluated version: the Friedman line, and the scapula blade line.

Friedman definition: *"For the determination of the glenoid version, a line is drawn between the anterior and posterior margins of the glenoid. The transverse axis of the scapula is determined by a line drawn from the midpoint of the glenoid fossa to the medial end of the image of the scapula; a line drawn perpendicular to this is defined as a line of neutral version. If the posterior margin of the glenoid was medial to this line of neutral version, then the condition was defined as retroversion of the glenoid cavity, and the angle between* *the line of neutral version and the line connecting the anterior and posterior margins of the glenoid was measured and recorded as a negative number of degrees. If, instead, the anterior margin was medial to the line of neutral version, the condition was defined as anteversion of the glenoid cavity, and the angle between the line of neutral version and the line connecting the anterior and posterior margins of the glenoid was measured and record as a positive number of degrees."* (JBJS 1992)

Scapula body method: The antero-posterior glenoid or version is the angle that is complementary to the one formed by the intersection of the scapular body axis and glenoid surface.

Version

Negative and positive reference of version: For simplicity, we chose to keep the positive and negative description as Friedman described: the anteversion is a positive number of degrees and retroversion is a negative number of degrees.

B2 glenoid: Three different reference lines have been measured: the neo-glenoid NG (posterior erosion surface), paleo-glenoid PG (original glenoid surface) and the intermediate-glenoid IG (line from anterior and posterior edge) (fig. 2). The intra-class correlation coefficient (ICC) is the statistics used for assessing the agreement between two evaluators for measurements. Correlation coefficients (r) and ICC between 0.70 and 0.79 were regarded as good; values between 0.80 and 0.89 were categorized as very good; and *r* values of 0.90 and greater were considered excellent. The significance level of 0.05 was used for the Student *T*-tests.

Group 1 (B2 Glenoid excluded)

Measurements

The average version using the scapula blade technique is -7.29 degrees and is -10.43 degrees for the Friedman technique. The average glenoid version is significantly higher using Friedman method for all three observers with a mean difference of +5.64 degrees, +2.74 degrees and +1.04 degrees respectively for observer A, B and C.

Reliability

For group 1, the intra-observer reliability (consistency) measured by the intra-class correlation (ICC) was excellent (>0.9) for the three observers for both methods. The intra-observer correlation (ICC) for the glenoid version was always slightly better for the Friedman method. The inter-observer correlation, or agreement, between observer A, B and C was excellent for glenoid version for both techniques with an ICC of 0.962 (CI 95%, 0.935-0.979) for the scapula body method, and with an ICC of 0.977 (0.961-0.987) for the Friedman value. Again the reliability seems to be a little bit higher with Friedman method, without being statistically significant.

Group 2 (B2 Glenoid)

Measurements

Two scapula reference lines were used: the Friedman method (FM) and the scapula body method (BM). Three glenoid reference lines were chosen and named: Paleo-glene (PG), intermediate glenoid (IG), and neo-glenoid (NG). A total of six different measurements of version were taken following the association of these methods: FM-PG, FM-IG, FM-NG, BM-

PG, BM-IG, BM-NG. The average glenoid versions were significantly different ($p<0.05$) between the two different scapula reference line measurement techniques and between three glenoid reference lines of glenoid surface for all three observers, with an average of -8.93° for PG, -21.84° for IG and -27.29° for NG with the scapula body technique (BM) and an average of -12.56° for PG, -25.55° for IG and -31.04° for NG with the Friedman method (FM). The neo-glenoid reference line reports the most severe retroversion measurement.

Reliability

In group 2, intra-observer reliability, or consistency, was very good or excellent for all reference line associations, with an ICC over 0.82. The inter-observer reliability, or agreement, was also very good or excellent for all methods with an ICC over 0.79.

The most reliable method for measurement of B2 glenoid version was the association of the Friedman line for the scapula axis and the intermediate glenoid line, with excellent intra-observer reliability (ICC > 0.957) and inter-observer reliability of 0.954.

Section III: Glenohumeral subluxation

The first method, named Scapula Method (SM), uses the scapula axis as a reference line, which is a line drawn from the medial border of the scapula body to the center of the glenoid. The percentage of the humeral head posterior to that line was assessed at the longest AP diameter of the head on a line perpendicular to the scapula axis (fig. 4). A percentage higher than 55% defined posterior subluxation.
The second method, named Mediatrice Method (MM), used the "mediatrice" line, drawn as a perpendicular line to glenoid joint surface passing through its middle. Again, the percentage of humeral head posterior to that line was measured at the larger AP diameter (fig. 3).

Reliability of both methods was obtained and compared using intra-observer reliability (consistency) and inter-observer reliability (agreement) report by intra-class correlation test (ICC). Correlation coefficients (r) and ICC between 0.70 and 0.89 were regarded as good, and r values of 0.90 and greater were considered excellent.

The humeral head subluxation in percentage was from 37% to 119% when the Scapula Method (SM) was used, and from 29% to 92% when the Mediatrice Method (MM) was used. For all three evaluators, there was a significant difference between the mean obtained by each method, with the mediatrice method always reporting smaller percentages: 73.5% (SD 15.1%) vs. 59.7% (SD 11.2%) $p<0.001$. Figures 3 and 4 illustrate this phenomenon with a drastic difference in ratio in this case. The mediatrice method gives 58% of subluxation and the scapular method showed 100% of subluxation.

The intra observer reliability (consistency) was very good or excellent using SM (ICC: 0.921, 0.841 and 0.912) and good to very good with MM (ICC 0.794, 0.796, 0.704). The inter-observer reliability (agreement) was very good for SM (ICC: 0.822 CI 95%: 0.703 to 0.889) and good for MM (ICC: 0.733 CI 95%: 0.654-0.799).

Our results show that measurements of subluxation have high reproducibly with the same surgeon and among surgeons when done in a systematic method. CT scans were used in this study because, compared to X-rays, the margins of the glenoid and humeral head necessary to determine the amount of subluxations are easier to define. Measurements of subluxations based on the scapular axis as defined by Friedman et al. allow for a high intra- and inter-observer reliability. The mediatrice method does allow for a still high, but slightly lower, reliability compared to subluxation measurements based on the scapular axis. Both methods could be used with high reliability to assess the influence of subluxation on postoperative results.

Several points regarding the measurements should be discussed. The osteology of the scapular blade is extremely variable, with some demonstrating a flat, more straight appearance and others with a large curve along the medial border. Surgeons must encourage the radiologist to include the entire scapula. Lastly, the presence of posterior erosion as seen in a Type B2 glenoid poses a difficult problem with the measurement of subluxation. The erosion has by definition destroyed the posterior margin of the glenoid. Guesswork regarding its location can lead to less precise measurements of the scapular axis and thus subluxation ratio.

Currently, there is no published data suggesting a threshold past which increased subluxation will lead to decreased function and patient satisfaction. Certainly, more research is warranted to investigate our treatment for posterior subluxation of the humeral head and determine if it is adequate. We believe this study, which shows a high reliability for measurements of subluxation, will spawn further research into this peculiar and unsolved problem in shoulder arthroplasty.

Both methods showed significant difference in assessing humeral head subluxation. The method using the scapula axis as a reference line is more reliable from a purely statistical point of view. Further research is essential to unravel the mystery of posterior subluxation and its influence on outcomes following shoulder arthroplasty.

CONCLUSION

This chapter underlines some important facts on the evaluation of glenoid wear, measurement of version and humeral head subluxation. First, the Walch classification is reliable and must be used for glenoid wear evaluation. Usage of the subgroups slightly decreases the reliability, but it is still very good. The glenoid version measurement must be done using the Friedman line as a reference. In cases of B2 glenoid, the intermediate glenoid must be chosen. To measure the retroversion, the Friedman line showed statistical advantage, but the clinical implication still needs to be studied. The normal value of subluxation according to this reference line needs to be found.

THE GLENOID IN THE FRONTAL PLANE: THE FAVARD AND THE HAMADA RADIOGRAPHIC CLASSIFICATIONS OF CUFF TEAR OSTEOARTHRITIS

L. FAVARD, G. ALAMI

The height of the subacromial space (also known as the acromiohumeral interval, AHI) has been known to be representative of the status of the rotator cuff [8]. It is generally accepted that an AHI of less than 7 mm, measured on an antero-posterior radiograph in neutral position, is significantly correlated with a large or massive tear of the rotator cuff, especially the supraspinatus and infraspinatus [1, 2]. The progressive decrease in subacromial space was analyzed by Hamada *et al.* [5] in their 1990 publication. They reported on a group of 22 patients with massive cuff tears treated nonoperatively, then they described a classification used today in most series reporting on the treatment of massive cuff tears. In the Hamada classification, stage IV is the only stage dedicated to glenohumeral involvement. When that point is reached, arthroplasty is generally indicated.

Later, Favard *et al.* [3] distinguished different types of glenoid wear associated with a massive cuff tear and proposed a classification of these types. Each of these two classifications concerning the glenoid in the frontal plane is an important contribution to therapeutic decision making and surgical technique. They have different yet complementary uses, which will be detailed in the following sections.

THE HAMADA CLASSIFICATION

This is a descriptive and pathophysiologic classification based on the analysis of a small cohort of patients. Hamada *et al.* distinguished five stages (Fig. 1). *Stage I* is a normal shoulder without narrowing of the subacromial space. *Stage II* involves a narrowing of the subacromial space, with an AHI of less than 6 mm, and usually corresponds to a massive and old cuff tear. The authors found that from the time the AHI became smaller than 5 mm, there was no longer a long-head-of-biceps tendon between the humeral head and acromion. *Stage III* involves acetabulization, defined as a concave deformity of the acromial undersurface. The contact between the humeral head and acromion

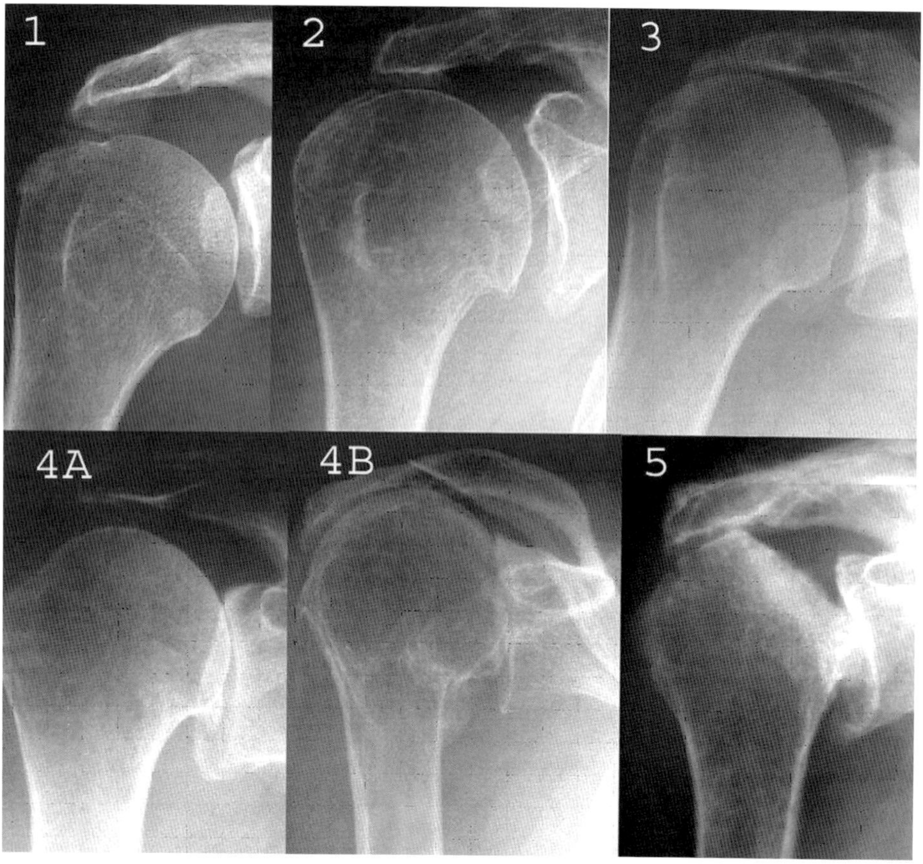

Fig. 1: Hamada classification

resulted in a new articulation, either by progressive ossification of the coracoacromial ligament or by wear due to friction between the undersurface of the acromion and the top of the head, which becomes rounded—or both. At this stage, no glenohumeral involvement would have occurred yet. *Stage IV* involves narrowing of the glenohumeral joint. Walch divided this stage into two groups: stage IV-A for eccentric wear or erosion at the superior part of the glenohumeral joint without acetabulization of the acromion, and stage IV-B for superior wear or erosion with acetabulization[(1)]. *Stage V* comprised features of the true cuff tear arthropathy described by Neer, with some humeral head collapse and bone destruction.

Classifying patients according to this system is not very difficult. One caveat, however, is that in stage III an increase in

[(1)] The goal of this specific sub-division was to emphasize the absence of a temporal relationship between acromial acetabularization and glenohumeral involvement—some patients pass directly from stage II to stage IV-A and then IV-B, while others pass through stages II and III before reaching stage IV-B.

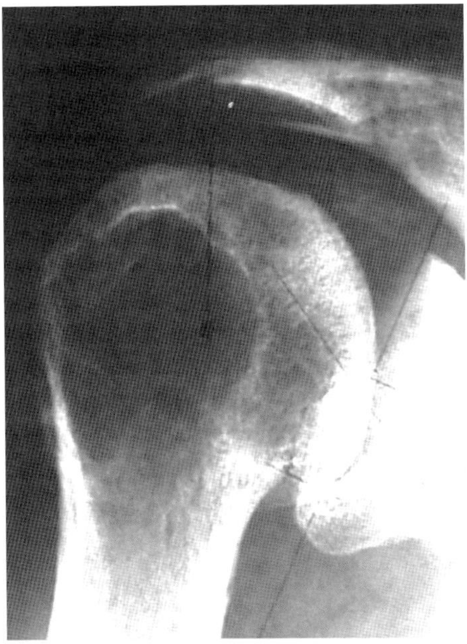

Fig. 2: Widening of subacromial space by an effusion

the subacromial space may occur if a large effusion distends the joint (Fig. 2). Usually, the correct diagnosis is still possible due to the concave appearance of the acromial undersurface.

In fact, it is with stages I and II that classification difficulties are most common. Indeed, through humeral rotation alone, a substantial artificial narrowing of the subacromial space can be caused, which is absent on radiographs in neutral position (Fig. 3). The space can also be increased due to an effusion in these earlier stages. Surprisingly, a subacromial space that is within normal limits in the standing position can be narrowed when the patient is supine. This has been described by Raillac [9] and is seen regularly on CT scans.

To find out whether there is a real difference between Hamada's stages I and II, we carried out a prospective study of massive cuff tears classified as stage I or II (Table I). No difference in age was present between the two groups. We found a significant difference in terms of fatty

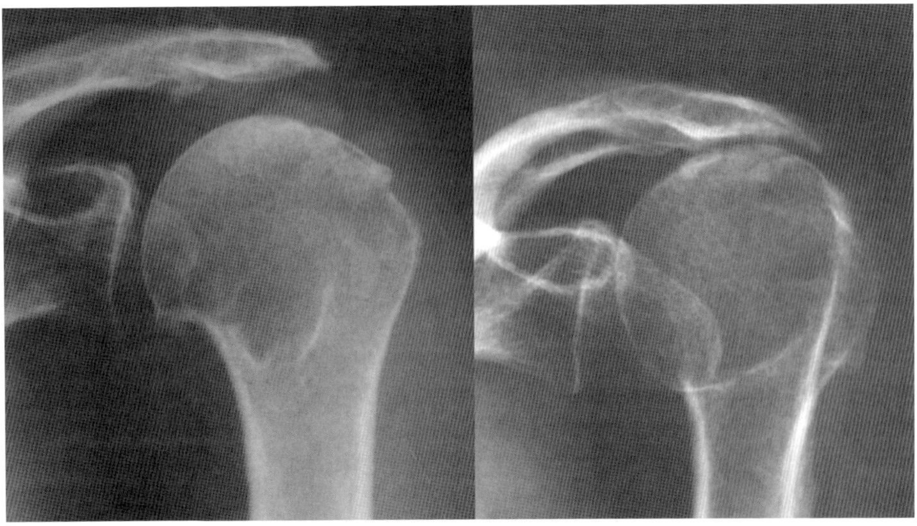

Fig. 3: Same shoulder in neutral and external rotation, demonstrating narrowing of subacromial space

HAMADA [5]	N	Age	Supra FI	Infra FI
1	26	60.2 ± 8.1	2.0 ± 0.9	2.1 ± 1.4
2	20	60.5 ± 5.3	2.8 ± 0.9	2.8 ± 1.2

Table I: Prospective comparison of stages I and II of Hamada classification. (FI, fatty infiltration; supra, supraspinatus; infra, infraspinatus.)

infiltration (FI) of the supraspinatus muscle [4]. There was no difference in FI of infraspinatus or subscapularis. The mean AHI of stage I was 9.0 mm on plain X-ray and 7.0 mm on CT scan. As for stage II, its mean AHI was 4.5 mm on plain X-ray and 3.7 mm on CT scan.

The practical usefulness of this classification is during the decision-making process regarding the timing of arthroplasty. Indeed, it appears that reverse shoulder arthroplasty (RSA) has significantly worse results in stages I and II than in the other stages [7]. For these early stages, antalgic, temporizing treatments such as biceps tenotomy can be considered, leaving RSA for stage-I and stage-II patients with a pseudoparalytic shoulder.

THE FAVARD CLASSIFICATION

This is a descriptive classification devised for choosing the correct treatment and anticipating technical difficulties. All stages of this classification involve glenohumeral cartilage disease (Fig. 4). ***Stage E0*** involves eccentric cartilage wear without subchondral-bone erosion. ***Stage***

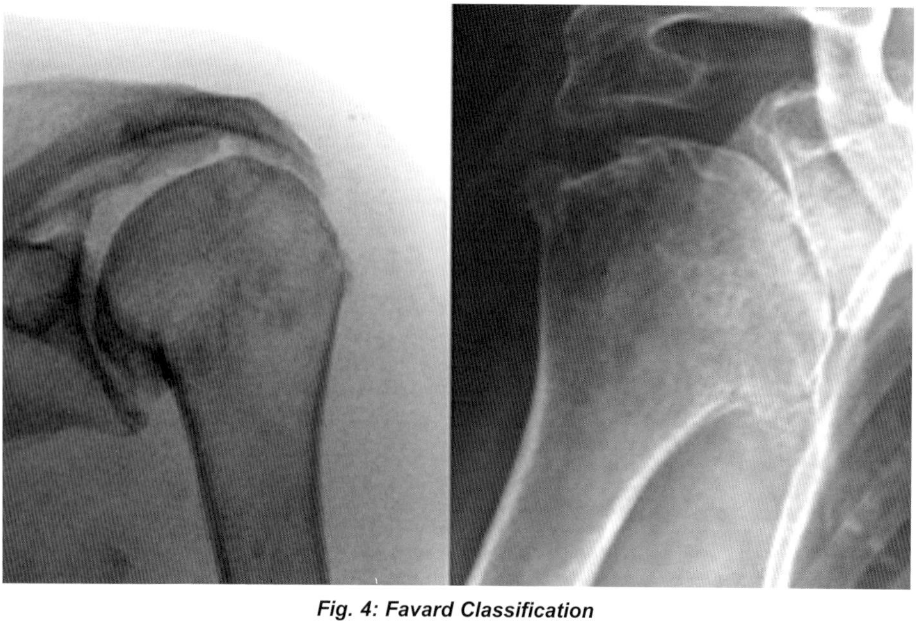

Fig. 4: Favard Classification

E1 involves concentric glenoid erosion. ***Stage E2*** involves eccentric erosion giving the glenoid a biconcave appearance. ***Stage E3*** involves advanced erosion with a large, proximally-facing concavity. Later on, after the discovery of some antero-inferior erosions associated with a massive cuff tear, ***stage E4*** was added (Fig. 5).

The value of stage E1 is to highlight the possibility of primary osteoarthritis that is unusually associated with a massive cuff tear (Fig. 6). Unlike in the other stages, it is likely that in stage E1 osteoarthritis would have preceded the cuff tear, and while still intact the cuff would have thus prevented the head from rising progressively. In the other stages, however, the cuff tear would have occurred first, explaining the eccentric (proximally migrated) head. That being said, radiographic narrowing of the subacromial space can be observed with primary osteoarthritis due to a posterior translation of the humeral head (Fig. 7).

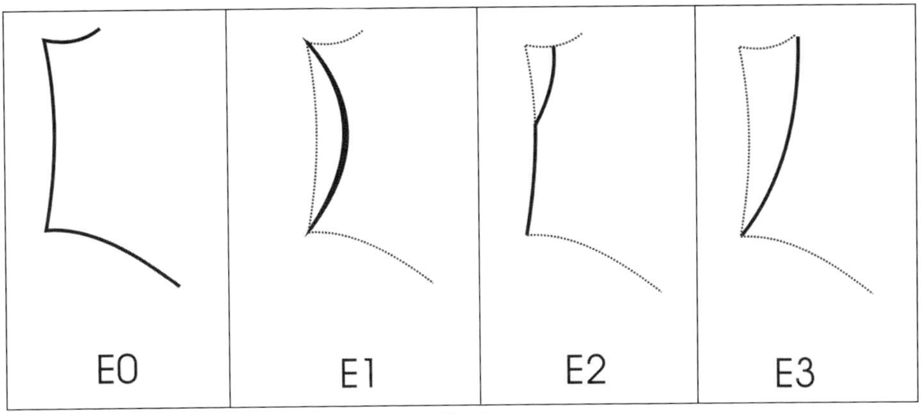

Fig. 5

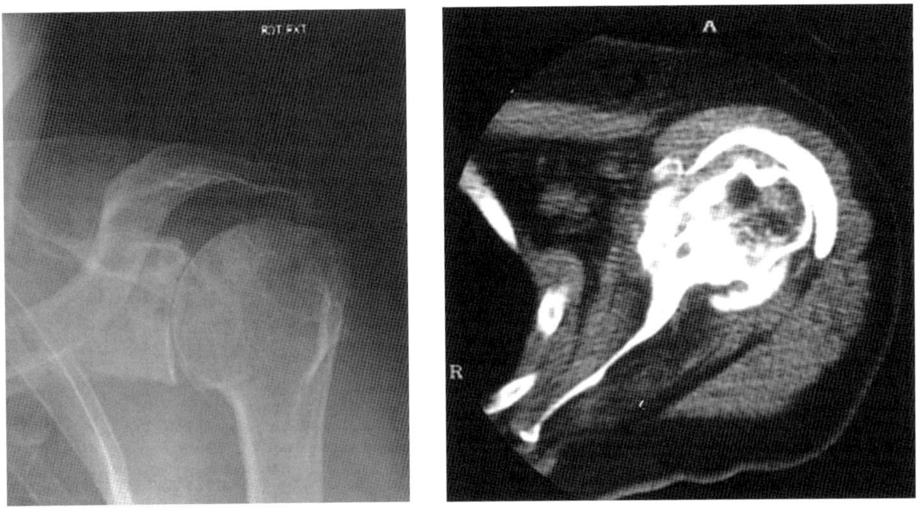

Fig. 6: Stage E1 of Favard classification; a non-traditional form of primary osteoarthritis associated with a massive cuff tear

Stages E2 and E3 are useful in the therapeutic decision-making process. Indeed, a comparative study of RSA and hemiarthroplasty [3] showed that hemiarthroplasty had significantly worse results with type-E2 glenoids. Moreover, a study of glenoid notching in RSA showed that stages E2 and E3 were the most vulnerable, while E4 was not [6]. The above findings lead us to recommend systematic glenoid bone grafting to correct the orientation of the glenoid base plate during RSA.

In conclusion, the classification of Hamada clarifies the point along the disease's natural history at which it is wise to consider RSA—that point is generally Hamada's stage III. When arthroplasty has been chosen, the classification of Favard allows the anticipation of technical difficulties and pitfalls in order to avoid scapular notching and rapid glenoid loosening.

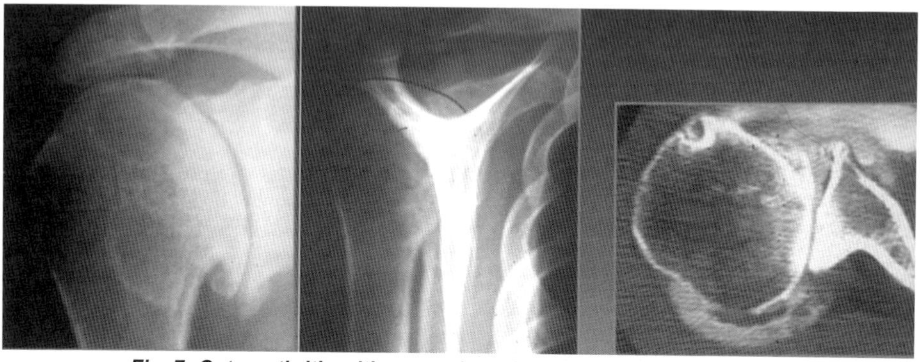

Fig. 7: Osteoarthritis with narrowing of subacromial space may be due to posterior translation of humeral head without cuff tear

REFERENCES

[1] BERNAGEAU J Roentgenographic assessment of the rotator cuff. *Clin Orthop Relat Res. 1990, 87-91.*

[2] COTTY P, F PROUST, P BERTRAND, B FOUQUET, P ROSSET, D ALISON, JP VALAT, P ROULEAU, J LAFFONT Rupture of the rotator cuff. Quantification of indirect signs in standard radiology and the Leclercq maneuver. *J Radiol 1988; 69: 633-8.*

[3] FAVARD L, S LAUTMANN, F SIRVEAUX, D OUDET, Y. KERJEAN, D HUGUET Hemiarthroplasty versus reverse arthroplasty in the treatment of osteoarthritis with massive rotator cuff tear. 2000 Shoulder Prostheses… two to ten years follow-up. BP Walch G, Mole D. *Montpellier, Sauramps Medical. 2001: 261-268.*

[4] GOUTALLIER D, JM POSTEL, J BERNAGEAU, L LAVAU, MC VOISIN Fatty muscle degeneration in cuff ruptures. Pre- and postoperative evaluation by CT scan. *Clin Orthop Relat Res. 1994 78-83.*

[5] HAMADA K, H FUKUDA, M MIKASA, Y KOBAYASHI Roentgenographic findings in massive rotator cuff tears. A long-term observation. *Clin Orthop Relat Res 1990, 92-6.*

[6] LEVIGNE C, P BOILEAU, L FAVARD, P GARAUD, D MOLE, F SIRVEAUX, G WALCH Scapular notching in reverse shoulder arthroplasty. *J Shoulder Elbow Surg. 2008;17: 925-35.*

[7] MOLE D, L FAVARD Excentered scapulohumeral osteoarthritis. *Rev Chir Orthop Reparatrice Appar Mot 2007; 93: 37-94.*

[8] NOVE-JOSSERAND L, C LEVIGNE, E NOEL, G WALCH The acromio-humeral interval. A study of the factors influencing its height. *Rev Chir Orthop Reparatrice Appar Mot 1996; 82: 379-85.*

[9] RAILHAC JJ, N SANS, A RIGAL, H CHIAVASSA, D GALY-FOURCADE, G RICHARDI, J ASSOUN, Y BELLUMORE, M MANSAT Strict anteroposterior radiography of the shoulder: value of the assessment of rotator cuff tears. *J Radiol 2001; 82: 979-85.*

RESULTS OF HEMIARTHROPLASTY IN PRIMARY OSTEOARTHRITIS

W.N. LEVINE

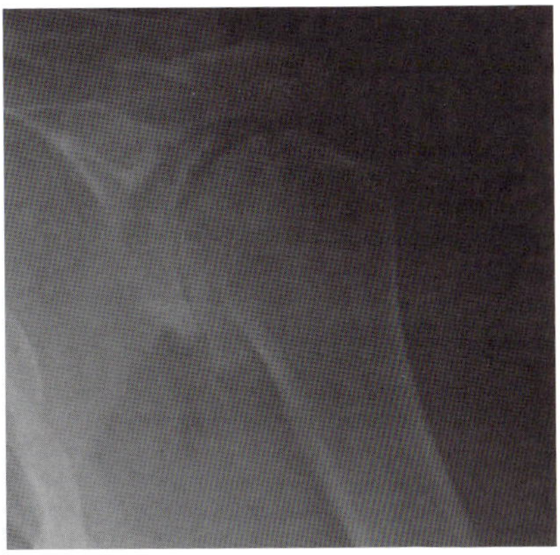

Overview
- *Treatment options*
- *Longitudinal study*
- *Literature review*
- *Final thoughts*

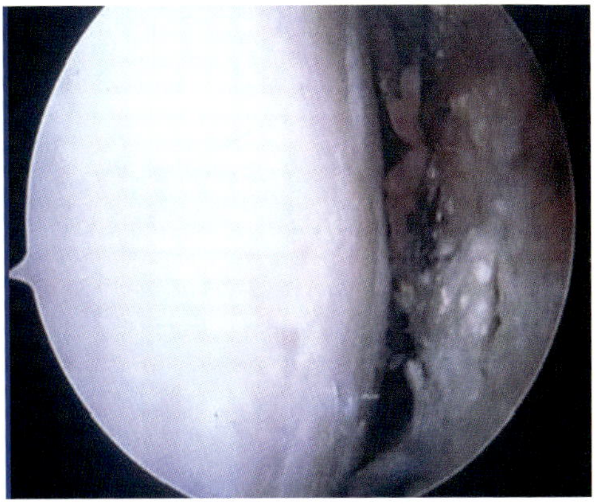

Options
- *Arthroscopy*
- *Resurfacing*
  - *+ biologic glenoid*
- *Standard Hemi*
  - *+ biologic*
- *TSA*

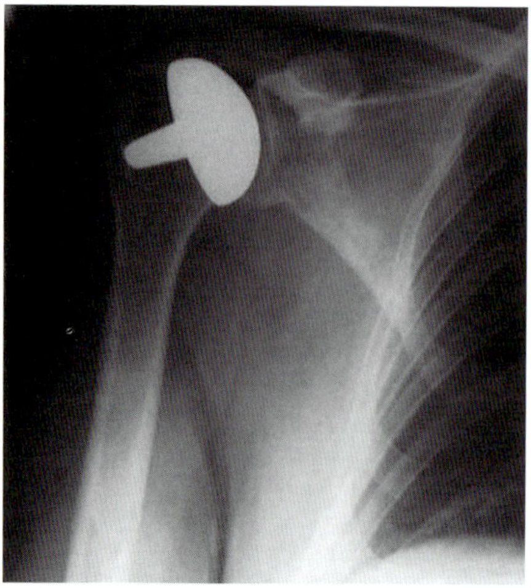

Options

- *Arthroscopy*
- ***Resurfacing***
  - *+ biologic glenoid*
- *Standard Hemi*
  - *+ biologic*
- *TSA*

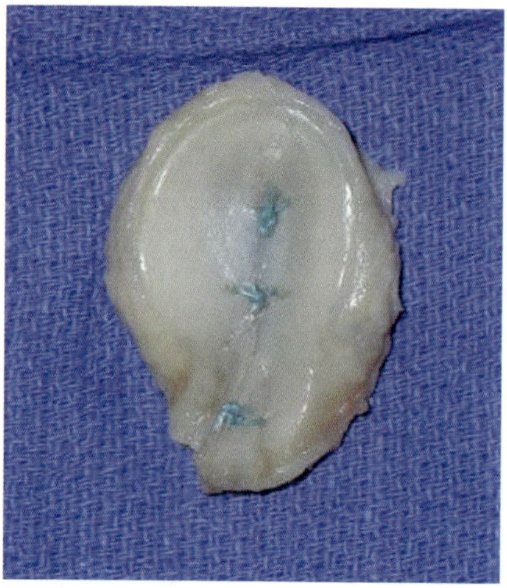

Options

- *Arthroscopy*
- ***Resurfacing***
  - ***+ biologic glenoid***
- *Standard Hemi*
  - *+ biologic*
- *TSA*

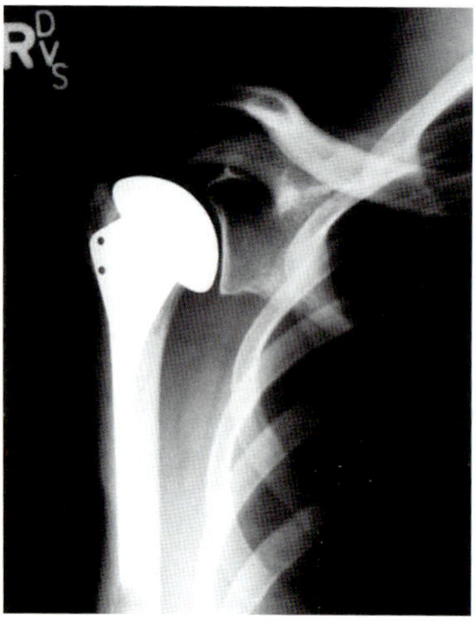

Options

- *Arthroscopy*
- *Resurfacing*
  - *+ biologic glenoid*
- ***Standard Hemi***
  - *+ biologic*
- *TSA*

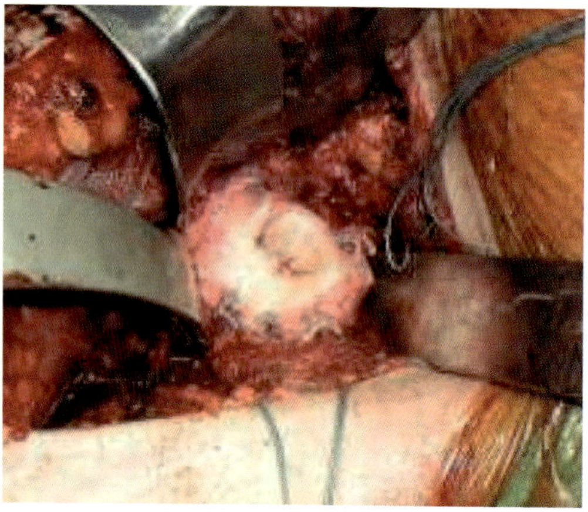

Options

- *Arthroscopy*
- *Resurfacing*
  - *+ biologic glenoid*
- ***Standard Hemi***
  - *+ **biologic***
- *TSA*

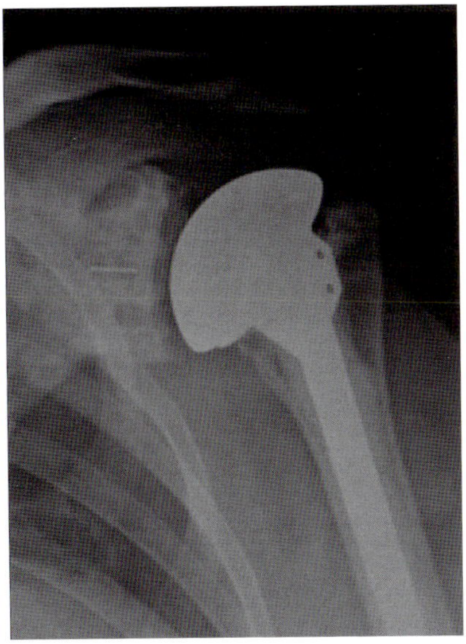

Options
- *Arthroscopy*
- *Resurfacing*
  - *+ biologic glenoid*
- *Standard Hemi*
  - *+ biologic*
- ***TSA***

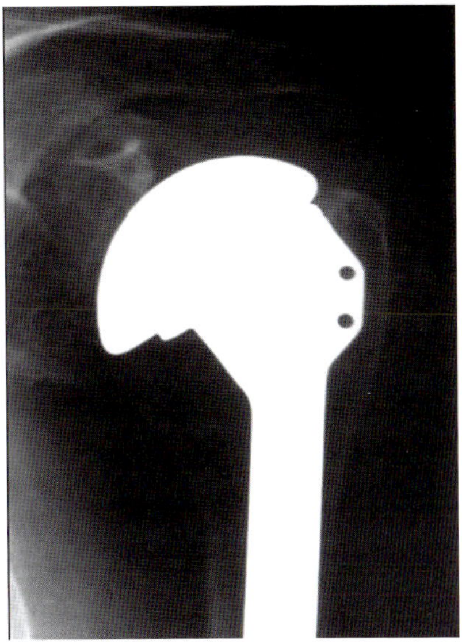

HHR Advantages
- *↓ Lateralization of joint line*
- *↓ Blood loss*
- *↓ OR time*
- *Avoid glenoid loosening*
- *? Bone sparing*

Hemiarthroplasty for glenohumeral osteoarthritis: Results correlated to degree of glenoid wear

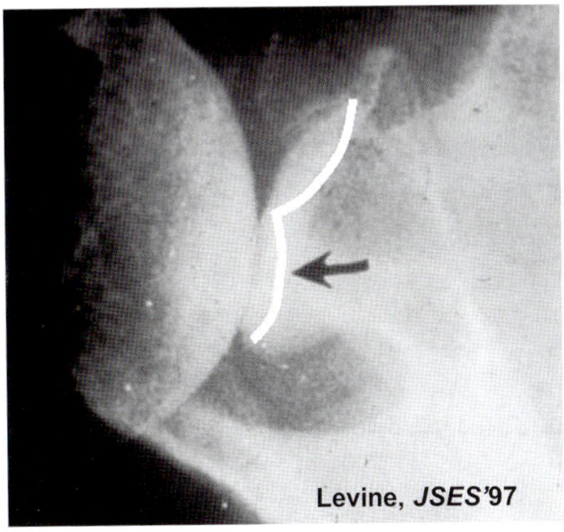

Original NYOH Series
- *31 Shoulders*
- *Avg age 56 (26-81)*
- *F/U **2.4** yrs (1.2-6)*
- *Sat. results **74**%*
  - *86% Concentric*
  - *63% Eccentric*

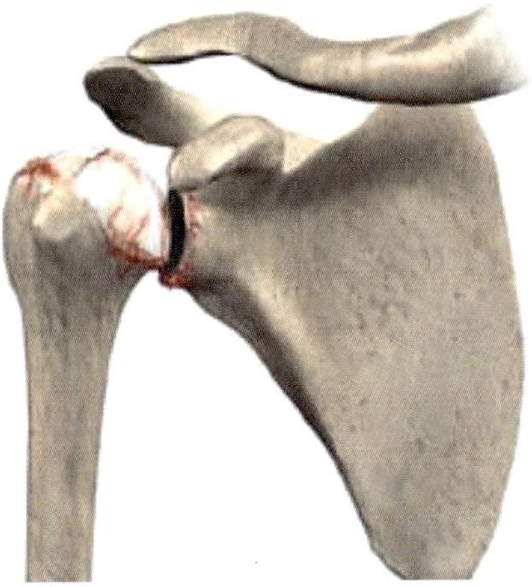

Purpose
- *Do HHR results **deteriorate** with time?*
- *Is HHR **inferior** to TSA for OA?*

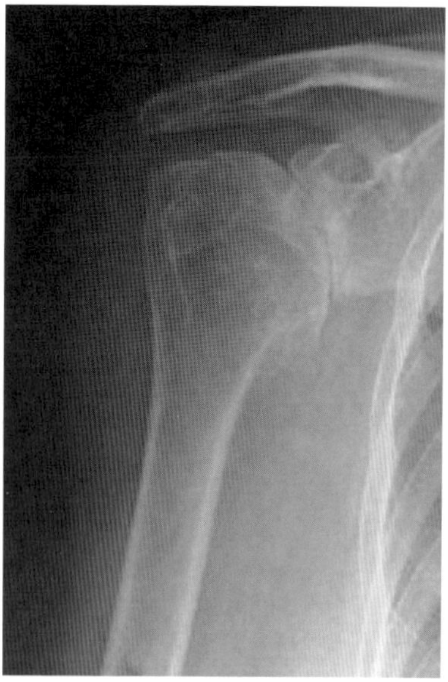

Methods

- *28 shoulders (27 pts)*
  - *3 died; 1 refused*
- *F/U **14.8** yrs (12.6-18.3)*
- *Average: **55.5** (26-78)*
- *Gender: 15M, 12F*
- *Glenoid Type: 12 Con, 16 Ecc*

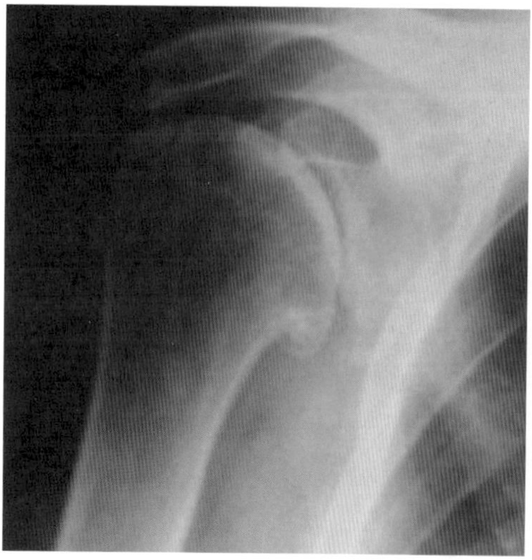

Indications

- *1° DJD – **9***
- *2° DJD – **19***
  - *Post-trauma 6*
  - *Instability 4*
  - *AVN 7*
  - *Other 2*

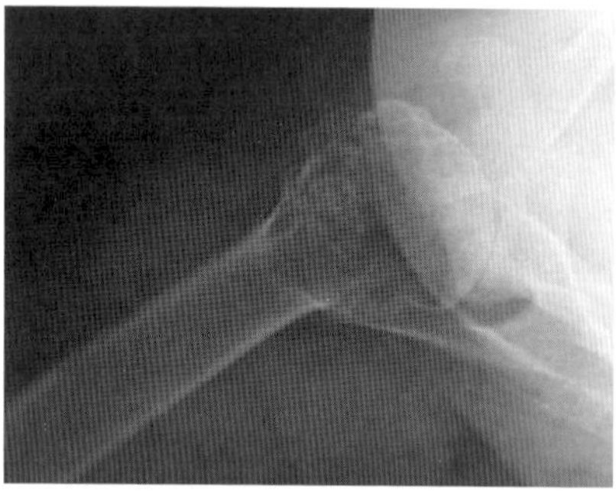

Results

All pts, n = 28

- *Average Follow-up Scores*
  - *Neer Sat **29%***
  - *Neer Ratings*
- *Excellent 4*
- *Good 4*
- *Fair 4*
- *Poor 16*

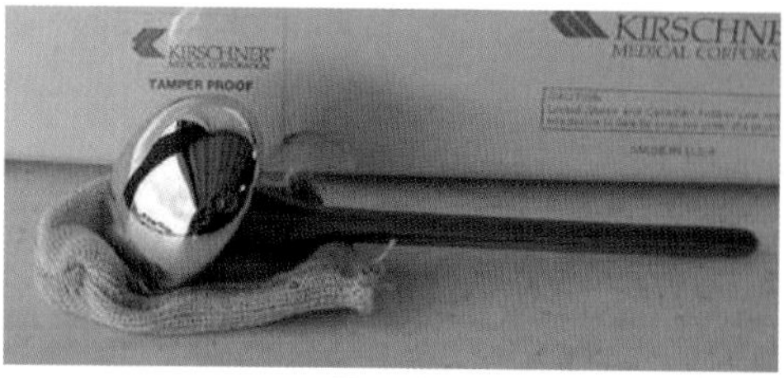

Results

Non-revised, n = 21

	Pre-op ROM	Post-op ROM	p-value
FF	104	**143.6**	<0.05
ER	20.7	**62.4**	<0.05
IR	gluteal	L5	0.186

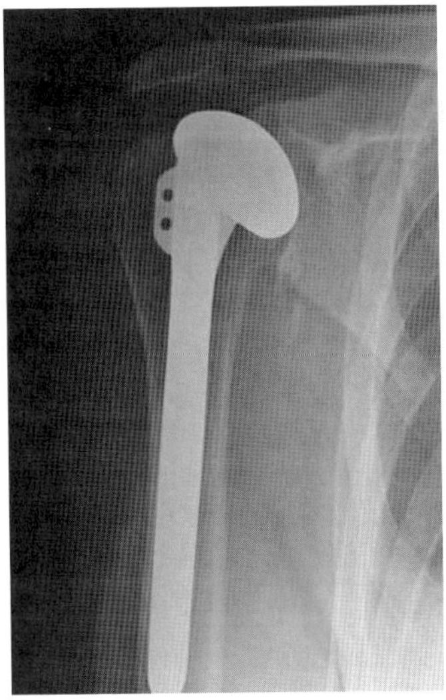

Results
Non-revised, n = 21

- *Average Follow-up Scores*
  - *ASES 70.59*
  - *SF-36 70.76*
  - *Euroqol 0.56*
  - *SST 8.24*
  - *Pai 2.29*

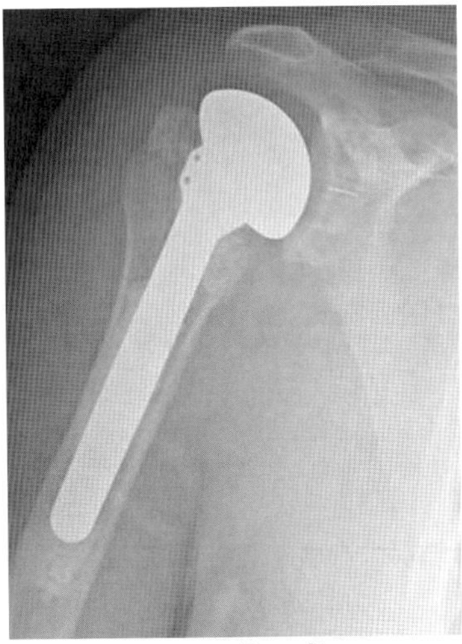

Results
Revisions, n = 7

- ***25**% overall*
  - *Concentric 3/12*
  - *Eccentric 4/16*
  - *Average revised **50.7***
  - *Average non-revised 56.9*
  - *Revision Indication **Pain***

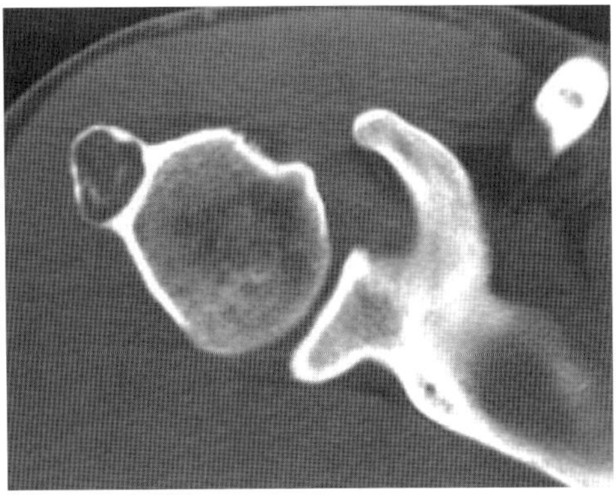

Results
Non-revised, n = 21

- *Concentric Better (p <0.05)*
  - *Euroqol*
  - *Neer Score*
  - *Neer Rating*

Results

	2.4 years n = 31	7.9 years n = 28	14.8 years n = 28
Overall	**74 %**	61 %	29 %
Concentric	**84 %**	67 %	42 %
Eccentric	**63 %**	56 %	19 %
1° OA	**80 %**		44 %
2° OA	**71 %**		21 %

Results

	2.4 years n = 31	**7.9 years n = 28**	14.8 years n = 28
Overall	74 %	**61 %**	29 %
Concentric	84 %	**67 %**	42 %
Eccentric	63 %	**56 %**	19 %
1° OA	80 %		44 %
2° OA	71 %		21 %

Results

	2.4 years n = 31	7.9 years n = 28	**14.8 years n = 28**
Overall	74 %	61 %	**29 %**
Concentric	84 %	67 %	**42 %**
Eccentric	63 %	56 %	**19 %**
1° OA	80 %		**44 %**
2° OA	71 %		**21 %**

Results
All pts, n = 28

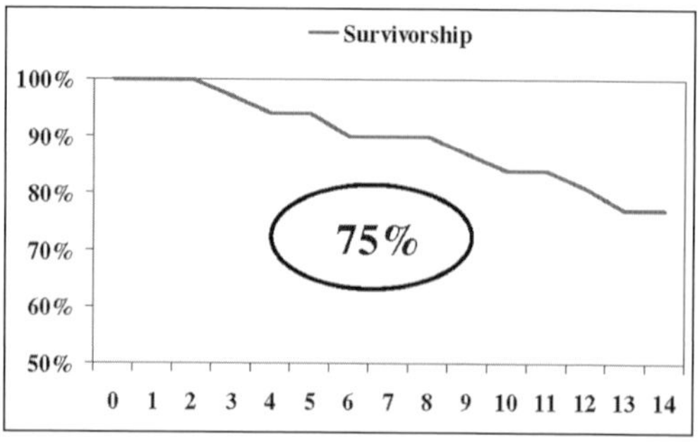

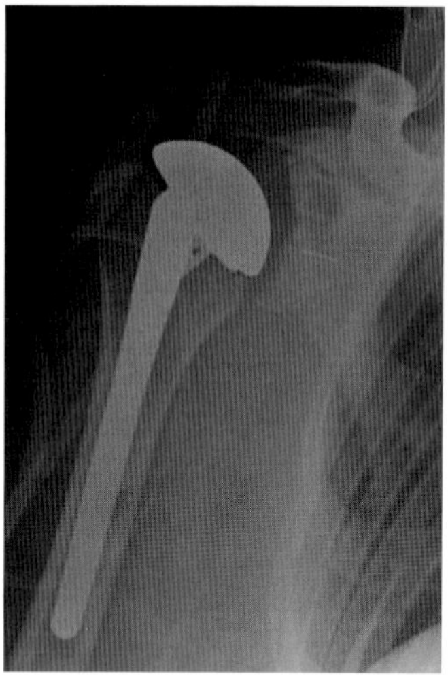

Conclusions
- ***29****% Satisfactory*
- *↓ results long term*
- *↑ short term rate HHR*
  - *TSA conversion*
- ***TSA*** *preferred to HHR for GH DJD in most pts*

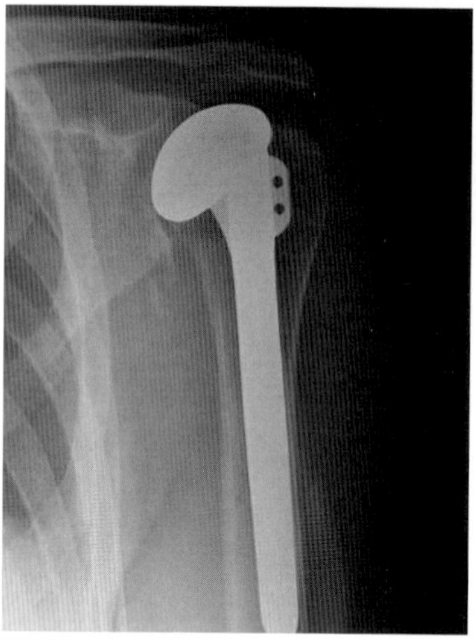

HHR Long-Term Results
- *Rispoli et al JBJS '06*
  - ***11.3*** *yr f/u*
  - ***25****% Revision rate*
  - ***58****% Neer Sat*
- *Wirth et al JBJS '06*
  - ***2.5*** *yr &* ***7.5*** *yr f/u*
  - ***All*** *pts* ***worse*** *in long term*

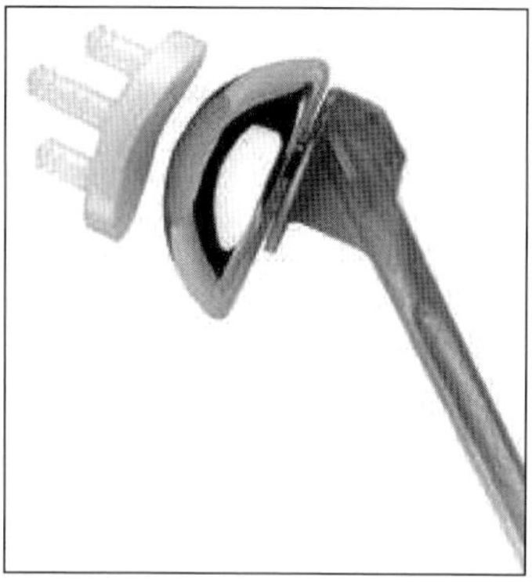

TSA vs HHR
- *Edwards et al JSES 2003*
  - ***2*** *yr f/u*
  - *TSA* ***superior*** *to HHR*
- *Sperling et al JSES '04*
  - ***16.8*** *yr f/u*
  - *TSA ↑ sat*
  - *TSA ↓ révision*

Outcomes

Hemiarthroplasty versus total shoulder prosthesis: Results of cemented glenoid components *(Mole et al., JSES 2006)*

- *705 TSA; 469 HHR*
- ***TSA>HHR*** *(independent age or cuff)*
  - *Post-op Functional Outcome*
  - *Post-op Patient Satisfaction*
- *↑ rate of radiolucent lines (**67.9%**)*

Cost effectiveness analysis of hemiarthroplasty and total shoulder arthroplasty (Mather et al., JSES 2010)

- *TSA Summary*
  - *Lower costs*
  - *Greater effectiveness*
  - *... therefore*
  - *More cost-effective!*

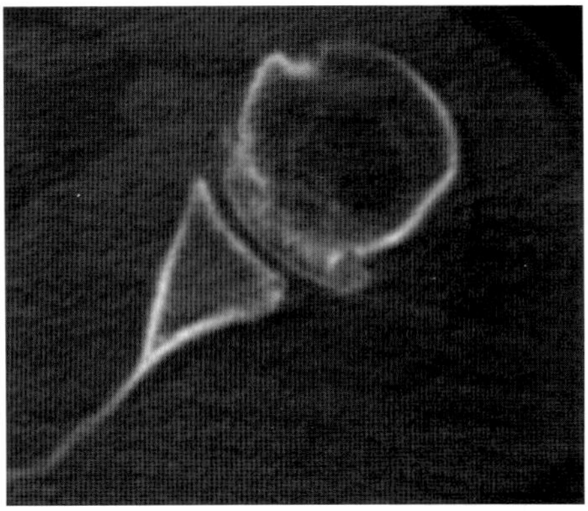

HHR Conversion to TSA

- *Sperling JBJS 1998*
  - *18 pts*
  - ***5.5** yr f/u*
  - ***40**% unsat*
- *Carroll JSES '04*
  - *16 pts*
  - ***5.5** yr f/u*
  - ***47**% unsat*

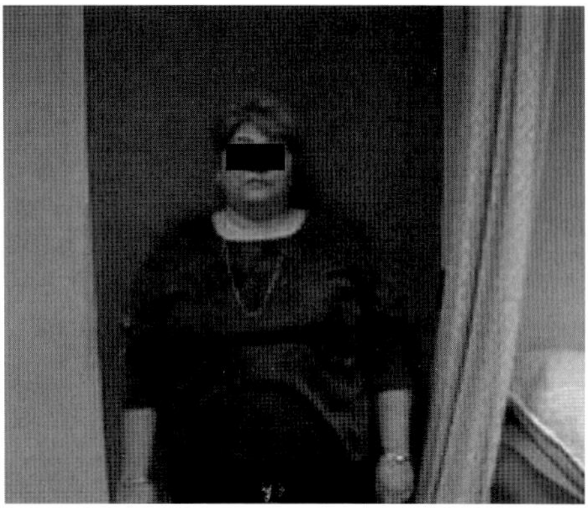

Summary

- *HHR (± biologic)*
  - *Theoretical advantages*
  - *Very little evidence*
- *TSA*
  - *Proven history*
  - *Patient satisfaction*

BIOLOGICAL RESURFACING FOR GLENOHUMERAL ARTHRITIS THEN AND NOW

W.Z. BURKHEAD J^R, S.G. KRISHNAN

Biological resurfacing of the glenoid in conjunction with hemiarthroplasty continues to be an important part of the armamentarium in the treatment of glenohumeral arthritis in young active patients on the Shoulder Service of the W.B. Carrell Memorial Clinic. The choice of bearing surfaces have evolved over the years beginning with autogenous capsule and fascia lata, transitioning to tendo Achilles allograft in the late 90's, and then to Dermal Matrix Allograft over the last 5 years. While it appeared in publication of the midterm results that tendo Achilles allograft was superior to autogenous capsule this was not a bearing surface issue but a subscapularis insertion weakness problem combined with the limitations of the 2nd generation humeral component which was used at that time leading to a component of subscapularis deficiency in a small number of patients (fig. 1).

Long-term follow-up of the initial cohort of 6 patients reported in 1995 reveals that the humeral component survivorship at an average of 19.5 years is 83.3%. Only 2 patients in this initial group have had subsequent surgery, one to remove a metal anchor centrally placed at the time of her initial surgery, the second patient was converted to a 3rd generation total shoulder arthroplasty 18 years after his

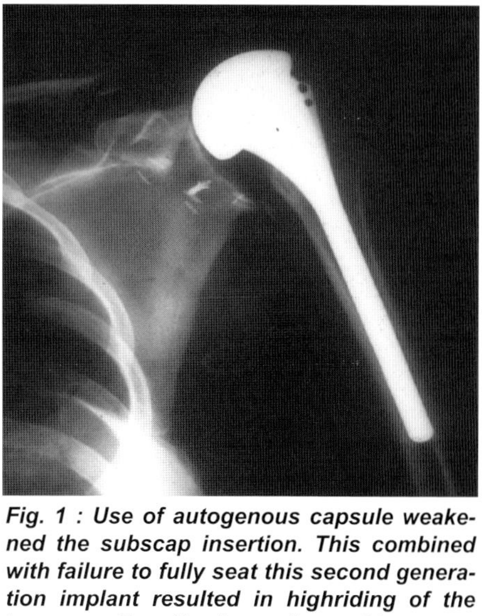

Fig. 1 : Use of autogenous capsule weakened the subscap insertion. This combined with failure to fully seat this second generation implant resulted in highriding of the humerus. Despite the radiographic appearance, the patient still enjoys satisfactory shoulder function, can saddle a horse, and carry hay 18 years post surgery.

initial surgery. The results have remained static for all of these years and continue to be good or excellent in four shoulders, satisfactory in 1. All patients were satisfied with the results of their operations and returned to active sports weight lifting manual labor and ranching.

Over the last 5 years the technique has evolved to include a 3rd generation humeral component combined with an allograft dermal matrix graft. The ability to balance the soft tissue provided by the newer stem combined with what appears to be a regenerative quality to the dermal matrix has enhanced our clinical results. The operation still is not without failures however with two patients developing symptomatic humeral loosening in three shoulders when uncemented stems were used. Biopsy of these patients has shown safranin O staining in chondral cells within the graft and on the surface of the bone. Similar findings have been reported by others after isolated arthroscopic resurfacing using the same material.

Newer techniques of biological resurfacing by other authors have emerged since our original description. The use of allograft lateral meniscus has been championed by some and most recently this has been used with a bulk fresh osteochondral humeral head allograft to accomplish an all biological total shoulder.

Not all authors report successful results with modifications of our original technique. The reasons for the differences in their results may be related to subtle but important technical differences, humeral component differences, or patient populations. It appears that younger (2nd and 3rd decade) patients who develop rapidly destructive arthritis after arthroscopic instability or SLAP repairs do not respond as well to any type of arthroplasty when compared to older (4th and 5th decade) who develop primary osteoarthritis or post reconstruction arthropathy 20 plus years after their index procedure.

The principles of Biological Resurfacing have not changed. They are as follows:

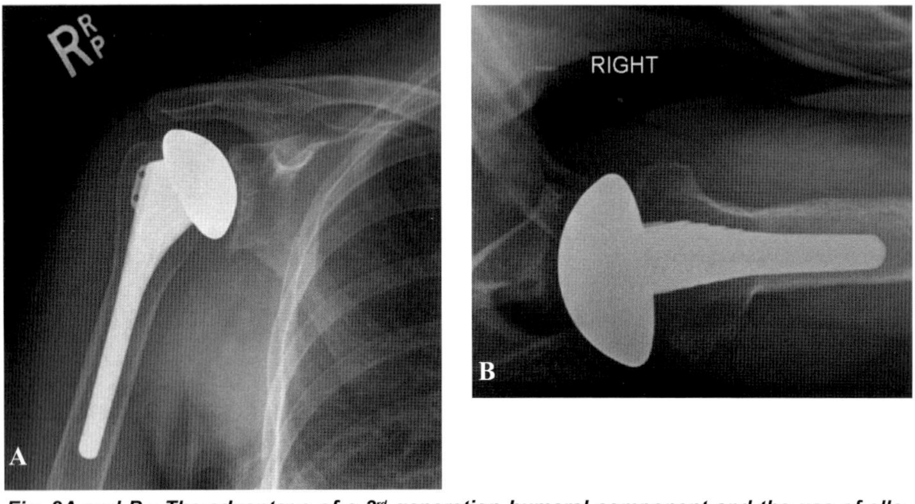

Fig. 2A and B : The advantage of a 3rd generation humeral component and the use of allograft dermal matrix as the bearing surface is illustrated in this 60 y/o woman 3 years postop. Note maintenance of joint space and lack of glenoid erosion is this well balanced shoulder.

1) Release of all contractures to return motion.

2) Glenoid surface preparation by reaming to normalize version but to preserve subchondral bone.

3) Deep drill holes past the subchondral plate to denervate the subchondral neural network decrease venous hypertension and allow pluripotential cells to come to the surface to repopulate the graft or create buds of fibrocartilage below the graft.

4) Application of a smooth wettable bearing surface to lower the coefficient of friction and to protect the embryonic tissue formed on the surface of the glenoid.

5) Anatomic humeral component placement that respects multi-plane offset, and allows matching of inclination of the head and shaft.

6) Careful subscapularis repair.

7) Early (days) protected passive range of motion.

8) Individualize positions of immobilization and rehabilitation based on stability testing and tissue quality at the termination of the procedure.

9) Close supervision "Orthotherapy".

REFERENCES

[1] BAILEY BN Dermal arthroplasty. *Hand, 3(2): 135-7, 1971.*

[2] BAILEY BN Dermal arthroplasty. *Ann Rheum Dis, 28(5): Suppl: 98-9, 1969.*

[3] BALL CM, GALATZ LM, YAMAGUCHI K Meniscal allograft interposition arthroplasty for the arthritic shoulder: Description of a new surgical technique. *Tech Shoulder Elbow Surg 2001:2: 247-54.*

[4] BHATIA DN, VAN ROOYEN KS, DUTOIT DF, DE BEER JF Arthroscopic technique of interposition arthroplasty of the glenohumeral joint. *The Journal of Arthroscopic & Related Surgery May 2006 Vol 22 issue 5 570.e1-570.e5.*

[5] BRISLIN KJ, SAVOIE FH, FIELD LD, RAMSEY JR Surgical treatment for glenohumeral arthritis in the young patient. *Tech Shoulder Elbow Surg 2004: 5(3): 165-69.*

[6] BROWN JE, MCGAW WH, SHAW DT Use of cutis as an interposing membrane in arthroplasty of the knee. *J Bone Joint Surg Am, 40-A(5): 1003-18, 1958.*

[7] BURKHEAD WZ Jr, HUTTON KS Biologic resurfacing of the glenoid with hemiarthroplasty of the shoulder. *Journal Shoulder Elbow Surg 1995: 4: 263-70.*

[8] BURKHEAD WZ Dissociation of metal backed glenoid components. *Presented at Closed Meeting of American Shoulder and Elbow Surgeons; 1990 Nov; Chicago.*

[9] COLONNA PC Congenital dislocation of the hip in older subjects: based on a study of 66 open operations. *J Bone Joint Surg Br 1932; 14: 277-98.*

[10] CHOSSEGROS C, GUYOT L, CHEYNET F, BLANC JL, CANNONI P Full-thickness skin graft interposition after temporomandibular joint ankylosis surgery. A study of 31 cases. *Int J Oral Maxillofac Surg, 28(5): 330-4, 1999.*

[11] DE BEER JF Personal Communication.

[12] DIMITROULIS G The use of dermis grafts after discectomy for internal derangement of the temporomandibular joint. *J Oral Maxillofac Surg, 63(2): 173-8, 2005.*

[13] DINES J, WARREN R, CRAIG E, DINES D Glenoid Revision in Failed Shoulder Arthroplasty. *Presented at Open Meeting of American shoulder and Elbow Surgeons; March 2006; Chicago.*

[14] DINES D Personal Communication

[15] ELHASSAN B, OZBAYDAR M, DILLER D, HIGGINS LD, WARNER JJ Soft-tissue resurfacing of the glenoid in the treatment of glenohumeral arthritis in active patients less than fifty years old. *J Bone Joint Surg 91(2):419-424, Feb 2009.*

[16] FROIMSON AI, SILVA JE, RICHEY D Cutis arthroplasty of the elbow joint. *J Bone Joint Surg Am, 58(6): 863-5, 1976.*

[17] HEY GROVES EW Reconstructive surgery of the hip. *Br J Surg 1927; 14: 486-517.*

[18] KALLIO KE Skin arthroplasty of the hip joint. *Ann Chir Gynaecol Fenn, 45(3): 181-92, 1956.*

[19] KELLEY JW, GROSS WM Dermal arthroplasty of the hip joint. *Plast Reconstr Surg, 23(5): 540-6, 1959.*

[20] KETTUNEN K Changes in the fresh autogenous whole-thickness skin graft used as interposition material in arthroplasty of the hip joint on cats; preliminary report. *Ann Chir Gynaecol Fenn, 45(3): 193-6, 1956.*

[21] KRISHNAN SG, BURKHEAD WZ, NOWINSKI RJ Humeral hemiarthroplasty with biologic resurfacing of the glenoid and acromion for rotator cuff tear arthropathy. *Tech Shoulder Elbow Surg 2004:5: 51-59.*

[22] KRISHNAN SG, NOWINSKI RJ, HARRISON DK, BURKHEAD WZ Humeral hemiarthroplasty with biologic resurfacing of the glenoid for glenohumeral arthritis: 2-15 year outcomes. *Accepted for publication J Bone Joint Surg Am.*

[23] MacAUSLAND WR Mobilization of the elbow by free fascia transplantation with report of thirty-one cases. *Surg Gynecol Obstet 1921: 33: 223-45.*

[24] MATSEN FA Prosthetics. Presented at Open Meeting of American Shoulder and Elbow Surgeons: *Biologics in Shoulder Surgery; 2006 Sept; Chicago.*

[25] MATSEN FA, CLARK JM, TITELMAN RM, GIBBS KM, BOORMAN RS, DEFFENBAUGH D, KORVICK DL, NORMAN AG, OTT SM, PARSONS IM, SIDLES JA Healing of reamed glenoid bone articulating with a metal humeral hemiarthroplasty: a canine model. *J Ortho Res, 23: 18-26, 2005.*

[26] McNICKLE AG, L'HEUREUX DR, PROVENCHER MT, ROMEO AA, COLE BJ Postsurgical glenohumeral arthritis in young adults. *Am J Sports Med 37(9): 1784-1791, Sep 2009, Epub June 9 2009.*

[27] MURPHY JB Ankylosis: arthroplasty-clinical and experimental. *Trans Am Surg Assoc 1904: 22: 215.*

[28] NAGAI S, MATSUI T, YUGE D, OKUMURA T Homogenous and heterogenous skin arthroplasty and the reconstruction of the suprapatellar bursa. *Pac Med Surg, 73(5): 317-9, 1965.*

[29] POPESCU V, VASILIU D Treatment of temporo-mandibular ankylosis with particular reference to the interposition of full-thickness skin autotransplant. *J Maxillofac Surg, 5(1): 3-14, 1977.*

[30] SATTERLEE C, VANI J Glenoid soft tissue resurfacing for cuff tear arthropathy. *Presented at Closed Meeting of American Shoulder and Elbow Surgeons; 1998 New York.*

[31] SMITH MG, TILLETT ED Anatomic study of humeral head retroversion and the relationship of the central axis of the humeral head to the bicipital groove. *Journal Shoulder Elbow Surg 1993:2.*

[32] SMITH-PETERSEN MN Arthroplasty of the hip. *J Bone Joint Surg Br 1939: 21B: 269-88.*

[33] SMITH-PETERSEN MN Evolution of mould arthroplasty of the hip joint. *J Bone Joint Surg Br 1948: 30B: 59-75.*

[34] TAUNTON MJ, McINTOSH AL, SPERLING JW, COFIELD RH Total shoulder arthroplasty with metal-backed, bone in-growth glenoid components. *Presented at Closed Meeting of American Shoulder and Elbow Surgeons; 2006 Sept; Chicago.*

[35] UUSPAA V Anatomical interposition arthroplasty with dermal graft. A study of 51 elbow arthroplasties on 48 rheumatoid patients. *Z Rheumatol, 46(3): 132-5, 1987.*

[36] Verneriel *Arch Med 1860.*

[37] WARNER JP

[38] WILLIAMS GR, FONT-RODRIGUEZ D, BAGHIAN S Soft-tissue interposition without hemiarthroplasty as an alternative for degenerative shoulder arthritis in young, active patients. *Presented at Closed Meeting of American Shoulder and Elbow Surgeons; 2002 Oct; Pebble Beach.*

ARTHROSCOPIC BIOLOGICAL RESURFACING OF THE GLENOID IN GLENOHUMERAL ARTHRITIS: TWO TO FIVE YEAR OUTCOMES OF A PILOT STUDY

J.F. DE BEER, D.N. BHATIA

PURPOSE AND BACKGROUND

In spite of the excellent results of shoulder arthroplasty for osteoarthritis of the shoulder, the problem of failure of the prostheses in time persists in the younger patient. The problem relates to the glenoid in most cases, with wear and loosening of the prosthetic glenoid [1]. The multitude of methods to try and evade this problem proves the existence thereof: hemi-arthroplasty, resurfacing of the humeral head and various biological implants [2, 3]. The problem of prostheses (hemiarthoplasty and resurfacing) is that the subscapularis has to be detached to insert them and this and the potential damage by the prostheses to the bones of the joint influence the results of revision at a later stage negatively.

In our quest to seek for less invasive alternative solutions for the younger patients with osteoarthritis of the shoulder joint, we developed the technique of attaching a biological graft to the glenoid using the arthroscopic technique and thus avoiding any damage to the subscapularis [4]. The reason for restricting it to the glenoid and not addressing the head of the humerus is simply that the technical difficulties of the latter procedure have not been overcome.

The purpose of this study was to analyze the intermediate-term results of an arthroscopic procedure to resurface the arthritic glenoid using an acellular human dermal scaffold.

METHODS

Between 2003 and 2005, thirty-two consecutive patients (32 shoulders, 22 males and 10 females, mean age 55.7 years) underwent an arthroscopic glenoid resurfacing for glenohumeral arthritis. The diagnoses included primary osteoarthrosis (27 patients), arthritis after arthroscopic reconstruction for anterior instability (1 patient), and inflammatory arthritis (3 patients). All shoulders were assessed clinically using the Constant and Murley score [5], and results graded according to Neer's criteria [6]. Statistical analysis was performed to determine significant parameters and associations.

SURGICAL TECHNIQUE

1. The patient is positioned in the lateral decubitus position.
2. Four portals are usually employed: two anterior and two posterior. This allows for adequate access and visualisation of joints which are usually very stiff.
3. A capsulotomy is advisable to achieve improved range of motion.
4. Though debridement of loose tissue is done and the long head of biceps is attended to as needed – often a tenotomy would be performed in the case of severe tendinitis.
5. The glenoid surface is inspected: if significant bi-concavity is present the surface would be burred down to neutral version. Micro-fracturing of the surface of the glenoid is performed with a burr to enable bone marrow to exude into the graft which will act as a scaffold for the ingrowth of cells.

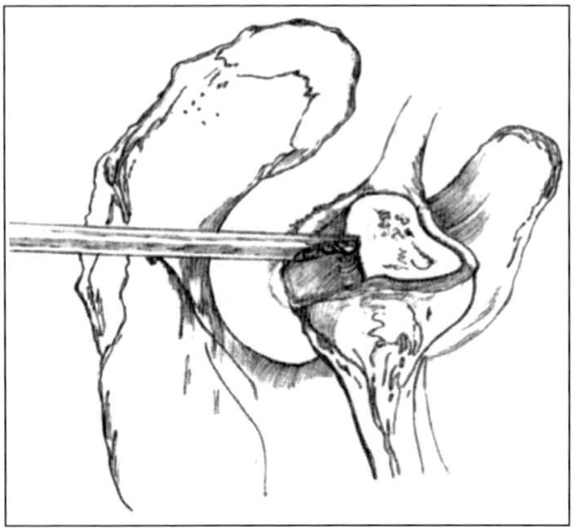

The biconcavity of the glenoid is eliminated using a burr

6. The glenoid dimensions are measured using a suture and graspers.
7. The biological graft is cut to size.
8. Several variations of the technique are possible. In the most recent modification, four anchors are inserted into the edge of the glenoid, antero-superior, antero-inferior, postero-superior and postero-inferior. The joint-side (JS) tail of each suture is brought out through the antero-inferior cannula and the four sutures are passed through the graft and their ends tied into “STIK” (Short Tail Interference Knots) [7].

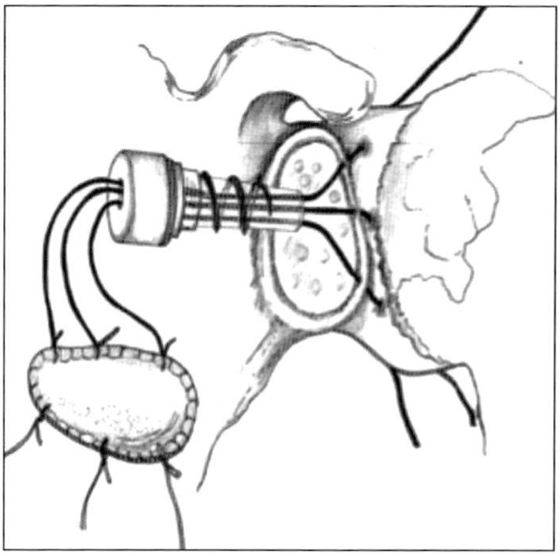

The sutures from the anchors are placed through the graft outside the joint

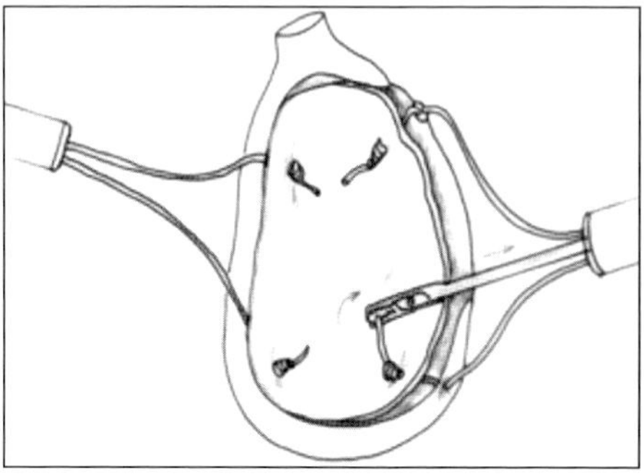

“STIK” knots work especially well for this purpose

9. By pulling on the outside (OS) tail of each suture, the graft is pulled into the joint after special care has been taken to verify the spatial orientation of the sutures.

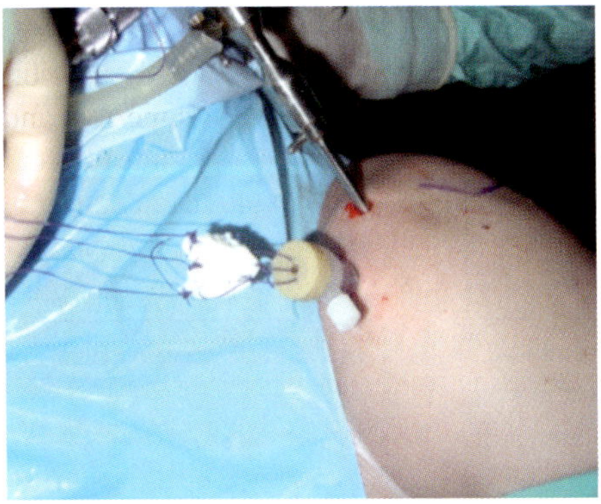

The graft is about to pulled into the joint

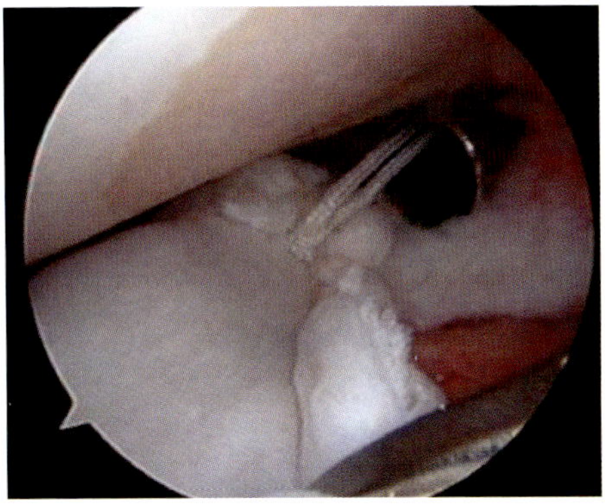

The graft being fixed to the surface of the glenoid

10. After arrival of the graft in the joint the short tails of the knots are retrieved and the sutures are all tied.

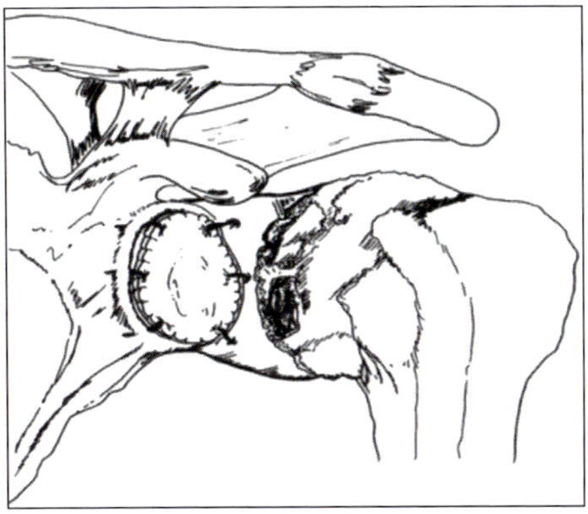

Resurfaced arthritic shoulder joint

11. Post-operatively the shoulder is immobilized for a period of 3 weeks and then gradually mobilized.

RESULTS

A significant improvement ($p < 0.0001$) in each parameter of the subjective evaluation component (severity of pain, limitation in daily living and recreational activities) of the Constant score was observed. The Constant and Murley score increased significantly ($p < 0.0001$) from a mean of 38.6% (range 26 to 63) pre-operatively, to 57.5 (range 19 to 84) at the final assessment. Overall, the procedure was considered as "successful outcome" in 23 patients (71.8%) and as a "failure" in 9 patients (28.1%). According to Neer's criteria, the result was categorized as excellent in 9 (28.1%), satisfactory in 14 (43.8%), and unsatisfactory in 9 (28.1%). Within the unsatisfactory group, there were 5 conversions to prosthetic arthroplasty. Overall, five complications included transient axillary nerve paresis, foreign body reaction to biological material, interlayer dissociation, mild chronic non-specific synovitis, and post-traumatic contusion. Dominance of affected extremity and generalized disease (diabetes, rheumatoid arthritis, generalized osteoarthritis) were associated with an unsatisfactory outcome ($p<0.05$).

CONCLUSIONS

Arthroscopic resurfacing of the glenoid using an acellular human dermal allograft scaffold is a minimally invasive therapeutic option for pain relief, functional improvement, and patient satisfaction, in glenohumeral osteoarthritis, in the intermediate term. Further prospective studies and a longer follow-up are necessary before this procedure can be routinely recommended for glenohumeral osteoarthritis. Revision to a prosthetic implant is a relatively uncomplicated procedure.

REFERENCES

[1] MATSEN FA III, BICKNELL RT, LIPPITT SB. Shoulder arthroplasty: The socket perspective. *J Shoulder Elbow Surg 2007; 16:s214-7.*

[2] KRISHNAN SG, NOWINSKI RJ, HARRISON D, BURKHEAD WZ. Humeral Hemiarthroplasty with Biologic Resurfacing of the Glenoid for Glenohumeral Arthritis. Two to Fifteen-Year Outcomes. *J Bone Joint Surg Am 2007; 89: 727-734.*

[3] BALL CM, GALATZ LM, YAMAGUCHI K. Meniscal allograft Interposition arthroplasty for the arthritic shoulder: Description of a new surgical technique. *Tech Shoulder Elbow Surg 2001; 2: 247-254.*

[4] BHATIA DN, van ROOYEN KS, de BEER JF. Arthroscopic technique of interposition arthroplasty of the glenohumeral joint. *Arthroscopy* 2006; *22:570.e1-5.*

[5] CONSTANT CR, MURLEY AHG. A clinical method of functional assessment of the shoulder. *Clin Orthop 1987; 214:160-4.*

[6] NEER CS, WATSON KC, STANTON FJ. Recent experience in total shoulder replacement. *J Bone Joint Surg Am 1982; 64:319-337.*

[7] DOPIRAK R, BOND JL, SNYDER SJ. Arthroscopic total rotator cuff replacement with an acellular human dermal allograft matrix. *Int J Shoulder Surg 2007; 1:7-15.*

HEMIARTHROPLASTY: LONG-TERM SURVORSHIP AND OUTCOMES

F. GADEA, G.B. ALAMI, J. KIDDER, M. PFAHLER, C. LÉVIGNE, L. FAVARD

INTRODUCTION

Since the study by Neer in 1955 [23], humeral hemiarthroplasty (HA) has been the subject of several cohort studies and meta-analyses. Essentially, HA is viewed as the procedure of choice in the following 3 cases: intact glenoid articular surface, glenoid bone stock too poor to allow glenoid component implantation [20], and young or active patients for whom the risk of long-term loosening is unacceptable [3]. For massive cuff tear arthropathy (CTA), HA is favored by some authors because of the risk of glenoid loosening by the rocking-horse effect [11, 22], although reverse arthroplasty is an increasingly employed solution for this pathology [14].

A number of reports comparing total shoulder arthroplasty (TSA) with HA claim clinical superiority of the total prosthesis in the short and medium term (2 to 5 years) [2, 3, 9, 10, 11, 26, 27]. Similarly, a comparison between TSA and HA survival curves without prosthesis removal has shown TSA to be superior in the short-to-medium term for primary osteoarthritis (OA) [27]. However, the long-term survival rate of a glenoid component remains controversial [6, 23, 30]. The risk of loosening and the decline in clinical results, along with the difficulty of revision surgery with a destroyed glenoid, all challenge the supposed advantage of TSA. Furthermore, for some etiologies such as rheumatoid arthritis (RA), the difference in clinical outcome with TSA is lost over time [29].

Although clinical outcomes with HA have been satisfactory, caution is required, as its rate of revision is substantial—between 5 and 10% depending on the report [12, 14, 20, 24]. Factors influencing glenoid erosion, which is the main cause of failure after HA, are numerous. Most influential are the preoperative factors of glenoid-wear type (concentric or excentric) and severity [4, 7, 15, 16, 18] — although these factors themselves have yet to be better studied.

The main focus of this study, however, are the long-term survivorship and outcomes of HA for the different original etiologies, in cases where the prosthesis has been in place for at least 8 years. We hypothesized that some etiologies give significantly better functional outcomes than others, and that when the right indications are chosen the prosthesis survival curves remain stable over time.

MATERIALS AND METHODS

Between May, 1988 and December, 1999, 409 consecutive patients (423 shoulders) were treated in 9 centers with the same nonconstrained, modular, and adaptable prosthesis – the Aequalis prosthesis (Tornier Inc., St Ismier, France). Exclusion criteria were: follow-up <8 years (except if a complication or revision occurred), prosthesis implanted during a revision arthroplasty, and tumor cases. The patients were divided into 8 groups according to etiology: ***1)*** fractures (150 cases), ***2)*** fracture sequelae (FS, 73 cases), ***3)*** primary OA (68 cases), ***4)*** CTA (43 cases), ***5)*** osteonecrosis (ON, 40 cases), ***6)*** RA (31 cases), ***7)*** instability (defined by arthropathy following frequent anterior dislocation, 6 cases), and ***8)*** miscellaneous etiologies (12 cases). Ninety-three patients were excluded because of inadequate follow-up and 98 were lost because of death, leaving 190 shoulders in 184 patients with follow-up of at least 96 months. The average follow-up was 135.6 months (96 to 142 months). Data on diagnosis, gender, age, and follow-up duration for reviewed patients is provided in Table I. Among the total 423 shoulders, 73 had complications. These cases were included in the analysis but were not analyzed with regard to follow-up length or complication type. All patients from the same center were not necessarily reviewed by the same examiner. Cases of conversion to TSA were counted as prosthesis removals, whether or not they

Table I: Characteristics of shoulders treated with hemiarthroplasty reviewed at a minimum of 8 years

Diagnosis	No. of shoulders/ no. of patients	No. of females/ no. of males	Age* (yr)	Duration of follow-up (mo.)
Fractures	52/51	37/14	67 ± 11	139.7
Fracture sequelae	34/34	26/8	59 ± 10	140.5
Cuff tear arthropathy	18/18	14/4	70 ± 9	141.9
Rheumatoid arthritis	14/12	12/0	41 ± 18	144.5
Osteonecrosis	20/18	9/9	46 ± 9	141.9
Primary osteoarthritis	42/41	26/15	66 ± 10	123.5
Instability	4/4	1/3	65 ± 6	128.7
Misc.	6/6	3/3	59 ± 11	115.5
ALL	190/184	128/56	61 ± 10 (16-85)	135.6 (96-209)

** Values are given as mean and standard deviation, with range in parentheses.*

involved stem replacement, stem removal, or arthrodesis. Prosthesis removal was analysed with survival curves generated using the Kaplan-Meier technique with 95% confidence intervals according to Rothman and Greenland. Prosthesis removal was the sole end-point examined. Survival curves were cumulative and segmented according to etiology. Moreover, comparisons of instantaneous survivorship were carried out with homogeneity tests.

Clinical assessment was carried out using the rating system of Constant and Murley [8]. The functional outcome was assessed by the change between the evaluations preoperatively and at last follow-up. We also analyzed the clinical results at last follow-up that were considered poor (with a Constant score <30). Because of the small number of arthritis after instability cases and the disparity of the miscellaneous etiologies (1 septic arthritis, 1 inflammatory arthritis, 1 neurologic arthropathy, 1 multi-directional instability, and 1 dysplasia), these two groups were not included in the outcome analysis.

Statistical analysis of the long-term results was performed using the Chi-squared test for comparison of nominal variables, Student's *t*-test for comparison of means with a Gaussian distribution, and the non-parametric Mann-Whitney and Kruskall-Wallis tests for means without Gaussian distribution.

RESULTS

At the time of review, 38 implants were considered removed, as defined above. Twenty-five were converted into TSA (17 of whom had a stem replacement), 2 had a stem replacement only, 10 had a stem removal without replacement, and 1 had an arthrodesis on the prosthesis. The overall survival rate, survival without removal being the end-point, was 88.7% at 10 years (Table II). Between 10 and 15 years, 5 prostheses were removed. The reason for removal was: glenoid wear for 3 of them (originally, 1 fracture, 1 ON, and 1 FS), an infection for 1 of them (from the fractures group) and a subscapularis lesion with anterior instability for another (also from the fracture group). Looking at specific etiologies (Table III), the survival-without-removal rate was low for CTA and FS and especially good (100%) for RA. For the other etiologies, it was around 95%.

The overall survival-without-removal curve shows two breaks. The first break occurs during the first 3 years and the second break after the 10th year (Fig. 1). During the first 3 years, 25 prostheses were removed: 10 for glenoid wear (3 primary OA, 3 FS, 2 CTA, 1 fracture, and 1 ON), 7 for infection (3 fractures, 3 FS, and 1 ON), 3 for stiffness without glenoid wear (1 FS, 1 persistent posterior dislocation, and 1 multi-directional instability), 3 for rotator cuff tear (with 2 subscapularis

Table II: Overall survival rate

	0 year	5 years	10 years	15 years
Number remaining	423	233	126	11
Survival rate	1	0.912	0.887	0.850

Table III: Survival rate as a function of etiology

	5 years			10 years	
Etiology	Shoulders at outset	Remaining shoulders	Survival rate	Remaining shoulders	Survival rate
Fractures	150	66	0.932	37	0.908
Fracture sequelae	73	43	0.816	25	0.768
Cuff tear arthropathy	43	25	0.985	14	0.815
Rheumatoid arthritis	31	16	1	11	1
Osteonecrosis	40	25	0.940	15	0.940
Primary osteoarthritis	68	46	0.949	19	0.949
Instability	6	5	1	3	1
Misc.	12	7	0.839	2	0.839

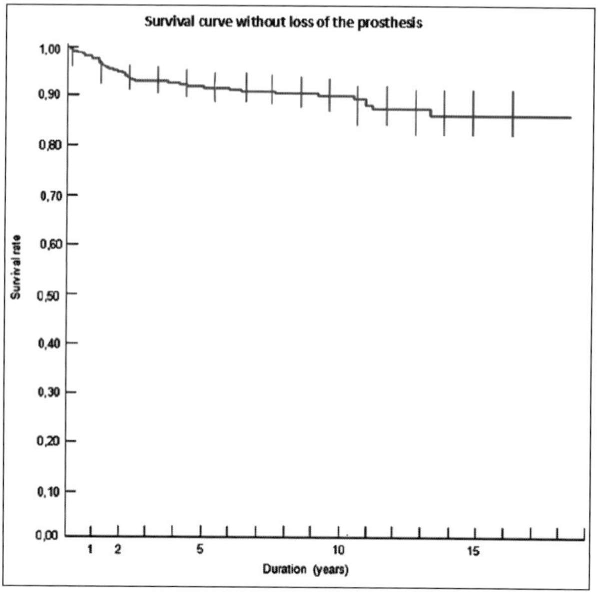

*Fig. 1 - Survival curve**
(end-point = survival without removal of prosthesis)
** Kaplan-Meier method, Rothman's 95% confidence intervals*

Survival curves according to etiology show that the majority of severe adverse events occurred early for primary OA (during the first 2 years), in the first 7 years (medium term) for fractures, continuously for FS, and in 2 periods for ON and CTA corresponding to the two breaks described previously (Fig. 2).

lesions), 1 for anterior dislocation, and 1 for tuberosity migration (originally from the fracture group; final treatment including a stem replacement). The reasons for prosthesis removal after 10 years have already been described above.

The comparison between preoperative and postoperative clinical status at a minimum of 8 years shows a significant improvement of all Constant score parameters for all etiologies (Table IV). The largest improvement was observed for primary OA and ON, while RA and FS were penalized by the poor improvement in mobility, and the outcomes of CTA were the worst, even though a moderate improvement was observed at the last follow-up (Fig. 3). The analysis of poor outcomes shows that the number of poor Constant scores was largest for CTA and fractures (Table V).

There were 73 complications in total, representing 17% of the initial population. Thirteen patients had two complications and 1 had more than two. For this patient (initially with primary OA), the three complications were a rotator cuff tear, a posterior dislocation, and glenoid erosion; this patient's HA was converted to a TSA 13 month after the index surgery. In fact, for this patient, who initially had a brachial plexus palsy, TSA had been originally planned, but difficulty with intra-operative glenoid exposure led to the change of plan.

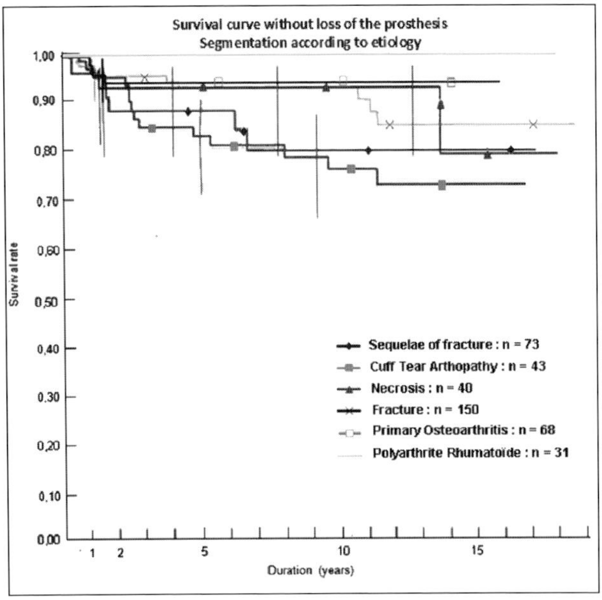

Fig. 2 - Survival curve* according to original etiology** (without instability or rheumatoid arthritis, for which no events occurred)

** Kaplan Meier method, Rothman's 95% confidence intervals*
*** p (Logrank test) = 0.09*

Table IV: Constant score means according to original etiology

	Primary osteoarthritis	Fractures**	Fracture sequelae	Osteonecrosis	Cuff tear arthropathy	Rheumatoid arthritis	Instability	Misc.
Preoperative Constant score	27±7		29.3±12,6	32.2±14.3	26.8±10.4	26.7±11.7	30.1±12.7	38.9±7.0
Pain	3.3		4.7	3.8	4.3	5.1	3.9	5.5
Activity	6.4		6	7.5	6	7.4	6.2	8.8
Mobility	13		13.6	17.6	13.9	12.3	13.5	19
Strength	4.3		5	3.3	2.6	1.9	6.5	5.6
Last follow-up Constant score	60.3±21.2	56.3±21.5	57.7±18	62.8±24.9	46.2±14.5	55.3±12.6	72.25±14.4	66.3±18.5
Pain	11.6	12	11.2	12.3	10.2	12.5	14.5	13.2
Activity	15.2	14	14.6	16.3	11	13.7	16.5	15.7
Mobility	27.3	24.1	24.8	32.5	22.3	22.2	33	27.5
Strength	7.7	6.2	7.1	9.2	2.7	6.8	8.5	10

** Values are given as mean and standard deviation*
*** For fractures, testing was not feasible preoperatively*

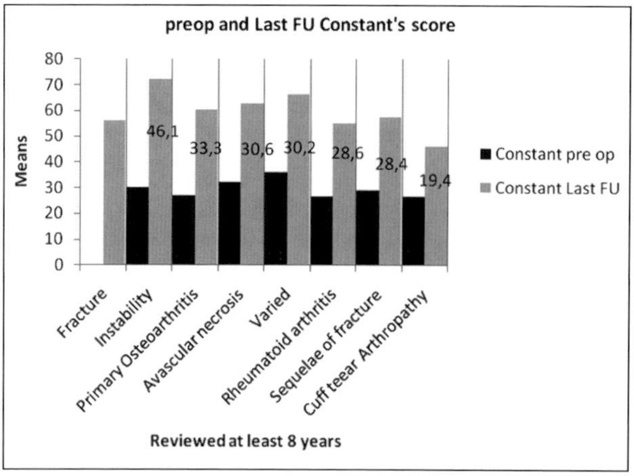

Fig. 3: Improvement between Constant score preoperatively and at last follow-up according to etiology

NB: For fractures, testing was not feasible preoperatively; values correspond to difference between Constant score preoperatively and at last follow-up

Table V: Poor outcomes, according to etiology*

	Primary osteoarthritis	Fractures	Fracture sequelae	Osteonecrosis	Cuff tear arthropathy	Rheumatoid arthritis	Instability	Misc.
Constant <30	9%	15%	6%	0%	11%	0%	0%	0%

** Values are given as a percentage out of the 190 shoulders reviewed at a minimum of 8 years*

The 5 most frequently observed complications were: glenoid wear, stiffness without glenoid wear, infection, tuberosity complications, and rotator cuff tear (Table VI). Looking at the time of occurrence of these complications showed that the majority appeared during the first 5 years, then after a relatively uneventful period a new critical period began from 10 years on (see Fig. 4). The distribution of the complications responsible for prosthesis removal shows that glenoid wear, infection, and stiffness usually led to prosthesis removal (Table VI).

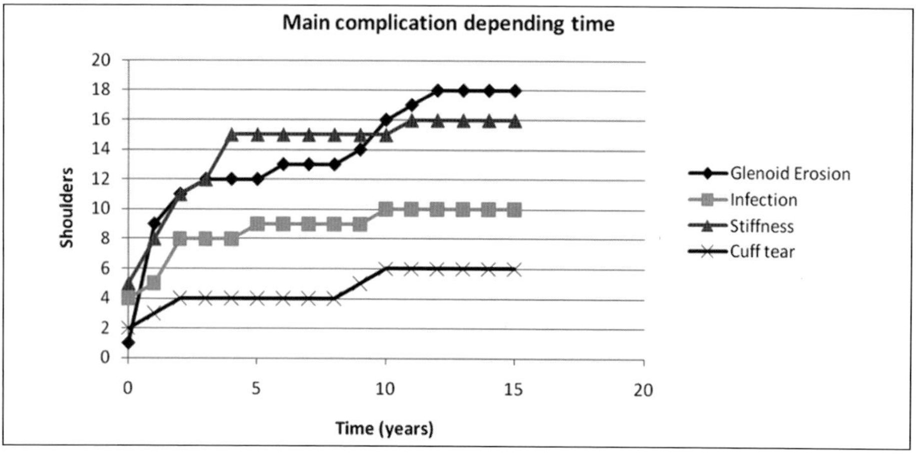

Fig. 4: Time to occurrence of main complication

Table VI: Distribution of complications and prosthesis removal according to etiology, regardless of follow-up length*

	Fractures	Fracture sequelae	Cuff tear arthropathy	Rheumatoid arthritis	Avascular necrosis	Primary osteoarthritis	Misc.	TOTAL
Glenoid wear	2/1	7/7	3/3		2/2	3/3	1	18
Stiffness	8	2/2	2/2	1		2	1	16
Infection	6/4	3/3			1/1			10
Tuberosity nonunion, malunion, or migration	7/1	1/1						8
Humeral fracture	3	3						6
Rotator cuff tear	2	1/1	1/1		1		1	6
Humeral loosening	1/1	1/1	1					3
Anterior dislocation	2							2
Posterior dislocation	1					1		2
Neurologic	1							1
Hematoma					1			1
TOTAL complication/removal	33(22%)/ 9(6%)	18(24.6%)/ 15(20.3%)	7(16.3%)/ 6(13.2%)	1(3.2%)/ 0	5(12.5%)/ 3(7.5%)	6(8.8%)/ 3(4.4%)	3(25%)/ 2(16.6%)	73(17.2%)/ 38(8.9%)

** The first figure is the number of complications, the second is the number of prosthesis removals*
*** The values in parentheses are the percentages out of the total 423 shoulders*

DISCUSSION

This study shows that long-term survivorship is related to etiology, but a higher survival rate does not always mean a very good functional result.

A few aspects of this study can be criticized. One is its multi-center design with numerous clinical examiners. Another is the high rate of loss to follow-up or death, although the elderly nature of the population makes that inevitable.

For primary OA, after the first 5 years, during which risk of prosthesis removal is high, survivorship and functional outcomes are good. Between 5 and 10 years, the survival rate remains stable around 92%. The mean Constant score was 60.3, including 9% with a Constant score <30. Haines *et al.* [15] have shown that the most common cause for revision in HA was glenoid pain and that was at a mean follow-up of 1.5 years. However, similar to ours, their survival rate was 90% at 10 years. Haines *et al.* highlighted the role of the rotator cuff, and their functional results were significantly better after TSA for patients with an intact rotator cuff.

For ON, this group's lower age compared to that of others etiologies (with the exception of RA) translates to a higher functional demand. The persistence over time of satisfactory function is therefore important for this group. In terms of the Constant score at last follow-up, our mean result of 62, with no scores below 30, was relatively quite good. In their series on the results of 71 HAs performed after ON, with a mean follow-up of 8.9 years,

Hattrup and Cofield [17] showed that a pain-free shoulder and good functional results were obtained in almost 90% of patients. Like ours, their survival rate was good (94% at 10 years), with only 3 revisions for a painful glenoid (performed in the first 2 years).

For RA, the survival rate was excellent (100% at 10 years) and the number of complications very low with only 1 reoperation for stiffness without prosthesis removal. That said, there was a lot of stiffness, even with a mean Constant score of 55, with a 28-point improvement. In a series reported by Sperling *et al.* [30], comparing HA and TSA with a mean follow-up of 12 years, HA had a high rate of prosthesis removal (7.4%) for painful glenoid arthritis. In our study, we did not have such a rate, and limited passive range of motion was well tolerated in the absence of pain.

For fractures, the survival rate at 5 years was similar to that of primary OA, but their survival continued to decline between 5 and 10 years. As far as functional outcome is concerned, this group's mean Constant score was 55 with a large standard deviation of 21.5, and it had the highest percentage (15%) of Constant scores <30. This disparity in functional results has already been reported by Antuna *et al.* [1] in a recent study (57 HAs, mean follow up of 10.6 years). But Antuna *et al.* still concluded that HA was a valid and predictable treatment option, as poor results are often the consequence of bad tuberosity reduction and fixation.

The CTA group had the study's worst functional results, with a poor improvement in Constant score (only 19.4) and 11% of cases having a Constant score <30. The survival rate of 81.5% at 10 years was not good either. In their series of 62 HAs with a minimum follow-up of 2 years, Favard *et al.* [11] showed that if the early postoperative Constant score was poor (46), it remained stable over time. The long-term results of our study agree with this observation and suggest that after the first 5 years the functional outcome does not deteriorate over time.

For FS, the functional results were fairly satisfactory. However, the survival rate was the worst of the series and continued to deteriorate over time, mainly because of painful glenoid erosion. In their short-term report on a series of FS, Boileau *et al.* [4] noted a high rate of revision (5.6%), mostly for late infections, and a poor postoperative Constant score in 33% of cases. With a mean follow-up of 19 months, they were not able to find any significant difference in outcome between 46 HAs and 26 TSAs. From these results, it can be deduced that poor clinical outcomes are poorly tolerated and lead to a relatively high rate of revision.

CONCLUSION

In the long term, we were able to identify 3 groups:

- Primary OA and ON, the results of which were the best, but which also need to be compared to those after TSA.
- Fractures and RA, which had a good survival rate – especially for RA – but for which functional outcomes were moderately satisfactory, mainly because of stiffness. Moreover, the complication rate for fractures was high, which calls for a great deal of attention to the prevention of infections and to the positioning of the tuberosities.

- Cuff tear arthropathy and FS, which we found not to be ideal indications for HA, as their functional results and survival rates were moderately satisfactory at 8 years. For CTA, these long-term results ought to ultimately be compared with those of reverse arthroplasty. For FS, except when the patient is young and the risk of loosening high, it seems wiser to consider a reverse prosthesis or a TSA.

Naturally, this study should be complemented with an analysis of predictive factors such as the radiographic appearance of glenoid wear preoperatively and postoperatively, the presence and characteristics of a rotator cuff tear, and the quality of the tuberosity reconstruction. This is the goal of the next study.

REFERENCES

[1] ANTUNA SA, SPERLING JW, COFIELD RH Shoulder hemiarthroplasty for acute fractures of the proximal humerus: A minimum five-year follow-up. *J Shoulder Elbow Surg 17 (2008), p. 202-9.*

[2] DE BEER MA. Hemi-versus total shoulder replacement a retrospective comparison. *J Bone Joint Surg Br 84 (Suppl I) (2002), p 77.*

[3] BOILEAU P, SINNERTON RJ, CHUINARD C, WALCH G. Arthroplasty of the shoulder. *J Bone Joint Surg Br. 88 (2006), p. 562-75.*

[4] BOILEAU P, TROJANI C, WALCH G, KRISHNAN SG, ROMEO A, SINNERTON R. Shoulder arthroplasty for the treatment of the sequelae of fractures of the proximal humerus. *J Shoulder Elbow Surg 10 (2001), p. 299-308.*

[5] BOILEAU P, WALCH G, NOËL, E., LIOTARD JP. Neer's shoulder prosthesis: outcomes according to etiology. *Revue du rhumatisme 61(1994), p 607-18.*

[6] BRYANT D, LITCHFIELD R, SANDOW M, GARTSMAN GM, GUYATT G, KIKLEY A. A comparison of pain, strength, range of motion, and functional outcomes after hemiarthroplasty and total shoulder arthroplasty in patients with osteoarthritis of the shoulder. A systematic review and meta-analysis. *J Bone Joint Surg Am. 87 (2005), p. 1947-56.*

[7] COFIELD RH, EDGERTON BC. Total shoulder arthroplasty: complications and revision surgery. *Instr Course Lect 39 (1990), p 449-62.*

[8] CONSTANT CR, MURLEY AH. A clinical method of functional assessment of the shoulder. *Clin Orthop Relat Res. 214(1987), p. 160-64.*

[9] CRAIG S, RADNAY MD, SETTER MD. Total shoulder replacement compared with humeral head replacement for the treatment of primary glenohumeral osteoarthritis: A systematic review. *J Shoulder Elbow Surg 16 (2007), p 396-402.*

[10] EDWARDS TB, KADAKIA NR, BOULAHIA A, KEMPF JF, BOILEAU P, NEMOZ C. A comparison of hemiarthroplasty and total shoulder arthroplasty in the treatment of primary glenohumeral osteoarthritis: outcomes of a multicenter study. *J Shoulder Elbow Surg 12 (2003), p 207-13.*

[11] FAVARD L, OUDET D, HUGUET D, SIRVEAUX F, MOLE D. Results of anatomical and reversed prosthesis in cuff tear arthropathy. In Boileau P, Walch G eds Prothèses d'épaule. Etat actuel. *Cahiers d'enseignement de la SOFCOT (2008), p 311-314.*

[12] FRANKLIN JL, BARRETT WP, JACKINS SE, MATSEN FA III. Glenoid loosening in total shoulder arthroplasty. Association with rotator cuff deficiency. *J Arthroplasty 3 (1988), p 39-46.*

[13] GARTSMAN GM, RODDEY TS, HAMMERMAN SM. Shoulder arthroplasty with or without resurfacing of the glenoid in patients who have osteoarthritis. *J Bone Joint Surg Am. 82 (2000), p 26-34.*

[14] GUERY J, FAVARD L, SIRVEAUX F, OUDET D, MOLE D, WALCH G. Reverse total shoulder arthropathy. Survivorship of eighty replacements followed for five to ten years. *J Bone Joint surg Am 88 (2006), p 1742-47.*

[15] HAINES JF, TRAIL IA, NUTTALL D, BIRCH A, BARROW A. The outcomes of arthroplasty in osteoarthritis of the shoulder. *J Bone Joint Surg Br. 88 (2006), p 496-501.*

[16] HASAN SS, LEITH JM, CAMPBELL B, KAPIL R, SMITH KL, MATSEN FA III. Characteristics of unsatisfactory shoulder arthroplasties. *J Shoulder Elbow Surg 11 (2002), p 431-41.*

[17] HATTRUP SJ, COFIELD RH. Osteonecrosis of the humeral head: results of replacement. *J Shoulder Elbow Surg 3 (2000), p. 177-82.*

[18] HETTRICH CM, WELDON E III, BOORMAN RS, PARSONS IM, MATSEN FA III. Preoperative factors associated with improvements in shoulder function after humeral hemiarthroplasty. *J Bone Joint Surg Am 86 (2004), p 1446-51.*

[19] IANNOTTI JP, NORRIS TR. Influence of preoperative factors on outcome of shoulder arthroplasty for glenohumeral osteoarthritis. *J Bone Joint Surg Am. 85 (2003), p 251-58.*

[20] KELLY JD, NORRIS TR. Decision making in glenohumeral arthroplasty. *J Arthroplasty 18 (2003), p 75-82.*

[21] LEVINE WN, DJURASOVIC M, GLASSON JM, POLLOCK RG, FLATOW EL, BIGLIANI LU. Hemiarthroplasty for glenohumeral osteoarthritis: outcomes correlated to degree of glenoid wear. *J Shoulder Elbow Surg 6 (1997), p 449-54.*

[22] LO IK, GRIFFIN S, FABER K, PATTERSON SD, LITCHFIELD RB, KIRKLEY A. Quality of life outcome following hemiarthroplasty or total shoulder arthroplasty in patients with osteoarthritis. A prospective, randomized trial. *J Bone Joint Surg Am. 87(2005).*

[23] NEER CSII. Indications for replacement of the proximal humeral articulation. *Am J Surg 89 (1955), p 901-7.*

[24] NORRIS TR, IANNOTTI JP. Functional outcome after shoulder arthroplasty for primary osteoarthritis: a multicenter study. *J Shoulder Elbow Surg 11 (2002), p 130-35.*

[25] ORFALY RM, ROCKWOOD CA, ESENYEL CZ, WIRTH MA. A prospective functional outcome study of shoulder arthroplasty for osteoarthritis with an intact rotator cuff. *J Shoulder Elbow Surg 12 (2003), p 214-21.*

[26] PARSONS IM, MILLETT PJ, WARNER JJ. Glenoid wear after shoulder hemiarthroplasty: quantitative radiographic analysis. *Clin Orthop Relat Res. 421 (2004), p.120-25.*

[27] ROTHMAN KJ. Estimation of confidence limits for the cumulative probability of survival in life table analysis. *J. Chronic Dis. 31 (1978), p 557-560.*

[28] SANDOW M, GARTSMAN G, KIRKLEY S. Total or hemiarthroplasty for OA shoulder: meta-analysis of trials. *J Bone Joint Surg Br 84 (Suppl III) (2002), p 256.*

[29] SMITH KL, MATSEN FA. Total shoulder arthroplasty versus hemiarthroplasty. Current trends. *Orthop Clin North Am. 29 (1998), p. 491-506.*

[30] SPERLING JW, COFIELD RH, ROWLAND CM. Neer hemiarthroplasty and Neer total shoulder arthroplasty in patients fifty years old or less: Long-term outcomes. *J Bone Joint Surg Am 80 (1998), p 464-73.*

[31] SPERLING JW, COFIELD RH, SCHLECK CD, HARMSEN WS. Total shoulder arthroplasty versus hemiarthroplasty for rheumatoid arthritis of the shoulder: Outcomes of 303 consecutive cases. *J Shoulder Elbow Surg 6 (2007), p 68-72.*

[32] TORCHIA ME, COFIELD RH, SETTERGREN CR. Total shoulder arthroplasty with the Neer prosthesis: long-term outcomes. *J Shoulder Elbow Surg 6 (1997), p. 495-505.*

PREDICTIVE FACTORS OF GLENOID EROSION

G. FAMA, F. SIRVEAUX, G. PAPE, F. GADEA, L. FAVARD

INTRODUCTION

Since Neer's work [16], the indications for shoulder arthroplasty have expanded significantly. Depending on the initial etiology or on the surgeon's convictions, the arthroplasty can be either a total shoulder arthroplasty (TSA) or a hemiarthroplasty (HA). Even though it is widely assumed that HA is preferable when the glenoid cartilage is intact, as in fractures or avascular necrosis (AVN) [2], no consensus exists regarding cases where the glenoid cartilage is damaged, as in osteoarthritis (OA) [15, 23] or rheumatoid arthritis (RA) [14, 21]. Those who prefer using TSA cite better clinical results [6, 9, 15] and argue that progressive deterioration has been observed with HA [4, 13, 19]. As for those preferring HA [12, 24], they view its results as differing little from those of TSA and argue that its patients have a generally low revision requirement and do not run the relatively frequent risk of glenoid loosening past the tenth year [4, 22].

To be sure, there are etiologies for which reported results with HA are not very satisfactory, such as fractures sequelae (FS) [3, 10] or cuff tear arthropathy (CTA) [1, 7]; but glenoid wear in those cases is not always major. Therefore, it seems that HAs do not all deteriorate inevitably over time. Moreover, most published studies only have medium-term follow-up, which prevents proper comparison between HA and TSA in the long-term.

It can be assumed that some etiologies are at risk of symptomatic glenoid erosion whereas others maintain an adequate glenoid or evolve towards asymptomatic glenoid erosion. This is why the goal of our study was to analyze a series of HA with a 5-year minimum follow-up, in order to estimate predictive factors of the occurrence of symptomatic glenoid erosion. Our hypothesis is that glenoid erosion depends mainly on the initial etiology and on the state of the rotator cuff, and that all glenoid erosion does not lead to bad results.

PATIENTS AND METHODS

This is a multi-center, European study including all consecutive Aequalis (Tornier) HA cases, both standard or fracture versions, implanted before January, 2000. Only prostheses implanted during a revision arthroplasty or for cases of tumors were excluded. A total of 399 patients (423 shoulders) were included. To evaluate glenoid erosion, we estimated that a minimum follow-up of 5 years was necessary. Of the 423 shoulders included initially, 86 patients died, with their prostheses in place, before the 5th year. Seventy-six were lost to follow-up, and 29 had an implant removal. Thus, 218 patients (232 shoulders) were reviewed at more than 5 years. This population is composed of 63 men (67 shoulders) and 155 women (165 shoulders), with a total of 14 patients operated on for both sides. The dominant shoulder was involved in 59% of cases. The mean age at surgery was 62.6 years (16-85), 65 years (16-85) for women and 56.5 years (30-81) for men ($p<0.001$).

Etiologies are detailed in Table I. Two etiology categories (Instability and Miscellaneous) are apart due to their heterogeneity and low numbers. They were not included in the results analysis according to etiology. Patient age at surgery was significantly lower for RA and AVN and higher for CTA. Preoperatively, the clinical evaluation of patients (Constant score and mobility) according to etiology (except for fractures, for which the examination was impossible) is described in Table I.

Table I: Number of shoulders, age, and preoperative Constant score according to etiology.

Etiology	N	Ct Preop.	Age
Miscellaneous	7	39.14 ± 6.39	56.71 ± 11.84
CTA	25	24.84 ± 9.83	71.44* ± 7.94
Fracture	66	.	68.29 ± 10.13
Instability	5	24.40 ± 16.68	66.00 ± 5.29
OA	46	28.41 ± 11.18	65.11 ± 11.22
AVN	25	31.00 ± 14.75	50.24 ± 12.15
RA	15	25.67 ± 11.46	43.67* ± 20.36
FS	43	28.19 ± 12.61	60.63 ± 10.77
Total/Mean	232	28.28 ± 12.19	62.64 ± 13.65

**$p<0.05$. (CTA, cuff tear arthropathy; OA, osteoarthritis; AVN, avascular necrosis; RA, rheumatoid arthritis; FS, fracture sequelae; Ct, Constant score.)*

The mean Constant score was 28.2 (2-64) and did not significantly differ among different etiologies. The average active anterior elevation was 83° (5°-170°). Nearly half of the patients had a passive anterior elevation below 90°. The surgical approach used was first mainly deltopectoral (98% of cases). On the glenoid side, 2 bone grafts and 2 "ream and run" cases were included. The retroversion of the humeral implant was documented in 156 shoulders with an average of 22°. The diameter and thickness of the humeral heads are reported on in Table II.

At the time of this review, clinical evaluation was assessed by Constant score [5] and range of motion (ROM). The radiographic evaluation was based on an antero-posterior view at 1 year postoperatively and from the last follow-up. On these radiographs, we analyzed the extent of erosion or glenoid wear and whether it was concentric or eccentric (fig. 1 and 2). The term "wear" is used to denote cartilage wear (joint-space narrowing without involvement of the subchondral bone). The term "erosion" is used in cases where the subchondral bone is involved as well. Using the above criteria enabled us to define 3 groups: no wear (group A), wear or erosion with concentric head (group B), and wear or erosion with eccentric head (group C). With no imaging to evaluate the cuff, we have considered that all proximally eccentric heads were associated with a rotator cuff tear.

Statistical analysis of the results was performed using the Chi-squared test for comparison of nominal variables, Student's *t*-test for comparison of means with a Gaussian distribution, and the non-parametric Mann-Whitney and Kruskall-Wallis tests for means without a Gaussian distribution.

Table II: Number, diameter, and thickness of humeral head.

N (on 219)	Diameter (mm)	Thickness (mm)
1	37	13
17	39	14
30	41	15
48	43	16
46	46	17
38	48	18
12	50	16
24	50	19
2	52	19
1	52	23

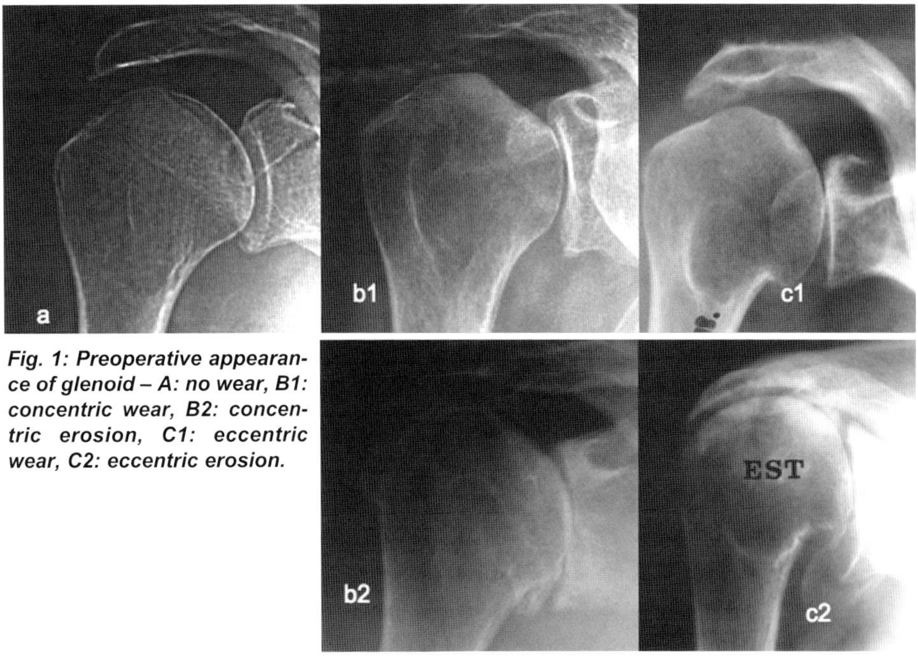

Fig. 1: Preoperative appearance of glenoid – A: no wear, B1: concentric wear, B2: concentric erosion, C1: eccentric wear, C2: eccentric erosion.

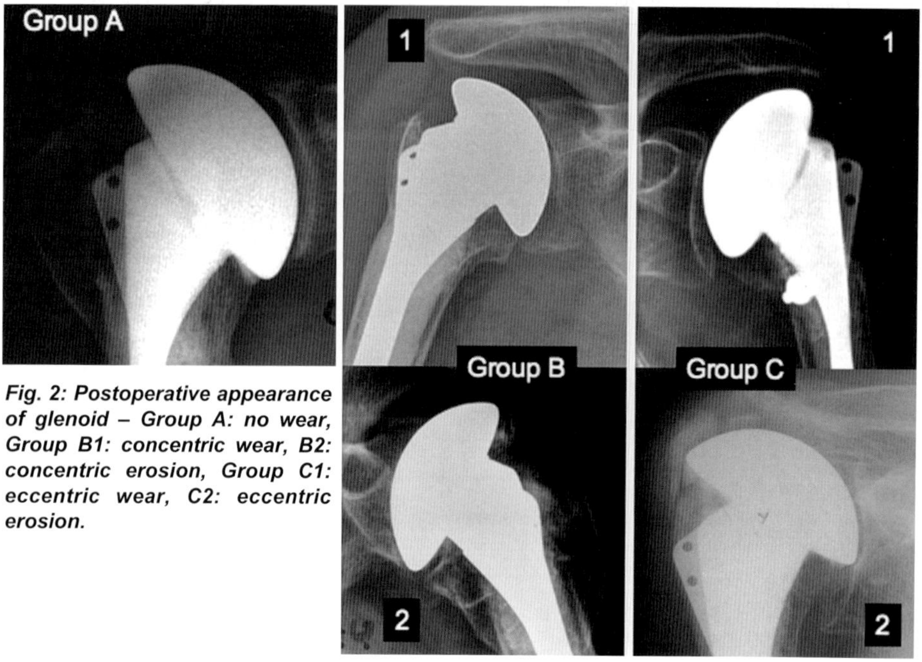

Fig. 2: Postoperative appearance of glenoid – Group A: no wear, Group B1: concentric wear, B2: concentric erosion, Group C1: eccentric wear, C2: eccentric erosion.

RESULTS

Patients were reviewed with a mean follow-up of 125 months (60-209). Rheumatoid arthritis had a significantly longer mean follow-up (139 months) than that of OA (120 months). Fifteen patients had complications after 5 years, 9 of whom required prosthetic removal at a mean follow-up of 108 months. The cause of those removals was stiffness (CTA and fracture) in 2 cases; loosening in 2, one of which was septic (1 fracture and 1 FS); and glenoid erosion (2 FS, 1 fracture, 1 AVN, 1 CTA) in 5. All the erosions were proximally eccentric because of a cuff tear or tuberosity migration, except in one case of AVN, which involved concentric erosion.

Results of the Constant score and its parameters are shown in Table III. Only CTA had significantly worse results. The difference observed according to etiology is less evident if we consider the weighted Constant score.

Radiographic results

Preoperatively, OA and RA were the etiologies with significantly ($p<0.001$) the most glenoid wear or erosion compared to AVN and fractures, which had significantly much less ($p<0.01$) (Table IV). Superior migration was significantly more frequent in the CTA group (100%). Postoperatively, group A comprised half of AVN cases, one-third of FS cases, and one-fourth of fracture cases. Where they occurred, erosion or wear mainly were concentric (group B) for OA, RA, and AVN, and they were eccentric (group C) for fractures, FS, and CTA.

Table III: Gain = gain between, preoperative and postoperative Constant score.

	F/U (mo.)	Pain	Activity	Mobility	Strength	Ct	W Ct	Gain
CTA	122.04 ± 39.38	8.26 ± 4.73	9.04 ± 4.94	18.2 ± 11.03	2.16 ± 2.32	39.57* ± 21.3	59.32 ± 33.6	13.24 ± 21.3
Fracture	125.39 ± 36.16	9.88 ± 5.61	11.5 ± 7	19.98 ± 13.03	4.97 ± 4.83	45.34 ± 28.35	64.30 ± 40.23	.
OA	120.52 ± 22.04	10.30 ± 5.23	13.56 ± 6.22	24.32 ± 12.12	6.82 ± 5.67	55.02 ± 26.54	76.67 ± 36.74	26.61 ± 29.58
AVN	131 ± 36.87	9.28 ± 6.03	12.28 ± 7.86	24.84 ± 15.18	6.96 ± 6.15	52.33 ± 32.88	60.5 ± 39.01	21.42 ± 30.71
RA	139.2* ± 33.22	12.57 ± 1.95	13.71 ± 1.94	21.93 ± 6.91	6.43 ± 6	55.28 ± 12.58	66.5 ± 28.14	29.07 ± 8.56
FS	125.30 ± 34.88	9.49 ± 5.36	12.21 ± 6.71	20.93 ± 13.05	5.79 ± 4.64	49.05 ± 26.75	63.42 ± 35.44	19.65 ± 24.75

$p<0.05$. (CTA, cuff tear arthropathy; OA, osteoarthritis; AVN, avascular necrosis; RA, rheumatoid arthritis; FS, fracture sequelae; Ct, Constant score; W Ct, weighted Constant score.)

Table IV: Appearance of postoperative glenoid erosion according to etiology

Etiology	Group C	Group B	Group A	N
CTA	13	10	0	23
Fracture	22	15	13	50
OA	9	29	0	38
AVN	1	11	11	23
RA	4	10	0	14
FS	13	10	14	37
N	65	87	38	190

Group A: no wear, group B: concentric wear or erosion, group C: eccentric wear or erosion. (CTA, cuff tear arthropathy; OA, osteoarthritis; AVN, avascular necrosis; RA, rheumatoid arthritis; FS, fracture sequelae.)

The presence of postoperative erosion was correlated with age: 57.28 years ± 11.53 on average for those with no wear or erosion, versus 63.47 years ± 15.46 for those with wear or erosion.

There was no correlation between the occurrence of erosion and the operated side. Nor was there a correlation between erosion and the diameter or thickness of the prosthetic head or with preoperative stiffness.

The Constant score as a function of glenoid status is presented in Table V. We notice that group C had a significantly worse Constant score than group A. This is related to the abundance in group C of CTA and FS (involving either a cuff tear or a tuberosity migration, respectively).

Regarding progression, glenoids that were intact preoperatively and those that remained intact postoperatively gave the best Constant scores (58.3). Those that were already eroded preoperatively had a commensurate Constant score (54.9). Those that were not worn preoperatively but became so had a significantly worse Constant score (42.2), due mainly to fractures. There was a significant variability in Constant score, for example 44 in the presence and 55 in the absence of rotator cuff tears. This mainly concerns CTA, fractures, and FS.

Table V: Constant score according to postoperative appearance of glenoid

	N	Pain	Activity	Mobility	Strength	Ct
Group C	64	9.25* ± 5.30	10.81* ± 5.93	18.98* ± 11.92	3.89* ± 4.37	43.05* ± 24.45
Group B	87	10.38 ± 4.85	12.92 ± 5.91	23.43 ± 11.49	6.37 ± 5.23	53.18 ± 24.27
Group A	38	11.29 ± 4.22	14.58 ± 5.75	27.39 ± 10.96	7.29 ± 5.51	61.33 ± 22.75

*Group A: no wear, group B: concentric wear or erosion, Group C: eccentric wear or erosion. *p<0.05. (Ct, Constant score.)*

DISCUSSION

With a mean follow-up of 125 months and minimum follow-up of 5 years, our study highlights a difference among results according to initial etiology, which proves to be an important predictive factor. Cuff tear arthropathy gave the worst results. The occurrence of glenoid erosion was a bad prognostic factor, especially if the glenohumeral space had been normal preoperatively. This was mainly the case for OA, for which preoperative glenoid wear does not translate to bad results, especially as far as pain is concerned. If wear or erosion occurred, concentricity was a good prognostic factor. In all cases, the presence of proximal eccentricity and a rotator cuff tear generally led to poor results.

This is a retrospective multi-center study with many patients who died or were lost to follow-up. However, the minimum follow-up of 5 years and mean follow-up of 125 months are substantial. Many series, especially those that are randomized, that reported on or compared results of HA, did not have such follow-up [9, 15] (Table VI). As shown in the study by Gadea *et al.* (reported in the previous chapter), most problems arise within the first 3 years, and that is the period during which revisions are reported in most other

Table VI: Follow-up of main published studies.

Authors	Etiology	Prothesis	Follow up	Results
Edwards 2003 [6]	OA	TSR vs. HA	43 mo	TSR > HA
Fox 2009 [8]	Varied	TSR	7.2 y	
Gartsmann 2000 [9]	OA	TSR vs. HA	34	TSR > HA
Haines 2006 [10, 14]	Varied	TSR vs. HA	5.1	HA = TSR
Levy 2004 [14]	RA	TSR and HA	6.5	HA = TSR
Lo 2005 [15]	OA	TSR vs. HA	24 mo	HA = TSR
Norris 2002 [17]	OA	TSR and HA	46 mo	HA = TSR
Orfaly 2003 [18]	OA	TSR vs. HA	4.3 y	TSR > HA
Sperling 2007 [21]	RA	TSR vs. HA	11.6 y	TSR > HA if intact cuff
Sperling 1998 [20]	Varied	TSR vs. HA < 50 y	12.3 y	TSR = HA

(OA, osteoarthritis; RA, rheumatoid arthritis; y, years.)

studies. Such a period is relatively short, which raises questions on the real nature of glenoid erosion. We think that in most cases it is related to rapid and poorly-tolerated eccentric migration [10], generally linked to a cuff tear or tuberosity migration. To us, it seemed more interesting to study, once this critical period has elapsed, the status of patients who retained their prostheses and the consequences of glenoid erosion that appears gradually over a long period of time.

It emerges that the occurrence of glenoid erosion has proven to be associated with worse results as far as functional results and pain are concerned [11]. This is even more obvious when the patient starts out with no erosion preoperatively and when the erosion is eccentric. Thus, in OA and RA, in which the erosion is mainly concentric, the results remain good [13]. This is consistent with Levine's ideas, except that we did not observe the same deterioration in the long term.

The best results were obtained in patients whose glenoid remained intact beyond 5 years, and this was mainly the case in AVN, as well as a few fractures and FS that did not deteriorate over time. Results were definitely worse when a rotator cuff tear or superior glenoid wear occur.

To conclude, once the critical first 3-year period is over, symptomatic glenoid erosion occurrence is due to:

- Etiology, with worse results in CTA, fractures, and FS than in RA, OA, and AVN.
- Transformation of a normal preoperative glenoid to a postoperative worn or eroded glenoid (as opposed to the results of glenoids that are already eroded preoperatively, which do not evolve much with time).
- Glenoid erosion or wear of an eccentric nature, which appears to be more painful, less mobile, and less strong, with a significantly lower Constant score.

REFERENCES

[1] ARNTZ CT, S JACKINS, FA MATSEN, 3rd Prosthetic replacement of the shoulder for the treatment of defects in the rotator cuff and the surface of the glenohumeral joint. *J Bone Joint Surg Am. 1993; 75: 485-91.*

[2] BOILEAU P, RJ SINNERTON, C CHUINARD, G. WALCH Arthroplasty of the shoulder. *J Bone Joint Surg Br. 2006; 88: 562-75.*

[3] BOILEAU P, C TROJANI, G WALCH, SG KRISHNAN A. Romeo and R. Sinnerton. Shoulder arthroplasty for the treatment of the sequelae of fractures of the proximal humerus. *J Shoulder Elbow Surg. 2001; 10: 299-308.*

[4] COFIELD RH Total shoulder arthroplasty with the Neer prosthesis. *J Bone Joint Surg Am. 1984; 66: 899-906.*

[5] CONSTANT CR, AH MURLEY. A clinical method of functional assessment of the shoulder. *Clin Orthop Relat Res. 1987, 160-4.*

[6] EDWARDS TB, NR KADAKIA, A BOULAHIA, JF KEMPF, P BOILEAU, C NEMOZ, G WALCH. A comparison of hemiarthroplasty and total shoulder arthroplasty in the treatment of primary glenohumeral osteoarthritis: results of a multicenter study. *J Shoulder Elbow Surg. 2003; 12: 207-13.*

[7] FIELD LD, DM DINES, SJ ZABINSKI, RF WARREN Hemiarthroplasty of the shoulder for rotator cuff arthropathy. *J Shoulder Elbow Surg. 1997; 6: 18-23.*

[8] FOX TJ, A CIL, JW SPERLING, J SANCHEZ-SOTELO, CD SCHLECK, RH COFIELD Survival of the glenoid component in shoulder arthroplasty. *J Shoulder Elbow Surg. 2009; 18: 859-63.*

[9] GARTSMAN GM, TS RODDEY, SM HAMMERMAN. Shoulder arthroplasty with or without resurfacing of the glenoid in patients who have osteoarthritis. *J Bone Joint Surg Am. 2000; 82: 26-34.*

[10] HAINES JF, IA TRAIL, D NUTTALL, A BIRCH, A BARROW. The results of arthroplasty in osteoarthritis of the shoulder. *J Bone Joint Surg Br. 2006; 88: 496-501.*

[11] IANNOTTI JP, TR NORRIS Influence of preoperative factors on outcome of shoulder arthroplasty for glenohumeral osteoarthritis. *J Bone Joint Surg Am. 2003; 85-A: 251-8.*

[12] KREPLER P, AH WANIVENHAUS, C WURNIG. Outcome assessment of hemiarthroplasty of the shoulder: a 5-year follow-up with 4 evaluation tools. *Acta Orthop. 2006; 77: 778-84.*

[13] LEVINE WN, M DJURASOVIC, JM GLASSON, RG POLLOCK, EL FLATOW, LU BIGLIANI. Hemiarthroplasty for glenohumeral osteoarthritis: results correlated to degree of glenoid wear. *J Shoulder Elbow Surg. 1997;6: 449-54.*

[14] LEVY O, L FUNK, G SFORZA, SA COPELAND. Copeland surface replacement arthroplasty of the shoulder in rheumatoid arthritis. *J Bone Joint Surg Am. 2004; 86-A: 512-8.*

[15] LO IK, RB LITCHFIELD, S GRIFFIN, K FABER, SD PATTERSON, A KIRKLEY. Quality-of-life outcome following hemiarthroplasty or total shoulder arthroplasty in patients with osteoarthritis. A prospective, randomized trial. *J Bone Joint Surg Am. 2005; 87: 2178-85.*

[16] NEER CS 2nd. Replacement arthroplasty for glenohumeral osteoarthritis. *J Bone Joint Surg Am. 1974;56: 1-13.*

[17] NORRIS TR, JP IANNOTTI. Functional outcome after shoulder arthroplasty for primary osteoarthritis: a multicenter study. *J Shoulder Elbow Surg. 2002; 11: 130-5.*

[18] ORFALY RM, CA ROCKWOOD Jr, CZ ESENYEL, MA WIRTH A prospective functional outcome study of shoulder arthroplasty for osteoarthritis with an intact rotator cuff. *J Shoulder Elbow Surg. 2003; 12: 214-21.*

[19] SANCHEZ-SOTELO J, RH COFIELD, CM ROWLAND. Shoulder hemiarthroplasty for glenohumeral arthritis associated with severe rotator cuff deficiency. *J Bone Joint Surg Am. 2001;83-A: 1814-22.*

[20] SPERLING JW, RH COFIELD, CM ROWLAND. Neer hemiarthroplasty and Neer total shoulder arthroplasty in patients fifty years old or less. Long-term results. *J Bone Joint Surg Am. 1998;80: 464-73.*

[21] SPERLING JW, RH COFIELD, CD SCHLECK, WS HARMSEN. Total shoulder arthroplasty versus hemiarthroplasty for rheumatoid arthritis of the shoulder: results of 303 consecutive cases. *J Shoulder Elbow Surg. 2007;16: 683-90.*

[22] TORCHIA ME, RH COFIELD, CR SETTERGREN. Total shoulder arthroplasty with the Neer prosthesis: long-term results. *J Shoulder Elbow Surg. 1997;6: 495-505.*

[23] WILLIAMS GR Jr, CA ROCKWOOD Jr Hemiarthroplasty in rotator cuff-deficient shoulders. *J Shoulder Elbow Surg. 1996;5: 362-7.*

[24] WIRTH MA, CA ROCKWOOD Jr Complications of total shoulder-replacement arthroplasty. *J Bone Joint Surg Am. 1996;78: 603-16.*

WHAT IS THE IDEAL ETIOLOGY AND PREOPERATIVE GLENOID STATUS FOR SHOULDER HEMIARTHROPLASTY?

L. FAVARD, D. MOLÉ, J.C. BALESTRO, C. TROJANI, G. ALAMI, F. GADEA

INTRODUCTION

Since Neer's early work [17], the indications for shoulder arthroplasty have expanded substantially. Depending on the original etiology and on the surgeon's convictions, the arthroplasty consisted of either total shoulder arthroplasty (TSA) or hemiarthroplasty (HA). Even though it is widely assumed that a HA is preferable when the glenoid cartilage is intact, as in fractures or osteonecrosis (ON) [3], no consensus exists regarding cases where the glenoid cartilage is damaged, as in osteoarthritis (OA) [16, 18, 22] or rheumatoid arthritis (RA) [15, 20]. Those who prefer using TSA cite better clinical results [5, 8, 11] and argue that progressive deterioration has been observed with HA [6, 14]. As for those who prefer HA [12, 23], they view its results as differing little from those of TSA and argue that its patients have a generally low revision requirement and do not run the relatively high risk of glenoid-component loosening past the tenth year [6, 21]. The reported results with HA for some etiologies are not very satisfactory—for instance for fractures sequelae (FA) [4] or cuff tear arthropathy (CTA) [1, 10]. Yet, glenoid wear in those cases is not always substantial.

Therefore, according these studies, it seems that HAs do not all deteriorate inevitably over time. Moreover, with the exception of those of Sperling *et al.* [19, 20], most published studies only have medium-term follow-up, which hinders proper comparison between HA and TSA in the long term.

In analyzing the outcomes of HA, two elements must be considered: *the rate of revision, and the clinical and radiographic long-term results*. Thus, for a certain indication, if long-term results of the prostheses that are still in place are good and the revision rate is low, it is a good indication. Otherwise, it is a bad one. As for indications for which the results are good but the revision rate is high, the cause of this high revision rate should be sought.

The aim of this study was to analyze the results and survivorship of a series of HAs with a minimum follow-up of 5 years, in order to delineate the best indications of HA, according to etiology. Our hypothesis is that an initially intact glenoid and rotator cuff would emerge as important prognostic factors.

PATIENTS AND METHODS

This is a multi-center, European study including all consecutive Aequalis HA cases, of both standard and fracture types, implanted before January, 2000. Only prostheses implanted during a revision arthroplasty or for cases of tumors have been excluded. Thus, 399 patients (423 shoulders) have been included. To evaluate the results we estimated that a minimum follow-up of 5 years was necessary. Of the 423 shoulders included initially, 86 patients died, with their prosthesis in place, before the 5th year. Seventy-six patients were lost to follow-up, and 29 had a prosthetic removal. Thus, 247 patients (261 shoulders) were reviewed or had a prosthetic removal past their 5th follow-up year. This population is composed of 72 men (76 shoulders) and 175 women (185 shoulders), so 14 patients had both shoulders operated on. The dominant shoulder was involved in 59% of cases. The mean age at surgery was 62.6 years (16-85).

The etiology distribution is presented in Table I. Because of the small number of arthritis-after-instability cases and the disparity of the miscellaneous etiologies, these two groups were not included in the outcomes analysis.

Preoperatively, the patients' clinical status was assessed with the Constant score [7] and separately with range of motion (ROM). The mean Constant score was 28.2 (2-64) and the mean active anterior elevation (AAE) was 83° (5-170). The approach used was mainly deltopectoral (98% of cases). On the glenoid side, 2 bone grafts and 2 "ream and run" cases were included. The retroversion of the humeral implant was documented in 156 shoulders with a mean of 22°.

At the time of review, the clinical evaluation was assessed with the Constant score and ROM. The radiographic evaluation was based on an antero-posterior view at 1 year postoperatively and from the last follow-up. On these radiographs, we ana-

Table I: Characteristics of each etiology

	N	Age	FU	Ct	Removal
CTA	29	71.65 ± 7.9	107.07 ± 52.7	36.13 ± 23.3	6
Fracture	73	68.50 ± 9.9	115.06 ± 47.2	41.33 ± 30	10
OA	49	64.49 ± 11.1	114.02 ± 33.4	52.73 ± 28.2	3
ON	27	50.74 ± 12.6	121.78 ± 48.6	50.24 ± 33.8	3
RA	15	43.66 ± 20.3	139.2 ± 33.2	55.28 ± 12.5	0
FS	54	60.63 ± 11.3	104.72 ± 52	42.65 ± 30	14

***CTA**, cuff tear arthropathy; **OA**, osteoarthritis; **ON**, osteonecrosis; **RA**, rheumatoid arthritis; **FS**, fracture sequelae; **N**, number; **FU**, follow-up; **Ct**, Constant score* lyzed the extent of erosion or glenoid wear and whether it was concentric or eccentric.

The term "wear" is used to denote cartilage wear (joint-space narrowing without involvement of the subchondral bone). The term "erosion" is used in cases where the subchondral bone is involved as well. Using the above criteria enabled us to define 3 groups: no wear *(group A)*, wear or erosion with a concentric head *(group B)*, and wear or erosion with an eccentric head *(group C)*. With no imaging to evaluate the cuff, we considered all proximally-eccentric heads as being associated with rotator cuff tears.

Analysis was done for each etiologic category. Prosthetic removals were analyzed with survival curves generated using the Kaplan-Meier technique, with a 95% confidence interval according to Rothman and Greenland. Only one end-point was examined: the survivorship until prosthetic removal. Statistical analysis of the results was performed using the Chi-squared test for comparison of nominal variables, Student's *t*-test for comparison of means with a Gaussian distribution, and the non-parametric Mann-Whitney and Kruskall-Wallis tests for means without a Gaussian distribution.

had a prosthetic removal at a mean follow-up of 49 months. Causes of these removals were infection in 4 (one late), aseptic loosening in 1, stiffness in 2, and proximal glenoid erosion in 3. Three were converted to TSA, 3 were converted to reverse shoulder arthroplasty (RSA), 3 had a stem removal without replacement, and 1 had an arthrodesis. The survival rate – survival without removal being the end-point – was 93% at 5 years and 91% at 10 years (Fig. 1). The overall survival-without-removal curve shows two breaks, occurring during the first 5 years and the second after 10 years. During the first 3 years 7 prostheses were removed, and after 10 years only 3 were removed.

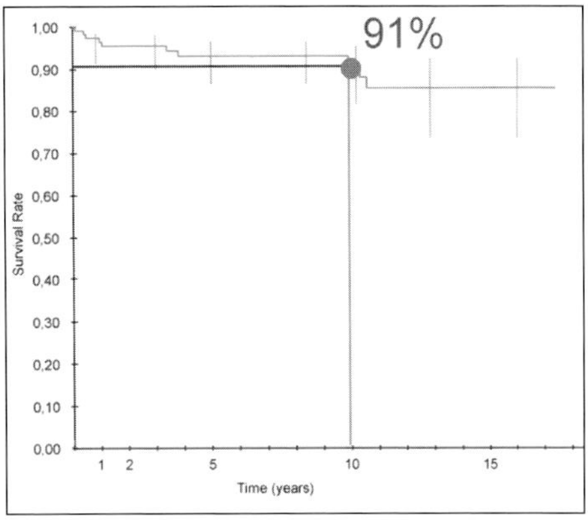

Fig. 1: Survival curve of fracture group.

RESULTS AND DISCUSSION

Fracture

Results

Seventy-three patients were reviewed with a mean follow-up of 115 months (1-209). The mean age at surgery was 68.5 years (39-85) (Table I). Ten patients

At the time of review, the mean Constant score was 41.3 (0-89) and the mean weighted Constant score was 58.6 (0-129). The AAE was 114 ° (30-180) and active external rotation (AER) was 18° (-20 to 80). Preoperatively, all glenoids had been intact. Postoperatively, the following distribution in glenoid status was found: 50% in group C, 27% in group B, and 23% in group A (Table II). The presence of erosion or wear after surgery did not correla-

Table II: Percentage and Constant score according to type of postoperative glenoid.

	CTA	Fracture	OA	ON	RA	FS
Group C	63% /35.53	50% / 37.59*	24% /42.80	4% /9.50	28% / 45	38% /38.33
Group B	37% /38.90	27% /55.73	76% /53.17	48% /56.18	72% / 58.20	33% /37.56
Group A	-	23% /54.42	-	48% /58.73	-	29% /61.36

***CTA**, cuff tear arthropathy; **OA**, osteoarthritis; **ON**, osteonecrosis; **RA**, rheumatoid arthritis; **FS**, fracture sequelae*

te with age, side operated, or prosthetic-head diameter or thickness. Proximal wear or erosion was associated with migration of the tuberosities in 70% of cases. The postoperative Constant score according to glenoid status is detailed in Table II. We found that patients in group C had a significantly worse Constant score than those in groups A or B, essentially because of lower strength and mobility sub-scores. No significant differences were found between groups A and B.

Discussion

With a mean follow-up of 115 months, the fractures group had a survival rate of 91% at 10 years. The mean Constant score was 41.3. The occurrence of proximal glenoid erosion was a poor prognostic factor and was almost always the result of tuberosity migration. However, when wear was concentric, there was no adver se effect on outcome, which was similar to that of intact glenoids. Most prosthetic removals occurred early and were caused by either infection or tuberosity migration. All these phenomena have already been widely reported in the literature [3], and they confirm the idea that fractures are a good indication for HA as long as the quality of *tuberosity fixation* is perfect.

In conclusion, our hypothesis was only partially confirmed: a rotator cuff tear – or, in the case of fractures, a tuberosity migration – is a poor prognostic factor. However, the occurrence of glenoid erosion is not a poor prognostic factor provided it is concentric.

Fracture Sequelae

Results

Fifty-four patients were reviewed with a mean follow-up of 105 months (3-185). The mean age at surgery was 60.6 years (24-80). Fourteen had a prosthetic removal at a mean follow-up of 41 months (Table I). The causes of these removals were 3 infections (all in the first 2 years), 1 aseptic loosening, and 10 glenoid erosions (5 concentric and 5 eccentric). Six were converted to TSA, 3 were converted to RSA, 4 had a stem removal without replacement, and 1 had an arthrodesis. The survival rate – survival without removal being the end-point – was 81% at 5 years and 76% at 10 years (Fig. 2). The overall survival-without-removal curve shows a stronger decline in survival during the first 3 years.

The comparison between preoperative and postoperative clinical status at a minimum of 5 years shows a significant improvement in Constant scores. At the time of review, the mean postoperative Constant score was 42.6 (0-84), as opposed to 26.7 (2-64) preoperatively. The AAE was 114° (30-180) and AER was 23° (-30 to 90). Preoperatively 76% of glenoids had been intact, while postoperative glenoid status was distributed as follows: 38% in group C, 33% in group B, and 29% in group A.

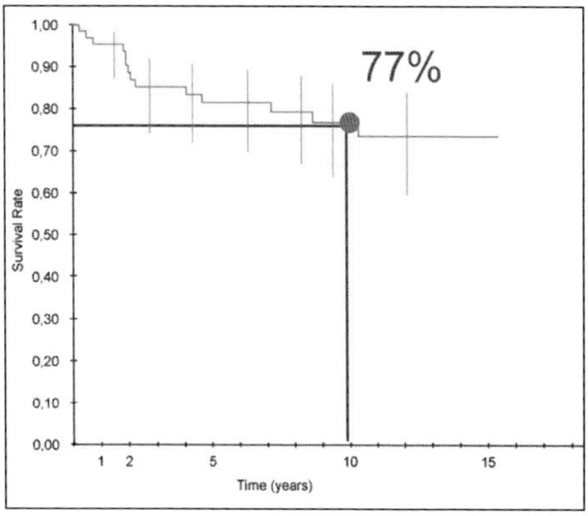

Fig. 2: Survival curve of fracture sequelae group.

Group B was associated with an older mean age (65 versus 57 years). However, no correlation was observed between glenoid status (i.e. group) and side operated, preoperative stiffness, or prosthetic-head diameter or thickness. Constant scores according to glenoid status are presented in Table II. We found groups B and C to have a significantly worse (38.3) Constant score than group A (61.3). No significant differences were found between group B and C.

Over time, glenoids that had been intact preoperatively and remained intact after surgery were those that gave the best Constant scores (60.2). Glenoids that had already been eroded preoperatively had a poor score (31.2), and those that had been intact and became worn after surgery did even more poorly (mean Constant score of 27.4).

Discussion

With a mean follow-up of 104 months, FS had a survival rate of 76% at 10 years and a mean Constant score of 42.6. The occurrence of eccentric or concentric glenoid erosion was a poor prognostic factor. This was either due to a rotator cuff tear or a poorly-tolerated symptomatic worn glenoid, especially when the age at surgery was over 65 years. Most prosthetic removals were due to eccentric or concentric glenoid erosion. When the glenoid was eroded preoperatively, results were not good.

All of the above confirms that FS are *not* a good indication for HA. This is in agreement with Hettrich *et al.* [13], who found that the use of HA for this etiology does not lead to good results. As concluded by Boileau *et al.* [4], it seems better to consider glenoid replacement whatever the preoperative status of the glenoid. Moreover, these authors concluded that RSA may also be useful depending on the type of FS. Perhaps one exception that can be made to the above conclusion is for younger patients, preferably those without glenoid erosion. That aside, the revision rate for FS was high, the clinical results fair, and glenoid erosion poorly tolerated. In conclusion, our hypothesis was again only partially confirmed. A rotator cuff tear is a poor prognostic factor. Here, however, a preoperatively intact glenoid is not a good prognostic factor, as even without a cuff tear a strong trend exists towards symptomatic erosion.

Cuff Tear Arthropathy

Results

Twenty-nine patients were reviewed with a mean follow-up of 107 months (9-190).

The mean age at surgery was 71.6 years (50-82) (Table I). Six patients had a prosthetic removal at a mean follow-up of 32 months. The cause of these removals was always eccentric glenoid erosion. One was converted to TSA and 5 to RSA. The survival rate – survival without removal being the end-point – was 98% at 5 years and 81% at 10 years (Fig. 3). The overall survival-without-removal curve shows two breaks, the first occurring during the first 2 years and the second after 5 years. During the first 2 years 4 prostheses were removed, and after 5 years 2 prostheses were removed.

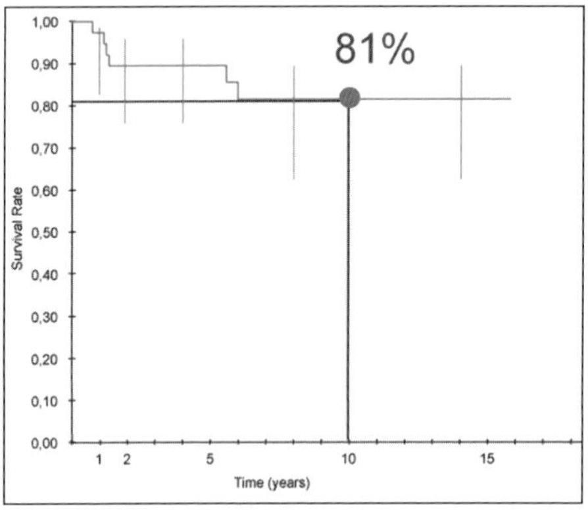

Fig. 3: Survival curve of cuff tear arthropathy group.

The comparison between preoperative and postoperative clinical status at a minimum of 5 years shows a significant improvement in Constant scores. At the time of review, the mean preoperative Constant score was 23.4 (9-49) and the mean postoperative Constant score was 36.1 (0-77). The AAE was 100° (20-170) and AER was 23.8° (-10 to 80). Preoperatively, 27% had had an intact glenoid, representing massive cuff tears without osteoarthritis (Hamada I and II). As for postoperative glenoid status, 63% were in group C and 37% were in group B.

No correlation was observed between glenoid status distribution and age, side operated, preoperative stiffness, or prosthetic-head diameter or thickness. Finally, no significant differences were found between groups B and C (Table II).

Discussion

With a mean follow-up of 107 months, the CTA survival rate was 81% at 10 years. Constant score and mobility results for this etiology were poor – the mean Constant score was 36.1. The occurrence of eccentric or concentric glenoid erosion did not change the outcome, but all these patients, by definition, had a massive cuff tear. Almost all prosthetic removals were due to symptomatic glenoid erosion. This series with long follow-up but few cases confirms the notion that HA has limited goals with this etiology [1]. In his study comparing the results of HA and RSA for patients with cuff tear arthropathy, Favard [9] observed better results for RSA for all criteria even beyond 5 years of follow-up. Only the AER was more limited with RSA. All this strongly suggests that it is better to consider RSA for this indication, except for younger patients for whom the need for revision is a concern.

In conclusion, our hypothesis was confirmed: with this etiology, rotator cuff tears and glenoid erosion are poor prognostic factors that produce limited results.

Osteonecrosis

Results

Twenty-seven patients were reviewed with a mean follow-up of 121 months (1-199). The mean age at surgery was 50 years (35-79) (Table I). Three had a prosthetic removal at a mean follow-up of 55 months. The cause of these removals was one infection and 2 glenoid erosions (one after subscapularis insufficiency). Two were converted to TSA, and 1 had a stem removal without replacement. The survival rate – survival without removal being the end-point – was 94% at 5 years and 94% at 10 years (Fig. 4). The overall survival-without-removal curve shows a progressive decline that is strongest during the first year.

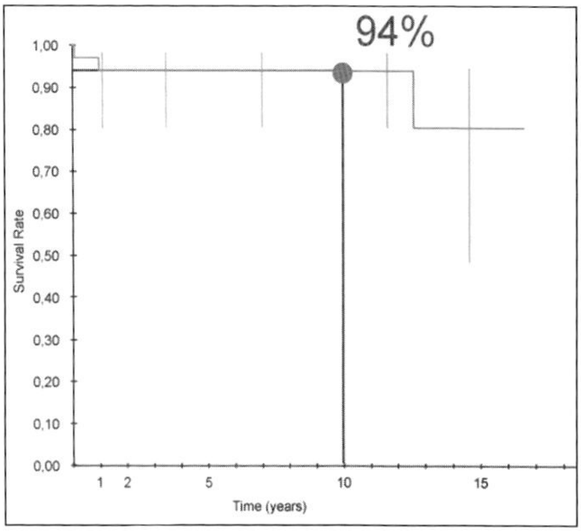

Fig. 4: Survival curve of osteonecrosis group.

The comparison between preoperative and postoperative clinical status at a minimum of 5 years shows a significant improvement in Constant scores (Table I). At the time of review, the mean postoperative Constant score was 50 (0-89), versus 32 (7-59) preoperatively. The AAE was 143° (30-180) and AER was 31° (0-90). Preoperatively, 90% had had an intact glenoid. Postoperatively, the aspect of the glenoid was as follows: 48% in group A, 48% in group B, and 4% in group C.

No correlation was observed between glenoid status distribution and age, operated side, preoperative stiffness, or prosthetic-head diameter or thickness. No significant differences – not even with regard to pain – were found between groups A and B (Table II).

Discussion

With a mean follow-up of 121 months, ON had a survival rate of 94% at 10 years. The mean Constant score was 58. There were few revisions, which occurred especially during the first year (due to infection and subscapularis insufficiency). The ROM was excellent. The occurrence of concentric wear did not significantly affect outcomes, pain included. These results agree with those reported in the literature [3, 13] and with the notion that HA is very good solution for ON without cuff tear particularly. Osteonecrosis is an even better indication when patients are young.

In conclusion, our hypothesis was confirmed in the case of ON: for this etiology, the absence of preoperative glenoid erosion and a rotator cuff tear gives good functional results.

Rheumatoid Arthritis

Results

Fifteen patients were reviewed with a mean follow-up of 139 months (65-201). The mean age at surgery was 43.6 years (35-79) (Table I). None had a prosthetic removal. Thus, the survival rate –survival without removal being the end-point – was 100% at both 5 and 10 years (Fig. 5). The comparison between preoperative and postoperative clinical status at a minimum of 5 years shows a significant improvement in Constant scores.

At the time of review, the mean postoperative Constant score was 55.2 (36-87), versus 25.6 (8-50) preoperatively. The AAE was 98° (30-160) and the AER was 22° (-5 to 90). Preoperatively, there had been no intact glenoids. Postoperatively, the glenoid status was as follows: 72% in group B and 28% in group C.

No correlation was observed between glenoid status and age, operated side, preoperative stiffness, or prosthetic-head diameter or thickness. In terms of functional results, no significant differences were found between Groups B and C, except with regard to the weighted Constant score (76.4% in group B and 41.7% in group C) (Table II).

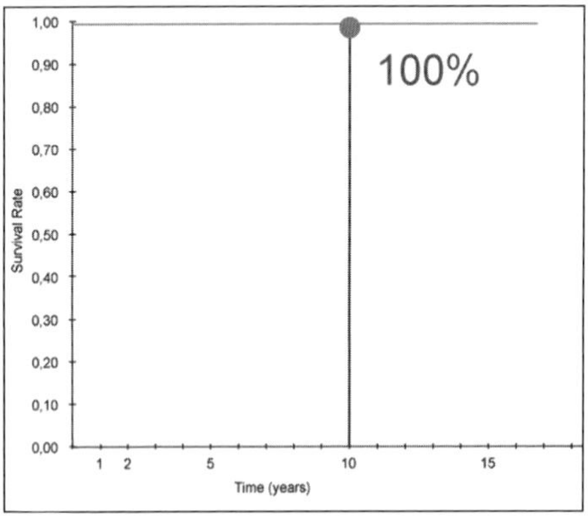

Fig. 5: Survival curve of rheumatoid arthritis group.

Discussion

With a mean follow-up of 139 months, the survival rate with RA was 100% at 10 years. The mean Constant score was 55. The ROM was limited but there was a number of young, juvenile-RA patients, who are notoriously stiff. The occurrence of eccentric wear correlated significantly with a worse weighted Constant score. The eccentric wear reflects the rotator cuff insufficiency, which is known to adversely affect results after TSA. The patients of this group were young with a substantial life expectancy. Revising their prostheses for loosening is often difficult due to the associated bone defects. Their risk of glenoid loosening over time is very high [2]. All this confirms the notion that HA is particularly indicated for this etiology, *even in the presence of a rotator cuff tear* and whatever the preoperative glenoid status.

In conclusion, our hypothesis was not confirmed in this case: with RA, even with preoperative glenoid erosion and a rotator cuff tear, the results are good. The only concern is the limited range of motion.

Osteoarthritis

Results

Forty-nine patients were reviewed with a mean follow-up of 114 months (12-179). The mean age at surgery was 64.5 years (30-80) (Table I). Three had a prosthetic removal, the cause of all 3 being glenoid erosion (one was associated with a cuff tear). All were converted to TSA. The survival rate – survival without removal being the end-point – was 95% at 5 years and 95% at 10 years (Fig. 6). The overall survival-without-removal curve shows a break during the first 2 years.

The comparison between preoperative and postoperative clinical status at a minimum follow-up of 5 years showed a significant improvement in Constant scores. At the time of review, the mean postoperative Constant score was 52.7 (0-93), versus 28.7 (5-49) preoperatively. The AAE was 130° (60-180) and the AER was 37° (-30 to 80). Preoperatively, there had been no intact glenoids. Postoperatively, the glenoid status was as follows: 76% in group B and 24% in group C.

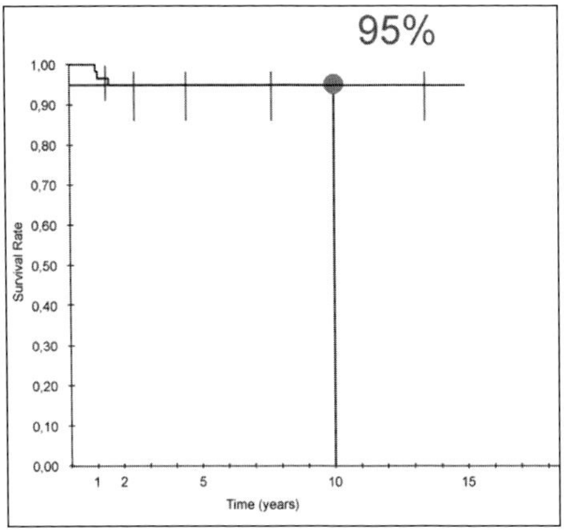

Fig. 6: Survival curve of osteoarthritis group.

Group B correlated with older age. In terms of functional results, there were no significant differences between Groups B and C, although the mean Constant score was better in group B (53 versus 43) (Table II). However, we did observe a difference using Walch's classification: A1 and B1 glenoids had significantly worse Constant scores than A2 or B2 glenoids.

Discussion

With a mean follow-up of 114 months, the survival rate was of 95% at 10 years. The mean Constant score was 52.7. There were few implant removals, which took place mostly during the first year. The ROM was good. The type of glenoid erosion did not significantly affect the outcome, pain included. However, the fact that Walch type-A1 and -B1 glenoids gave worse results may be due to a lower initial congruence between the prosthetic head and the glenoid, causing uneven pressure distribution, whereas Walch type-A2 and -B2 glenoids offered a larger contact surface. All these findings strongly suggest that HA should be offered for OA with an intact rotator cuff, particularly in younger patients and particularly for Walch type-B2 glenoids, which are difficult to manage with TSA.

In conclusion, here again our hypothesis was not confirmed. Finally, our results interestingly suggest more advanced preoperative glenoid erosion as being a good prognostic factor in OA.

REFERENCES

[1] ARNTZ CT, S JACKINS, FA MATSEN, 3rd Prosthetic replacement of the shoulder for the treatment of defects in the rotator cuff and the surface of the glenohumeral joint. *J Bone Joint Surg Am. 1993;75: 485-91.*

[2] BETTS HM, R ABU-RAJAB, T NUNN, AJ BROOKSBANK Total shoulder replacement in rheumatoid disease: a 16- to 23-year follow-up. *J Bone Joint Surg Br. 2009;91: 1197-200.*

[3] BOILEAU P, RJ SINNERTON, C CHUINARD, G WALCH Arthroplasty of the shoulder. *J Bone Joint Surg Br. 2006; 88: 562-75.*

[4] BOILEAU P, C TROJANI, G WALCH, SG KRISHNAN A. Romeo and R. Sinnerton. Shoulder arthroplasty for the treatment of the sequelae of fractures of the proximal humerus. *J Shoulder Elbow Surg. 2001;10: 299-308.*

[5] BRYANT D, R LITCHFIELD, M SANDOW, GM GARTSMAN, G GUYATT, A KIRKLEY. A comparison of pain, strength, range of motion, and functional outcomes after hemiarthroplasty and total shoulder arthroplasty in patients with osteoarthritis of the shoulder. A systematic review and meta-analysis. *J Bone Joint Surg Am. 2005; 87: 1947-56.*

[6] COFIELD RH Total shoulder arthroplasty with the Neer prosthesis. *J Bone Joint Surg Am. 1984;66: 899-906.*

[7] CONSTANT CR, AH MURLEY. A clinical method of functional assessment of the shoulder. *Clin Orthop Relat Res. 1987, 160-4.*

[8] EDWARDS TB, NR KADAKIA, A BOULAHIA, JF KEMPF, P BOILEAU, C NEMOZ, G WALCH. A comparison of hemiarthroplasty and total shoulder arthroplasty in the treatment of primary glenohumeral osteoarthritis: results of a multicenter study. *J Shoulder Elbow Surg. 2003; 12: 207-13.*

[9] FAVARD L, S LAUTMANN, F SIRVEAUX, D OUDET, Y. KERJEAN, D HUGUET Hemiarthroplasty versus reverse arthroplasty int the treatment of osteoarthritis with massive rotator cuff tear. 2000 Shoulder Prostheses… two to ten years follow-up. B.P. Walch G, Mole D. *Montpellier, Sauramps Medical. 2001: 261-8.*

[10] FIELD LD, DM DINES, SJ ZABINSKI, RF WARREN. Hemiarthroplasty of the shoulder for rotator cuff arthropathy. *J Shoulder Elbow Surg 1997;6: 18-23.*

[11] GARTSMAN GM, TS RODDEY, SM HAMMERMAN. Shoulder arthroplasty with or without resurfacing of the glenoid in patients who have osteoarthritis. *J Bone Joint Surg Am. 2000;82: 26-34.*

[12] GOLDBERG SS, LU BIGLIANI. Hemiarthroplasty for the rotator cuff-deficient shoulder. Surgical technique. *J Bone Joint Surg Am. 2009; 91 Suppl 2 Pt 1: 22-9.*

[13] HETTRICH CM, E WELDON 3rd, RS BOORMAN, IM PARSONS, FA MATSEN 3rd. Preoperative factors associated with improvements in shoulder function after humeral hemiarthroplasty. *J Bone Joint Surg Am. 2004;86-A: 1446-51.*

[14] LEVINE WN, M DJURASOVIC, JM GLASSON, RG POLLOCK, EL FLATOW, LU BIGLIANI. Hemiarthroplasty for glenohumeral osteoarthritis: results correlated to degree of glenoid wear. *J Shoulder Elbow Surg. 1997;6: 449-54.*

[15] LEVY O, L FUNK, G SFORZA, SA COPELAND. Copeland surface replacement arthroplasty of the shoulder in rheumatoid arthritis. *J Bone Joint Surg Am. 2004;86-A: 512-8.*

[16] LO IK, RB LITCHFIELD, S GRIFFIN, K FABER, SD PATTERSON, A KIRKLEY. Quality-of-life outcome following hemiarthroplasty or total shoulder arthroplasty in patients with osteoarthritis. A prospective, randomized trial. *J Bone Joint Surg Am. 2005;87: 2178-85.*

[17] NEER CS 2nd. Replacement arthroplasty for glenohumeral osteoarthritis. *J Bone Joint Surg Am. 1974;56: 1-13.*

[18] RADNAY CS, KJ SETTER, L CHAMBERS, WN LEVINE, LU BIGLIANI, CS AHMAD. Total shoulder replacement compared with humeral head replacement for the treatment of primary glenohumeral osteoarthritis: a systematic review. *J Shoulder Elbow Surg. 2007;16: 396-402.*

[19] SPERLING JW, RH COFIELD, CM ROWLAND. Neer hemiarthroplasty and Neer total shoulder arthroplasty in patients fifty years old or less. Long-term results. *J Bone Joint Surg Am. 1998;80: 464-73.*

[20] SPERLING JW, RH COFIELD, CD SCHLECK, WS HARMSEN. Total shoulder arthroplasty versus hemiarthroplasty for rheumatoid arthritis of the shoulder: results of 303 consecutive cases. *J Shoulder Elbow Surg. 2007;16: 683-90.*

[21] TORCHIA ME, RH COFIELD, CR SETTERGREN. Total shoulder arthroplasty with the Neer prosthesis: long-term results. *J Shoulder Elbow Surg. 1997;6: 495-505.*

[22] WILLIAMS GR, Jr, CA ROCKWOOD Jr Hemiarthroplasty in rotator cuff-deficient shoulders. *J Shoulder Elbow Surg. 1996;5: 362-7.*

[23] WIRTH MA, CA ROCKWOOD Jr. Complications of total shoulder-replacement arthroplasty. *J Bone Joint Surg Am. 1996;78: 603-16.*

LONG-TERM RESULTS OF A FLAT-BACK POLYETHYLENE GLENOID COMPONENT IN PRIMARY OSTEOARTHRITIS – A MULTI-CENTER STUDY

G. WALCH, A. YOUNG, F. GOHLKE, R. PHILIPPE, L. FAVARD, P. BOILEAU

ABSTRACT

Background

The goal of this study was to analyze the long-term outcome of the flat-back glenoid component. Our hypothesis was that the rates of radiologic loosening and glenoid revision increase with time, but also that these outcomes could be influenced by specific pre-operative factors.

Methods

Between 1991 and 2003, in nine European centers, 308 shoulder arthroplasties were performed for primary osteoarthritis using a flat-backed, cemented, all-polyethylene, keeled glenoid component. Kaplan-Meier survivorship analysis was performed with glenoid revision for loosening and radiologic glenoid loosening as end-points. Clinical outcome was assessed with the Constant score, patient satisfaction score, and range of movement.

Results

At a mean of 10.3 years, the rate of radiologic glenoid loosening was 44% and revision was performed for glenoid loosening in 9.1%. Glenoid component survival with end-point being revision surgery for glenoid loosening was 99.1% at 5 years, 94.5% at 10 years and 79.4% at 15 years. Glenoid survivorship with end-point being radiologic loosening was 99.2% at 5 years, 80.3% at 10 years and 33.6% at 15 years. The mean Constant score improved significantly ($p<0.0001$) from 26.8 points preoperatively to 57.6 points at last follow-up, with all components improving significantly ($p<0.0001$). Active forward elevation improved from a mean of 85.3° to 125.0° ($p<0.0001$) and external rotation improved from a mean of 7.0 to 30.3° ($p<0.0001$). 75.7% of patients were either satisfied or very satisfied, 20% uncertain and 4% disappointed.

Conclusions

While we have demonstrated satisfactory early results using a flat-back glenoid design, there was a marked progression of radiolucent lines and glenoid loosening with increasing duration of follow-up. Therefore, we recommend that any future studies reporting radiologic outcomes of a new glenoid design must report follow-up of at least 5 to 10 years. In addition to length of follow-up, we also found that younger patient age and curettage technique of glenoid preparation were correlated with glenoid loosening.

INTRODUCTION

In 2001, a multicenter study was organized in Nice in order to analyze the mid term results of the Aequalis total shoulder arthroplasty (TSA) [10]. With an average follow-up of 44 months (24-110), 319 cases with a cemented, all-polyethylene flat-back, keeled component were reported. The rate of radiologic loosening was 11.5% and the rate of revision was 1.3%. In 2005, a radiographic comparison of flat-back and convex-back glenoid components in total shoulder arthroplasty showed at 2 years of follow-up a higher radiolucent-line (RLL) score with the flat-back compared to the convex-back [32].

The goal of this study was to analyze the long-term results of the flat-back glenoid in a large multi-center European study with a single aetiology: primary glenohumeral osteoarthritis. Our hypothesis was that the rate of radiologic loosening and glenoid revision would increase with time, but also that other specific preoperative factors, such as age at surgery, glenoid shape, gender, and dominance, could also significantly influence the radiographic evolution of the glenoid component.

MATERIALS AND METHODS

Between September, 1991 and December, 2003, 308 total shoulder arthroplasties were performed for primary glenohumeral osteoarthritis, as described by Neer [25], in nine European centers (Table 1).

Table I: Number of Aequalis total shoulder arthroplasties implanted between 1991 and 2003 for primary gleno-humeral osteoarthritis with a keeled PE glenoid flat-back component in 9 European centers

	Number of cases reviewed with X-rays > 5y fu	Questionnaire alone	Death (fu <5y)	Lost to follow-up	Total number of cases operated on 1991-2003
Lyon 1 - France	100	4	4	3	111
Nice - France	12	2	1	0	15
Heidelberg - Germany	35	1	3	3	42
Lyon 2 - France	12	0	2	2	16
Wurzburg - Germany	16	1	4	5	26
Marseille - France	5	0	6	6	17
Bordeaux - France	7	0	8	16	31
Nancy - France	17	1	4	6	28
Tours - France	13	0	5	4	22
TOTAL	217	9	37	45	308

In an effort to obtain a pure series of primary osteoarthritis, shoulders with an inflammatory arthropathy, post infectious arthropathy, neurologic problem, osteonecrosis (post-traumatic, idiopathic) or post-traumatic arthritis were excluded. Additional exclusion criteria included any shoulder with a history of shoulder trauma (fracture or soft-tissue injury), instability (surgically or non-surgically treated), or prior shoulder surgery. Lastly, shoulders with marked rotator cuff pathology as indicated by acromiohumeral arthritis or by the presence of a massive rotator cuff tear seen on preoperative imaging, or at the time of surgery, were excluded.

All shoulder arthroplasties were performed with the third generation Aequalis prosthesis (Tornier, Montbonnot, France). The glenoid component used was a keeled, ultra-high-molecular-weight, all-polyethylene flat-back in all cases. Cases operated on with a metal-back glenoid or convex-back, keeled glenoid component were excluded from this series, as well as cases with bone grafting of the glenoid.

Forty-five prostheses were lost to follow-up and had incomplete charts, leaving 263 TSAs performed in 247 patients (16 bilateral prostheses) who are the basis of this study and were included in the Kaplan-Meier survivorship analysis with end-points being glenoid revision for glenoid loosening and radiologic glenoid loosening [19]. 226 TSA in 210 patients, for which complete preoperative and operative records were available with minimum follow-up of 5 years (mean, 124.1 months; range 61 to 219) or until revision, were included in the clinical analysis. Complete sets of radiographs were available for 217 shoulders and were the basis of the radiographic analysis. The mean age at the time of operation was 66.9 years (range 40-90). There were 182 females (69.2%) and 81 males (30.8%). The right shoulder was involved in 157 cases (59.8%) and the dominant shoulder in 60.2% of cases.

CLINICAL ANALYSIS

All patients in this series were evaluated preoperatively with a Constant score consisting of four individual scores for pain (15 points), activity (20 points), active mobility (40 points), and strength (25 points) [8]. The absolute constant score was subsequently adjusted for age and sex. In addition, active preoperative mobility for forward flexion in the plane of the scapula and external rotation at the side was recorded (Table II).

The postoperative evaluation was performed on all shoulders at the time of the latest follow-up or immediately before the revision and consisted of a Constant score, mobility evaluation and a subjective patient assessment graded by asking the patients to rate their outcome as very satisfied, satisfied, uncertain, or disappointed. Additionally, a subjective shoulder value (SSV) was determined by asking the patient to score their shoulder as a percentage of a normal shoulder [16].

Table II: Comparison of preoperative and postoperative clinical results

	Preoperative	Postoperative	P value
Pain ± std dev (15 points)	3.7 + 2.1	11.1 + 4.2	<0.0001
Activity ± std dev (40 points)	6.9 + 2.8	14.7 + 5	<0.0001
Mobility ± std dev (40 points)	13 + 5.7	26.4 + 9.8	<0.0001
Strength ± std dev (25 points)	3 + 3.3	5.8 + 4	<0.0001
Total Constant Score ± std dev (100 points)	26.8 + 10.3	57.6 + 20	<0.0001
Adj Constant Score (%) **± std dev**	36.2% + 13.8	83% + 29.6	<0.0001
AFE ± std dev (degree)	85.3° + 27.4	125° + 37.3	<0.0001
External Rotation at side ± std dev (degree)	7°± 6.5	30.3° + 21.8	<0.0001
Subjective results		Very Satisf 130 (57.5%) Satisfied 42 (18.6%) Uncertain 45 (19.9%) Disappointed 9 (4%)	
SSV (%)		70.9% + 24.4	

AFE = Active Forward Elevation ; SSV= Subjective Shoulder Value (%)

RADIOGRAPHIC ANALYSIS

The preoperative, initial postoperative and most recent radiographs were evaluated. Anteroposterior (AP) views in neutral, internal, and external rotation, and an axillary view were systematically performed under fluoroscopic control. Radiographs at the latest follow-up were assessed by three authors, two of them being involved in the operations, and one independent observer. The radiographs were evaluated to determine the presence of glenohumeral subluxation, a periprosthetic lucent line, and a shift in the position of the components. Glenohumeral subluxation was evaluated according to Torchia & Cofield [35] on the AP view in neutral rotation. The presence of periprosthetic radiolucent lines around the glenoid component and the humeral component were evaluated. Glenoid radiolucencies were scored according to Molé [24] (0 points for no radiolucency to 18 points for radiolucencies exceeding 2 mm in 6 zones). A score of 0 to 6 points is considered to indicate no loosening, 7 to 12 points indicates possible loosening, and 13 to 18 points indicates definite loosening. Any migration or shift of the component received by convention a score of 18 points and was also considered as a definite radiological loosening whatever the radiolucent lines score.

A preoperative Arthro-CTscan was available in 170 shoulders (65%) and an MRI in 35 cases (14%) allowing for analysis of the glenoid shape in the horizontal plane and the state of the rotator cuff tendons. A partial tear of the supraspinatus tendon was present in 19 cases (7.2%) and a full-thickness tear in 19 cases (7.2%). No infraspinatus or subscapularis tears were detected. The shape of the glenoid was assessed according to the classification of Walch *et al.* [36]: 48 type A1, 48 type A2, 36 type B1, 51 type B2, and 4 type C. The glenoid was not classified in 18 cases.

OPERATIVE TECHNIQUE

All the procedures were done through a deltopectoral approach. The subscapularis was tenotomized at the level of the anatomical neck in 233 cases (88.6%), it was detached from the lesser tuberosity in 29 cases (11%), and an osteotomy of the lesser tuberosity was performed in one case.

An associated subacromial decompression was performed in 4 cases (1.6%), a supraspinatus tendon repair in 6 cases (2.3%), and a tenotomy or tenodesis of the long head of the biceps in 136 cases (52.3%).

Resection of the humeral head was performed at the level of the anatomical neck after removal of osteophytes under direct vision. The goal was to respect the original inclination and retroversion of each individual. The characteristics of the humeral implants used are outlined in Table III. The average mismatch between the glenoid and humeral diameter of curvature was 11 ± 3.06mm. The humeral stem was cemented in 250 cases and press-fit in 13 cases.

Two techniques of glenoid preparation were used according to surgeon preference: the curettage technique as described by Neer [26], (which consists of removing the cancellous bone with a curette and doing anchorage hall superiorly and inferiorly before cementing the keel), was used in 164 cases (62.4%); and the compaction technique as described by Gazielly [14-15] was used in 96 cases

Table III: Characteristics of the Prostheses used

Inclination		
125°	55 cases	(21%)
130°	90 cases	(34.4%)
135°	82 cases	(31.3%)
140°	33 cases	(12.6%)

Head Size	
39/4	0.4%
41/15	3.5%
43/16	18.9%
46/17	30.1%
48/18	18.9%
50/16	11.2%
50/19	13.9%
52/23	1.2%

Glenoid Size	
Small	23.1%
Medium	50.6%
Large	24.7%
No Info	1.5%

(36.5%). In 1.1% of cases the technique used was uncertain or not recorded.

STATISTICAL ANALYSIS

Differences among subgroups were tested by ANOVA for the quantitative variables, followed by post-hoc Bonferroni tests or Kruskal-Wallis tests (quantitative variables not normally distributed) or by Chi-squared tests or Fisher's exact test (qualitative variables). Correlations between quantitative variables were analyzed by the Spearman correlation coefficient. Survivorship analysis was performed according to the method of Kaplan-Meier with right censored data for no event or missing data.

RESULTS

Complications and revisions

A postoperative complication was observed in 62 cases (23.5%), as shown in Table IV, and 38 of these (14.4%) necessitated a revision surgery. 24 cases (9.1%) were revised for glenoid loosening. The revision was performed at a mean follow-up of 122.7 months. The mean age at operation in this subgroup of glenoid revisions was significantly younger than that observed in the full series (60.4 years vs-66.9 years; $p<0.01$). With the numbers available, we could not detect an association between the need for revision and gender or dominant arm.

The 14 revisions that were done for a reason other than painful glenoid loosening included: two cases of humeral fracture distal to the stem three cases of loosening of press-fit humeral stems (revisions were performed at 5, 7 and 8 years after the initial surgery); two cases of posterior dislocation (revised one and 10 years after surgery), two with traumatic subscapularis rupture (repaired at two and three months after surgery), one anterior dislocation (revised at 3 years), two infections (revised at 3 months), two cases of severe stiffness (revised during the first post-operative year).

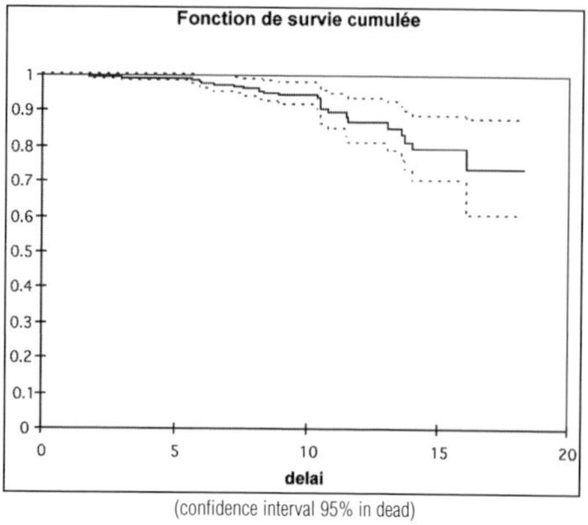

Fig. 1: Survivorship of Flat back keeled glenoid component with end point being revision surgery for glenoid loosening.

The estimated survival rate with end-point being revision surgery for glenoid loosening was 99.1% [95% Confidence Interval (CI) 98; 100] at 5 years, 94.5% [95% CI

Table IV: Complications and revisions

	Complications	Revisions
Glenoid loosening revised	24 (9.1%)	24 (9.1%)
Rotator cuff tear	16 (6%)	
Subscapularis tear	7 (2.6%)	2 (0.7%)
Humeral loosening revised	3 (1.1%)	3 (1.1%)
Posterior dislocation	3 (1.1%)	2 (0.7%)
Fracture of distal humerus	3 (1.1%)	2 (0.7%)
Infection	2 (0.7%)	2 (0.7%)
Stiffness	2 (0.7%)	2 (0.7%)
Anterior dislocation	1 (0.4%)	1 (0.4%)
Persistent neurologic complication	1 (0.4%)	
TOTAL	**62 (23.5%)**	**38 (14.4%)**

91.4; 97.7] at 10 years, and 79.4% [95% CI 70.3; 88.5] at 15 years (fig. 1).

Clinical results

After exclusion of the 37 patients deceased before completing the 5-year follow-up, 226 patients were available for clinical follow-up. Table I outlines the results of the postoperative evaluation. Highly significant improvements from preoperative values were seen in every parameter of the Constant score ($p<0.0001$ for all parameters). Subjectively 76% (196) of patients were either satisfied or very satisfied, 20% were uncertain, and 4% were disappointed.

Radiographic analysis

After exclusion of the patients with only a questionnaire (9 cases), 217 cases were available for the radiographic analysis. All patients who underwent revision surgery, regardless of the cause, were included in the radiographic analysis, including those revised for glenoid loosening. The radiographs taken immediately before the revision were used for this analysis. The average value of glenoid RLL was 11.3 ± 6.4. No radiologic loosening, defined by a RLL score between 0 and 6 (Fig. 4), was observed in 73 cases (33.6%) (Fig. 5); a possible radiologic loosening, defined by a RLL score between 7 and 12, was observed in 45 cases (20.7%); and definite radiologic loosening, defined by RLL score >12, was observed in 99 cases (45.6%) (Fig. 6 & 7). Survivorship of the glenoid component with end point being radiologic loosening (i.e. RLL score >12) was 99.2% (98.08; 100) at 5 years, 80.3% (74.5; 86.1) at 10 years and 33.6% (24.06; 43.07) at 15 years (Fig. 2).

The influence of the postoperative delay was analyzed and was found statistically significant ($p<0.0001$) (Fig. 3): the longer the follow-up, the higher the RLL score. The mean age at time of surgery was significantly lower in cases of loosening (64.4 years) versus those without loosening (68.3 years) ($p=0.0005$). The influence of surgical technique used for preparation of the glenoid keel on RLL score was also

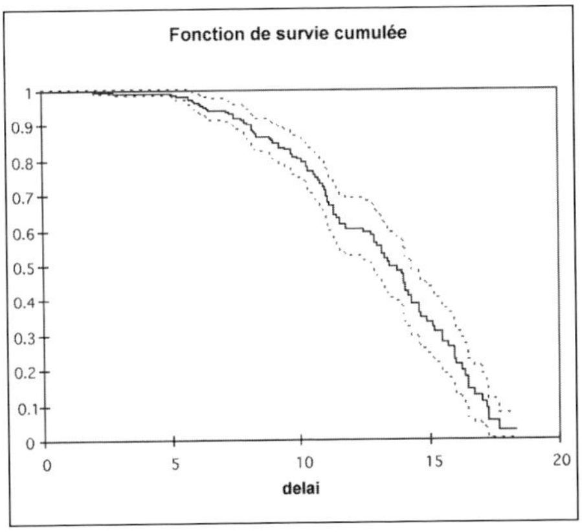

Fig. 2: Survivorship of flat-back keeled glenoid component with end-point being glenoid loosening with a RLL score > 12.

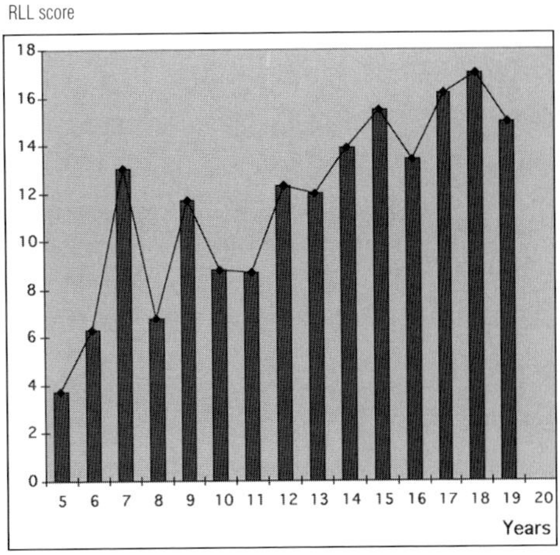

Fig. 3: Influence of follow-up on postoperative RLL score.

analyzed (60% of the patients had a curettage technique; whereas 40% had a compaction technique), the duration of follow-up was not statistically different between the two techniques (120 vs. 125 months). The compaction technique was significantly better with a mean RLL score of 9.5 versus 12.6 for the curettage technique ($p<0.001$). The percentage of definite radiologic loosening increased from 32.1% with the compaction technique to 58.9% with the curettage ($p=0.0001$). Finally, upward migration of the humeral head was also statistically correlated with RLL score ($p<0.0001$).

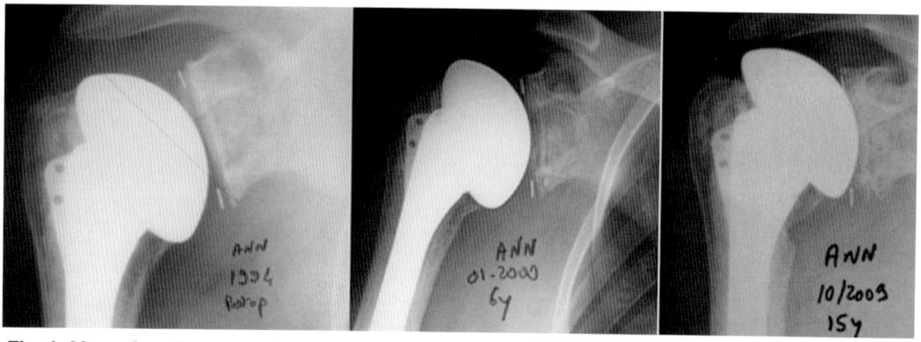

Fig. 4: 68 y.o. female operated on in 1994 (A) at 6y (B) and 15y (C) postop, the RLL score is 5 points.

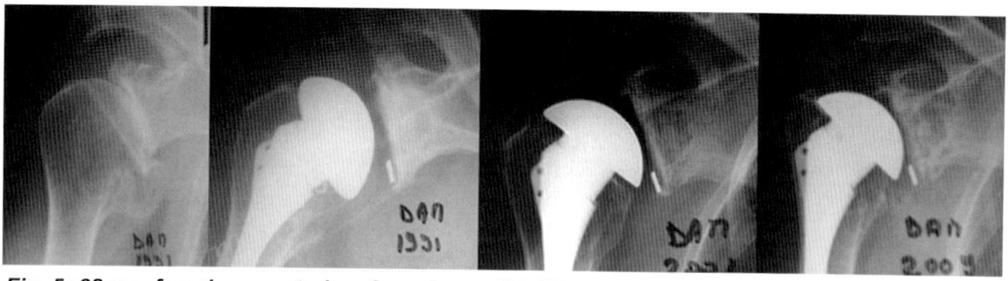

Fig. 5: 62 y.o. female operated on for primary OA (A) in 1992, postop (B), 10y (C), and 18y (D) follow-up. The RLL score is 10 at final follow-up (note the subsidence of the non cemented humeral stem at 18y follow-up).

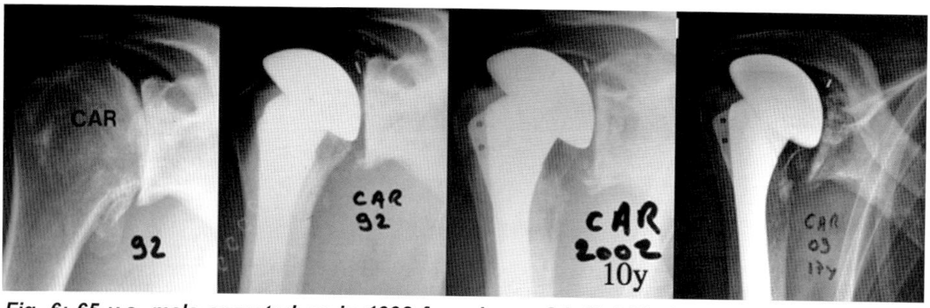

Fig. 6: 65 y.o. male operated on in 1992 for primary OA (A &B). Control X-rays show progressive loosening between 8y follow-up (C) and 17 y follow-up (D); superior tilt and upward migration of the humeral head.

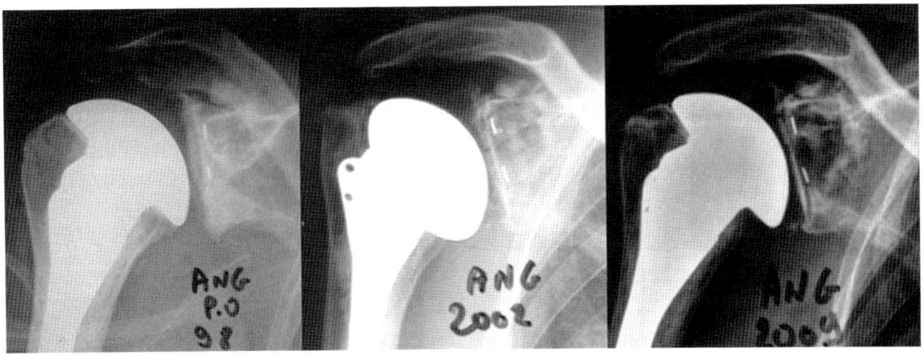

***Fig. 7:** 68 y.o. female operated on in 1998 (A). At 4y the RLL score is <6 whereas it is 18 points at 11y.*

With the numbers available, we found that gender, preoperative shape of the glenoid, dominance, and mismatch did not influence statistically glenoid loosening.

Regarding the influence of radiologic loosening on clinical results, we found highly significant correlations ($p<0.0001$) between radiological loosening and all of the following: pain, activity, mobility, active forward elevation, total Constant score, adjusted Constant score, subjective assessment, and the SSV. There was no statistically significant variations between the group "no radiologic loosening" and the group "possible radiologic loosening", whereas the difference was highly significant when comparing "definite radiologic loosening" versus the other two groups (Table V).

Superior subluxation of the prosthetic humeral head was observed in 41.8% of cases, graded as: mild in 35 cases (16%), moderate in 27 cases (12.4%), and severe in 30 cases (13.4%).

***Table V:** p value between radiolucent line score and clinical results*

RLL score	0 – 6 vs 7 – 12	0 – 6 vs >12	7 – 12 vs >12
Pain	p= 0.4	p<0.0001	p<0.0001
Activity	p=0.25	p<0.0001	p<0.0001
Mobility	p=1	p<0.0001	p=0.0002
Strength	p=1	p=0.0025	p=0.025
Constant score	p=1	p<0.0001	p<0.0001
Adj. Constant score	p=0.98	p<0.0001	p<0.0001
AFE	p=1	p<0.0001	p<0.0001
Subjective	p=0.32	p<0.0001	p<0.0001

DISCUSSION

Glenoid loosening is recognized to be the weak link of TSA with cemented polyethylene glenoids. The reported frequency of glenoid RLL at the bone-cement interface varies between 22% and 95% [1, 7, 11, 26, 28], and they are often observed in the immediate postoperative radiographs [13, 22]. Cementing techniques have evolved in an attempt to reduce the incidence of radiolucent lines, and while reduced rates have been reported [27], Sperling and Cofield [30] demonstrated that even with modern cementing techniques, a radiolucent line was present in the immediate postoperative follow up in 59% of the cases. We have previously reported [33] that the compaction technique for glenoid keel preparation was better than the curettage technique in decreasing the rate of early postoperative RLL, but no cementing technique was able to avoid RLL. Importantly, a number of authors have shown that this phenomenon evolves over with time [1, 3, 5, 7, 20, 32, 34, 38, 39] and influences the clinical results [35, 29, 31].

Radiologic loosening is not clearly defined in the literature. While we used a RLL score greater than 12 as proposed by Molé [24], other authors utilize different definitions. For example, Sperling and Cofield [23], defined radiologic loosening, referred to as a "glenoid at risk," when 2 of 3 independent observers identified a shift or a migration of the glenoid component, or if there was a complete bone-cement RLL of at least 1.5 mm in diameter. In the literature, the incidence of radiologic loosening varies from 0 to 15% after 3 years, increasing to 24 and 44% after 9 years [20, 37]. In our series it was 45.6% at an average of 10 years of follow-up. Because of the oblique orientation of the glenoid fossa, measurements of the RLL using plain radiographs are prone to error and under-report the true incidence [39]. Even with standardization of techniques and the systematic use of fluoroscopic control, we observed marked variability in the radiographs obtained, likely contributed to by individual patient differences in scapular mobility and anatomy. It was possible that only gross loosening, with an obvious component shift, or severe radiolucencies could be detected by plain radiography. Yian *et al.* [39] demonstrated that plain radiography under-reported the rate of radiolucencies by more than 30% when compared with computed tomography. Furthermore, they demonstrated that the overall reproducibility of scoring based on computed tomography was higher than that using plain radiographs.

The incidence of revision for glenoid loosening was 9.1% in our series, and the revised patients were younger (60 y.o.) than the patients with definitive radiologic loosening who did not undergo revision (67 y.o.) ($p<0.01$). The revisions were performed at an average time of 123 months after the index surgery. In the literature, the revision rate of all-polyethylene, keeled glenoid components was 8.5% for Kahn-Bunker [21] and 5.6% for Torchia Cofield [37] with a similar follow-up, whereas it was 4.2% for Iannotti-Norris [18] with three times less follow up. Clearly, postoperative follow-up duration is essential to appropriately analyze the incidence of glenoid loosening and revision. With end-point being revision surgery for glenoid loosening we observed 99.1% survivorship at 5 years, 94.5% at 10 years, and 79.4% at 15 years. Results reported by Fox-Cofield [12], with a survivorship free of revision for Cofield 2 all-polyethylene, keeled prostheses were 99% at 5 years, 94% at 10 years, and 89% at 15 years, support our recommendation that a minimum follow-up of 5 to 10 years is mandatory for any new glenoid design hoping to prove any improvement in radiologic outcome.

In 2003, we stopped using the flat-back glenoid component in favour of a convex-back design. This change was brought about following a comparative study we performed that demonstrated lower early radiolucencies associated with the convex component compared to the flat-back design [32].

Besides the duration of follow-up and the technique of glenoid preparation, which we have shown in this study to be highly significant, other factors that have been reported to be associated with the development of glenoid loosening are as follow's :

- ***Patient age:*** Operative age was significantly lower in cases of glenoid loosening (64 vs 68 years) in our series, while Fox *et al.* [12] also recently reported a trend toward lower rates of revision in patients aged 65 or older. This positive correlation most likely suggested that greater activity in younger patient groups was a contributing factor for glenoid radiologic loosening and glenoid revision.
- ***Patient gender:*** While gender was not correlated in our series with glenoid loosening, Fox *et al.* [12] reported an increased risk of revision with males. Other authors [30, 23] have not found statistical relationships. Edwards reported, on the contrary, increased radiologic loosening in females (2010).
- ***Rotator cuff tears:*** Reported by Franklin Matsen [2] to result in a typical pattern of glenoid loosening through the "rocking horse" mechanism. No patient had a preoperative massive tear in our series. However, using moderate and severe postoperative proximal migration of the humeral component as evidence of secondary rotator cuff tear [4, 9], 61 cases (23.2%) were identified having a massive tear. For these patients we found a positive relationship with the RLL score of the glenoid ($p<0.0001$).
- ***Glenoid shape and posterior static instability:*** Type B1 and B2 glenoids, as seen on preoperative CT scans, were reported in our 2001 multi-center study as risk factors for glenoid loosening. In this series they were not found to have statistical influence. However, it was possible that the absence of a correlation was due to the fact that all of the severe cases were treated by glenoid reconstruction with bone graft and therefore excluded from this study.
- ***Glenohumeral mismatch:*** The mismatch between the radius of curvature of the humeral head and the glenoid was not found to be a prognostic factor in this study, however we believe this was due to conformity amongst the surgeons in choosing a mismatch within our previous recommendations of between 6 and 10 mm [37]. The average value of the radial mismatch in this study was 5.6 mm.
- ***Etiology:*** post-traumatic arthritis and rheumatoid arthritis have been shown to have a much higher risk of glenoid loosening and revision because of poor bone quality, cuff insufficiency, or malunions of the tuberosities. Our study was limited to primary glenohumeral osteoarthritic, and therefore likely represented the "best-case scenario" for total shoulder arthroplasty.

Our results in this study for glenoid loosening with the flat-back component at 10 years were inferior to those reported by Khan *et al.* [21] and Raiss *et al.* [28] using the same prosthesis. Clearly, there are more important factors than the initial fit of the back of the glenoid component that influenced the occurrence of radiologic loosening. There are a number of limitations with this study, including the multicenter design, with different surgeons and consequently variations in surgical technique. However, the prosthesis used was the same and this study design allowed us to report on a large number of patients. As we have already mentioned, plain radiographs likely under-report the true incidence of radiolucencies and CT scan is a more accurate method. Also, we used an indirect method of assessing the presence of massive cuff tearing, however the accuracy of this method has been validated by numerous studies [9, 21, 31.

In conclusion, the flat-back all-polyethylene, cemented glenoid component demonstrated a radiologic loosening rate of 45.6% at an average of 10 years and a revision rate of 9.1%. The curettage technique, which sacrificed good bone, and a younger age at operation were demonstrated as significant negative prognostic factors. Glenoid loosening had a definite influence on all objective and subjective criteria of clinical outcome and continues to be the main problem affecting the longevity of non-constrained TSA with cemented, all-polyethylene, keeled glenoid components.

REFERENCES

[1] AMSTUTZ HC, THOMAS BJ, KABO JM, DOREY FJ The Dana total shoulder arthroplasty. *J Bone Joint Surg [Am] 1988; 70: 1174-82.*

[2] BARRETT WP, FRANKLIN JL, JACKINS SE, WYSS CR., MATSEN FA III. Total shoulder arthroplasty. *J Bone Joint Surg [Am] 1987 : 69: 865-72.*

[3] BARRETT WP, THORNHILL TS, THOMAS WH, GEBHART EM, SLEDGE CB Nonconstrained total shoulder arthroplasty in patients with polyarticular rheumatoid arthritis. *J Arthroplasty 1989; 4: 91-6.*

[4] BOYD AD Jr, ALIABADI P, THORNHILL TS Postoperative proximal migration in total shoulder Arthoplasty. Incidence and significance. *J Arthroplasty 1991; 6: 31-7.*

[5] BOYD AD Jr, THOMAS WH, SCOTT RD, SELDGE CB, THORNILL TS Total shoulder arthroplasty versus hemiarthroplasty. Indications for glenoid resurfacing. *J Arthroplasty 1990; 5: 329-36.*

[6] BRENNER BC, FERLIC DC, CLAYTON ML, DENNIS DA Survivorship of unconstrained total shoulder arthroplasty. *J Bone Joint Surg [Am] 1989; 71: 1289-96.*

[7] COFIELD RH. Total Shoulder Arthroplasty with the Neer prosthesis. *J Bone Joint Surg [Am] 1984; 66: 899-906.*

[8] CONSTANT CR, MURLEY AHG A clinical method of functional assessment of the shoulder. *Clin Orthop 1987; 214:160-4.*

[9] DEUTSCH A, ALTCHEK DW, SCHWARTZ E, OTIS J, WARREN RF Radiologic measurement of superior displacement of the humeral head in the impingement syndrome. *J Shoulder Elbow Surg 1996; 5: 186-93.*

[10] EDWARDS TB, KADAKIA NR, BOULAHIA A, KEMPF JF, BOILEAU P, NEMOZ C *et al.* A comparison of hemiarthroplasty and total shoulder arthroplasty in the treatment of primary glenohumeral osteoarthritis: results of a multicenter study. *J Shoulder Elbow Sur 2003; 12: 207-13.*

[11] FIGGIE MP, INGLIS AE, FIGGIE HE, 3rd SOBEL M, BURSTEIN AH, KRAAY MJ Custom total shoulder arthroplasty in inflammatory arthritis. Preliminary results. *J Arthroplasty. Mar 1992; 7(1): 1-6.*

[12] FOX TJ, CIL A, SPERLING J, SANCHEZ-SOTELO J, SCHLECK C, COFIELD RH Survival of the glenoid component in shoulder arthroplasty. *J. Shoulder Elbow Surg (2009) 18, 859-63.*

[13] GARTSMAN GM, ELKOUSY HA, WARNOCK KM, EDWARDS TB, O'CONNOR DP. Radiographic comparison of pegged and keeled glenoid components. *J Shoulder Elbow Surg. May-Jun 2005; 14(3): 252-57.*

[14] GAZIELLY DF Comment je scelle un implant glénoïdien en polyéthylène convexe à quille avec ma technique de compaction d'os spongieux. *Maitrise Orthopédique Numéro 162; Mars 2007; pp. 6-11.*

[15] GAZIELLY DF, ALLENDE C, PAMELIN E Results of cancellous compaction technique for glenoid resurfacing. Presented at the 17th Congress of the European Society for Surgery of the Shoulder and the Elbow. *Heidelberg, September 24-27, 2003.*

[16] GILBART MK, GERBER C. Comparison of the subjective shoulder value and the Constant score. *J Shoulder Elbow Surg. Nov-Dec 2007; 16(6): 717-21.*

[17] HAINES JF, TRAIL IA, NUTTALL D, BIRCH A, BARROW A The results of arthroplasty in osteoarthritis of the shoulder. *J Bone Joint Surg [Br] 2006; 88-B: 456-501.*

[18] IANNOTTI JP, NORRIS TR Influence of preoperative factors on outcome of shoulder arthroplasty for osteoarthritis. *J Bone Joint Surg. 2003 Feb; 85-A(2): 251-8.*

[19] KAPLAN EL, MEIER P Nonparametric estimation from incomplete observations. *J Am Stat Assoc 1958; 53: 457-81.*

[20] KELLY IG, FOSTER RS, FISHER WD Neer Total shoulder replacement in rheumatoid arthritis. *J Bone Joint Surg [Br] 1987; 69: 723-6.*

[21] KHAN A, BUNKER TD, KITSON JB Clinical and radiological follow-up of thc Aequalis third generation cemented total shoulder replacement. A minimum ten year study. *J Bone Joint Sur [Br] 2009; 91-B: 1594-600.*

[22] LAZARUS MD, JENSEN KL, SOUTHWORTH C, MATSEN FA, 3rd The radiographic evaluation of keeled and pegged glenoid component insertion. *J Bone Joint Surg Am. Jul 2002; 84-A(7): 1174-82.*

[23] MILETI J, BOARDMAN ND 3rd, SPERLING JW, COFIELD RH, TORCHIA ME, O'DRICOLL SW, ROWLAND CM Radiographic analysis of polyethylene glenoid components using modern cementing techniques. *J Shoulder Elbow Surg. 2004 Sep-Oct; 13(5): 492-8.*

[24] MOLÉ D, ROCHE O, RIAND N, LÉVIGNE C, WALCH G Cemented glenoid components: results in osteoarthritis and rheumatoid arthritis. In: Walch G, Boileau P, eds. Shoulder Arthroplasty. *Berlin: Springer, 1999: 163-71.*

[25] NEER CS II. Replacement arthroplasty for glenohumeral osteoarthritis. *J Bone Joint Surg [Am] 1974; 56: 1-13.*

[26] NEER CS II, WATSON KC, STANTON FJ Recent experience in total shoulder replacement. *J Bone Joint Surg [Am] 1982; 64: 319-37.*

[27] NORRIS BL, LACHIEWICZ PF. Modern cement technique and the survivorship of total shoulder arthroplasty. *Clin Orthop Relat Res. Jul 1996(328): 76-85.*

[28] RAISS P, ALDINGER PR, KASTEN P, RICKERT M, LOEW M Total Shoulder replacement in young and middle aged patients with glenohumeral osteoarthritis. *J Bone Joint Surg [Br] 2008; 90-B: 764-9.*

[29] SOJBJERG JO, FRICH LH, JOHANNSEN HV, SNEPPEN O Late results of total shoulder replacement in patients with rheumatoid arthritis. *Clin Orthop Relat Res. 1999 Sep;(366): 39-45.*

[30] SPERLING JW, COFIELD RH, ROWLAND CM minimum fifteen year follow-up of Neer hemiarthroplasty and total shoulder arthroplasty in patients aged fifty years or younger. *J Shoulder Elbow Surg. 2004 Nov-Dec; 13(6): 604-13.*

[31] STEWART MP, KELLY IG. Total shoulder replacement in Rheumatoid disease:7- to 13- year follow-up of 37 joints. *J Bone Joint Surg [Br] 1997 Jan; 79(1): 68-72.*

[32] SZABO I, BUSCAYRET F, EDWARDS TB, NEMOZ C, BOILEAU P, WALCH G Radiographic comparison of flat back and convex-back glenoid components in total shoulder arthroplasty. *J Shoulder Elbow Surg. 2005 Nov Dec;14(6): 636-42.*

[33] SZABO I, BUSCAYRET F, EDWARDS TB, NEMOZ C, O'CONNOR DP, BOILEAU P, WALCH G Radiographic comparison of two glenoid preparation techniques in total shoulder arthroplasty. *Clin Orth 2005; 431: 104-10.*

[34] THROCKMORTON TW, ZARKADAS PC, SPERLING JW, COFIELD RH Pegged versus keeled glenoid components in total shoulder arthroplasty. *J Shoulder Elbow Surg. Feb 2010.*

[35] TORCHIA ME, COFIELD RH, SETTERGREN CR Total shoulder arthroplasty with the Neer prosthesis: long term results. *J Shoulder Elbow Surg 1997; 6: 495-505.*

[36] WALCH G, BADET R, BOULAHIA A, KHOURY A Morphologic study of the glenoid in primary glenohumeral osteoarthritis. *J Arthroplasty 1999; 14: 756-60.*

[37] WALCH G, EDWARDS TB, BOULAHIA A, BOILEAU P, MOLÉ D, ADELEINE P The influence of glenohumeral prosthetic mismatch on glenoid radiolucent lines: results of a multicenter study. *J Bone Joint Surg [Am] 2002 Dec; 84-A(12): 2186-91.*

[38] WIRTH MA, ROCKWOOD CA Jr Complications of total shoulder replacement arthroplasty. *J Bone Joint Surg [Am] 1996; 78: 603-16.*

[39] YIAN EH, WERNER CM, NYFFELER RW, PFIRRMANN CW, RAMAPPA A, SUKTHANKAR A, GERBER C Radiographic and computed tomography analysis of cemented pegged polyethylene glenoid components in total shoulder replacement. *J bone Joint Surg [Am] 2005 Sept; 87(9): 1928-36.*

RESULTS OF THE CONVEX BACK CEMENTED KEELED GLENOID COMPONENT IN PRIMARY OSTEOARTHRITIS

MULTICENTRIC STUDY WITH A FOLLOW-UP > 5 YEARS

G. WALCH, A. YOUNG, B. MÉLIS, D. GAZIELLY, M. LOEW, P. BOILEAU

ABSTRACT

Background

The aim of this paper was to assess the results of third generation total shoulder arthroplasty with an all-polyethylene, convex back glenoid component. Our hypothesis was that the rate of loosening would be lower than that reported in the literature for earlier designs.

Methods

Between 1996 and 2003, in five European centers, 333 shoulder arthroplasties were performed for primary osteoarthritis using a third generation anatomic prosthesis with a convex backed cemented all polyethylene keeled glenoid component. Kaplan Meier survivorship analysis was performed with glenoid revision for loosening and radiological glenoid loosening as end points. Clinical outcome was assessed with the Constant score, patient satisfaction score, subjective shoulder value and range of movement.

Results

At a mean of 7.5 years, the rate of radiological glenoid loosening was 18.9% and revision was performed for glenoid loosening in 0.6%. Glenoid survival with end point being revision surgery for glenoid loosening was 99.7% at 5 years and 98.3% at 10 years. Glenoid survivorship with end point being radiological loosening was 99.7% at 5 years and 51.5% at 10 years. The mean Constant score improved significantly ($p<0.0001$) from 31.4 points preoperatively to 67.6 points at last follow-up or immediately before revision, with all components of the Constant score improving significantly ($p<0.0001$). Mean active forward elevation improved from 94.9° to 146.6° ($p<0.0001$) and mean external rotation improved from 9.0 to 35.3° ($p<0.0001$). 93.5% of patients were either satisfied or very satisfied. The average subjective shoulder value was 79.5%.

Discussion-Conclusions

Our results compare favorably with the literature regarding glenoid loosening and survival of the glenoid component free of revision for glenoid loosening. It will be difficult to improve on these results at 5 years, and probably 10 years, therefore innovations in this field will need to wait for more than 10 years to prove any superiority. Likewise, the incidence of radiological loosening was minimal at 5 years, however clearly increased between 5 and 10 years follow-up, demonstrating the progressive nature of radiolucent lines and need for greater than 5 year follow-up to adequately assess the radiological outcome of glenoid components.

INTRODUCTION

Designed and first time implanted by Charles S. Neer in the early 1970s, the all-polyethylene keeled glenoid component is still used nowadays.

The incidence of radiolucency at the bone cement interface reported in the literature is high, ranging from zero to 100% [1, 2, 14], the rate of radiological loosening between zero and 44% [20, 25], whereas the rate of revision has been reported to be up to 8.1% [23]. Neer's original design [17] has undergone multiple changes over the years in an attempt to decrease the rate of radiolucent lines (RLL) and radiological loosening, including: shape of the back surface (flat, convex or metal back); glenoid preparation (curettage or compaction); cementing technique (simple packing or pressurization); conformity between the radius of curvature of the head and the glenoid (conforming or mismatch); fixation (pegged or keeled); and shape (oval or pear-shaped). However, despite many trials and controversies, several authors came back to all polyethylene keeled glenoid components. Reported survivorship established by Cofield et al of the Neer cemented, all-polyethylene glenoid component ranges from 83 to 93% at 10 years and 73 to 87% at 15 years [7, 21, 22, 25].

The aim of this paper was to assess the results of a third generation total shoulder arthroplasty with an all-polyethylene, convex back glenoid component with a minimum follow-up of 5 years. Our hypothesis was that the rate of loosening would be lower than that previously reported in the literature.

MATERIAL AND METHODS

Between 1996 and 2003, in four European centers, 396 shoulder arthroplasties were performed for primary glenohumeral osteoarthritis as described by Neer [17] using a third generation anatomic prosthesis with a convex backed cemented all polyethylene keeled glenoid component (Table 1). In all cases the same unconstrained, cemented, third generation implant (Aequalis: Tornier Inc, Minneapolis) was used. The modular humeral component with eccentric heads and variable inclination was used with a keeled, convex back, ultra high molecular weight all- polyethylene glenoid component. Cases operated on with a metal back glenoid or a flat back keel glenoid were excluded from this series as well as cases that underwent an associated bone graft of the glenoid.

An attempt was made to callback all patients. Sixty-three cases were either lost to follow-up or did not want to come back and had an incomplete chart that did not allow considering them for inclusion in the database leaving 333 for inclusion in

Tableau I : Multicenter data of Aequalis Total Shoulder Arthroplasties implanted between 1996 and 2003 for Primary Glenohumeral Osteoarthritis Keeled PE Glenoid Component Convex Back

	Number of Shoulders reviewed with X-Ray FU>5y	Questionnaire alone	Death < 5y FU	Lost to follow-up or did not want to come back <5y FU	Total number of shoulders operated on 1996-2003
Center 3 - Lyon - France	133	4	5	25	167
Center 4 - Nice - France	84	5	10	15	114
Center 2 - Heidelberg/Wurzburg Germany	46	1	5	8	60
Center 1 - Genève - Switzerland	38	0	2	15	55
TOTAL	301	10	22	63	396

the study. From this series, survivorship curves of the glenoid were constructed according to the Kaplan-Meier method [13]. Twenty-two patients died before a follow-up of 5 years. Ten patients sent a questionnaire and refused to perform the radiography leaving 311 shoulders for the clinical study and 301 shoulders for the radiographic analysis with a follow-up of more than 5 years, average 89.5 months (range 61 to 152 months). Thirty-eight patients were operated on both shoulders (11.4%). The mean age of the patients in this series was 69.3 years (range 35 to 90). There were 68.5% women and 60.7% of the prosthesis where performed in right shoulders. The dominant shoulder underwent replacement in 61.1% of cases.

Clinical analysis

All patients in this series were evaluated preoperatively with a Constant score, consisting of four individual scores for pain (15 points), activity (20 points), active mobility (40 points), and strength (25 points), that was subsequently adjusted for age and sex [4]. In addition, active preoperative mobility for forward flexion in the plane of the scapula and external rotation with the arm at the side was recorded. Table II shows the results of the preoperative evaluation.

The postoperative evaluation consisted of the Constant score, the adjusted Constant score, measurement of the same mobility parameters evaluated preoperatively, and a subjective patient result graded as very satisfied, satisfied, uncertain or disappointed. In addition, patients were asked to rate their shoulder as a percentage of a normal shoulder and recorded as the subjective shoulder value (SSV) [11].

Radiographic analysis

Radiographic evaluation consisting of antero-posterior views in neutral, internal and external humeral rotation and an axillary view, were performed preoperatively, immediately postoperatively and at the latest follow-up. These films were evaluated to assess for glenoid periprosthetic

Table II : Statistical comparison of preoperative and postoperative clinical data

	Preoperative	Postoperative	P value
Pain ± std dev (15 points)	3.8 + 2.6	12.7 + 3	<0.0001
ADL ± std dev (20 points)	7.2 + 3.10	16.9 + 4.7	<0.0001
Mobility ± std dev (40 points)	15.9 + 7.8	31 + 8.8	<0.0001
Strength ± std dev (25 points)	4.5 + 5.4	7.6 + 3.9	<0.0001
Total Constant score ± std dev (100 points)	31.4 + 13.3	67.6 + 17.6	<0.0001
Adjusted Constant score % ± std dev	42.7 % + 17.6	97.3% + 26.5	<0.0001
AFE (degrees) **± std dev**	94.9° + 28.2	146.6° + 27.1	<0.0001
ER1 (degrees) **± std dev**	9° + 16.4	35.3° + 19.5	<0.0001
SSV (%) **± std dev**		79.5% ± 19.2	
Subjective results		Very Satisf = 221 (71%) Satisfied = 70 (22.5%) Uncertain = 13 (4.2%) Disappointed = 7 (2.2%)	

AFE: Active forward elevation; ER1: Active external rotation with elbow at side; SSV: subjective shoulder value

radiolucencies, evidence of glenoid component loosening, and proximal migration of the humerus. Radiographs were systematically assessed by three authors, two of them being involved in the operation and the third person being an independent observer.

Glenohumeral subluxation was evaluated according to Torchia & Cofield on the AP view in neutral rotation [25]. Glenoid radiolucencies were scored according to Molé (0 point for no radiolucency to 18 points for radiolucencies exceeding 2 mm in 6 zones). A score of 0 to 6 points was considered to indicate no loosening, 7 to 12 points was possible loosening, and 13 to 18 points was considered definite loosening [16]. Any migration or shift of the component received by convention a score of 18 points.

A preoperative Arthro-CT was available in 269 cases (80.8%) and MRI or Arthro-MRI in 47 cases (14.1%), allowing analysis of the glenoid shape in the horizontal plan and the state of the rotator cuff tendons. A partial articular side tear of the supraspinatus was present in 8.7% of the cases (29 cases) and a complete full thickness tear in 7.2% (24 cases). Glenoid shape in the horizontal plane has been classified according to the Walch classification (26): Type A1 (86 cases 27.2%), type A_2 (91 cases 28.8%), type B_1 (61 cases, 19.3%), type B_2 (73 cases, 23.1%); and type C (4 cases, 1.2%). It was not possible to classify the glenoid shape in one case (0.3%).

Operative technique

All of the procedures were done through a deltopectoral approach. The subscapularis was tenotomized at the level of the anatomical neck in 280 cases (84.1%), it was detached from the lesser tuberosity in 50 cases (15%), and an osteotomy of the lesser tuberosity was performed in 3 cases. An associated subacromial decompression was performed in two cases, a supraspinatus tendon repair in 6 cases, and a tenotomy or tenodesis of the long head of the biceps in 266 cases (85.5%). The cut of the humeral head was performed at the level of the anatomical neck after resection of the osteophytes under direct vision. The goal was to respect the original inclination and retroversion of each individual. The characteristics of the humeral implants used are outlined in Table III. The average mismatch between the glenoid and humeral radius of curvature was 5.9 mm (range 0-8.5). The humeral stem was cemented in 320 cases and press fitted in 13 cases. The cement used was high viscosity in 74.5% and low viscosity in 25.5%. Regarding glenoid preparation, there were different techniques used in different centers. In Center 1, the surgeon [9, 10] did not ream the articular surface and compacted the cancellous bone in the slot with a special compactor (38 cases) in order to keep the maximum glenoid bone stock. In Center 2, no reaming was used, but a curettage technique according to Neer [17] was used to prepare the glenoid slot (46 cases). In the third and fourth centers, generous reaming was performed in an attempt to achieve optimal seating of the glenoid component and a normal version of the glenoid component. The reaming technique was more aggressive in center 4 than in the center 3, but it was not possible to objectively quantify this except that the percentage of small glenoids used in center 4 was 3 times more frequent (36% of the cases) than in center 3 (12.9%) and perforation of the anterior cortex with leak of cement was almost systematic in the fourth center. Excessive reaming decreases the amount of available glenoid bone surface area for support and also decreases the depth of bone for the keel slot. Compaction technique was used in both centers. The cement used for the glenoid was more often high viscosity in 247 cases (74%) than low viscosity in 86 cases (25.8%).

Table III : Characteristics of the prosthesis used

Humeral inclination		Size of humeral head	
125° :	12.9% (45)	39/14 :	1.1%
130° :	29.8% (104)	41/15 :	6%
135° :	41% (143)	43/16 :	25.5%
140° :	16.3% (57)	46/17 :	25.2%
		48/18 :	20.9%
		50/16 :	4%
		50/19 :	12%
		52/23 :	1.4%
Diameter of humeral stem		**Size of the Glenoid**	
6mm :	14% (49)	Small :	20.4% (71)
9mm :	58.7% (205)	Medium :	56% (195)
12mm :	23.8% (83)	Large :	23.6% (82)
15mm :	1.4%(5)		

Statistical analysis

The differences among subgroups were tested by ANOVA for the quantitative variables, followed by post-hoc Bonferroni tests or Kruskal-Wallis tests (quantitative variables not normally distributed) or by chi-square tests for Fisher exact test (qualitative variables). The correlations between quantitative variables were analyzed by the Spearman correlation coefficient. Survivorship analyses were performed according to the method of Kaplan-Meier [13] with right censored data for no event or missing data.

RESULTS

Among the 333 prosthesis available, twenty-two died before having 5 year follow-up leaving 311 shoulder arthroplasties with a full clinical follow-up. Ten of them refused to perform follow-up radiographs leaving only 301 prostheses available for the radiological study with a follow-up greater than 5 years, average 89.5 months (range 61-152).

Complications and revisions

Eight revisions (2.5%) were performed (Table IV) at an average follow-up of 4.3 years (range 1 to 9). Two patients had painful glenoid loosening at 44 and 108 months postoperatively respectively and were revised to a reverse shoulder arthroplasty. Survivorship of the glenoid component with the end point being revision surgery for glenoid loosening, was: 99.7% at 5 years (95% CI 99;100) and 98.3% at 10 years (95% CI 99;100) (fig. 1).

Two patients were revised for infection at 12 and 84 months after surgery respectively. One underwent one stage exchange of the anatomic prosthesis and the other had a two stage revision with reverse shoulder arthroplasty. Two patients had an open arthrolysis for postoperative stiffness and in both cases the prosthesis was retained. An additional case was revised at 92 months postoperatively for a massive secondary rotator cuff tear and was revised with a reverse shoulder arthroplasty.

Besides these 8 patients that were revised, an additional 19 cases (6.1%) had a complication not requiring revision surgery. Twelve patients (3.8%) presented with a symptomatic massive rotator cuff tear (supra + infraspinatus) diagnosed clinical-

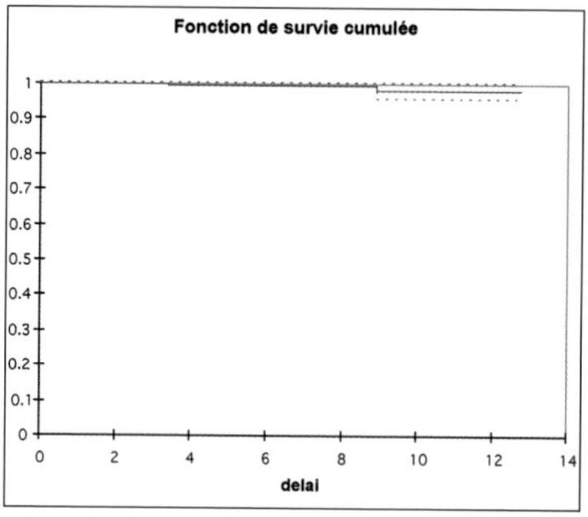

Fig. 1 : Survivorship of the convex back glenoid in Primary GH Osteoarthritis with end point being Glenoid revision (95% Confidence interval in red)

Table IV : Complications and revisions

	Complications	Revisions
Massive rotator cuff tear	13 (4.2%)	1 (0.3%)
Subscapularis tear	6 (1.9%)	
Infections	2 (0.6%)	2 (0.6%)
Glenoid loosening	2 (0.6%)	2 (0.6%)
Stiffness	3 (0.9%)	3 (0.9%)
Humeral diaphysis fracture	1 (0.3%)	
TOTAL	**27 cases (8.7%)**	**8 cases (2.5%)**

ly and radiologically with upward migration of the humeral head. Six patients were diagnosed with a postoperative subscapularis tear (1.9%) and were not reoperated on. One had a traumatic humeral fracture at the tip of the prosthesis and was treated non-operatively, with healing of the fracture after 4 months.

Clinical results

Table II depicts the results of the postoperative evaluation. Highly significant improvements were seen in every parameter of the Constant score ($p<0.0001$). Subjectively, 291 (93.5%) were either very satisfied or satisfied with their results, whereas 4.2% (13 cases) were disappointed and 2.2% (7 cases) were unhappy. The average Subjective Shoulder value was 79.5% ± 19.2.

Radiological results

At the time of latest follow-up or immediately before revision, the glenoid radiolucent line score was established. The average score was 6.45 + 6.1 (range 0–18 points). Fifty-seven cases (18.9%) had radiological loosening with a RLL score > 12. Among them, 47 had either a migration or a shift of the glenoid component: 7 had a superior tilt, 9 had a posterior tilt and 31 had subsidence (fig. 3). A possible loosening with the score between 7–12 was observed in 39 cases (12.9%), whereas no loosening with a RLL < 6 was present in 205 cases (68.1%). Survival of the glenoid with radiological loosening as the end point was 99.7% at 5 years with 95% confidence Interval (99;100) and 51.5% (CI 95% 39.5;53.6) at 10 years (fig. 2).

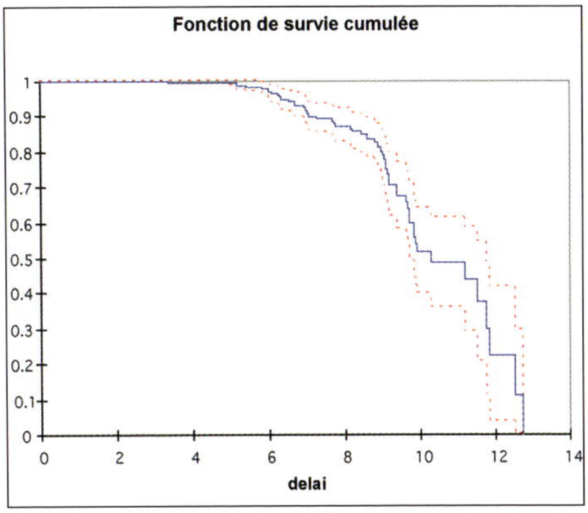

Fig. 2 : Survivorship of the convex back glenoid in Primary GH Osteoarthritis with end point being Glenoid radiological loosening (Radiolucent line score >12) (95% Confidence interval in red)

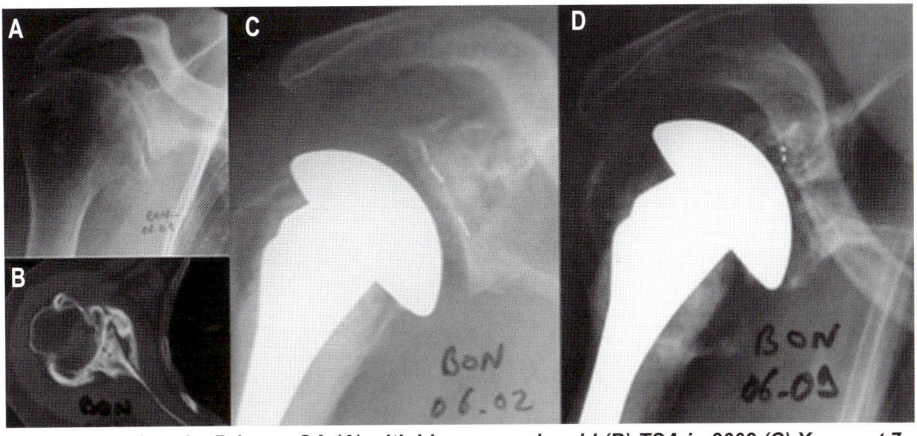

Fig. 3: 68 yo female, Primary OA (A) with biconcave glenoid (B) TSA in 2002 (C) X-rays at 7y follow-up (D) showing subsidence of the glenoid component

On the last follow up radiographs, 11.6% (35 cases) of the prostheses had an ossification: moderate in 9.7% and severe in 1.9% of cases. Some degree of superior gleno-humeral subluxation was seen in 17.6%: mild superior subluxation in 25 cases (8.3%), moderate in 22 cases (7.3%) and severe in 6 cases (2%).

Correlations with the RLL Score

The average radiolucent line score increased with duration of follow-up (fig. 4), and the influence of follow-up was statistically significant (<0.002). Other factors that we found influencing RLL score were the dominant side (p=0.0003) and the surgical center (p=0.0072). With the number of cases available, preoperative lesions of the supraspinatus, preoperative shape of the glenoid, age at operation, and gender did not reach significance. The RLL was found to significantly correlate with: pain, adjusted constant score, subjective assessment and SSV (p<0.0001); activity and total constant score (p=0.0003). By classifying the RLL score into 3 categories (no loosening, possible loosening and radiological loosening), we observed again statistically significant differences between the centers (p=0.01) and with the clinical results (Table V).

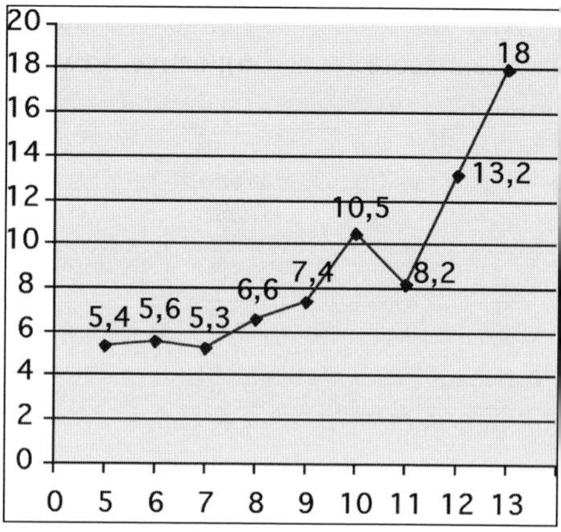

Fig. 4: RLL scores according to the duration of follow-up (FU) (p=0.01)

Correlations with glenoid component migration

A possible influence of the surgical technique (Center) on the migration of the glenoid component was observed especially for subsidence (Table VI) (fig. 5). With an identical average follow-up, the incidence of subsidence was 9.8% and 21.4% in Centers 3 and 4 (reaming performed) versus 0% in Centers 1 and 2 (no reaming performed) (fig. 6). Migration of the glenoid component at the latest follow-up or just before revision had a strong influence on the clinical results: pain (p<0.0001);

Table V : p value between radiolucent line score and clinical results

RLL score	0 – 6 Vs 7 – 12	0 – 6 Vs >12	7 – 12 Vs >12	ANOVA
Pain	p= 1	p<0.0001	p<0.0005	p<0.0001
Activity	p=1	p<0.0001	p<0.0002	p<0.0001
Mobility	p=0.98	P=0.0045	p=0.40	P=0.0063
Strength	p=1	p=0.025	p=0.25	P=0.053
Constant Score	p=0.5	p<0.0001	P=0.02	p<0.0001
Adj. Constant Score	p=0.85	p<0.0001	P=0.057	p<0.0001
AFE	p=1	p<0.003	p<0.066	P=0.004
Subjective	p=0.46	P=0.0001	P=0.22	P=0.0002

activity of daily living (p<0.001); total Constant score (p<0.006); active forward elevation (p=0.04); and subjective results (p<0.0001).

Table VI : Migration of the glenoid component at the last follow-up (FU>5y) Difference according to the centers p=0.0008

	n	FU Months	Reaming	NO Migration	Sup. Tilt	Post. Tilt	Subsidence
Center 1	38	101.5 ± 27.7	0	84.6%	5.1%	10.3%	
Center 2	39	74.3 ± 12.4	0	94.9%	5.1%		
Center 3	133	87.3 ± 18.4	++	87.2%	0.7%	2.3%	9.8%
Center 4	84	94.5 ± 20.2	+++	71.4%	2.4%	3.5%	21.4%

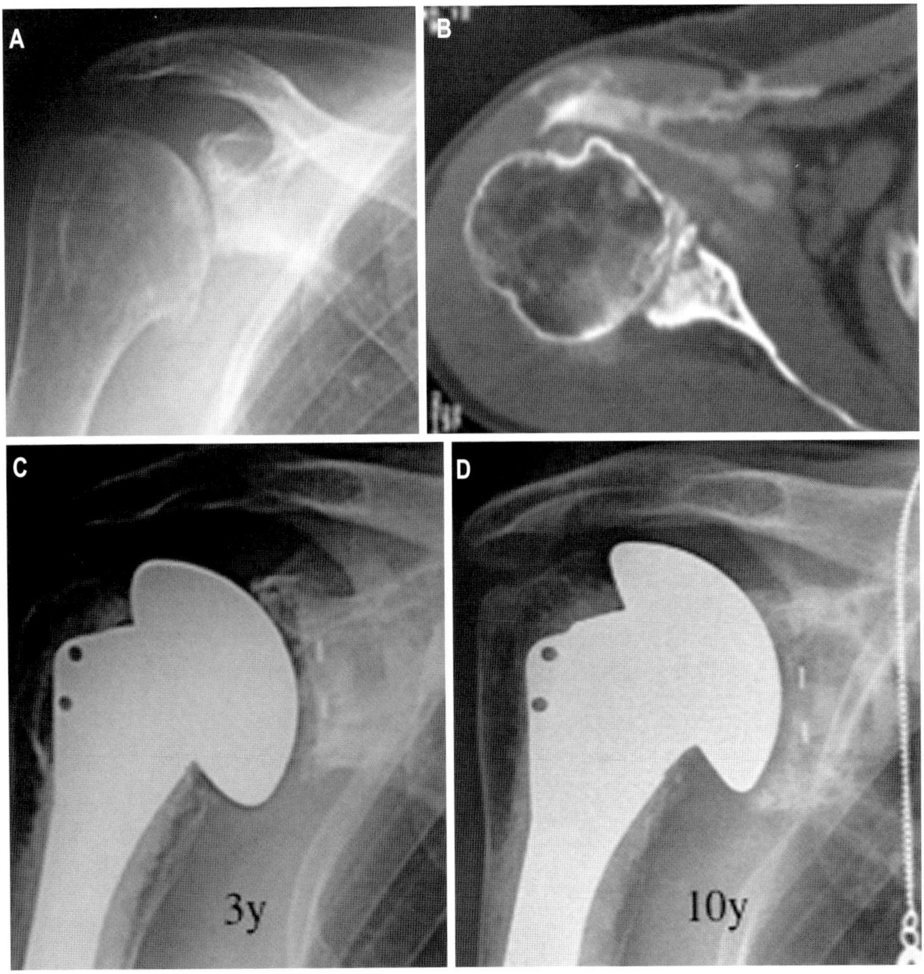

Fig. 5: 72 yo female, Primary OA (A) with concentric glenoid (B) TSA with generous reaming of the glenoid (C). X-ray at 10y follow-up showing subsidence of the glenoid component

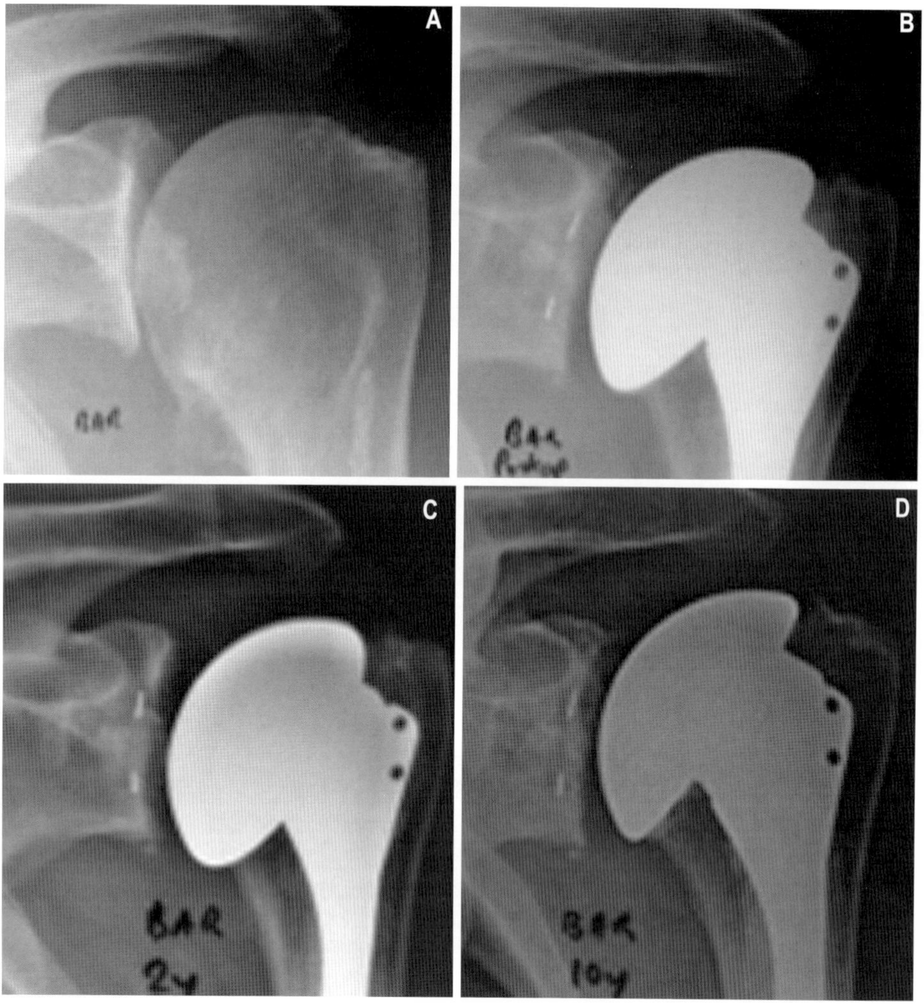

Fig. 6: 68yo male, Primary OA (A), TSA in 1999 (B), X-rays at 2y (C) and 10y (D) with a radiolucent line score of 2points

DISCUSSION

This study demonstrates satisfactory clinical results with dramatic improvements in each parameter of the Constant Score and active range of motion. The rate of complications, at an average follow up of 7.5 years, was 8.7% with only 2.5% needing revision surgery. This rate of complications is lower than the incidence reported in our previous multicenter study of Nice in 2001, where we had a 19% rate of complications [28]. Bohsali *et al.* [1] in a meta-analysis of complications in 2540 shoulders after total shoulder arthroplasty reported a rate of complications of 15.8% at 5.3 years. Chin and Cofield in 2006 reported an incidence of 9.2% in 431 total shoulder arthroplasties implanted between 1990 and 2000 [3]. Our series compares favorably with the literature regarding the rate of complications. In the present study, the survival of the glenoid component free of revision for glenoid loosening was 99.7% at 5 years and 98.3% at 10 years. This compares favorably with the survivorship of total shoulder arthroplasty, excluding infection, reported by Sperling and Cofield of 97% at 10 years using the Neer II prosthesis [21]. More recently, although not restricted to the single diagnosis of primary osteoarthritis, they reported survival rates of different types of glenoid components free of revision for any cause, including: 94% at 10 years for the Cofield 2 all-polyethylene keeled glenoid; 96% at 10 years for the Neer II glenoid; and 95% at 10 years overall for cemented polyethylene glenoid designs [7]. The 99% survival at 5 years of 358 Cofield 2 all-polyethylene pegged components was comparable to the results of this multicenter study investigating an all-polyethylene keeled convex back glenoid component design. Unfortunately, no other studies are available in the literature regarding the pegged design to know whether this modification of Neer's original design, i.e. peg versus keel, will be of significant benefit or not in the long-term [6, 8, 15, 18, 26].

Considering end point being revision for glenoid loosening, it will be difficult to report better results than those presented in this multicenter study at 5 years and probably also at 10 years. Therefore, any innovations in this field must wait for more than 10 years to prove any superiority in terms of glenoid survival. If, however, we consider the radiolucent lines and the appearance of radiological loosening, then the rates we observed were different. Whereas Cofield and Sperling did not report on this kind of survivorship in their recent paper [7] our study showed 99.7% survival at 5 years and a marked drop to 51.5% at 10 years. Again, these very good results at 5 years make it extremely difficult to assess a new design (eg. peg) with less than 5 years follow-up. However, clearly the incidence of radiological loosening markedly increased between 5 and 10 years follow-up, thereby proving the evolutive nature of radiolucent lines. Of the three factors we found that had a statistically significant influence on the RLL (ie. length of follow up, dominant side, surgical technique from each Center), of particular interest was the last one. The rate of migration of the glenoid and especially the subsidence was clearly different between centers and the likely important contributing factor was the reaming. Following the recommendation of Collins *et al.* [5], two surgeons reamed the glenoid with a motorized reamer in order to have the best conformity between the bone and the convex back of the glenoid component and in order to re-establish a normal version of the articular surface. Whereas the radiological results observed during the first 5 years were not worrying, between 5 and 10 years as many as 21% of the glenoid components subsided in Center 4 where the surgeon was the more aggressive for reaming (fig. 5). Other authors have reported increased glenoid component migration in cases of glenoid erosion that was corrected with reaming, however a clear explanation was not provided with the authors hypothesizing that incomplete re-alignment was potentially responsible [19]. An earlier study by the same group demonstrated that the presence of glenoid erosion was predictive of increased risk of loosening and, like us, suggested that reaming of the subchondral bone may cause structural weakness [12]. This finding was important because it showed that the longevity of glenoid component fixation depended on the degree of osseous support provided by the subchondral bone. Therefore, rather than to try to obtain the best fit between the surfaces of the bone and component, it is probably better to preserve as much as possible the subchondral bone and to increase the coverage of the glenoid component on the underlying cortical bone. Most of the forces across the glenohumeral joint are a combination of shear and compressive forces, better resisted by cortical than cancellous bone, making preservation of the underlying subchondral bone or sclerotic bone crucial. This finding has renewed our preference for using a keeled type of glenoid component that minimizes removal of the important subchondral bone. This is in contrast to the widespread current popularity of pegged designs, based on the belief that early fixation is more stable [18] and there are less early postoperative radiolucencies [6, 8, 15], despite there being no reported proof that the long term results are better. In a recent study from the Mayo Clinic [26], the authors investigated 50 pegged versus 50 keeled glenoid components and reported no difference in clinical or radiographic outcomes at intermediate-term follow-up. We have concerns regarding the amount of subchondral bone that is removed during insertion of some pegged glenoids, especially in 4 or 5 peg designs, and the possible influence on long-term results. Surgeons should be careful in using such prostheses before radiological studies prove that the results are at least as good as keeled glenoids at 10 years. Furthermore, although we have demonstrated excellent results in this study using a convex back component and have previously reported improved radiographic results with convex back compared to flat back glenoid components [24], there may be situations depending on the shape of the glenoid when a flat back, or other geometry, would be preferable because less (or no) reaming is required.

There are several potential weaknesses of our study including its multicenter nature with different surgeons and different techniques making it difficult to assess other preoperative factors. It was possible that the influence of different surgical techniques was overriding and meant that other important factors remained hidden. On the other hand, the greater number of cases made available by different centers allowed for comparison of the influence of specific technical factors like reaming. Another weakness was the very large variation that we observed with the quality of the axillary views. We discovered with this study that it was extremely difficult to standardize the technique for obtaining this particular image. Even in the same specialized surgical Center, the technique used was sometimes found to be different. In some axillary views, focal osteolysis was evident beneath the flange suggesting the possibility of chemical reaction to polyethylene wear debris at the component bone interface (fig. 7). Besides the mechanical loosening of the glenoid component, demonstrated by subsidence or shift of the component on plain radiographs, it was possible that chemical osteolysis could have been responsible for some glenoid loosening. We propose further efforts be made to standardize radiographic assessment when reporting results of the glenoid component in total shoulder arthroplasty.

In conclusion, the results of this multicentric study confirm the low complication rates and excellent survival of the glenoid component in total shoulder arthroplasty performed using a third generation prosthesis with a convex back cemented all-polyethylene keeled glenoid. It will be difficult to improve on these results at 5 years, and probably 10 years, therefore any innovations in this field will need to wait for more than 10 years to prove any superiority. Likewise, the incidence of radiological loosening was minimal at 5 years, however clearly increased between 5 and 10 years follow-up. Improved radiological outcomes were observed with preservation of subchondral bone by performing no or only minimal reaming.

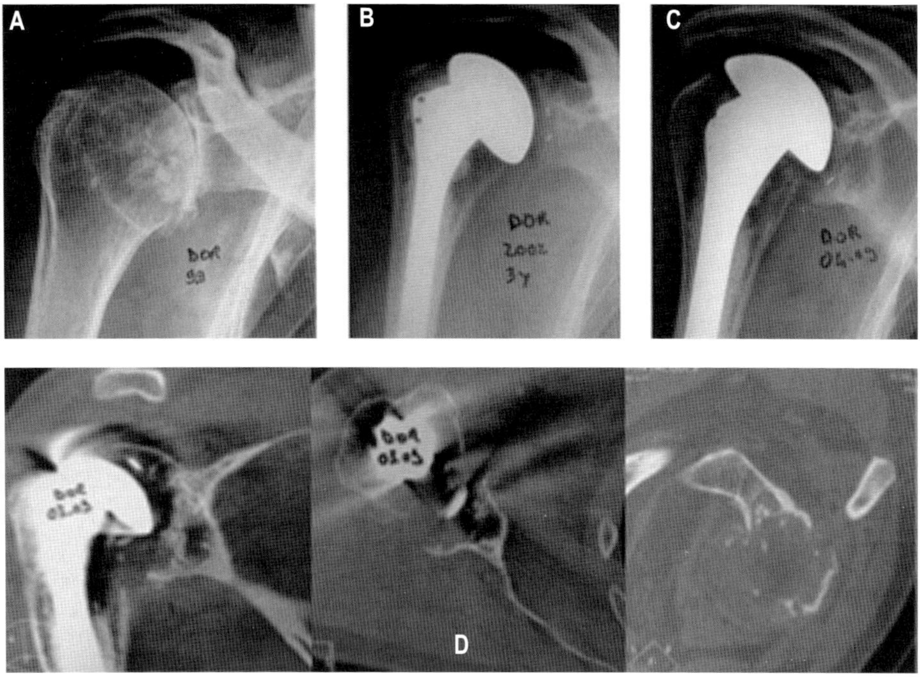

Fig. 7: 65yo male, Primary OA (A) operated on in 1999; Control X-rays at 3y f-up (B) without abnormality. At 10y f-up, X-ray shows osteolysis of the glenoid with superior tilt of the glenoid component (C). CT scan confirmed gross glenoid loosening with osteolysis (? chemical) of the glenoid (D).

REFERENCES

[1] BOHSALI KI, WIRTH MA, ROCKWOOD CA Complications of total shoulder arthroplasty. *J Bone Joint Surg [Am] 2006;88-A: 2279-92.*

[2] BREMS J. The glenoid component in total shoulder arthroplasty *J Shoulder Elbow Surg. 1993;2: 47-54*

[3] CHIN PY, SPERLING JW, COFIELD RH, SCHLECK C. Complication of total shoulder arthroplasty: are they ewer or different? *J Shoulder Elbow Surg 2006;15: 19-22*

[4] CONSTANT CR, MURLEY AH A clinical method of functional assessment of the shoulder. *Clin Orthop 1987; 214: 160-4.*

[5] COLLINS D, TENCER A, SIDLES J, MATSEN F Edge displacement and deformation of glenoid componentsin response to eccentric loading- the effect of preparation of the glenoid bone. *J Bone Joint Surg Am 1992 ;74: 501-7.*

[6] EDWARDS TB, LABRIOLA JE, STANLEY RJ, O'CONNOR DP, ELKOUSY HA, GARTSMAN GM. Radiographic comparison of pegged and keeled glenoid components using modern cementing techniques: A prospective randomized study *J Shoulder Elbow Surg 2010;19: 251-7.*

[7] FOX TJ, FOX TJ, CIL A, SPERLING JW, SANCHEZ-SOTELO J, SCHLECK CD, COFIELD RH. Survival of the glenoid component in shoulder arthroplasty. *J Shoulder Elbow Surg. Nov-Dec 2009;18(6): 859-63.*

[8] GARTSMAN GM, ELKOUSY HA, WARNOCK KM, EDWARDS TB, O'CONNOR DP. Radiographic comparison of pegged and keeled glenoid components. *J Shoulder Elbow Surg. May-Jun 2005;14(3): 252-7.*

[9] GAZIELLY DF. Comment je scelle un implant glénoïdien en polyéthylène convexe à quille avec ma technique de compaction d'os spongieux *Maitrise Orthopédique Numéro 162; Mars 2007; pp. 6-11.*

[10] GAZIELLY DF, ALLENDE C, PAMELIN E Results of cancellous compaction technique for glenoid resurfacing. Presented at the 17th Congress of the European Society for Surgery of the Shoulder and the Elbow. *Heidelberg, September 24-27, 2003.*

[11] GILBART MK, GERBER C. Comparison of the Subjective Shoulder Value and the Constant score *J Shoulder Elbow Surg 2007 ;16 : 717-21.*

[12] HAINES JF, TRAIL IA, NUTTALL D, BIRCH A, BARROW A. The results of arthroplasty in osteoarthritis of the shoulder. *J Bone Joint Surg [Br] 2006; 88-B: 496-501.*

[13] KAPLAN EL, MEIER P Nonparametric estimation from incomplete observations. *J Am Stat Assoc 1958;53: 457-81.*

[14] KLEPPS S, CHIANG AS, MILLER S, JIANG CY, HAZRATI Y, FLATOW EL. Incidence of early radiolucent glenoid lines in patients having total shoulder replacements *Clin Orthop Relat Res 2005; 435: 118-125.*

[15] LAZARUS MD, JENSEN KL, SOUTHWORTH C, MATSEN FA, 3rd The radiographic evaluation of keeled and pegged glenoid component insertion. *J Bone Joint Surg Am. Jul 2002; 84-A(7): 1174-82.*

[16] MOLÉ D, ROCHE O, RIAND N, LÉVIGNE C, WALCH G Cemented glenoid components: results in osteoarthritis and rheumatoid arthritis. In: Walch G, Boileau P, *eds. Shoulder Arthroplasty. Berlin: Springer, 1999:163-71.*

[17] NEER CS II. Replacement arthroplasty for glenohumeral osteoarthritis. *J Bone Joint Surg [Am] 1974; 56:1-13.*

[18] NUTTALL D, HAINES JF, TRAIL II. A study of the micromovement of pegged and keeled glenoid components compared using radiostereometric analysis. *J Shoulder Elbow Surg. May-Jun 2007;16(3 Suppl): S65-70.*

[19] NUTTALL D, HAINES JF, TRAIL IA. The effect of the offset humeral head on the micromovement of pegged glenoid components – a comparative study using radiostereometric analysis. *J Bone Joint Surg [Br] 2009;91-B: 757-61.*

[20] RAISS P, ALDINGER PR, RICKERT M, LOEW M Total shoulder replacement in young and middle-aged patients with glenohumeral osteoarthritis. *J Bone Joint Surg [Br] 2008; 90-B:764-9.*

[21] SPERLING JW, COFIELD RH, ROWLAND CM Minimum fifteen-year follow-up of Neer hemiarthroplasty and total shoulder arthroplasty in patients aged fifty years or younger. *J Shoulder Elbow Surg 2004;13: 604-13.*

[22] SPERLING JW, COFIELD RH, ROWLAND CM Neer hemiarthroplasty and Neer total shoulder arthroplasty in patients fifty years old or less: long-term results. *J Bone Joint Surg [Am] 1998; 80-A:464-73.*

[23] STEWART MPM, KELLY IG Total shoulder replacement in rheumatoid disease: 7- to 13-years follow-up of 37 joints. *J Bone Joint Surg [Br] 1997;79-B: 68-72.*

[24] SZABO I, BUSCAYRET F, EDWARDS TB, NEMOZ C, BOILEAU P, WALCH G. Radiographic comparison of flat-back and convex-back glenoid components in total shoulder arthroplasty. *J Shoulder Elbow Surg. Nov-Dec 2005;14(6): 636-42.*

[25] TORCHIA ME, COFIELD RH, SETTERGREN CR Total shoulder arthroplasty with the Neer prosthesis: long term results. *J Shoulder Elbow Surg 1997;6: 495-505.*

[26] THROCKMORTON TW, ZARKADAS PC, SPERLING JW, COFIELD RH. Pegged versus keeled glenoid components in total shoulder arthroplasty. *J Shoulder Elbow Surg 2010 (epub ahead of print).*

[27] WALCH G, BADET R, BOULAHIA A, KHOURY A Morphologic study of the glenoid in primary glenohumeral osteoarthritis. *J Arthroplasty 1999;14: 756-60.*

[28] WALCH G, BOILEAU P Presentation of the multicenter study in "2000 Shoulder Prostheses… two to ten year follow-up" Walch G., Boileau P., Molé D. *ed Sauramps medical, Montpellier 2001 pp 11-20.*

A 10 YEAR RADIOLOGICAL COMPARISON OF TWO ALL-POLYETHYLENE GLENOID COMPONENT DESIGNS A PROSPECTIVE TRIAL

P. COLLIN, A. TAY, B. MELIS, P. BOILEAU, G. WALCH

INTRODUCTION

From its birth, shoulder arthroplasty has continued to evolve in an attempt to achieve the goals of its pioneers: the recreation of normal anatomy, restoration of function and prosthesis endurance. In 1972, Charles Neer successfully achieved his goal of an unconstrained total shoulder arthroplasty for glenohumeral osteoarthritis with the introduction of a polyethylene glenoid [1]. More than two decades later, it was recognised that there was a greater variability and a complex nature of the morphology of the normal shoulder; this varies from patient to patient and even within an individual from side to side [2]. The limitations of the previous monobloc, and then modular designs lead to the development of "anatomical" prostheses [3, 4].

Glenoid design has evolved with these changes. The introduction of the glenoid component yielded superior functional results [5, 6, 7, 8]. Clinical follow-up studies have revealed that radiolucencies at the glenoid cement-bone interface are common, increase with time, and are associated with poor clinical function and can progress to frank loosening. There remains no consensus on the optimal all-polyethylene glenoid design, whether it should be keeled or pegged. With regards to the backside geometry, convex designs were introduced, with biomechanical studies reporting that this geometry transmitted forces more in compression and were resistant to shear forces compared to flat back designs [9, 10]. Furthermore, a convex glenoid may help improve the implantation technique by limiting reaming and bone loss.

Today, where out of all the patients who have a major joint replacement, those who have a TSR have the lowest mean age [11] the importance of improving the survivorship of total shoulder replacement is evident. This entails responsibility for the thorough assessment of prosthesis designs and changes that are implemented. This is the first long term *in-vivo* evaluation of the effect of two glenoid backside designs have on the presence and progression of radiolucencies and loosening.

MATERIALS & METHOD

A retrospective study was performed on a prospective series of primary total shoulder arthroplasty performed by the 2 senior authors, to evaluate two types of cemented glenoid components. A single shoulder arthroplasty system was used, the Aequalis primary shoulder prosthesis. All patients underwent sugery for primary osteoarthritis, as described by Neer [12, 1] between 1997 and 1999. To ensure an exclusive series of primary osteoarthritis, shoulders with the diagnosis of inflammatory arthropathy, osteochondromatosis, postinfectious arthropathy, skeletal dysplasia, and neurologic problems were excluded. Furthermore, shoulders with a history of trauma (fracture or soft-tissue injury), instability (treated surgically or nonsurgically), or prior shoulder surgery were excluded. Any shoulders with marked rotator cuff pathology defined by the presence of acromio-humeral arthritis, a massive rotator cuff tear or a rotator cuff tear involving the infraspinatus were further excluded.

Patients with glenoid bone erosion requiring bone grafting at the time of arthroplasty were also excluded.

To be included within this study, a complete preoperative radiographic evaluation, including an anteroposterior radiograph, as well as computer tomographic arthrography, for analysis of the rotator cuff and glenoid morphology had to been performed. Patients were required to have had an immediate postoperative anteroposterior radiograph (within 3 days of surgery) and a 2-year postoperative anteroposterior radiograph available. At the 10-year follow up, radiographs were repeated. All radiographs in this series were performed via a standardized fluoroscopic technique, such that the X-ray beam was perpendicular to the plane of the implant-bone interface, determined by use of a wire marker embedded in the polyethylene as described by Kelleher *et al.* [11].

In total, 66 arthroplasties performed in 63 patients met the criteria for inclusion for a first 2-year study, published in 2005 [13]. For this study, we examined the same population. Four patients were lost to follow-up and 5 deceased. Fifty-four patients remained (56 arthroplasties). The mean age at the time of surgery was 66.7 (range, 43-83 years). There were 23 men and 31 women. The operation involved the dominant side in 31 cases. Of the 54 patients, 2 underwent bilateral arthroplasty. All patients had complete records with an average of 10-years follow-up.

Glenoid morphology was determined by the classification of Walch *et al.* [29] as follows: A1 in 29 cases, A2 in 1 case, B1 in 9 cases, B2 in 15 cases, and C in 2 cases.

All patients underwent primary total shoulder arthroplasty using the Aequalis prosthesis (Tornier Inc, Minneapolis, MN). Seven different sizes of prosthetic humeral head diameter, varying between 39 mm and 50 mm, were used, and 3 different sizes of glenoid components were used with radii of curvature of 27.5 mm, 30 mm, and 32.5 mm.

The flat-back and convex-back, ultra-high-molecular-weight all-polyethylene, pear-shaped glenoid components were compared in this study. They are produced with a keel that is 4 mm thick and 15 mm in length, and designed for cementation into the medullary canal of the glenoid. The dimensions of the keel are the same for both flat-back and convex-back glenoids and across all component sizes.

The manufacturer's recommendation states that a preferential association exists for this prosthetic system (head sizes 39/14 and 41/15 are best coupled with a small glenoid, head sizes 43/16 and 46/17 are best coupled with a medium glenoid, and head sizes 48/18, 50/16, and 50/19 are best coupled with a large glenoid). However, the system permits the use of any humeral head size with any glenoid size, resulting in a radial prosthetic mismatch between 0 and 12 mm [23]. An identical surgical technique was used in all patients. All patients during this study-period underwent glenoid bone preparation including reaming of the glenoid surface and compaction of the cancellous bone as described by Gazielly (fig. 2) [14]. With this technique, rather than removing cancellous bone, the glenoid component was implanted after the cancellous bone was compacted with a glenoid punch of the same dimensions as the keel. All the humeral components were fixed with cement CMW1 (DePuy, Warsaw, USA) whereas the glenoid components were fixed with CMW2.

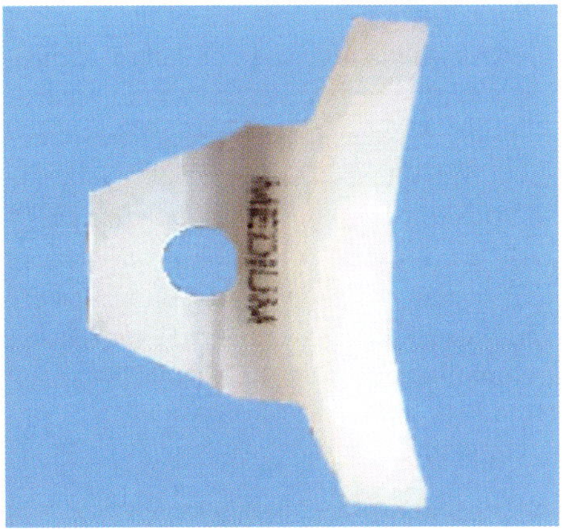

Fig. 1A: Flat-back component

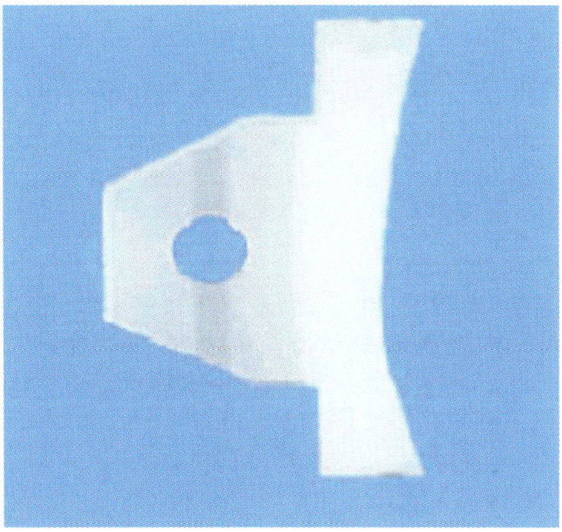

Fig. 1B: Convex-back component

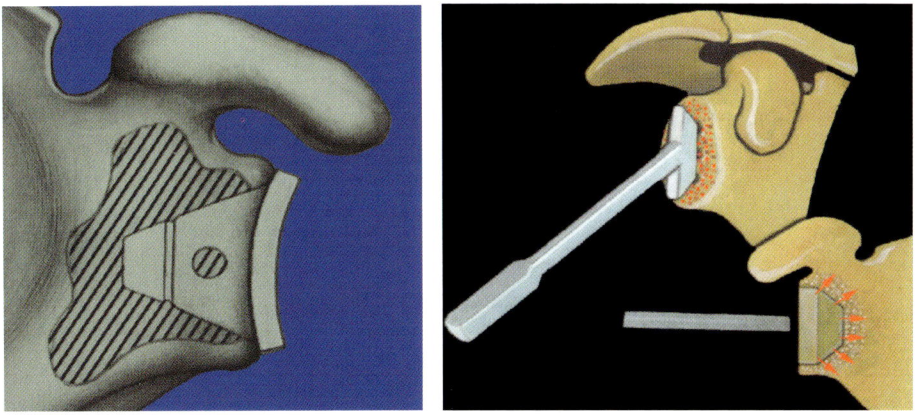

Fig. 2: Compaction technique

The type of glenoid implant was selected at the time of the procedure according to the surgeon's preference. The first group (33 shoulders) underwent glenoid resurfacing with the cemented flat-back, polyethylene glenoid component (Fig. 1A). The second group (28 shoulders) underwent glenoid resurfacing with the cemented convex-back, polyethylene glenoid component (Fig. 1B).

No statistically significant differences existed between the groups with regard to follow-up, patient age, gender, hand dominance, rotator cuff condition, glenoid morphology, or glenohumeral prosthetic mismatch.

Three observers evaluated the radiographs (AP view in internal, neutral, external rotations) with specific emphasis on identifying the presence and progression of radiolucent lines at the bone-cement interface. The extent of radiolucent lines, whether complete or incomplete and whether affecting the faceplate (the portion of the glenoid implant perpendicular to the keel), the keel, or both-was analyzed. Glenoid radiolucencies were scored according to the previously validated system of Molé (Fig. 3) *et al.* [15] by use of anteroposterior radiographs (0 points for no radiolucency to 18 points for radiolucencies exceeding 2 mm in 6 zones). A numeric value was assigned to each zone as determined by the thickness of the radiolucent line in that zone-0 points for no radiolucent line, 1 point for a radiolucent line less than 1 mm, 2 points for a radiolucent line at least 1 mm but less than or equal to 2 mm, or 3 points for a radiolucent line more than 2 mm. The scores for each zone were added to yield the total radiolucent line score (Fig. 3). In addition, the radiolucent line scores were also calculated in the 3 zones of the keel and in the 3 zones of the faceplate by use of the same method, creating the keel radiolucent line score and the faceplate radiolucent line score. We separated the scores into 3 groups: ***1)*** 0 to 6 points: no radiological loosening, ***2)*** 6 to 12 points: possible radiological loosening and ***3)*** >12 points: definite radiological loosening.

As the Molé's technique of scoring has already been validated during the first study [13], no attempt was made to calculate intra -inter observer variability of the radio lucent lines assessment.

The 2 groups of patients with different glenoid implants were compared regarding the presence and extent of radiolucent lines (complete or incomplete and whether affecting the faceplate or keel), the radiolucent line score, the progression of radiolucent lines around the entire glenoid component, the progression of radiolucent lines around the keel, and the progression of radiolucent lines behind the faceplate.

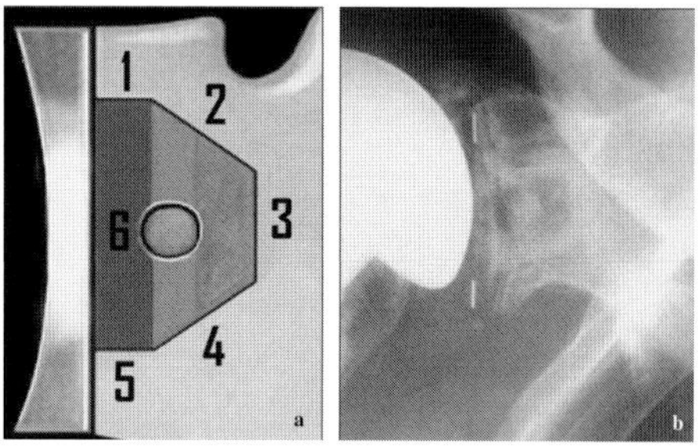

RL / Zone	< 1 mm (1 point)	1 to 2 mm (2 points)	> 2 mm (3 points)	RL Score
1		X		2
2		X		2
3				
4		X		2
5			X	3
6	X			1

Fig. 3: Molé score

We compared the X-rays immediately post operative, at 2 years and at the 10 year last follow up.

In addition, factors that could potentially contribute to the development of radiolucent lines (patient gender, patient age, patient hand dominance, condition of the rotator cuff, glenoid morphology, component size, Mismatch) were analyzed. We also analyzed the Constant-Murley [16] score at the last follow-up.

Radiolucent line scores at follow-up were studied as a discrete variable with three groups: no loosening (0-6), moderate (7-12) and severe (>12). The Chi^2 test or Fisher's exact test were used on contingency tables to study the link between radiolucent line score at follow-up and age at surgery (as a discrete variable), dominance, initial radiolucent line score, glenoid component type, passive external rotation and passive anterior elevation. A one-way analysis of variance was performed to compare means for Constant score with follow-up radiolucent line as a factor. Significance was set at $p < 0.05$.

RESULTS

On the 10-year postoperative radiographs, the mean total radiolucent line score was 9.75, in the flat-back group and 8.33 in the convex-back group. (Wilcoxon, p= 0.2412) The mean keel radiolucent line score was 5.03 in the flat-back group and 4.17 in the convex back group, the mean faceplate radiolucent line score was 4.72 in the flat-back group and 4.17 in the convex-back group these differences were not statistically significant. With the number of patients available in this study, no significant differences were seen on RLL scores, between the 2 groups with 10 year follow up.

The mean Constant score was 63 (0-89), with a mean of 60 (0-89) for the flat-back glenoid and 67(20-89) for the convex glenoid. (Student p= 0.1835).

Five patients had been reoperated: two for isolated glenoid loosening, one for posterior dislocation and glenoid loosening, one for secondary massive rotator cuff tear and upward migration of the humeral head, and one for subscapularis tendon tear. For those patients, if the glenoid was revised, the score preceding the revision was used.

We separated the patients into 3 groups of total RLL score, where (0-6) is no loosening, (7-12) possible loosening and (>12) definitive radiological loosening. The total results were no loosening in 25 cases (Fig. 4b, 5) (45 %), possible in 11 (20 %) and definitive in 20 (35 %) (Fig. 6, 7). With regard to the type of glenoid implant, in the flat back group: (0-6) 12 cases, (7-12) 9 cases, and (>12-) 11 cases. For the convex group: (0-6) 13 cases, (7-12) 2 cases, and (>12-) 9 cases. No significant differences were seen between the 2 groups with the numbers available. (Chi^2 p= 0.16, Fisher's exact p=0.17).

Nor did we find differences when we compared the keel scores and the face plate scores in both groups. We analysed the factors potentially contributing to the development and progression of radiolucent lines in the total population for the mean RLL and in each group (none, possible and definitive radiological loosening). Four factors were found to be significant.

1) The presence of RLL on the immediate post-op X-rays and at 2-year follow-up (Fishers exact, p = 0,018).
2) The age at surgery (<60 years old vs >60 years old) was significant

(Fisher's exact p= 0.03), age had a statistically significant influence on the 10 years follow-up radiolucent lines scores. Younger people (under 60 years at the implantation) had significantly more loosening ("loosening" or "radiolucent lines"?).

3) Patient hand dominance was significant (Fisher's exact p = 0.017).

4) Glenoid implant loosening had a significant impact on the Constant score (p=0.006). A mean score of 71 for a RLL between the no loosening (0-6) group and 51 for the radiological loosening (>12-) group.

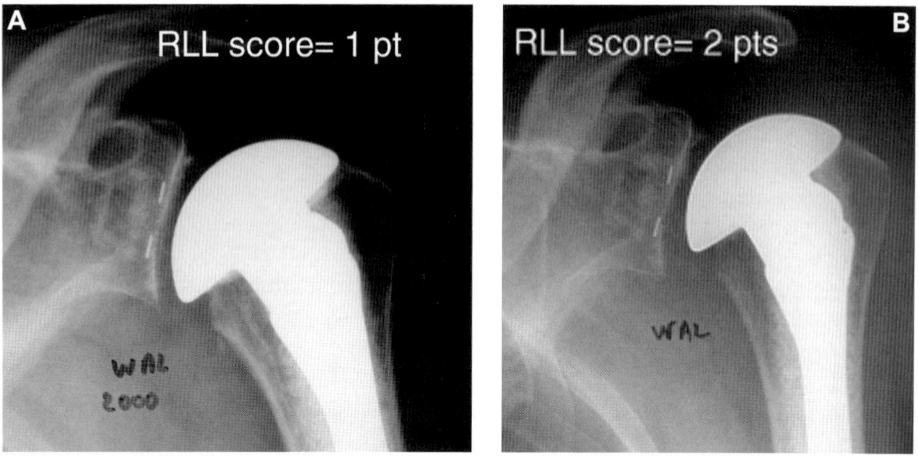

Fig. 4: A) Case N-1 convex-back: RLL 1 at 2 years; B) Case N-1 convex-back: RLL 2 at 10 years

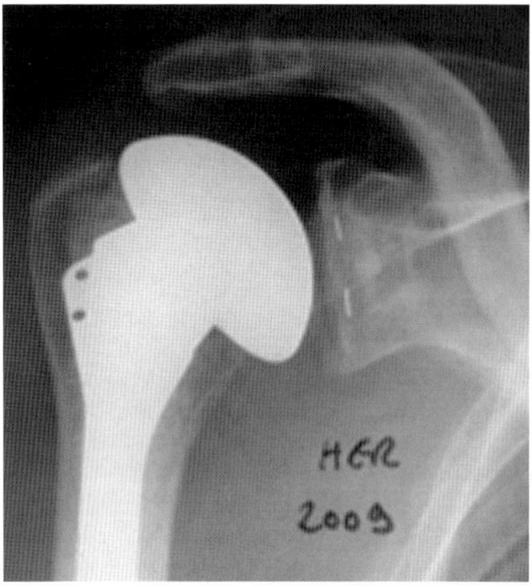

Fig. 5: Flat back component: RLL < 6 at 11 years follow up.

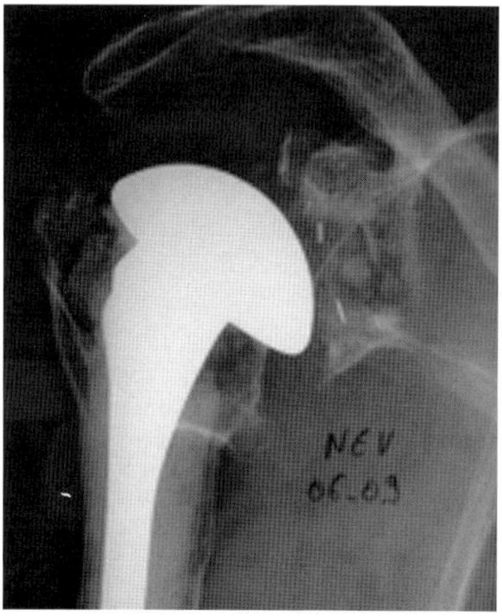

Fig. 6: Convex-back component with a RLL at 14 at 11 years follow-up

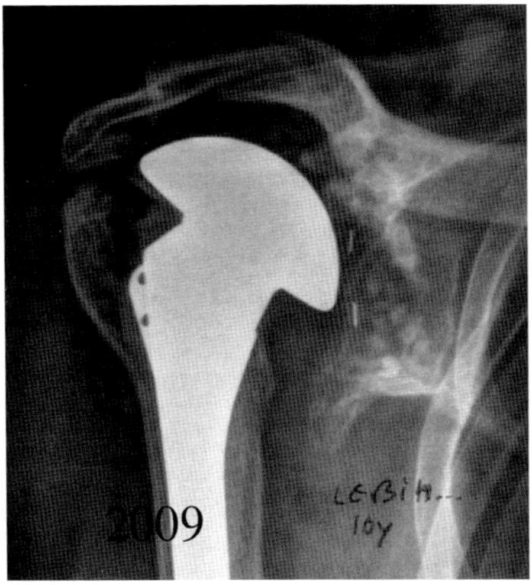

Fig. 7: Flat-back component with a RLL at 18 at 10 years Follow-up

Patient gender, the presence of rotator cuff tear, glenoid morphology did not statistically influence the frequency and size of the 10 year glenoid radiolucencies in the total population.

At 10 years follow-up; the results according to the type of glenoid design were not statistically significant. Thus, if we consider the total population (56 shoulders), the quality of the initial fixation, age at surgery (under 60) and hand dominance were significant factors for loosening. This loosening had a negative effect on the Constant Score at the last follow-up.

DISCUSSION

The literature demonstrates ongoing concerns with the problem of long-term glenoid component survivorship [17, 18, 19, 3, 20, 21, 22, 23, 24]. Glenoid loosening remains the most common reason for failure and revision surgery. This study evaluates the long-term follow-up of two glenoid component designs, and the effect on radiolucent lines and their progression. The initial study at 2 years reported that the flat-back glenoid demonstrated greater RLL than the convex-back glenoid design. This result was in keeping with biomechanical studies of glenoid component design, where a more conforming back-side geometry is preferential [10]. Less reaming of the subchondral glenoid is required at implantation and the geometry allows for better congruency and distribution of shear forces. In this study at 10 years, there has been progression of the mean RLL scores in both glenoids, from 2 years to 10 years the flat back glenoid RLL score increased from 4.19 to 9.78, and the convex glenoid 3.23 to 8.33. These results show that there is no statistical difference of the RLL scores between the two glenoid designs at 10 years ($p>0.05$). This was an unexpected finding given the initial 2 year results.

There has been no other study in the literature that has compared two types of glenoid backside designs and the effect on long-term radiolucent line development. It would be interesting to compare to other series. It is possible that backside geometry may have a role in RLL in the early period, but the development of RLL at the glenoid-bone interface remains multifactorial and on the longer term, other factors may have a greater influence.

Among these factors we can confirm that the presence of a RLL immediately post operatively and at 2 years predicts further progression. This indicates that good surgical technique at the time of glenoid implantation is crucial (fig. 4 A and B). Key factors in glenoid preparation are minimising the removal and reaming of glenoid bone and to achieve a stable platform to cement the glenoid component [25]. In this study, all glenoids were implanted with careful attention to these two details, using an impaction bone saving technique described by Gazielly [14]. Despite this, 31 glenoids (55%) had moderate to severe RLL in our study at 10 years.

Patient demand for good function is important; this is reflected that in younger patients and shoulder arthroplasties in the dominant limb were seen to have a greater progression of RLL [26]. We did not see a difference between the genders, which have been previously reported [27, 28]. Other authors have also reported that the development of rotator cuff tears following surgery influence the development of RLL, but this was not found in this series.

With regard to the glenoid morphological type as described by Walch [29], we expected to see that the preoperative glenoid morphology would influence glenoid component loosening. However, with the number of cases available in this study, the glenoid type did not appear to predispose to loosening. In this study we excluded the glenoids with severe erosion that required bone graft; we recognised this as a limitation of our study design. Even though there is no evidence in our study or in the literature, that glenoid morphology affects glenoid implant survival, we still maintain that this is likely and our population size is too small to identify a difference.

Loosening of the glenoid component results in deterioration of clinical function. The progression of RLL in our study correlates with declining Constant scores. The group of patients with definite radiological evidence of glenoid loosening, reported the worse functional results, and 3 (5.36%) of them required revision surgery. This rate is comparable to other series of cemented glenoids [5, 18, 19, 20, 30, 31].

This study of shoulder arthroplasties should demonstrate a true representation of the long term effect of the backside glenoid component geometry on the development of RLL. It has a robust design with a mean follow-up period of ten years in a prospective population, where only two surgeons with a standardised technique performed the surgery. However limitations still remain. Despite the standardisation of radiographic techniques for evaluation of RLL, this is an imperfect technique for identifying radiolucencies. X-ray analysis is also prone to observer variation, which we have tried to limit in our methods by using the average of three examiners. Due to the multifactorial nature of glenoid loosening, the sample size is too small to clearly identify all factors that influence glenoid loosening.

This study shows that the back side geometry of the glenoid component does not affect the rate of RLL or loosening at 10 years. The problem of glenoid component loosening is clearly multifactorial and it is evident that good implantation technique and the functional demand have an important effect on component survival. Our study furthermore illustrates the importance of long term follow up in arthroplasty, in ensuring an accurate picture of clinical outcome.

We have seen that at 10 years, the two types of glenoids (flat-back and convex-back) show no difference in the presence of RLL. However, there are important factors identified in the progression of RLL in the population as a whole. These are the early presence of RLL, patient age at surgery and hand dominance. Furthermore, we have seen that the progression of RLL has a detrimental effect on the clinical outcome.

REFERENCES

[1] NEER CS Replacement arthroplasty for glenohumeral osteoarthritis. *J Bone Joint Surg Am 1974, 56, 1-13.*

[2] PEARL ML Proximal humeral anatomy in shoulder arthroplasty: Implications for prosthetic design and surgical technique. *J Shoulder Elbow Surg 14, 2005. 99S-104S.*

[3] WALCH G & BOILEAU P Prosthetic adaptability: a new concept for shoulder arthroplasty. *J Shoulder Elbow Surg 1999. 8, 443-51.*

[4] BOILEAU P & WALCH G Adaptability and modulation in shoulder prosthesis. *Acta Orthop Belg 61 Suppl 1995. 1, 49-61.*

[5] IANNOTTI JP & NORRIS TR Influence of preoperative factors on outcome of shoulder arthroplasty for glenohumeral osteoarthritis. *J Bone Joint Surg Am 2003. 85-A, 251-58.*

[6] GARTSMAN GM, RODDEY TS, HAMMERMAN SM Shoulder arthroplasty with or without resurfacing of the glenoid in patients who have osteoarthritis. *J Bone Joint Surg Am 2000. 82, 26-34.*

[7] EDWARDS TB, KADAKIA NR, BOULAHIA A, KEMPF J, BOILEAU P, NEMOZ C, & WALCH G. A comparison of hemiarthroplasty and total shoulder arthroplasty in the treatment of primary glenohumeral osteoarthritis: results of a multicenter study. *J Shoulder Elbow Surg 2003. 12, 207-13.*

[8] BRYANT D, LITCHFIELD R, SANDOW M, GARTSMAN G M, GUYATT G & KIRKLEY A. A comparison of pain, strength, range of motion, and functional outcomes after hemiarthroplasty and total shoulder arthroplasty in patients with osteoarthritis of the shoulder. A systematic review and meta-analysis. *J Bone Joint Surg Am 2005. 87, 1947-56.*

[9] ANGLIN C, WYSS UP, NYFFELER RW, GERBER C Loosening performance of cemented glenoid prosthesis design pairs. *Clin Biomech (Bristol, Avon) 2001. 16, 144-150.*

[10] ANGLIN C, WYSS UP, PICHORA DR Mechanical testing of shoulder prostheses and recommendations for glenoid design. *J Shoulder Elbow Surg 2000, 9, 323-31.*

[11] BREMS JJ Complications of shoulder arthroplasty: infections, instability, and loosening. *Instr Course Lect 2002. 51, 29-39.*

[12] II, NC Glenohumeral arthroplasty. *In: Shoulder reconstruction. 1990, p. 146-271.*

[13] SZABO I, BUSCAYRET F, EDWARDS TB, NEMOZ C, BOILEAU P, WALCH G Radiographic comparison of flat-back and convex-back glenoid components in total shoulder arthroplasty. *J Shoulder Elbow Surg 2005. 14, 636-42.*

[14] BOILEAU P, MOLÉ DWG Technique of glenoid resurfacing 1999.

[15] MOLÉ D, ROCHE O, RNLCWG () Cemented glenoid component: results in osteoarthritis and rheumatoid arthritis. *Berlin: Springer-Verlag; 1999. p. 163-71.*

[16] CONSTANT CR, MURLEY AH A clinical method of functional assessment of the shoulder. *Clin Orthop Relat Res, 1987. 160-4.*

[17] BOILEAU P, AVIDOR C, KRISHNAN SG, WALCH G, KEMPF J, MOLE D. Cemented polyethylene versus uncemented metal-backed glenoid components in total shoulder arthroplasty: a prospective, double-blind, randomized study. *J Shoulder Elbow Surg 2002. 11, 351-59.*

[18] TORCHIA ME, COFIELD RH, SETTERGREN CR Total shoulder arthroplasty with the Neer prosthesis: long-term results. *J Shoulder Elbow Surg 1997. 6, 495-505.*

[19] NORRIS TR, IANNOTTI JP Functional outcome after shoulder arthroplasty for primary osteoarthritis: a multicenter study. *J Shoulder Elbow Surg 2002. 11, 130-35.*

[20] HAINES JF, TRAIL IA, NUTTALL D, BIRCH A BARROW, A The results of arthroplasty in osteoarthritis of the shoulder. *J Bone Joint Surg Br 2006. 88, 496-501.*

[21] GODENECHE A, BOILEAU P, FAVARD L, LE HUEC J, LEVIGNE C, NOVE-JOSSERAND L, WALCH G, EDWARDS TB Prosthetic replacement in the treatment of osteoarthritis of the shoulder: early results of 268 cases. *J Shoulder Elbow Surg 2002. 11, 11-18.*

[22] COFIELD RH Total shoulder arthroplasty with the Neer prosthesis. *J Bone Joint Surg Am 1984. 66, 899-906.*

[23] CHIN PYK, SPERLING JW, COFIELD RH, SCHLECK C Complications of total shoulder arthroplasty: are they fewer or different? *J Shoulder Elbow Surg 2006. 15, 19-22.*

[24] BUCKINGHAM BP, PARSONS IM, CAMPBELL B, TITELMAN RM, SMITH KL, MATSEN FA Patient functional self-assessment in late glenoid component failure at three to eleven years after total shoulder arthroplasty. *J Shoulder Elbow Surg 2005. 14, 368-74.*

[25] COLLINS D, TENCER A, SIDLES J, MATSEN Fr Edge displacement and deformation of glenoid components in response to eccentric loading. The effect of preparation of the glenoid bone. *J Bone Joint Surg Am 1992, 74, 501-7.*

[26] FOX TJ, CIL A, SPERLING JW, SANCHEZ-SOTELO J, SCHLECK CD, COFIELD RH (Survival of the glenoid component in shoulder arthroplasty. *J Shoulder Elbow Surg 2009, 18, 859-63.*

[27] MEROLLA G, CAMPI F, PALADINI P, LOLLINO N, FAUCI F, PORCELLINI G. Correlation between radiographic risk for glenoid component loosening and clinical scores in shoulder arthroplasty. *Chir Organi Mov 93 2009. Suppl 1, S29-34.*

[28] EDWARDS TB, LABRIOLA JE, STANLEY RJ, O'CONNOR DP, ELKOUSY HA, GARTSMAN GM Radiographic comparison of pegged and keeled glenoid components using modern cementing techniques: a prospective randomized study. *J Shoulder Elbow Surg 2010. 19, 251-57.*

[29] WALCH G, BADET R, BOULAHIA A, KHOURY A Morphologic study of the glenoid in primary glenohumeral osteoarthritis. *J Arthroplasty 1999. 14, 756-60.*

[30] DESHMUKH AV, KORIS M, ZURAKOWSKI D, THORNHILL TS Total shoulder arthroplasty: long-term survivorship, functional outcome, and quality of life. *J Shoulder Elbow Surg 2005. 14, 471-79.*

[31] MEROLLA G, PALADINI P, CAMPI F, PORCELLINI G. Efficacy of anatomical prostheses in primary glenohumeral osteoarthritis. *Chir Organi Mov 2008. 91, 109-15.*

RESULTS OF UNCEMENTED, METAL-BACKED GLENOID IMPLANTS: A NORTH AMERICAN EXPERIENCE

R.H. COFIELD, M.J. TAUNTON

BACKGROUND

There is a long but fairly small history of the use of metal-backed bone ingrowth, anatomic glenoid components. In 1975 Pilliar, Cameron, and McNab developed a variety of porous surface layered prosthetic devices including a shoulder replacement [1]. This device was slightly more constrained than the typical shoulder arthroplasty with bone ingrowth surfaces on both the glenoid and the humeral components. Reports of the device were issued in 1987 by McElwain and English [2] and later by Weiss [3]. In both these studies clinical and radiographic outcomes were reasonable. Burkhead from Dallas, Texas, presented information about a different design of bone ingrowth metal-backed glenoid component at several meetings, but a clinical series was never published. Wallace from Australia reported on a comparison between metal-backed ingrowth prostheses and those cemented in position. The radiographic findings were better with the cementless type of implant, but some complications were identified [4], Boileau and co-authors in 2002 published a second series comparing cemented polyethylene components with uncemented metal-backed components, and again recognized difficulties with the metal-back design [5]. So, in summary, the clinical results of this type of glenoid implant were often reasonably favorable, but issues were identified including a higher frequency of instability, component dissociation, and a suggestion that wear rates may be increased leading to osteolysis and loosening.

In the early 1980's we became interested in the potential for this type of design and developed a type of glenoid component that would allow for bone ingrowth. This first component design was used clinically between 1984 and 1987. A report was published in 1992 [6]. Yet, again, the component performed reasonably well clinically, but there were some problems identified.

During this same period engineering studies were undertaken. A finite element analysis showed that this type of component created significant stress transfer to the cortices of the scapula, and this was a substantial change from the native glenoid or an all-polyethylene cemented component [7]. As a side line to this study, it was recognized that there were also increased stresses in the polyethylene portion of this component. Material testing was performed on this component along with others using a standard polyurethane model [8]. The force to distract the metal-backed bone ingrowth component with screws from the native glenoid was much in excess of that required to extract all-polyethylene components. However, in detailed analysis it was recognized that the mode of failure shifted from component fatigue in the polyethylene designs to failure of the synthetic glenoid model, seemingly indicating, as one might anticipate, that metallic elements are quite strong – not necessarily that fixation is more secure.

An additional study was performed for radiographic assessment of ingrowth total shoulder arthroplasty, and the findings were quite favorable with only 4 of 62 glenoid components showing adverse radiographic features [9].

PATIENT STUDY

The above background suggested that we should continue to explore the use of metal-backed bone ingrowth glenoid components. Between 1989 and 1998, 124 bone ingrowth total shoulder arthroplasties were placed. These shoulders represent the basis of this study. A more limited study of many patients in this group, focusing on the diagnosis of osteoarthritis, was reported in the Journal of Bone and Joint Surgery, American Volume in 2008 [10]. In these 124 shoulders, mean clinical follow-up was 9.4 years, ranging from 2 to greater than 15 years for shoulders not undergoing revision surgery. In this expanded group the average patient age was 62 years. There were 63 men and 56 women. The diagnoses were osteoarthritis in 83, rheumatoid arthritis in 21, traumatic arthritis in 10, cuff tear arthropathy in 6, and osteonecrosis in 4.

The surgical procedure demanded precision in fitting the components against the bones, and instruments were developed to allow this to occur both for the humeral and glenoid sides of the arthroplasty (fig. 1).

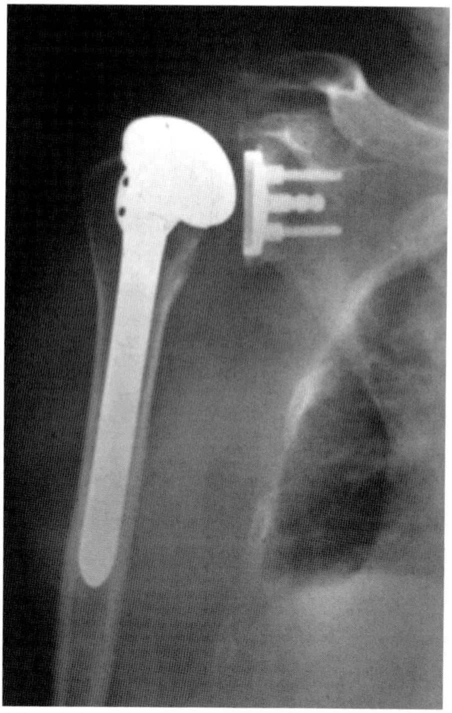

Fig. 1 : Two month postoperative radiograph of a total shoulder arthroplasty using both bone ingrowth components for the glenoid and the humerus. With the instrumentation it was possible to achieve exact fitting of the implants to the bones.

Sadly, there were too many complications and too great a need for revision surgery. Instability developed in 32 shoulders, rotator cuff tearing in 20, glenoid metal wear in 41, clinical or radiographic glenoid loosening in 42, clinical or radiographic humeral loosening in 20, humeral fracture in 2, wound healing problems in 1 and postoperative pulmonary emoblism in 1.

Forty shoulders underwent revision surgery often for a combination of features including rotator cuff tearing, instability or component wear or loosening, with component related problems dominating the revision scene (fig. 2). Component survival free of revision or removal was 85% at five years and 75% at 10 years.

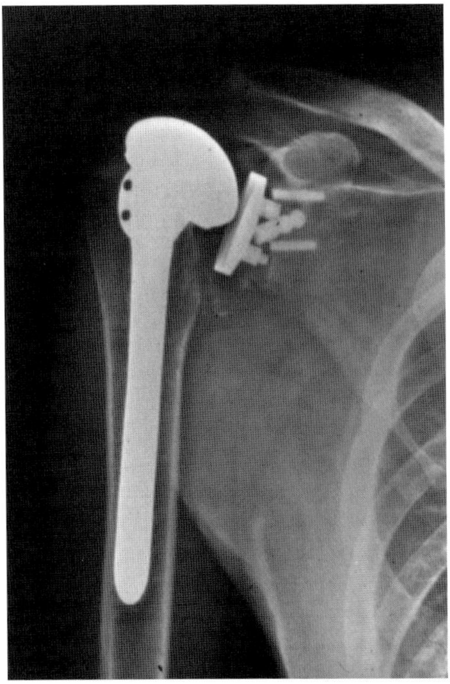

Fig. 2 : Radiograph of a bone ingrowth glenoid component showing osteolysis beneath the ingrowth tray and stress fracturing of the fixation screws and central glenoid peg. There is also lysis of the humeral calcar and the endosteal surface of the humeral shaft.

There were no identifiable patient, disease, or surgical characteristics associated with failure, either clinically or radiographically ($p<0.0001$).

Thankfully, the clinical outcomes of those not undergoing revision surgery were favorable with pain on a 1-5 scale being reduced from 4.6 to 1.9, active elevation improving from a mean of 103 degrees to a mean of 137 degrees, external rotation improving from a mean of 31 degrees to a mean of 58 degrees, and internal rotation improving from L5 to L1. All changes were statistically significant ($P = 0.0001$). Concerning patient satisfaction, 92% felt they were much better or better. Applying the Neer result rating, 89% had an excellent or satisfactory outcome.

However, the radiographic findings in this non-revised group of 84 shoulders continued to be worrisome with moderate or severe clinical instability in 18, glenoid metal wear in 10, and polyethylene wear in 18, the glenoid component being “at risk” for clinically important loosening in 31 and the humeral component being “at risk” for clinically important loosening in 11. If one combined the component revision data with the radiographic data of the unrevised components with metal wear, a glenoid component at risk or humeral component at risk, the survival rate dropped to 80% at 5 years and 48% at 10 years.

The high number of revision procedures needed was seemingly polyethylene and metal wear related – and accelerates with time. In the absence of the need for revision surgery the clinical measures were positive but the radiographic changes continued to be negative. In conclusion we would very seldom use this type of glenoid component. Situations where it's use might be considered would include focal glenoid bone loss preventing the use of a cemented component – such as in patients with scapular dysplasia and secondary osteoarthritis, or select revision surgical cases with moderate central glenoid bone loss.

RECOMMENDATIONS

Given our experience it would be hard to support the use of this type of glenoid component with the current bearing surfaces. We have returned to cemented all-polyethylene glenoid component designs, including pegged designs. We are making use of the precise instrumentation developed for the bone ingrowth metal-backed glenoid component and have incorporated advanced cement techniques. We continue to use an ingrowth humeral component but have altered the design to include a more extended ingrowth surface. Again, the precision instruments continue to be used. By adopting this methodology between 1995 and 2004, we placed 279 all-polyethylene glenoid components. Only one component has needed to be revised. During that same period of time, we used 713 bone ingrowth stems and only one of these had required revision surgery at the time of last review.

REFERENCES

[1] PILLIAR RM, CAMERON HU, MACNAB I. Porous surface layered prosthetic devices. *Biomed Eng 1975; 10: 126-31.*

[2] McELWAIN JP, ENGLISH E. The early results of porous-coated total shoulder arthroplasty. *Clin Orthop 1987; 218: 217-24.*

[3] WEISS AP, ADAMS MA, MOORE JR, WEILAND AJ. Unconstrained shoulder arthroplasty. A five-year average follow-up study. *Clin Orthop 1990; 257: 86-90.*

[4] WALLACE AL, PHILLIPS RL, MacDOUGAL GA, WALSH WR, SONNABEND DH. Resurfacing of the glenoid in total shoulder arthroplasty. A comparison, at a mean of five years, of prostheses inserted with and without cement. *J Bone Joint Surg 1999; 81A(4): 510-8.*

[5] BOILEAU P, AVIDOR C, KRISHNAN SG, WALCH G, KEMPF JF, MOLE D. Cemented polyethylene versus uncemented metal-backed glenoid components in total shoulder arthroplasty: a prospective, double-blind, randomized study. *J Shoulder Elbow Surg 2002; 11: 351-9.*

[6] COFIELD RH, DALY PJ. Total shoulder arthroplasty with a tissue-ingrowth glenoid component. *J Shoulder Elbow Surg 1992; 1: 77-85.*

[7] STONE KD, GRABROWSKI JJ, COFIELD RH, MORREY BF, AN KN. Stress analyses of glenoid components in total shoulder arthroplasty. *J Shoulder Elbow Surg 1999; 8: 151-8.*

[8] FUKUDA K, CHEN CM, COFIELD RH, CHAO EY. Biomechanical analysis of stability and fixation strength of total shoulder protheses. *Orthopedics 1988; 11: 141-9.*

[9] SPERLING JW, COFIELD RH, O'DRISCOLL SW, TORCHIA ME, ROWLAND CM. Radiograph assessment of ingrowth total shoulder arthroplasty. *J Shoulder Elbow Surg 2000; 9: 507-13.*

[10] TAUNTON MJ, McINTOSH AL, SPERLING JW, COFIELD RH. Total shoulder arthroplasty with a metal-backed bone-ingrowth glenoid component. Medium to long-term results. *J Bone Joint Surg 2008; 90A: 2180-8.*

RESULTS OF UNCEMENTED, METAL-BACK GLENOID IMPLANTS: THE UK EXPERIENCE

W.A. WALLACE

INTRODUCTION

In 2000 we reported in a paper presented to BESS a study of the survival of glenoid components over a 10 year period from 1989 to 1998. During that period the Nottingham Shoulder & Elbow Unit carried out a total of 514 Primary Shoulder Arthroplasties were performed. Of these, 222 or 43% were Total Shoulder Arthroplasties (TSAs) using an uncemented glenoid component. The 1 to 10 year (mean=4 years) results were for uncemented glenoid replacements of a Biomodular & Nottingham design. We reported, in this study the survival of the glenoid implants only and the following survival curve demonstrated a 66.7% survival of glenoid implants at 10 years (Fig. 1).

A significant problem of glenoid component loosening was revealed. The glenoid components prior to 1997 were designed with a titanium in-growth surface only, but the introduction of Hydroxy-Apatite (HA) coating to the back side of the metal glenoid baseplate in 1997 appeared to improve the early survival. This was reported in our paper on: "Improvements in survival of the uncemented Nottingham Total Shoulder prosthesis: a prospective comparative study" (Rosenberg, Neumann, Modi, Mersich and Wallace 2007). We showed in this paper that the survival of HA coated glenoid components (Fig. 2) had improved to 93% at 4 years (Fig. 3).

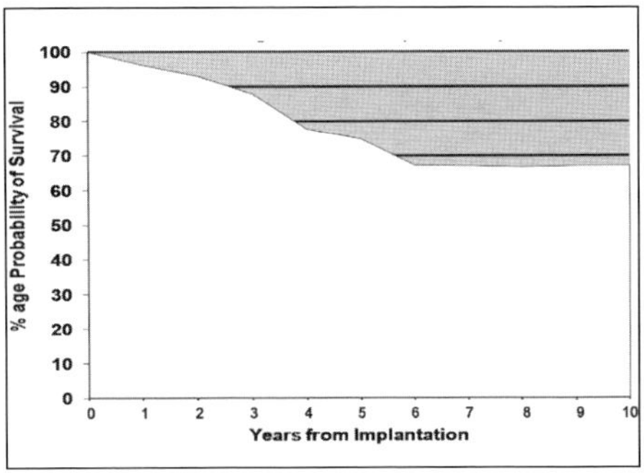

Fig. 1: Survival Curve for Uncemented Glenoid Components in Nottingham after TSR (1989-99).

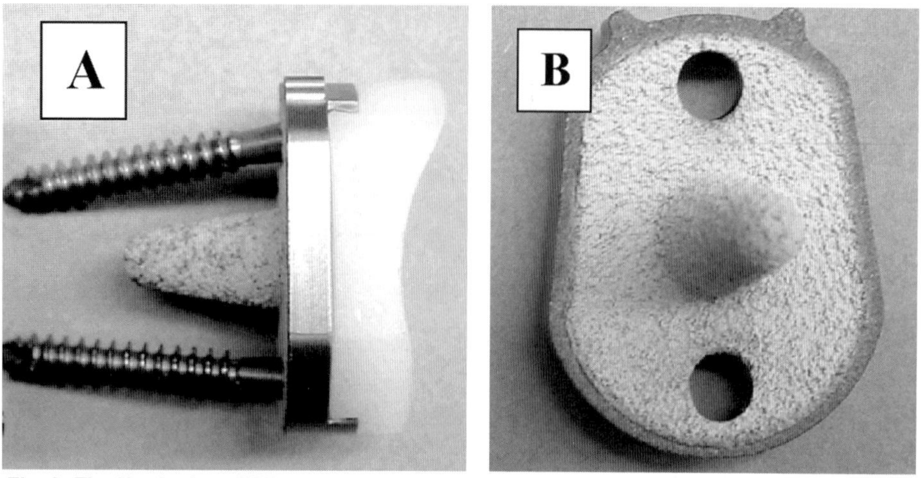

Fig. 2: The Nottingham TSR total shoulder arthroplasty prosthetic design with glenoid base-plate coated with hydroxyapatite. (A) A lateral view of the base-plate with fixation screws and with mounted polyethylene liner. (B) A view on the bone interface side of the base-plate covered by hydroxyapatite.

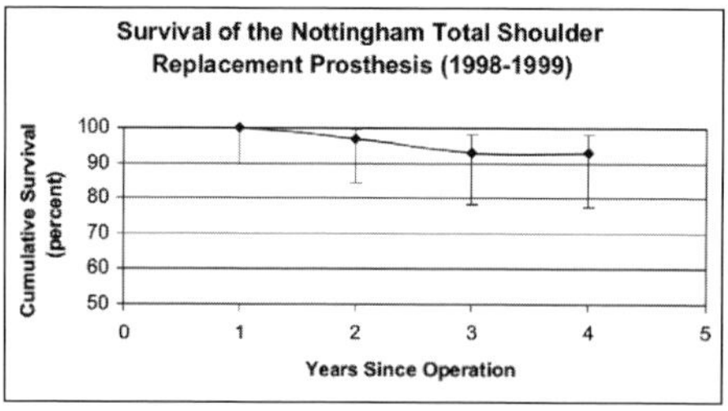

Fig. 3: This Survival Curve shows the survival of the current Nottingham TSR glenoid component with a hyroxyapatite coated glenoid baseplate (vertical bars represent 95% confidence intervals) from 1998-1999 – analysed in 2004.

MATERIALS AND METHODS

All patients who had Primary Total Shoulders under the implanted from 1997 to 2010 under the care of the senior author (WAW) were subjected to a case-note review. The survival of the glenoid component only was analysed. For cases where the patient's care was transferred to another surgeon, the patient's status was obtained through personal contact and email communication.

RESULTS

The outcomes are tabulated in Table 1 below. From this data a Kaplan-Meier Glenoid Survival has been developed. This is shown in Table 2 & Figure 4 below.

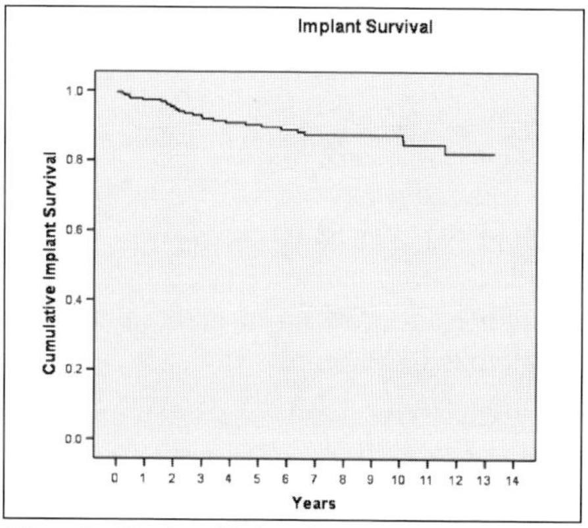

Fig. 4: Kaplan-Meier Glenoid Survival for Primary TSRs - Uncemented Glenoid Components – 1997 to 2010 (n=235).

Nottingham Uncemented Glenoid Components - Primary TSRs only												
		Pathology requiring TSR				Causes for Glenoid Revision						
Year	Total Uncemented Glenoids inserted	Primary OA	Secondary OA	RA	Other	Glenoid Disassembly	Deep Infection	Loosening ? Low grade infection	Technical Errors	Bearing wear	Other (not glenoid related)	Total Glenoid Revisions
1997	22	13	1	6	2	1	0	1	0	0	0	2
1998	20	13	2	4	1	1	1	0	0	0	1	3
1999	21	11	0	8	2	1	0	1	1	0	0	3
2000	25	13	4	7	1	0	1	2	1	1	0	5
2001	18	9	3	6	0	0	0	1	0	0	0	1
2002	11	7	3	1	0	1	0	0	0	0	1	2
2003	10	7	1	2	0	1	0	0	0	0	0	1
2004	12	9	3	0	0	0	0	0	0	0	1	1
2005	21	16	1	3	1	1	0	0	0	0	0	1
2006	14	12	0	2	0	1	0	1	0	0	0	2
2007	21	19	1	1	0	1	0	0	0	0	0	1
2008	21	17	0	4	0	1	0	0	1	0	0	2
2009	13	11	1	1	0	1	0	0	0	0	0	1
2010	6	5	0	1	0	0	0	0	0	0	0	0
Totals	**235**	**162**	**20**	**46**	**7**	**10**	**2**	**6**	**3**	**1**	**3**	25
%age	**100.0**	**68.9**	**8.5**	**19.6**	**3.0**	**4.3**	**0.9**	**2.6**	**1.3**	**0.4**	**1.3**	**10.6**

Table 1: Outcome from Uncemented Glenoid Components – 1997 to 2010 (n=235).

Time	Survival rate	Failure rate
1 year	97.4%	2.60%
2 years	95.1%	4.90%
3 years	92.0%	8.00%
4 years	90.9%	9.10%
5 years	90.2%	9.80%
6 years	88.8%	11.20%
7 years	87.3%	12.70%
8 years	87.3%	12.70%
9 years	87.3%	12.70%
10 years	87.3%	12.70%
11 years	84.5%	15.50%
12 years	82.1%	17.90%
13 years	82.1%	17.90%
14 years	82.1%	17.90%

Table 2: Glenoid Survival Outcome from 235 Total Shoulder Replacements

CONCLUSION

This is the largest survival analysis of uncemented glenoid components which has been reported. The major ongoing problem is disassembly. In October 2009, Biomet UK withdrew the Nottingham uncemented glenoid component in order to deliver a more stable upgraded version. However to date this has not yet been brought on to the market.

REFERENCE

ROSENBERG N, NEUMANN L, MODI A, MERSICH IJ, WALLACE WA (2007) Improvements in survival of the uncemented Nottingham Total Shoulder prosthesis: a prospective comparative study. *BMC Musculoskeletal Disorders 2007, 8:76 doi:10.1186/1471-2474-8-76*

LONG-TERM RESULTS AND SURVIVAL OF UNCEMENTED METAL-BACK GLENOID IMPLANTS IN PRIMARY GLENOHUMERAL OSTEOARTHRITIS

G. MOINEAU, A. GODENÈCHE, N. MORIN SALVO, B. MÉLIS, C. LÉVIGNE, L. FAVARD, D. MOLÉ, M. CARLES, G. WALCH, P. BOILEAU

SUMMARY

Introduction

The aim of this study was to assess the results of anatomical total shoulder prostheses with metal-back glenoid components in primary gleno-humeral osteoarthritis. We hypothesized that glenoid resurfacing with a MB implant would not be acceptable in the long term because of loosening and/or accelerated polyethylene (PE) wear.

Methods

Multi-center retrospective cohort study of patients with primary osteoarthritis treated between 1994 and 1999 using a non-constrained anatomic total shoulder arthroplasty with an uncemented metal-back glenoid component. Outcomes were assessed both clinically (mobility and Constant score) and radiologically (PE wear, loosening, instability). A prosthetic survival curve was constructed with the end point defined as either partial or complete revision and using 100% confidence intervals.

Results

158 patients with 165 TSA were included. The mean age at surgery was 68 years [35-89]. 109 TSA (66%) had one or more postoperative complications. The most frequent complication was polyethylene wear or dissociation in 87 cases (53%). 66 patients (40%) were re-operated upon, including 61 revision procedures (37%). Problems relating to the glenoid component accounted for revision in 54 cases including 21 cases of loosening and 33 cases of PE wear or dissociation without loosening. Seven revisions and 5 reoperations were secondary to soft tissue problems including 9 subscapularis tendon ruptures or insufficiency. The rate of prosthetic survival was respectively 60% [44-71%] and 46% [32-54%] at 10 and 12 years. The 104 patients, who retained their prostheses were assessed at a mean duration of 102 months following surgery [24-191]. There were statistically significant improvements in all measures of active range of motion and in all parameters of the Constant score. The mean active anterior elevation and external rotation were respectively 137° ± 33° and

33° ± 17°. The Constant score was 65 ± 18 points and 94 ± 26% when adjusted for age and gender.

Conclusion: Glenoid resurfacing using a metal-back glenoid component is not a viable long-term therapeutic option. At 12 years follow-up, only 46% of the prostheses were still in place. PE wear is the main limiting factor in the use of MB implants in shoulder replacement.

INTRODUCTION

Total shoulder arthroplasty (TSA) has proven to be a beneficial treatment for patients with primary glenohumeral osteoarthritis (OA) presenting with shoulder stiffness and pain. However, long-term fixation of the glenoid component remains an unsolved problem and loosening of cemented polyethylene (PE) glenoid components represent an important cause of failure in TSA [10, 11, 14]. To reduce glenoid lucent lines, uncemented fixation with porous coated or tissue-ingrowth components have been developed with the hope of achieving more stable fixation to the bone and a corresponding increase in implant survival [2, 5-7, 14, 18]. In a prior prospective randomized study, we found that metal-backed (MB) glenoid components had higher rates of complications, loosening and revision than cemented full PE implants [3]. Other authors have recently reported the long-term results of TSA with uncemented MB glenoid components: they also found high rates of glenoid loosening and failure [4, 8, 12, 15, 16]. The aim of this study was to assess the medium to long-term clinical and radiological results of TSA with MB glenoid components in primary OA and to determine the survival rate of this implant. We hypothesized that glenoid resurfacing with a MB implant would not be acceptable in the long term because of loosening and/or accelerated PE wear.

MATERIAL AND METHODS

This is a continuous retrospective multicenter cohort study of patients, with a single aetiology (primary OA), treated with an unconstrained anatomical TSA with uncemented bone-ingrowth MB glenoid component.

Inclusion and Exclusion Criteria

The inclusion criteria were: (1) TSA for the treatment of primary OA implanted by a senior shoulder surgeon; (2) glenoid resurfacing using the same uncemented MB glenoid component (Aequalis shoulder prosthesis, Tornier Inc, Houston, TX, USA); (3) minimum clinical and radiological follow-up of 2 years. The exclusion criteria included: (1) TSA for all others aetiologies; (2) Glenoid resurfacing using cemented full PE glenoid component; (3) follow-up less than 2 years.

Patient Population

Between 1994 and 1999, 178 TSA were implanted for the treatment of primary OA in five orthopaedics centres; 13 patients died or were lost to follow-up leaving 165 TSA. 158 patients (115 females and 43 males) were available for evaluation. At the time of shoulder arthroplasty, the mean age was 68 years [35-89]. Seven patients had surgery on both sides. The dominant arm was operated in 105 cases (64%).

Preoperative Radiographic Status

The presence of primary OA was confirmed in all patients on true antero-posterior [AP], axillary and lateral radiographs. 150 patients (90%) had preoperative CT arthrograms and 5 patients (3%) had preoperative MRI scans to evaluate the status of glenoid bone stock, the presence of rotator cuff tears and the fatty infiltration of the rotator cuff muscles. According to the Walch classification, the glenoid morphology was identified as type A in 72 cases (44%), type B in 75 cases (45%) and type C in 8 cases (5%), [19]. According to the Goutallier classification [9], the global fatty degeneration index [GFDI], evaluated on CT-arthrogram was less than one for 45 shoulders (27%) and one or more in 105 patients (64%).

Operative Technique and Implants

A deltopectoral approach was used in all patients. The subscapularis tendon and anterior capsule were divided at the medial edge of the lesser tuberosity in 154 cases (93%) (i.e. simple tenotomy); the tendon and capsule were detached with a fleck osteotomy of the lesser tuberosity in 11 cases (7%). The long head of the biceps was tenodesed in 86 cases (52%). There were 15 partial tears (9%) and 11 full thickness tears of the supraspinatus (7%).

A third generation anatomical, unconstrained, modular and adaptable humeral component with an uncemented, bone-ingrowth MB glenoid implant (Aequalis shoulder prosthesis, Tornier Inc, Houston, TX, USA) was used in all cases [1, 2]. All stems except two were cemented. The thickness of the glenoid component was 7 mm (3 mm for the metal tray and 4 mm for the PE insert). Two expansion-screws with 3 petals achieved the initial stability of the MB component. The MB component was hydroxyapatite-coated and had a porous surface to allow bone ingrowth (fig. 1). A cancellous bone graft was performed under the tray in 20 cases and a structural bone graft was performed in 2 cases.

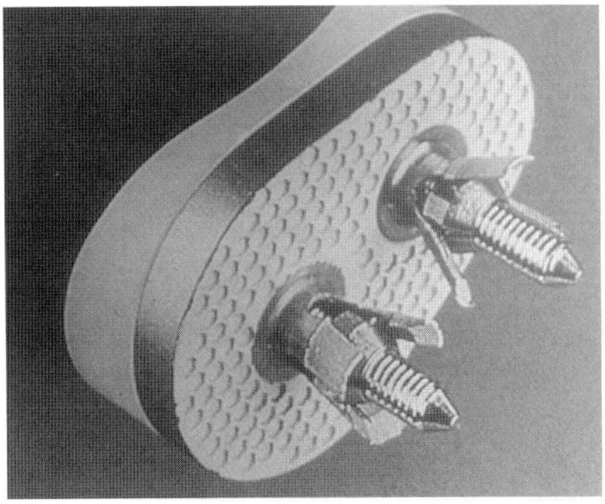

Fig. 1: Uncemented, bone-ingrowth Metal-Back glenoid implant (Aequalis shoulder prosthesis, Tornier Inc, Houston, TX, USA).

Clinical Assessment

Pre- and post-operative assessment included measurement of the active ranges of motion (anterior elevation, external rotation, internal rotation), the Constant score and the normalized Constant score calculated as a percentage of the normal reference value adjusted for age and gender. At the last follow-up, the Subjective Shoulder Value (SSV) was evaluated. Subjective results were also evaluated with the help of the question: are you very satisfied, satisfied, disappointed or dissatisfied with the result obtained with this procedure?

Radiographic Assessment

The immediate postoperative radiographic assessment included: *1)* glenoid vertical positioning as high, centered and low; ***2)*** glenoid vertical tilt as superior, vertical (no tilt) and inferior; ***3)*** expansion screws problems (fracture or not open); ***4)*** humeral reconstruction as anatomic or not.

The postoperative radiographic assessment at last follow up or before revision included: ***1)*** glenoid radiolucent lines in 5 zones (no, <1 mm, [1 mm-2 mm], >2 mm) to calculate the radiolucent lines score [14] (fig. 2); ***2)*** glenoid component migration or tilt (superior, inferior, medialization, anterior or posterior); ***3)*** petal and or tray fractures; ***4)*** PE wear as no, partial or complete (metal/metal contact); ***5)*** luxation or subluxation (anterior or posterior); ***6)*** superior humeral migration; ***7)*** humeral lucent lines in 8 zones (fig. 3).

Definitions

Glenoid loosening was considered to be present if there was either glenoid component migration, a petal or tray fracture or a glenoid radiolucent lines score >10 points [14] (fig. 2).

Polyethylene wear was considered to be present if the thickness between the humeral head prosthesis and the tray of the glenoid implant decreased between postoperative and last follow up on A/P and/or axillary views. PE wear was said to be complete if metal/metal contact was

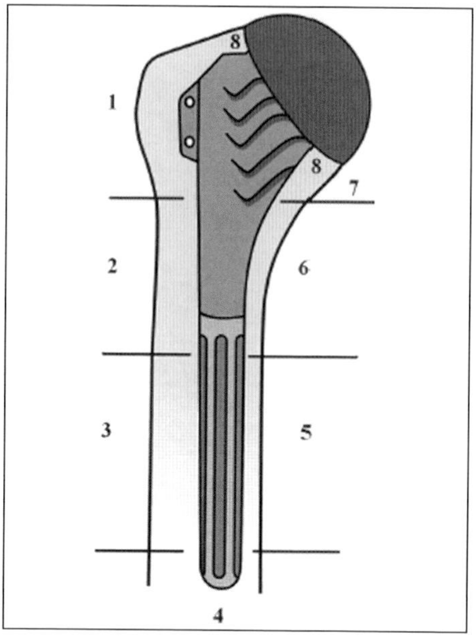

Fig. 3: Humeral radiolucent lines were analyzed on X-ray in 8 zones.

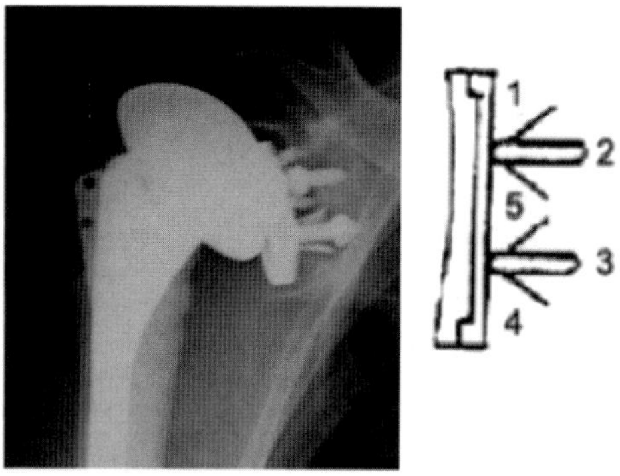

zone	RLL Thickness			points
	< 1 mm	1 – 2 mm	>2 mm	
1			×	3
2			×	3
3			×	3
4			×	3
5			×	3
			total	15/15

Fig. 2: Radiolucent lines were quantified in 5 zones taking into account their thickness. The maximum radiolucent line score was 15 points. Glenoid components with a score superior to 10 points was considered to be loose.

observed either on x-rays or CT scan images (fig. 4) and partial if a space between the humeral head prosthesis and tray component was still visible.

PE dissociation was diagnosed either on x-rays, CT scan images or intraoperatively during revision or reoperation procedures (fig. 4). Only complete PE wear or PE dissociation were considered as complications.

A Subscapularis tear or insufficiency was diagnosed on clinical examination at review in cases of positive lift off test or intraoperatively during revision or reoperation procedures.

A Supraspinatus tear or insufficiency was diagnosed on the A/P radiographic view if there was superior migration of the humeral head or intraoperatively during revision or reoperation procedures. Anterior or posterior instability was diagnosed on the axillary view and/or on CT scan images, if there was posterior or anterior subluxation or luxation of the humeral component (fig. 4).

A revision was defined as surgery with partial or total exchange or removal of the prosthesis.

A reoperation was defined as surgery for a soft tissue problem without exchange of the prosthesis.

Statistical analysis

The distribution of data was analysed with the d'Agostino-Pearson test. The pre- and post-operative data were analyzed for statistically significant differences between means; paired data was compared using a paired *t*-test and unpaired results were compared with the Mann-Whitney test (MWT). The Chi-squared test (Chi2) and Fisher's exact test (FET) for small numbers were used to compare categorical data. The significance level was set at $p=0.05$.

A prosthetic survival curve was constructed with the end point defined as revision of TSA and using 100% confidence intervals (maximal confidence intervals 100% if all patients deceased or

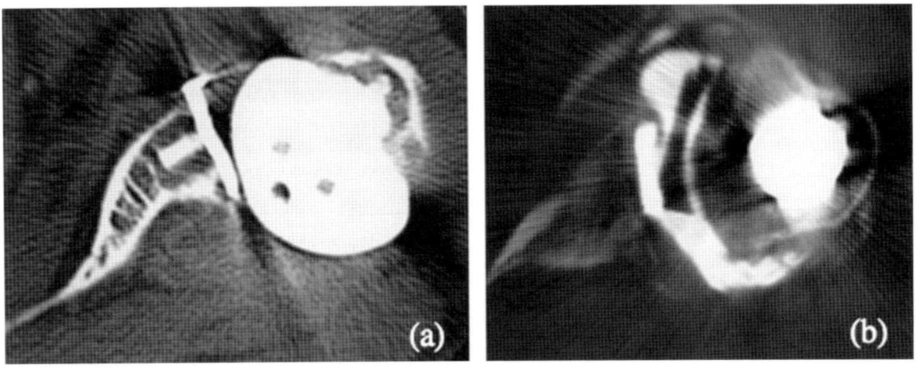

Fig. 4: Example of complete PE wear diagnosed on CT Scan with metal-metal contact (a). Notice posterior wear with recurrence of posterior humeral subluxation. Example of PE dissociation diagnosed on arthro-CT (b).

lost to follow up were considered as not revised and minimal confidence interval 100% if all patients deceased or lost to follow up were considered as revised).

RESULTS

Complications

One hundred and nine TSAs had one or more complication (66%). The complications are summarized in table 1. The two most frequent complications were PE wear or dissociation and glenoid component loosening, occurring respectively in 53% (87/165) and 19% (32/165) of cases. These two complications were rarely found in isolation, rather in association with prosthetic instability, subscapularis tears or insufficiency or supraspinatus tears (table 2). Subscapularis tears or insufficiency were present in 11% of cases (18/165) while supraspinatus tears were also present in 11% of cases. Sixty-six patients required further surgery (40%). A revision was required in 61 (37%) and reoperation was required in 5 patients (3%).

Table 1: Postoperative complications [n=109/165 TSA – (66%)]

Postoperative Complications	Number (%)
PE wear or dissociations	87 (53%)
Glenoid Loosening	32 (19%)
Prosthetic Instability	31 (19%)
- Anterior	6 (4%)
- Posterior	25 (15%)
Subscapularis rupture or insufficiency	18 (11%)
Supraspinatus tear	18 (11%)
Deep infection	2 (1%)
Shoulder stiffness	2 (1%)
Postoperative humeral fracture	1 (<1%)

Revision surgery

Of those arthroplasties experiencing a complication, 61 required a revision procedure. The types of revision procedure are summarized in table 2. Of those patients with isolated soft tissue failures, even if there was no glenoid implant failure, 7 were revised. Five of these arthroplasties were converted to a reverse shoulder arthroplasty because of prosthetic instability and/or a cuff insufficiency problem. One patient had a prosthetic bipolar exchange in combination with subscapularis repair, and the remaining patient had a prosthetic exchange performed for deep infection.

Table 2: Revision surgery procedures

Type of revision	Number of cases (/165)
Conversion to RSA	18 (11%)
Humeral and glenoid replacement	15 (7%)
New glenoid reimplantation - With Humeral head replacement (n=7)	15 (7%)
Glenoid removal & iliac crest bone graft - With Humeral head replacement (n=4)	7 (4%)
Glenoid removal	4 (2%)
New PE inserted on MB	1 (<1%)

Glenoid Implant Failures [n=93 (56%)]

These failures included loosening with or without PE wear in 32 cases (19%) and total PE wear or dissociation without loosening in 61 cases (37%). As already mentioned, glenoid implant failures were often associated with others complications (table 3).

Of the 32 patients with loose glenoid components (fig. 5 & 6), 22 (13%) required further surgery. The mean interval

Table 3: Glenoid implant failures (n=93) and associated complications

	Associated Complications	Number of revisions and reoperations
PE wear Without Loosening **(n= 61)**	Instability (n=14): Post (n=12) – ant (n=2)	**35 (21%)**
	Cuff tears (n=11): subscapularis ruptures (n=8)	
	Deep infection (n=1)	
	Humeral loosening (n=1)	
Glenoid loosening (n=32)	PE wear (n=26)	**22 (13%)**
	Instability (n=7): post (n=6) – ant (n=1)	
	Cuff tears (n=4): subscapularis ruptures (n=2)	
	Stiffness (n=2)	

between primary surgery and revision for glenoid loosening was 86 months [17-141]. Six patients had expansion screw problems (fractured or not open) on immediate postoperative X-ray. Two others patients had early glenoid loosening (in the 2 first years) without expansion screw problems on the immediate postoperative X-ray.

Among the 61 PE failures without glenoid loosening, there were 6 dissociations and 55 cases of total PE wear with metal on metal contact (fig. 4 & 7). Revision was performed in 35 cases (21%). The mean interval between primary surgery and revision for PE wear or dissociation was 78 months [6-152].

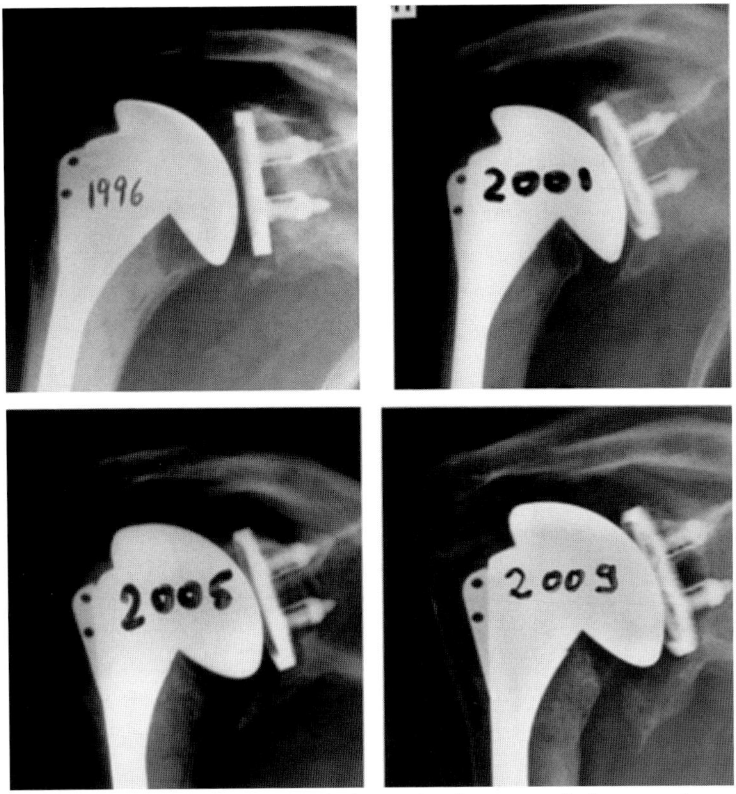

Fig. 5: A rare complication: early loosening because of absence of opening of the metallic petals (i.e. absence of primary fixation) leading to progressive medialization and PE wear.

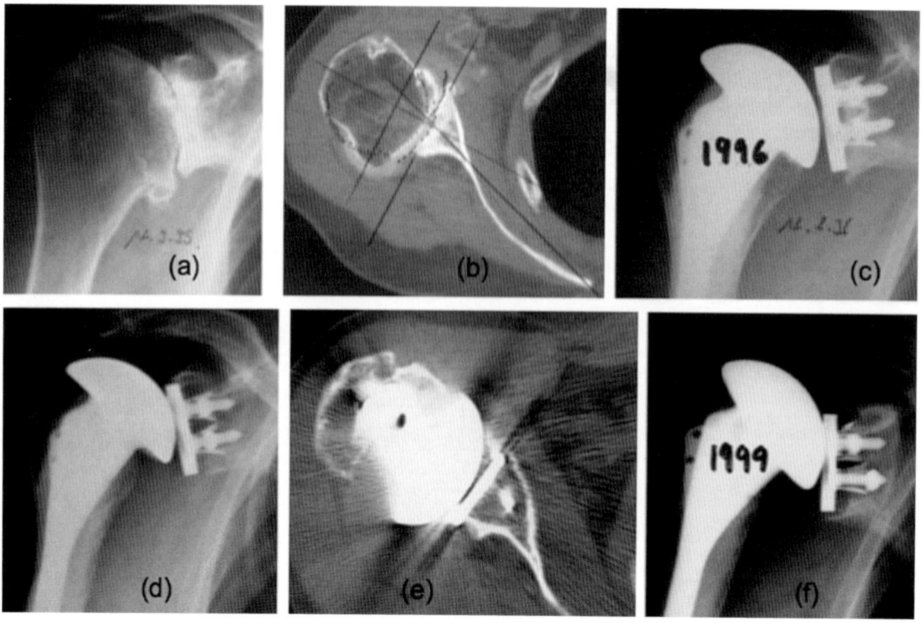

Fig. 6: Example of combined "mechanical" and "biological" loosening secondary to recurrence of posterior subluxation in a B2 glenoid with PE wear debris. Patient with osteoarthritis and glenoid type B2 (a & b) treated by TSA with MB implant (c). At 2 years follow-up, on X-ray (d) there was a recurrence of posterior subluxation (confirmed on CT scan image (e)) leading to eccentric load on PE an accelerated PE wear. At 3 years FU, glenoid component was completely loose. This loosening was associated with humeral proximal lysis in zone 7 and 8 (f) and complete PE wear.

Isolated Soft Tissue Failures without glenoid implant failures [n=16 (10%)]

These failures included all problems without glenoid implant failures. There were 16 TSAs (10%) consisting of 10 cases of prosthetic instability often associated with subscapularis or supraspinatus ruptures or insufficiency, 2 isolated subscapularis tears, 2 rotator cuff tears, one humeral shaft fracture and one deep infection (table 4). The soft tissue failures required 7 revisions (4%) and 2 reoperations. The mean interval between primary surgery and revision or reoperation was 43 months [1-71].

Table 4: Isolated soft tissue complications without glenoid implant failure (n=16) and complications

	Associated Complications and reoperations	Number of revisions
Prosthetic Instability (n=10) Posterior (n=7) Anterior (n=3)	subscapularis ruptures (n=6) supraspinatus tears (n=1)	7
Subscapularis tears or insufficiency (n=2)		1
Supraspinatus tears (n=2)		
Deep infection (n=1)		1
Postoperative humeral fracture		0

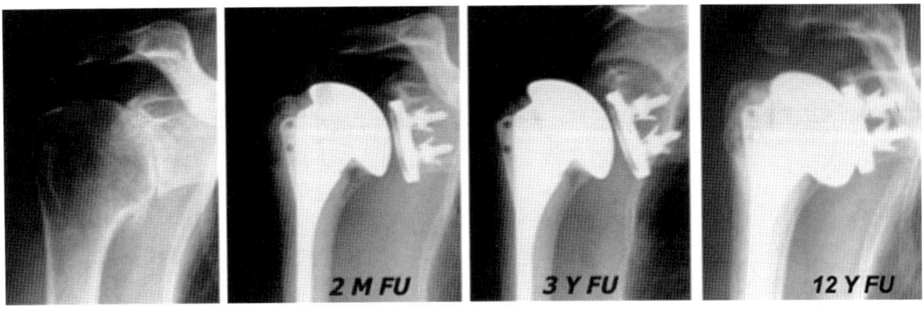

Fig. 7: Example of evolution of PE wear with times: at 12 y follow-up, complete PE wear (metal/metal contact) without glenoid loosening.

Radiological results on the humeral side

Radiolucent lines on the humeral side were diagnosed in 65 cases (39%). They were more frequent in zones 8, 7 and 1 (table 5 - fig. 3 & 6). Radiolucent lines and osteolysis of proximal humerus in zones 7 and 8 were significantly more frequent in the subgroup of patients with complete PE wear with or without glenoid loosening than in the subgroup of patients without PE wear ($p < 0,05$ FET).

Prosthetic survival curve

The rate of prosthetic survival (end point = revision) was 60% [44-71%] and 46% [32-54%] at 10 and 12 years respectively (fig. 8).

Functional results

The functional results are summarized in table 6. They were evaluated in the 104 shoulders that still retained their implant at the last follow-up. The mean follow up was 102 months [24-191]. There were statistically significant improvements in all measures of active range of motion and in all parameters of the Constant score (fig. 9). The mean postoperative SSV was 78% [range 40- 100%]. Of the patients who had their TSA in place, 76% (79/104) were still satisfied or very satisfied with their result.

Table 5: RLL around the humeral component (in 8 zones)

Humeral RLL	All patients	Patients with PE wear	Patients without PE wear
Zone 1	**10**	**6**	**4**
Zone 2	3	2	1
Zone 3	2	2	1
Zone 4	2	2	0
Zone 5	2	2	0
Zone 6	2	2	0
Zone 7	**24**	**19**	**5**
Zone 8	**65**	**47**	**18**

Table 6: Functional results in the 104 patients with TSA still in place at last FU (102 months [24-191])

	Preoperative	Postoperative	P Value (test)
Active Mobility			
Active Anterior Elevation (°)	88 ± 26 (30 to 170)	140 ± 27 (70 to 180)	< 0.0001 (MWT)
Active External Rotation (°)	5 ± 15 (-30 to 50)	35 ± 19 (-10 to 70)	< 0.0001 (MWT)
Constant Score			
Pain / 15 points	4.2 ± 1.8 (0 to 8)	12.5 +/- 3.1 (4 to 15)	< 0.0001 (MWT)
Activities / 20 points	7.2 ±- 2.7 0 to 14	15.9 ±- 4.5 (3 to 20)	< 0.0001 (MWT)
Range of motion / 40 points	13.6 ± 6.5 (0 to 28)	29.4 ± 9 (4 to 40)	<0.0001 (MWT)
Strength / 25 points	2.7 ± 3.1 (0 to 14)	7.1 ± 4.8 (0 to 25)	<0.0001 (MWT)
Absolute Constant Score /100 points	**27.6 ± 10.2 (6 to 52)**	**64.9 ± 17.8 (17 to 96)**	<0.0001 (MWT)
Adjusted Constant Score (%)	38 ± 24 (9 to 73)	94 ± 25.8 (20 to 136)	<0.0001 (MWT)

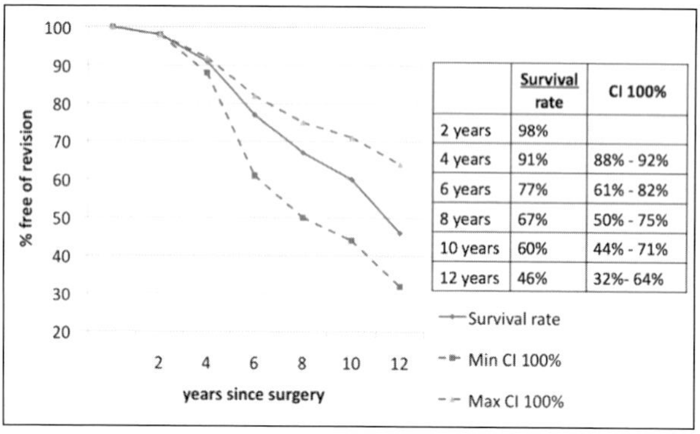

Fig. 8: Survival curve of TSA with uncemented MB implant in primary OA. The end point was partial or total revision of shoulder prosthesis component. Max CI 100% if all patients deceased or lost of follow up were considered as not revised. Min CI 100% if all patients deceased or lost of follow up were considered as revised.

Prognostic Factors

No correlation was found between the occurrence of complications and/or revision and the following parameters: gender, dominant or non dominant side, supraspinatus tears, rotator cuff muscle fatty infiltration, postoperative glenoid positioning, humeral component positioning and humeral head size.

There were more complications and more revisions in the subgroup of type B glenoids but these differences were not significant. Posterior subluxation at last follow-up was significantly more frequent in the type B glenoid subgroup (16/75) than in the type A subgroup (4/72) (p=0,007). Revisions in type B glenoid subgroup were earlier than in the type A subgroup (p=0,05) (table 7).

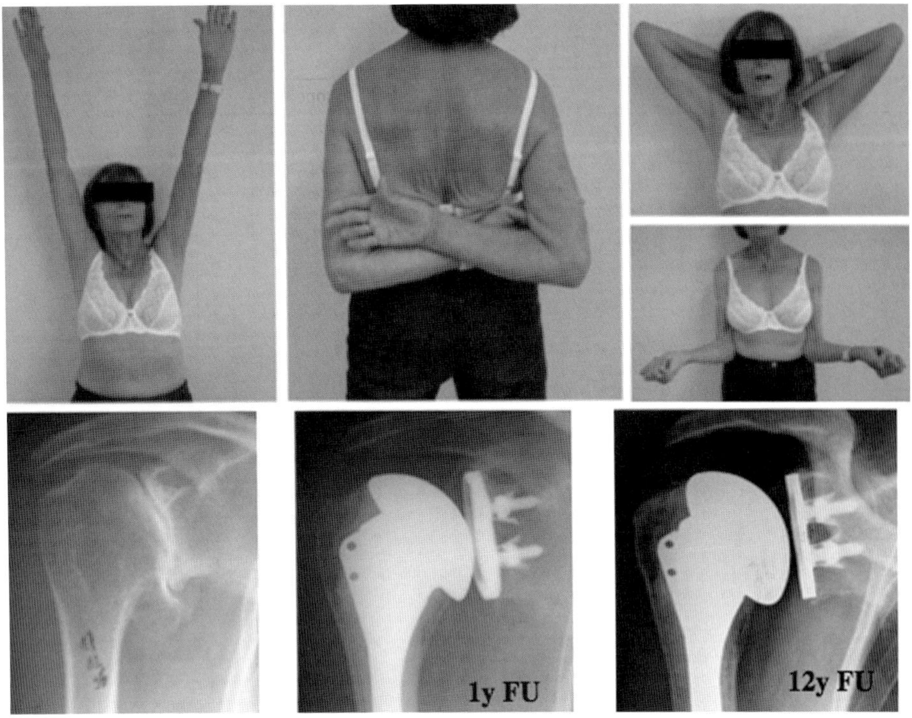

Fig. 9: Example of good clinical and radiological results at 12 y follow-up: minimal PE wear and secure bone fixation of the MB implant (no radiolucent line).

Table 7: Influence of glenoid type on complication, prosthetic posterior instability and revision rates

	Glenoid type A n=72	Glenoid type B N=75	P value (Test)
Complications (Nb)	42 (58%)	54 (72%)	0,15 (Chi2)
Revisions (Nb)	22 (30%)	33 (44%)	0,13 (Chi2)
Postoperative posterior instability	4 (5,5%)	16 (21%)	0,007 (FET)
Delay of revision (months)	92 [31-141]	73[17-152]	0,05 (t-test)

Patients with complications were younger (66.7 y [35-83]/70.9 y [43-89]) than patients without complications (p=0.03). Revised patients were younger (65.3 [35-80]/69,7 [43-89]) than those not revised (p=0.005).

DISCUSION

The results of this study confirm our hypothesis: TSA with MB glenoid resurfacing in primary OA is not acceptable in the long term because of accelerated polyethylene wear and glenoid loosening. We found an unexpected 10% (16/165) rate of isolated soft tissue complications without glenoid implant failure. Indeed, respectively at 10 and 12 years follow-up, 40 and 54% of the prostheses had already been revised. At the last follow-up, 56% of the patients (93/165) had experienced glenoid component failure including glenoid loosening in 32 cases and PE wear or dissociations in 61 cases.

There is a paucity of studies that address the results of uncemented glenoid MB component in TSA [3-7, 12, 13, 15, 16, 18]. Most reports are of small series with short follow-up [8, 12, 15, 16]. The results of these studies report a survival rate at 10 years of between 72 and 85% (end point = revision) and are summarized in table 8. Our 10-years survivorship was 60%; this lower survival rate can be partially explained by the higher rate of PE wear found in our series. The PE thickness of our implant was less than in other implant designs, specifically in the middle of the PE insert because of the use of flat metal-back tray.

We did not find any prognostic factors for complication and/or revision except age at surgery. Our high rate of complications (66%) probably explains the absence of real prognostic factors. In contrast to Martin [12], we did not find any influence due to male gender. In our previous study [3], MB glenoid components were revised in three patients with a type B2 glenoid, as a result of recurrent posterior humeral subluxation. This study at long-term follow-up shows a higher rate of revision and complications in patients with type B glenoids but this difference was not significant. However, revision surgery was performed at an earlier stage in patients with type B glenoids. The recurrence of posterior instability promotes glenoid implant failure and was more frequent in our series in patients with type B glenoids (table 7).

Table 8: Published series of TSA with glenoid MB implant. (RLL = Radiolucent Lines; PE = Polyethylene; TSA = Total Shoulder Arthroplasty; POA = Primary Osteoarthritis)

References	Number TSA – Number POA	Type of implant	Nb of Glenoid Loosening (GL) and PE wear	Radiological failure criteria	End points	Survival rate (%) and delay
Martin SD. JBJS Am. 2006 [11]	140 TSA – 70 POA	Kirschner II-C	- 16 GL (with 9 PE wear) were revised - 21 TSA had radiological failure not revised	- Screw or tray fracture - Migration or shift of the implant - Progressive RLL ≥ 2 mm in 2 or 3 zones around keel or consecutive zones.	Partial or total revision	85% at 10 years
					Radiological failure	76% at 10 years
Taunton MJ, Cofield RH. JBJS Am. 2008. [15]	83 TSA – 74 POA	Cofield 1 MB	- 9 GL and 15 PE wear were revised - 30 PE wear and 50 TSA had radiological failure	- Migration or tilt of the implant - Complete RLL and some parts of it was ≥ 1.5 mm for glenoid component - RLL ≥ 2 mm in 3 or more zones for humeral implant	Partial or total revision	78,5 % at 10 years
					Revision and /or radiological failure	51,9 % at 10 years
Fox TJ, Cofield RH. JSES 2009 [7]	316 TSA – 227 POA	Cofield 1 MB	- 24 GL and 23 PE wear were revised		Revision	79% at 10 years 67% at 15 years
Rosenberg N, Wallace AW. BMC Musculo. Dis. 2007. [14]	90 TSA – 48 POA	Biomodular	- 13 GL and 9 PE wear or dissociation were revised		Revision	72% at 10 years

This study confirms our initial concern [3]. Accelerated PE wear was the major complication encountered with MB implants (53%) in our series. It can be related to at least 5 factors, as explained in our previous study: ***1)*** Insufficient thickness of the PE insert (4 mm at the periphery but 3.2 mm in the center) compared to a standard full PE cemented glenoid component (5 mm); ***2)*** The excessive thickness of the glenoid component in MB glenoid may over-tension the soft tissues and increase load on the glenoid; ***3)*** The rigidity resulting from the metal back may also be responsible for accelerated wear of the PE insert due to changes in load transference; ***4)*** Recurrent posterior instability leads to posterior eccentric loading on the PE surface responsible for accelerated posterior PE wear; ***5)*** subscapularis ruptures or insufficiency (and cuff tears) result in eccentric loading and instability in a similar manner to that for recurrent posterior instability.

Glenoid loosening of MB implants is also a concern. It is important to differentiate glenoid loosening into 2 types: ***1)*** the absence of primary fixation (i.e. mechanical loosening), in cases where the petals have fractured or failed to open on the immediate postoperative X-rays or in cases where early loosening has occurred (fig. 5); ***2)*** loosening as a result of PE wear debris and osteolysis (i.e. biological loosening) (fig. 6).

Both glenoid loosening and accelerated wear of PE were often associated with soft tissue problems (subscapularis tear or insufficiency, supraspinatus tear) and/or prosthetic instability. Supraspinatus tears associated with proximal migration of the humerus are equivalent to the aging process of the rotator cuff in the elderly. Subscapularis tears or insufficiency are direct consequences of the anterior arthrotomy and arthrolysis performed during prosthetic implantation. Repair of the subscapularis after tenotomy is difficult, especially at the inferior part, which is mainly muscular. We have switched to using a technique of fleck osteotomy of the subscapularis from the lesser tuberosity instead of tenotomy. We have also become less aggressive in performing the subscapularis release as an extensive release performed as part of "soft tissue balancing" undoubtedly results in the denervation of part of the muscle-tendon unit. Finally, the high rate of prosthetic instability found in the present series is a concern. Posterior instability may be observed in two circumstances: ***1)*** in cases of recurrent posterior subluxation in type B2 glenoids and ***2)*** in cases of subscapularis tears or insufficiency. Anterior instability is also a consequence of subscapularis tear or insufficiency.

There are some limitations to our study. It is a retrospective multicenter cohort study and there is no control group. The true prevalence of subscapularis failures is probably underestimated. In contrast to previous published series, the present study has several notable strengths. Firstly, the group of TSA is homogenous with a single diagnosis, primary OA. Secondly, the number of cases is relatively large. Thirdly, the inclusion and exclusion criteria were strictly respected and all patients were reviewed with a minimum follow up of 2 years. Fourthly, the dropout rate was extremely low for a clinical study, with only 13 patients (13/178) lost to follow up or died in the study period.

In conclusion, TSA with metal-back glenoid resurfacing is not a viable long-term therapeutic option for the treatment of primary OA because of unacceptable rates of glenoid component failure requiring revision. At 12 years follow-up, 54% of the prostheses had been revised either for glenoid loosening (n=21), complete wear of PE without loosening (n=33) or isolated prosthetic instability (n=10). Complete wear of PE with or without MB glenoid loosening is the principal complication, present in 53% (87/165) of cases. PE wear appears to be the main limiting factor for the use of MB implants in anatomical shoulder replacement. Such a high rate of PE wear confirms the presence of high shearing forces on the glenoid component surface in anatomical shoulder replacement.

REFERENCES

[1] BOILEAU P, WALCH G. The three-dimensional geometry of the proximal humerus: Implications for surgical technique and prosthetic design. *J Bone Joint Surg 1997;79-B, 5, 857-65.*

[2] BOILEAU P, AVIDOR C, WALCH G. Prothèse totale d'épaule avec un implant glenoiddien métallique non-scellé: etude prospective de 354 implants suivis à plus de 2 ans. In: 2000 shoulder prostheses two to ten years follow-up. G. Walch, P. Boileau, D. Molé. *Sauramps medical, Montpellier, 2001:p 489-507.*

[3] BOILEAU P, AVIDOR C, KRISHNAN SG, WALCH G, KEMPF JF, MOLÉ D. Cemented polyethylene versus uncemented metal-backed glenoid components in total shoulder arthroplasty: a prospective, double-blind, randomized study. *J Shoulder Elbow Surg 2002;11: 351-9.*

[4] CHEUNG EV, SPERLING JW, COFIELD RH. Polyethylene insert exchange for wear after total shoulder arthroplasty. *J Shoulder Elbow Surg. 2007;16: 574-8.*

[5] COFILED RH. Uncemented total shoulder arthroplasty: a review. *Clin Orthop 1994; 307:86-93.*

[6] COFIELD RH, DLAY P. Total shoulder arthroplasty with a tissue ingrowth glenoid component. *J Shoulder Elbow Surg 1992;1: 77-85.*

[7] FALUDI DD, WEILAND AJ. Cementless total shoulder arthroplasty: preliminary experiences with thirteen cases. *Orthopaedics. 1983;6: 413-7.*

[8] FOX TJ, CIL A, SPERLING JW, SANCHEZ-SOTELO J, SCHLECK CD, COFIELD RH. Survival of the glenoid component in shoulder arthroplasty. *J Shoulder Elbow Surg 2009;18: 859-63.*

[9] GODENÈCHE A, BOILEAU P, FAVARD L, LE HUEC JC, LÉVIGNE C, NOVÉ-JOSSERAND L, WALCH G, EDWARDS B. Prosthetic replacement in the treatment of osteoarthritis of the shoulder. Eraly results of 268 cases. *J Shoulder Elbow Surg 2002;11: 11-8.*

[10] GOUTALLIER D, POSTEL JM, GLEYZE P, LEGUILLOUX P, VAN DRIESSCHE S. Influence of cuff muscle fatty degeneration on anatomic and functional outcomes after simple suture of full-thickness tears. *J Shoulder Elbow Surg 2003;12: 550-4.*

[11] KEMPF JF, WALCH G, LACAZE F. Results of shoulder arthroplasty in primary glenohumeral osteoarthritis. In: Walch G, Boileau P, editors. Shoulder arthroplasty. *Berlin: Springer-Verlag; 1999. P 141-6.*

[12] MARTIN SD, ZURAKOWSKI D, THORNHILL TS. Uncemented Glenoid Component in Total Shoulder Arthroplasty – Survivorship and outcomes. *J Bone Joint Surg Am. 2006;87: 1284-92.*

[13] Mc ELWAIN JP, ENGLISH E. The early results of porous-coated total shoulder arthroplasty. *Clin Orthop Relat Res. 1987;218: 217-24.*

[14] MOLÉ D, ROCHE O, RIAND N, *et al.* Cemented glenoid component: results in osteoarthritis and rheumatoid arthritis. In: Walch G, Boileau P, *editors. Shoulder arthroplasty. Berlin: Springer-Verlag; 1999. P 163-71.*

[15] ROSENBERG N, NEUMANN L, MODI A, MERSICH IJ, WALLACE AW. Improvements in survival of the uncemented Nottingham Total Shoulder prosthesis: a prospective comparative study. *BMC Musculoskeletal Disorders 2007;76: 1-11.*

[16] TAUNTON MJ, McINTOSH AL, SPERLING JW, COFIELD RH. Total Shoulder Arthroplasty with a Metal-Backed Bone-Ingrowth Glenoid Component – Medium to Long-term results. *J Bone Joint Surg Am. 2008;90: 2180-8.*

[17] TORCHIA ME, COFIELD RH, SETTERGEN CR. Total shoulder arthroplasty with the Neer prosthesis: long-term results. *J Shoulder Elbow Surg 1997;6: 495-505.*

[18] WALCH G, BOILEAU P, RIAN N. Results of a new uncemented glenoid component. In: Walch G, Boileau P, *editors. Shoulder arthroplasty. Berlin: Springer-Verlag; 1999. P 173-6.*

[19] WALCH G, BADET R, BOULAHIA A, KHOURY A. Morphologic study of the glenoid in primary glenohumeral osteoarthritis. *J Arthroplasty 1999;14: 756-60.*

FACTORS FOR PROPER EXPOSURE, PREPARATION AND CEMENTING TECHNIQUE OF THE GLENOID IMPLANT

M. LOEW, D. GAZIELLY, P. RAISS, G. PAPE

Proper implantation technique and a standardised cementing technique in the case of all-polyethylene glenoid components seems to be crucial for good function and long-term stability of the implant.

Exposure of the glenoid, especially in deformities of type B2 and C in Walch's classification, is a surgical challenge, which frequently leads to malpositioning of the implant, particularly at the posterior surface. Subperiostal subscapularis release at its humeral insertion and a 360-degree capsulotomy adjacent to the glenoid cavitiy can facilitate proper access to the working area.

Gazielly in 2003 introduced the cancellous compaction technique for glenoid replacement, without reaming of the medullary keel slot, leading to primary implant stability.

In a report on 30 shoulder arthroplasties 32 months after implantation, radiolucent lines were absent in 33%, incomplete in 53%, and complete in 14%.

Cementing technique has changed distinctly in the last decade, starting from simple manual stuffing to a sophisticated vacuum and pressurisation technique. Factors related by the patient seem to play a major role in glenoid stability as much as design considerations do.

It has been proposed that bone mineral density has an influence on cement penetration in hip and knee arthroplasty. The hypotheses of an experimental study, performed in our institution, is the existence of a negative correlation between bone mineral density (BMD) and cement penetration in cemented glenoid components, and that implant design has an influence on cement penetration and on primary stability of the implants.

The BMD of ten pairs of fresh frozen scapulas was measured. Micro-CT scans in three different sections were analyzed after implantation of cemented keeled and pegged glenoid components. Cement penetration was analyzed and correlated with BMD. Pull-out strength testing was performed to analyze primary stability.

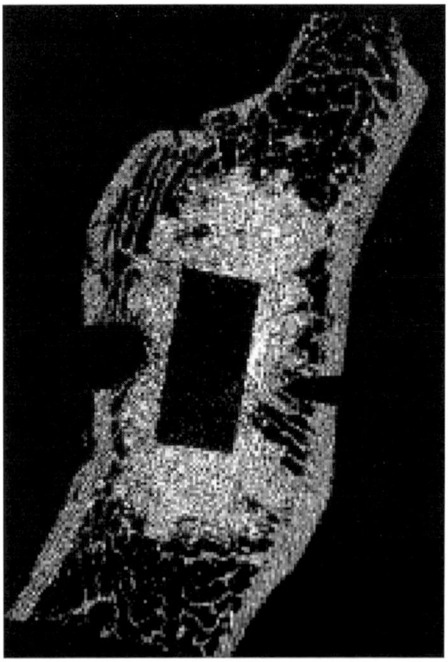

Fig. 1: Cement penetration in keeled glenoids

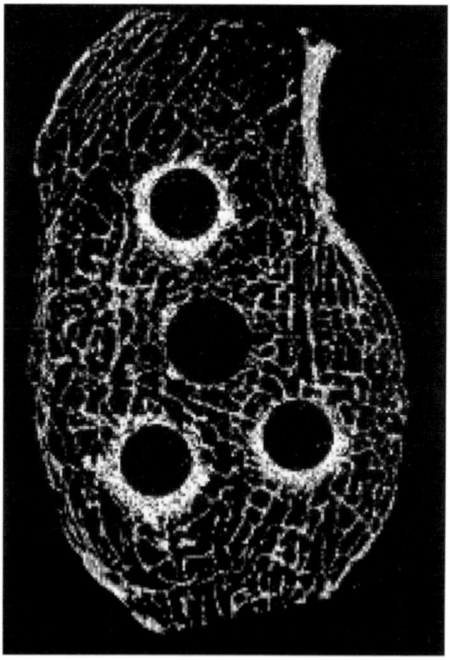

Fig. 2: Cement penetration in pegged glenoids

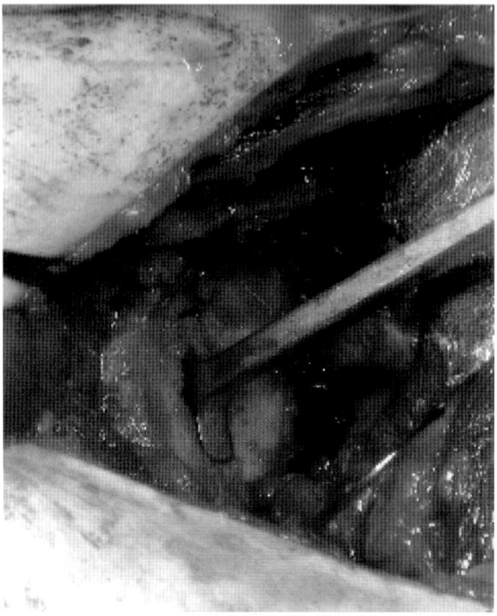

Fig. 3: Cement pressurization with a syringe

The overall peak BMD was 0.6 g/cm^2 (range 0.33-0.98). A strong negative correlation between overall BMD and mean cement penetration was found for the pegged group (r^2 = -0.83; $p<0.003$) and for the keeled group (r^2 = -0.81; $p<0.005$). Mean cement penetration was 78.4 (range 60.6-94.2) mm^2 in the keeled group and 113.9 (range 78.2-143.4) mm^2 in the pegged group ($p<0.0001$). In all cases the components were pulled-out of the cement mantle whereas the bone-cement interfaces remained intact. The mean pull-out strength was 1093N (764 - 1343N) for keeled and 884N (650 - 1264N) for pegged components ($p<0.05$).

Bone mineral density is negatively correlated to cement penetration into the glenoid. Implant design (pegged vs. keeled) has an influence on cement penetration with higher areas for pegged implants. In contrast, pull-out strength is higher in the keeled group. However, the failure mechanism in all implants (pegged and keeled) takes place uniformly at the implant-cement interface. Therefore, one could suppose that a modern cementing technique *in vivo*, leading to deep bonding between bone and cement, is crucial to prevent loosening in the long-term. Finally, the findings of this study might be helpful to the right choice of implant, especially in the elderly patient with osteoporotic bone.

RADIOGRAPHIC COMPARISON OF PEGGED AND KEELED GLENOID COMPONENTS USING MODERN CEMENTING TECHNIQUES:

A PROSPECTIVE RANDOMIZED STUDY

T.B. EDWARDS, J.E. LABRIOLA, R.J. STANLEY,
D.P. O'CONNOR, H.A. ELKOUSY, G.M. GARTSMAN

Background
Modern cementing techniques have improved glenoid fixation, reduced glenoid lucency seen with keeled components, and may eliminate differences attributable to glenoid design. The purpose of this study was to determine the effect of glenoid design on immediate and follow-up radiographic lucency of pegged and keeled glenoid components, using modern cementing techniques.

Material and methods
Fifty-three total shoulder arthroplasties were performed in patients with primary glenohumeral osteoarthritis. Patients were randomized prospectively to receive either a pegged or keeled glenoid component. Three raters graded radiographic glenoid lucencies.

Results
On immediate radiographs, there was no significant difference in the rate of glenoid lucency between pegged (0%) and keeled (15%) glenoid components (P = .128). However, after an average of 26 months, the rate of glenoid lucency was significantly higher in patients with keeled components (46%) compared to patients with pegged components (15%) (P = .003).

Conclusion
Even with modern cementing techniques, pegged glenoid components remain radiographically superior to keeled glenoid components.

Level of evidence
Level I, Randomized Clinical Trial, Treatment study.

Keywords
Shoulder; arthroplasty; reconstruction; adult; osteoarthritis; cement; component loosening.

Glenoid loosening is the most common indication for revision total shoulder arthroplasty [9, 11, 12, 16, 25, 31, 32] and loosening has been correlated with the development of glenoid radiographic lucency [2, 3, 5, 14, 20, 27]. In a study by Torchia *et al*, early radiolucent lines were present in 93% of glenoid components that eventually developed radiographic loosening, whereas similar lines were present in only 44% of glenoid components that did not develop radiographic loosening [27].

Several biomechanical, animal, and retrospective studies have implicated glenoid design in the development of glenoid lucency, stating the superiority of pegged over keeled glenoid components [15, 16, 18, 28, 31]. In a prospective, randomized study with early cementing techniques, Gartsman et al also demonstrated the superiority of pegged glenoid components in the immediate postoperative period [8]. On postoperative radiographs, the rate of lucency was significantly higher in patients with keeled components (39%) than the rate of lucency (5%) observed with pegged components, $P = .026$ [8].

Modern cementing techniques, however, have improved glenoid fixation and have reduced the rate and extent of glenoid lucency seen with keeled components [15, 20, 24, 26]. Utilizing improved cementing techniques including burr curettage, lavage, glenoid drying, and cement pressurization, Norris and Lachiewicz found a lower frequency of radiolucent lines on immediate postoperative radiographs than previously reported with older techniques [24]. After an average follow-up period of 5 years, a decrease in early radiolucent lines was associated with improved survivorship (97% at 5 years, 93% at 8 years) and a low rate of component loosening (6%) [24]. Szabo *et al.* demonstrated improved radiolucent line scores using glenoid preparation and cementing with compaction of the cancellous bone of the glenoid compared to burr curettage [26]. On immediate postoperative radiographs, glenoids prepared with the compaction technique had a lower rate of glenoid lucencies around the keel (11%) than the glenoids prepared with the curettage technique (38%) [26]. Furthermore, the glenoids prepared with the compaction technique showed a decreased rate of progression of the radiolucent lines after 2 years of follow-up [26]. With these modern cementing techniques, the difference in glenoid lucency between pegged and keeled glenoid components may be minimized or eliminated.

The purpose of this study was to determine the effect of glenoid design on the immediate and mid-term follow-up radiographic lucency of pegged and keeled glenoid components using modern cementing techniques. With improved glenoid preparation and cementing techniques, our hypothesis was that there would be minimal or no difference in radiographic lucency between pegged and keeled glenoid components on immediate and follow-up radiographs.

MATERIALS AND METHODS

Subjects

The study was approved by our institutional review board. Patients were recruited to participate by their surgeon and indicated their willingness to participate by signing informed consent. This study was a prospective, randomized trial. The patients were not told which glenoid component design they had received. Patients undergoing total shoulder arthroplasty were included in this study if they had a diagnosis of primary glenohumeral osteoarthritis and a glenoid that did not require bone grafting. In addition, all patients in this study had a complete preoperative radiographic assessment, including an anteroposterior radiograph and computed tomographic arthrography, for evaluation of the rotator cuff and morphologic features of the glenoid. Glenoid morphology was classified according to the classification of Walch *et al.* [29].

To maintain a pure series of patients with primary osteoarthritis, patients with an inflammatory arthropathy in their shoulder (rheumatoid arthritis, systemic lupus erythematosis, ankylosing spondylitis), osteochondromatosis, acromegaly, Paget's disease, postinfectious arthropathy, skeletal dysplasia, neurologic problems (Charcot arthropathy, Parkinson's disease), and osteonecrosis were excluded. Patients with a history of shoulder trauma (fracture or soft tissue injury), instability (surgically or nonsurgically treated), or prior shoulder surgery also were excluded. Finally, patients with marked rotator cuff disorders of their shoulder, as indicated by acromiohumeral arthritis, a massive rotator cuff tear, or a rotator cuff tear involving the infraspinatus or subscapularis, also were excluded because the etiology of their shoulder disease might not have been primary glenohumeral osteoarthritis.

A power analysis conducted prior to the study (5 X 2 Chisquare test, 1-tailed $\alpha = 0.05$, $\beta \leq 0.20$), $\Delta^2 = 0.14$, $\pi_0 = 0.20$, $V[\pi 0] = 0.02$) determined that at least 18 patients per group would be required to identify an average difference of 1 lucency grade (see below) between the pegged and keeled glenoid components to obtain a power of greater than 80%. Fifty patients (53 shoulders) with average age of 69 ± 11 years were enrolled in this study. The additional shoulders (beyond 18 in each group) were enrolled to ensure the study would have sufficient power should patients be lost to follow-up. Twenty-six shoulders were randomized to receive a pegged glenoid component and 27 shoulders were randomized to receive a keeled glenoid component; all patients received the component to which they were randomized. A simple randomization technique using a random numbers table (odd = pegged, even = keeled) with glenoid component type placed in sealed envelopes was employed. The design of the glenoid component, pegged versus keeled, was determined by opening a randomly selected envelope immediately preoperatively without any specific indication.

Surgical procédure

Fifty-three total shoulder arthroplasties were performed on patients with primary glenohumeral osteoarthritis who agreed to participate in this study over a 1-year period from December of 2004 to December of 2005. All patients in this series underwent primary total shoulder arthroplasty by a single surgeon using the Aequalis prosthesis (Tornier, Mont Bonnot, France). A standard deltopectoral approach was employed in all cases. A subscapularis tenotomy was performed at the anatomic neck of the humerus. The subscapularis tendon was mobilized by releasing the glenohumeral ligaments and glenohumeral capsule. Next, the humeral head was dislocated and peripheral osteophytes were removed. The humeral head cut was made along the anatomic neck of the humerus. The humerus was prepared to accept a press fit prosthesis. Six different size prosthetic humeral head diameters, varying between 39 and 50 mm, were used.

Attention was then turned toward implantation of the glenoid component. Following creation of a centering hole, the glenoid face was prepared with a concentric reamer chosen in relation to the glenoid component size. Four different size glenoid components were used with radii of curvature of 23.5, 26.5, 28, and 30.5 mm. The goal of reaming was to remove any residual articular cartilage, correct deformity detected on the preoperative computed tomographic arthrography, and create a congruent base for the convex back glenoid component. Glenoid biconcavity was corrected to physiologic version as judged by when the surgeon had corrected the biconcavity through reaming.

In 27 shoulders, a keeled glenoid component was used. The convex-back, polyethylene, pear-shaped glenoid component used 252 T.B. Edwards et al. in this study was equipped with a keel that is 4 mm thick and 15 mm in length and designed for cementation into the medullary canal of the glenoid. The dimensions of the keel are the same for all glenoid component sizes. During glenoid preparation, the keel slot was created using a drill and instrumented guides to assure proper size and position of the slot. The glenoid keel slot was prepared using the "compaction" technique developed by Gazielly and described by Boileau *et al.* [3] Rather than removing cancellous bone, the glenoid component was implanted after the cancellous bone was compacted with a glenoid punch of the same dimensions as the keel. In 26 shoulders, a pegged glenoid component with 1 central peg and 3 peripheral pegs was used. A peripheral hole drill guide was inserted into the previously made centering hole and the 3 peripheral holes were drilled to the same dimensions as the pegs. The pegged component has small flutes cut into the pegs to allow for interdigitation of the cement. Furthermore, the back of the component is textured to allow further interdigitation, as the cement extrudes out of the drilled holes and contacts the back of the component during component impaction. The interdigitation of cement in the cancellous bone and in the texturing of the pegs and back of the component hold the component in place.

Cementing was performed with modern pressurization techniques [24]. The prepared glenoid was cleansed of blood and bone fragments with saline solution lavage followed by sponge drying [6]. Cement was introduced under pressure using a catheter tip syringe. No cement was placed between the back of the glenoid component and the glenoid bone. The glenoid component was then impacted, further pressurizing the cement into the cancellous bone, and manually held until the cement polymerized. The final humeral component was placed, the subscapularis was closed using transosseous and transtendinous sutures, and the wound was closed in layers.

Postoperatively, the patients were placed in a standard sling. After 1 week, aquatic therapy rehabilitation was initiated to begin shoulder range of motion in elevation, extension, horizontal adduction, internal rotation, and external rotation [19]. External rotation was limited to neutral for 4 weeks. After at least 5 weeks of hydrotherapy, if acceptable range of motion was gained, patients graduated to a self-directed land based program. Strengthening exercises were not prescribed.

Radiographic lucency

Radiographs were obtained within 7 days of the surgical procedure and then yearly during the follow-up period. All radiographs in this series were obtained using a standardized fluoroscopic and magnification controlled technique to ensure that the x-ray beam was perpendicular to the plane of the bone-implant interface, as determined by the use of a wire embedded in the polyethylene [13]. Radiographic lucency of the keeled glenoid components was graded according to criteria previously described by Franklin *et al.* [7] and the pegged components were graded according to the modification described by Lazarus *et al.* [18]. The keeled and pegged components were graded between 0 and 5. A grade of 0 or 1 was considered negligible glenoid lucency (Tables I and II).

The radiographs were analyzed with a digital radiographic viewer (SwissVision Workstation; SwissRay, East Brunswick, NJ), which allowed manipulation of the image for optimal evaluation, thus obviating imprecisions related to image magnification as may occur with plain film radiographs [10]. The uncompressed DICOM images were viewed on high-resolution monitors at a single viewing station in the clinic under standard flourescent ambient lighting and free from glare. Any radiolucencies were measured with the digital caliper within the radiographic viewer. The radiographs were evaluated by 3 raters who independently graded the radiographs for each of the patients in this study. All immediate postoperative radiographs were evaluated by each rater at a single sitting within a single day; the follow-up radiographs were also evaluated by each rater at a single sitting on a different day to avoid "side-by-side" comparisons of a patient's 2 radiographs. The final lucency grade used in data analysis was the grade assigned independently by at least 2 of the 3 raters (ie, a single discordant grade was ignored). In no case did all 3 raters disagree on the lucency grade.

Table I: Grading system for keeled glenoid components

1 Radiolucency - at inferior and/or - superior flange
2 Incomplete - radiolucency at keel
3 Complete - radiolucency (≤ 2 mm wide) - around keel
4 Complete - radiolucency (≥ 2 mm wide) - around keel
5 Gross loosening

Table II: Grading system for pegged glenoid components

1 Incomplete - radiolucency around 1 or 2 pegs
2 Complete - radiolucency (≤ 2 mm wide) - around 1 peg only, - with or without - incomplete radiolucency around 1 other peg
3 Complete - radiolucency (≤ 2 mm wide) - around 2 or more pegs
4 Complete - radiolucency (≥ 2 mm wide) - around 2 or more pegs
5 Gross loosening

Statistical analysis

The Chi-squared test was used to evaluate the effect of glenoid component design on immediate and follow-up radiographs. Chi-squared tests were also used to evaluate whether glenoid component groups differed with respect to age, gender, shoulder dominance, humeral head size, glenoid component size, mismatch of radius of curvature between the glenoid and humeral components, or glenoid morphology. Chi-squared tests were also used to evaluate whether age, gender, shoulder dominance, glenoid morphology, humeral head size, glenoid component size, or glenohumeral mismatch were related to immediate and follow-up postoperative radiolucency of the glenoid component. Statistical significance was set at $P = .05$. Interobserver reliability was evaluated using intraclass correlation coefficients of Shrout and Fleiss type, which estimates the consistency of the composite lucency scores for these 3 raters.

RESULTS

Table III lists the demographic data for the patients returning for follow-up who received pegged and keeled glenoid components. Patient gender ($P = .381$), age ($P = .098$), shoulder dominance ($P = .244$), glenoid morphology ($P = .066$), humeral head size ($P = .221$), glenoid component size ($P = .121$), glenohumeral mismatch ($P = .055$), and length of follow-up ($P = .933$) did not differ significantly between patients who received pegged glenoid components and patients who received keeled glenoid components.

Table III: Demographic data for patients with pegged and keeled glenoid components

	Pegged	Keeled	
Number	21	26	
Average age (years)	71.8 ± 10.4	66.3 ± 11.6	P = .098
Dominant side	13	11	P = .244
Gender:			P = .381
Male	13	12	
Female	8	14	
Glenoid morphology [27]:			P = .066
A1	9	16	
A2	5	0	
B1	1	2	
B2	6	7	
C	0	1	
Humeral head size:			P = .221
39	1	3	
41	3	2	
43	2	9	
46	6	7	
48	5	4	
50	4	1	
Glenoid size:			P = .121
S	1	3	
M	5	9	
L	9	13	
XL	6	1	
Mismatch	7.9 ± 1.8	7.0 ± 1.1	P = .055

Immediate radiographic lucency

Fifty-one patients (96%) returned for immediate postoperative radiographs, including 26 patients in the keel group (96%) and 25 patients in the pegged group (96%). Figure 1 shows the lucency grades for the pegged and keeled glenoid components. In the immediate postoperative period, there was no significant difference in the rate of glenoid lucency (of at least grade 2) between the pegged (0%) and keeled (15%) glenoid components, $P = .128$.

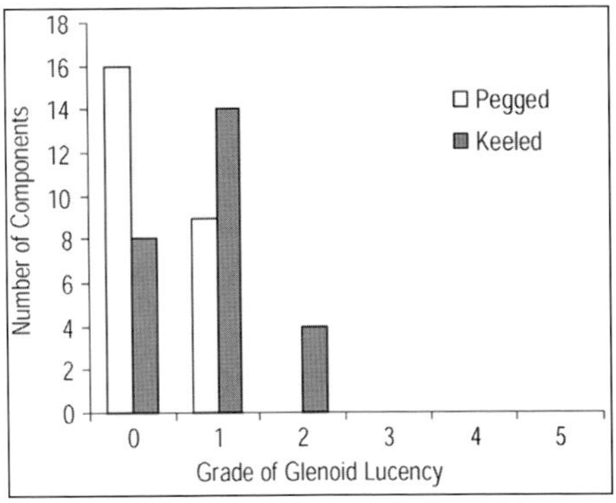

Fig. 1: Grades of glenoid lucency for pegged and keeled glenoid components on post-operatve radiographs. In the immediate postoperative period, there was no significant difference in the rate of glenoid lucency (of at least grade 2) betwen the pegged (0%) and keeled (15%) glenoid components, P = .128.

Furthermore, patient gender ($P = .168$), age ($P = .133$), shoulder dominance ($P = .361$), glenoid morphology ($P = .395$), humeral head size (P = .291), glenoid component size ($P = .234$), and glenohumeral mismatch ($P = .493$) were not significantly related to the glenoid component lucencies.

Follow-up radiographic lucency

Forty-seven patients (89%) returned for follow-up evaluation (average 26 months; range, 12-38), including 26 patients in the keel group (96%) and 21 patients in the pegged group (81%). Two patients in the keel group had failure of their component (see below) and are not included in the radiolucent line evaluation, leaving 24 patients in the keel group. Of the 5 patients in the pegged group who did not return for the follow-up evaluation, 2 were deceased (implant was in place and had not been revised at time of death), 2 had returned to practice as surgeons and reported no substantial problems, and 1 could not be located. Figure 2 shows the lucency grades for the pegged and keeled glenoid components. After an average follow-up of 26 months, the rate of glenoid lucency (of at least grade 2) was significantly higher in patients with a keeled glenoid component (46%) compared to patients with a pegged glenoid component (15%), $P = .003$.

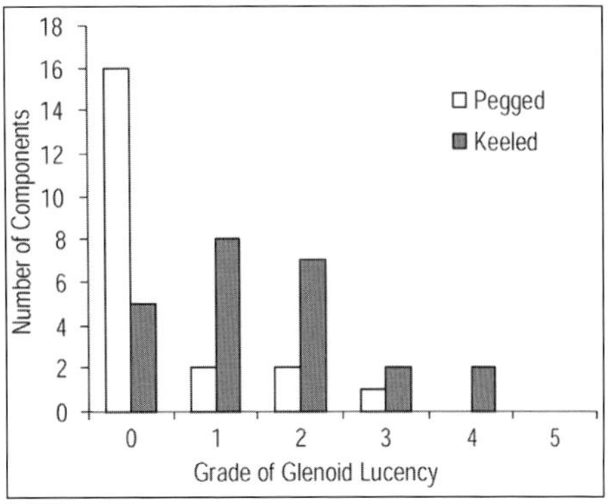

Fig. 2: Grades of glenoid lucency for pegged and leeled glenoid components on follow-up radiographs. After an average follow-up of 26 months, the rate of glenoid lucency (of at least grade 2) was significantly higher in patients with a keeled glenoid component (46%) compared to patients with a pegged glenoid component (15%), P = .003.

Glenoid lucency progressed (at least 1 grade) between postoperative radiographs and follow-up radiographs in 29% of patients, including 10 patients with keeled glenoid components (42%) and 3 patients with pegged glenoid components (14%). The rate of progression and the final grade of glenoid lucency were higher in patients with keeled glenoid components compared to patients with pegged glenoid components ($P = .044$; Fig. 3).

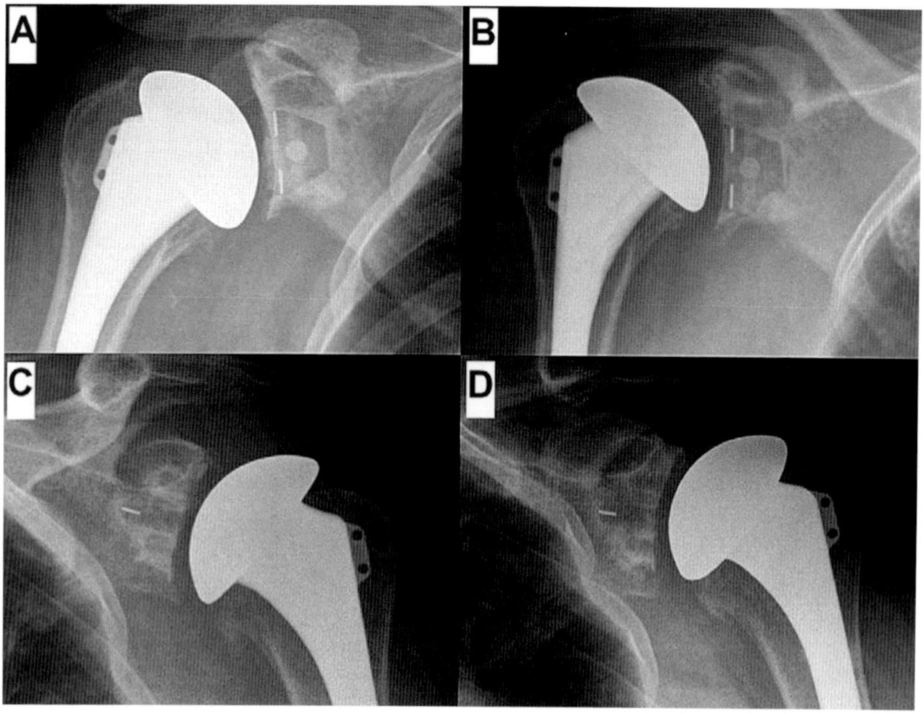

Fig. 3: A) Postoperative radiograph of a keeled glenoid component (grade 0 lucency). B) Twelve-month follow-up radiograph of the same keeled component demonstrating grade 3 lucency. C) Postoperative radiograph of a pegged glenoid component (grade 0 lucency). D) Three-year follow-up radiograph of the same pegged component demonstrating grade 0 lucency.

Glenoid lucency was not significantly related to patient age (P = .174), shoulder dominance (P = .615), glenoid morphology (P = .333), or glenohumeral mismatch (P = .923). Glenoid lucency was related to gender on follow-up radiographs (P = .011). Females had a significantly (38%) higher rate of glenoid lucency than males in patients with pegged glenoid components (38% vs 0%, P = .049). Females also had a 27% higher rate of glenoid lucency than males in patients with keeled glenoid components; but, with the numbers available, this difference did not reach statistical significance (57% vs 30%, P = .240). Increasing glenoid lucency was also related to smaller head size (P = .004) and smaller glenoid size (P = .002); however, females received a smaller head size (P < .001) and glenoid size (P < .001) than males, and component size was not related independently to the rate of glenoid lucency after accounting for this gender disparity in component size.

Failures

Over the follow-up period, total shoulder arthroplasties in 2 patients with keeled glenoid components failed, whereas there were no failures in patients with pegged glenoid components. One patient failed secondary to a posterior dislocation and was revised to a reverse total shoulder arthroplasty. The second patient failed secondary to fracture of the glenoid component following a fall. This patient was treated with removal of the fractured glenoid component and bone grafting of the glenoid.

Inter-rater reliability and agreement

On the immediate postoperative radiographs, the lucency grades had good reliability (0.70) and all 3 raters were in complete agreement for 80% of the lucency grades. On the follow-up radiographs, the lucency grades had good reliability (0.85) and all 3 raters were in complete agreement for 82% of the lucency grades.

DISCUSSION

This study evaluated the effect of glenoid design on the immediate and mid-term radiographic lucency of pegged and keeled glenoid components using modern cementing techniques. Although there were no significant differences in rates of glenoid lucency in the immediate postoperative period, pegged glenoid components had significantly less glenoid lucency than keeled glenoid components after an average follow-up of 26 months. We had hypothesized that with improved glenoid preparation and cementing techniques, there would be no difference in radiographic lucency between pegged and keeled glenoid components on postoperative and follow-up radiographs. Our results partially support our hypothesis. The use of modern cementing techniques, including glenoid compaction and cement pressurization, was able to minimize differences in glenoid lucency seen between pegged and keeled glenoid components in the immediate postoperative period. However, these results were not sustained. As follow-up increased, patients with keeled glenoid components had a significantly higher rate of glenoid lucency than patients with pegged glenoid components. Even with modern cementing techniques, pegged glenoid components were radiographically superior to keeled glenoid components.

Using a similar study design and radiographic lucency grading system, Gartsman et al found glenoid lucencies in 39% of patients with keeled glenoid components and 5% of patients with pegged glenoid components on postoperative radiographs [8]. The current study demonstrated a lower rate of postoperative glenoid lucency in both keeled (15%) and pegged (0%) glenoid components. The lower rates of glenoid lucency seen in this study may be attributable to modern cementing techniques, including glenoid compaction and cement pressurization. The rate of glenoid lucency seen with the keeled components in this study is similar to the rates seen in other studies that have used modern cementing techniques. For example, Mileti *et al* showed immediate glenoid lucency in 14% of keeled glenoid components and Szabo *et al* showed immediate glenoid lucency in 11% of keeled components, which increased to 17% after 2 years of follow-up [20, 26].

Radiographic lucencies seen with both pegged and keeled components increased as follow-up increased; however, the rate of progression and the final grade of glenoid lucency were greater in patients with keeled glenoid components. Length of follow-up was similar between the 2 glenoid groups. Patient age, glenoid morphology, and glenohumeral mismatch were unrelated to glenoid lucency and thus could not have contributed to the higher rate of lucency in the keeled components. Glenoid mismatch in particular has been shown in prior work to be related to the prevalence of radiolucent lines, which increase risk of component loosening [23, 30]. In particular, radiolucencies are worse when mismatch is less than 6 cm 30; all subjects in the current study had glenoid mismatch of 6 cm or greater, which may explain the lack of its effect on glenoid lucency. Furthermore, the length of follow-up in these previous studies was considerably longer than in the current study. It is possible that mismatch may lead to greater lucency or component failure, as time from surgery increases in our patients.

Previous studies have also documented progression of radiolucent lines with increased follow-up, with rates varying from 6% to 76% [4, 5, 20, 22, 24]. As previously stated by Neer, progression of radiolucent lines is the most concerning finding and may be used to identify glenoid components that are at risk for loosening [21]. Therefore, patients receiving keeled glenoid components in this study may be more at risk for glenoid loosening than patients receiving pegged glenoid components. The scope of this paper did not include investigation of mechanical, biological, or histological mechanisms that are potentially related to presence of radiolucent lines. Our results show some clinical manifestations of the previous biomechanical research demonstrating the ability of pegged glenoid components to better resist displacement forces, as compared to keeled components [1, 29].

As follow-up increased, 2 patient variables became significantly related to glenoid lucency. First, female patients were shown to have higher rates of glenoid lucency than male patients. This gender difference had not been seen in previous studies and may be related to increased rates of osteoporosis in female patients compared to male patients. In addition, smaller humeral head size and smaller glenoid size were associated with higher rates of glenoid lucency. This affect appears to be secondary to the fact that females received smaller component sizes. Future studies are needed to define the association between gender and glenoid lucency; and to develop treatment strategies to decrease the rate of glenoid lucency seen in female patients.

One advantage of this study was its design. Our inclusion and exclusion criteria were formulated to allow us to study a relatively pure series of patients with primary glenohumeral osteoarthritis. With a prospective, randomized study design, we were able to create 2 groups of patients that did not significantly differ from one another except in glenoid component design, to control for variables that are known to affect glenoid lucency, and to minimize the effect of unknown confounding variables. In addition, we eliminated selection bias of the operating surgeon.

One limitation of this study is in its radiographic evaluation and the limited scoring systems available for grading periglenoid radiolucencies. Although we followed protocols and grading systems that had been used by other authors, there is no clear correlation between the radiographic score assigned to a pegged component and the same score given to a keeled component [8, 18]. In fact, the scoring systems may be biased in favor of the pegged components. For example, an incomplete radiolucency around the keel of a glenoid component receives a grade of 2, whereas a similar incomplete radiolucency around a peg only receives a grade of 1. Future studies may help to refine the grading criteria for better comparison between pegged and keeled glenoid components. Another limitation of this study is that the raters could not be blinded to glenoid component design. Our study, however, did demonstrate a high level of interobserver consistency in radiographic evaluation.

CONCLUSION

This study supports the results of previous biomechanical, animal, retrospective, and prospective studies [8, 15-18, 28, 31]. Even with modern cementing techniques, pegged glenoid components remain radiographically superior to keeled glenoid components. In patients with primary glenohumeral osteoarthritis, the use of pegged glenoid components for total shoulder arthroplasty decreases the rate of glenoid lucency. Additional studies are needed to investigate the long-term radiographic and clinical significance of these findings.

DISCLAIMER

Two authors (TBE and GMG) acknowledge that they are consultants for Tornier and have received research and educational support from Tornier. None of the other authors have received financial renumeration related to or in support of this work. This study was approved by the Texas Orthopedic Hospital Institutional Review Board, as protocol #TOH040.

REFERENCES

[1] ANGLIN C, WYSS UP, NYFFELER RW, GERBER C. Loosening performance of cemented glenoid prosthesis design pairs. *Clin Biomech 2001;16: 144-50.*

[2] BARRETT WP, FRANKLIN JL, JACKINS SE, WYSS CR, MATSEN FA III. Total shoulder arthroplasty. *J Bone Joint Surg Am 1987; 69A:865-72.*

[3] BOILEAU P, AVIDOR C, KRISHNAN SG, WALCH G, KEMPF J, MOLE D. Cemented polyethylene versus uncemented metal-backed glenoid components in total shoulder arthroplasty: A prospective, doubleblind, randomized study. *J Shoulder Elbow Surg 2002; 11: 351-9.*

[4] BOILEAU P, MOLE´ D, WALCH G. Technique of glenoid resurfacing in shoulder arthroplasty. In: Walch G, Boileau P, editors. Shoulder arthroplasty. *Berlin: Springer-Verlag; 1999. p. 147-62.*

[5] COFIELD RH. Total shoulder arthroplasty with the Neer prosthesis. *J Bone Joint Surg Am 1984; 66A: 899-906.*

[6] EDWARDS TB, SABONGHY EP, ELKOUSY H, WARNOCK KM, HAMMERMAN SM, O'CONNOR DP, *et al.* Glenoid component insertion in total shoulder arthroplasty: Comparison of three techniques for drying the glenoid before cementation. *J Shoulder Elbow Surg 2007; 16: 107S-10.*

[7] FRANKLIN JL, BARRETT WP, JACKINS SE, MATSEN FA III. Glenoid loosening in total shoulder arthroplasty. Association with rotator cuff deficiency. *J Arthroplasty 1988; 3:39-46.*

[8] GARTSMAN GM, ELKOUSY HA, WARNOCK KM, EDWARDS TB, O'CONNOR DP. Radiographic comparison of pegged and keeled glenoid components. *J Shoulder Elbow Surg 2005; 14: 252-7.*

[9] HASAN SS, LEITH JM, CAMPBELL B, KAPIL R, SMITH KL, MATSEN FA III. Characteristics of unsatisfactory shoulder arthroplasties. *J Shoulder Elbow Surg 2002; 11: 431-41.*

[10] HAVIG MT, KUMAR A, CARPENTER W, SEILER JG. Assessment of radiolucent lines about the glenoid: an in vitro radiographic study. *J Bone Joint Surg Am 1997; 79A: 428-32.*

[11] HAWKINS RJ, BELL RH, JALLAY B. Total shoulder arthroplasty. *Clin Orthop Relat Res 1989; 242: 188-94.*

[12] IBARRA C, DINES DM, McLAUGHLIN JA. Glenoid replacement in total shoulder arthroplasty. *Orthop Clin North Am 1998; 29: 403-13.*

[13] KELLEHER IM, COFIELD RH, BECKER DA, BEABOUT JW. Fluoroscopically positioned radiographs of total shoulder arthroplasty. *J Shoulder Elbow Surg 1992; 1: 306-11.*

[14] KELLY IG, FOSTER RS, FISHER WD. Neer total shoulder replacement in rheumatoid arthritis. *J Bone Joint Surg Br 1987; 69B: 723-6.*

[15] KLEPPS S, CHIANG AS, MILLER S, JIANG CY, HAZRATI Y, FLATOW EL. Incidence of early radiolucent glenoid lines in patients having total shoulder replacements. *Clin Orthop Relat Res 2005; 435: 118-25.*

[16] LACROIX D, MURPHY LA, PRENDERGAST PJ. Three-dimensional finite element analysis of glenoid replacement prostheses: a comparison of keeled and pegged anchorage systems. *J Biomech Eng 2000; 122: 430-6.*

[17] LACROIX D, PRENDERGAST PJ. Stress analysis of glenoid component designs for shoulder arthroplasty. *Proc Inst Mech Eng [H] 1997; 211: 467-74.*

[18] LAZARUS MD, JENSEN KL, SOUTHWORTH C, MATSEN FA III. The radiographic evaluation of keeled and pegged glenoid component insertion. *J Bone Joint Surg Am 2002; 84A: 1174-82.*

[19] LIOTARD JP, EDWARDS TB, PADEY A, WALCH G, BOULAHIA A. Hydrotherapy rehabilitation after shoulder surgery. *Tech Shoulder Elbow Surg 2003; 4: 44-9.*

[20] MILETI J, BOARDMAN ND III, SPERLING JW, COFIELD RH, TORCHIA ME, O'DRISCOLL SW, *et al.* Radiographic analysis of polyethylene glenoid components using modern cementing techniques. *J Shoulder Elbow Surg 2004; 13: 492-8.*

[21] NEER C. Glenohumeral arthroplasty. In: Neer C, editor. Shoulder reconstruction. *Philadelphia: WB Saunders; 1990. p. 143-269.*

[22] NEER C, WATSON K, STANTON J. Recent experience in total shoulder replacement. *J Bone Joint Surg Am 1982; 64A: 319-37.*

[23] NHO SJ, ALA OL, DODSON CC, FIGGIE MP, WRIGHT TM, CRAIG EV, *et al.* Comparison of conforming and nonconforming retrieved glenoid components. *J Shoulder Elbow Surg 2008; 17: 914-20.*

[24] NORRIS BL, LACHIEWICZ PF. Modern cement technique and the survivorship of total shoulder arthroplasty. *Clin Orthop Relat Res 1996; 328: 76-85.*

[25] SKIRVING AP. Total shoulder arthroplasty - current problems and possible solutions. *J Orthop Sci 1999; 4: 42-53.*

[26] SZABO I, BUSCAYRET F, EDWARDS TB, NEMOZ C, O'CONNOR DP, BOILEAU P, *et al.* Radiographic comparison of two glenoid preparation techniques in total shoulder arthroplasty. *Clin Orthop Relat Res 2005; 431:104-10.*

[27] TORCHIA ME, COFIELD RH, SETTERGREN CR. Total shoulder arthroplasty with the Neer prosthesis: long-term results. *J Shoulder Elbow Surg 1997; 6: 495-505.*

[28] TRAIL IA, NUTTALL D. The results of shoulder arthroplasty in patients with rheumatoid arthritis. *J Bone Joint Surg Br 2002; 84B: 1121-5.*

[29] WALCH G, BADET R, BOULAHIA A, KHOURY A. Morphologic study of the glenoid in primary glenohumeral osteoarthritis. *J Arthroplasty 1999; 14: 756-60.*

[30] WALCH G, EDWARDS TB, BOULAHIA A, BOILEAU P, MOLE D, ADELEINE P. The influence of glenohumeral prosthetic mismatch on glenoid radiolucent lines: results of a multicenter study. *J Bone Joint Surg Am 2002; 84: 2186-91.*

[31] WIRTH MA, KORVICK DL, BASAMANIA CJ, TORO F, AUFDEMORTE TB, ROCKWOOD CA Jr. Radiologic, mechanical, and histologic evaluation of 2 glenoid prosthesis designs in a canine model. *J Shoulder Elbow Surg 2001; 10: 140-8.*

[32] WIRTH MA, ROCKWOOD CA Jr. Complications of total shoulderreplacement arthroplasty. *J Bone Joint Surg Am 1996; 78A: 603-16.*

PEGGED VERSUS KEELED GLENOIDS: A RETROSPECTIVE STUDY

R.H. COFIELD, T.W. THROCKMORTON

BACKGROUND

Several authors have evaluated the early radiographic appearance of keels versus pegs. Lazarus in 2002 found that there were worse cementing grades in keels than in pegs on the early postoperative films [1]. Similarly, Gartsman found that there were many more lucencies on early films surrounding keels than surrounding pegs [2]. In a more recent study by Barwood, only 7 of 69 pegged glenoid components had radiolucent lines on the early x-rays [3]. Thus, these radiographic reviews of early postoperative x-rays tended to favor the pegged type glenoid component fixation.

On radiostereometric analysis Nuttall found a greater maximum total point movement on keeled components versus pegged components [4]. Rahme found rotation greater than 2 degrees equal between keeled and pegged components [5].

On biomechanical testing using finite element analysis, Lecroix found the pegs were better with normal bone, and the keel was better with weaker bones such as in those with rheumatoid arthritis [6]. Roche, on biomechanical testing of one keeled and one pegged component with eccentric loading of 100,000 cycles, found that each glenoid remained firmly fixed [7].

Finally, in our registry analysis of survival from removal or revision of the glenoid component we could not find much of a difference between keeled and pegged components [8]. Of 497 keeled components followed for an average of 6.7 years, the Kaplan-Meier five year survival was 99%; the 10 year survival was 94%. Of 358 pegged components followed for an average of 2.3 years, the five year survival was 99%. It is too early to know what the 10 year survival would be for that type of component.

Thus, there is rather mixed and incomplete literature on this subject. We developed a study the purpose of which was to document the early radiographic and intermediate-term clinical and radiographic results of both types of implants [9].

PATIENTS AND METHODS

We identified shoulders that had undergone total shoulder arthroplasty for primary osteoarthritis, had greater than 2 years of clinical and radiographic follow-up, had radiographs performed at our institution, and had surgery between 1991 and 2005. One hundred and seventy-one such shoulders were identified. This group was narrowed chronologically to 50 early pegged glenoid components and 50 later placed keeled components, to equalize the length of radiographic and clinical follow-up. The average age of these patients was 69.4 years in the keeled group and 67.8 years in the pegged group. The sexes were quite even between the two groups, as was the age.

The pegged and keeled components were identical except for their attachments to bone. There were three sizes of each. Each had a 2 mm radial mismatch. The pegged component had three in-line pegs. Both components had a convex back surface with texturing. Both components had shallow rings on the keels or pegs to assist in cement fixation, and both components were sterilized in gas. A set of instruments was developed for precise fitting of the glenoid components, be they keeled or pegged (fig. 1). The cement technique was refined to include, in addition to the meticulous bone preparation, preserving a portion of the subchondral plate plus lavage, drying, cement compression by vacuum mixing, pressurization of the cement within the glenoid row and use of a holding instrument (fig. 2).

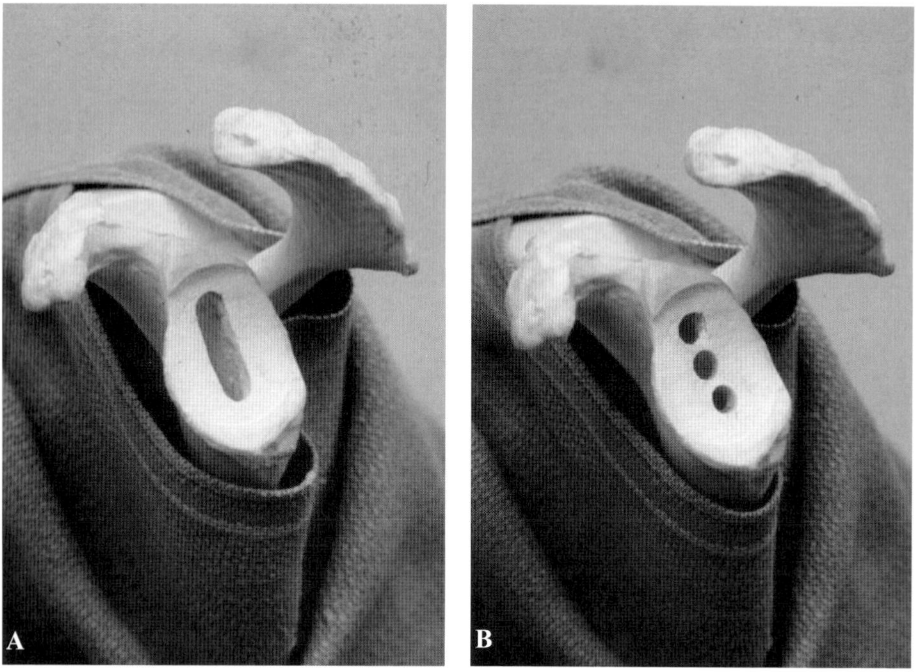

Fig. 1: Plastic bone models illustrating the preparation of the bone for the keeled (A) and for the pegged components (B).

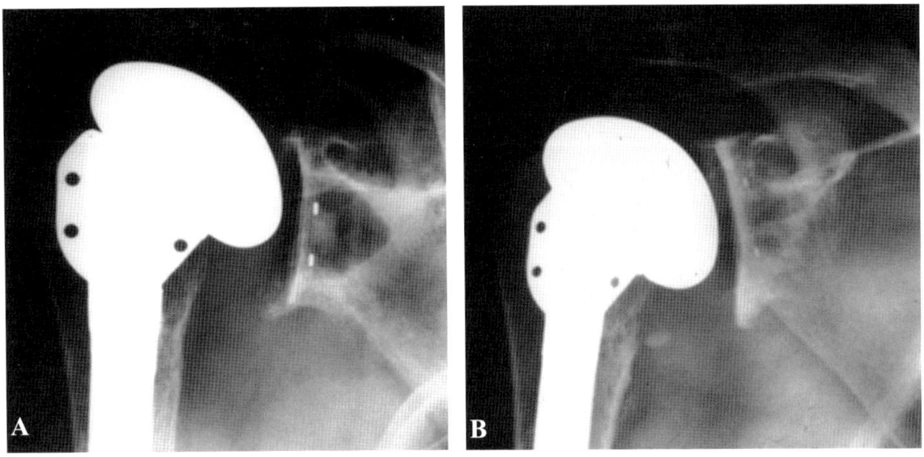

Fig. 2: Early postoperative radiographs illustrating the glenoid fixation on a fluoroscopically positioned spot views for the keeled component (A) and for the pegged component (B).

Radiographs taken included preoperative views, initial postoperative views and views at final follow-up. The films obtained were 40 degree posterior oblique films in internal and external rotation, an axillary view and a fluoroscopically guided spot view of the glenoid. The mean radiographic follow-up for the keeled components was 51.3 months (range 24-90 months), and for the pegged group was 45.7 months (range 27-98 months) ($p = 0.15$). The radiographic evaluation was by the consensus of four surgeons. Lucent lines were evaluated in millimeters. A shift in component position was assessed between the initial postoperative and final follow-up films. The films were analyzed for glenohumeral subluxation and for the degree and pattern of arthritic involvement by the Mayo [10] and the Walch systems [11]. Each component, be it keeled or pegged, was divided into five zones, one and five on the undersurface of the face plate, two, three, and four on either the keel or the pegs of the components (fig. 3).

A component was termed "at risk" for clinically symptomatic loosening if there was a circumferential radiolucency, some part of which was 1.5 mm in width or greater, or there was a change in implant position between the initial postoperative and final follow-up films.

A number of variables were assessed for associations. These included gender, operative side, rotator cuff tearing (all were small to medium in size with 6 in the keeled group and 2 in the pegged groups), subluxation (anterior, posterior or superior), glenoid erosion (by the Mayo or Walch systems), glenoid cement perforation, glenoid lucency, humeral lucency, glenoid shift and glenoid "at risk".

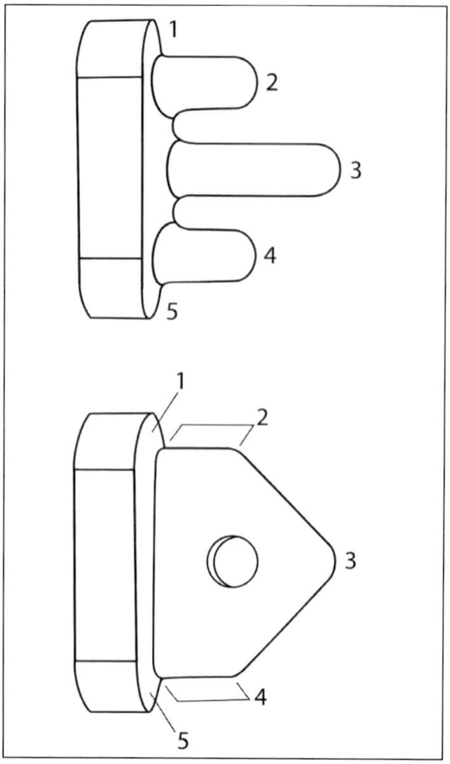

Fig. 3: Zone system used to compare lucent lines surrounding the pegged or keeled components. Zones 1 and 5 represent the area under the face plate. Zone 2 represents the upper peg or superior portion of the keel. Zone 3 represents the central peg or central portion of the keel, and Zone 4 represents the lower peg or lower portion of the keel. We also identified Zones 2, 3, and 4 as respectively representing the upper column, the middle column or the lower column for cement fixation.

RESULTS

Clinical data showed there was no difference in any parameter between the keel and peg groups. In the keel group pain changed from preoperatively at 4.6 (on a 1-5 scale) to 1.7. In the peg group this changed from 4.6 to 1.5. Active forward elevation in the keel group improved from 104 degrees to 150 degrees and in the peg group from 97 degrees to 147 degrees. External rotation in the keel group improved from 29 degrees to 58 degrees and in the peg group improved from 25 degrees to 53 degrees. Internal rotation in the keel group improved from L5 to L1 and in the peg group improved from the sacrum to L1. All improvements were significant at the $p < 0.001$ level. All comparisons between the keeled and the pegged groups were nonsignificant at the $p > 0.05$ level. There were three complications in each group. In the keeled group there was one case each of symptomatic glenoid loosening, posterior instability, and delayed onset neuropathic pain. In the pegged group there was one case each of anterior instability, posterior instability, and brachial neuropraxia that resolved.

On the initial postoperative films only five components had lucent lines that extended beyond the face plate (Table 1). Again, there were no significant differences between the keel and peg groups ($p = 0.37$).
On the final follow-up films there were again no significant differences ($p = 0.94$) (Table 2). There were four components at risk in the keel group and six in the peg group.

Table 1: Lucent Lines on Initial Postoperative Films*

	Keel	Peg
None	39	34
Face plate only	10	12
1 column		2
2 columns	1	2

* no significant differences p = 0.37

Table 2: Lucent Lines and "At Risk" status on Final Follow-up Films*

	Keel	Peg
None	11	13
Face plate only	22	19
1 column	11	12
2 columns	2	0
3 columns	0	0
At risk†	4	6

* no significant differences p = 0.37
† complete lucent line, some part being 1.5 mm or thicker or a change in component position

In assessing the association between the various variables mentioned, none proved to be statistically significant for the entire group, for either subgroup or for being at risk.

CONCLUSIONS

- There is a low frequency of early lucent lines (5 of 100)
- Changes occur over time
- Changes are not a continuum but bipolar
  - 88 good (none, face plate only or one column)
  - 12 bad (2 column, 3 column or shift)
- There were no differences between keeled or pegged components, clinically or radiographically

REFERENCES

[1] LAZARUS MD, JENSEN KL, SOUTHWORTH C, MATSEN FA 3rd. The radiographic evaluation of keeled and pegged glenoid component insertion. *J Bone Joint Surg 2002; 84A(7)1174-82.*

[2] GARTSMAN GM, ELKOUSY HA, WARNOCK KM, EDWARDS TB, O'CONNOR DP. Radiographic comparison of pegged and keeled glenoid components. *J Shoulder Elbow Surg 2005; 14(3)252-7.*

[3] BARWOOD S, SETTER KJ, BLAINE TA, BIGLIANI LU. The incidence of early radiolucencies about a pegged glenoid component using cement pressurization. *J Shoulder Elbow Surg 2008; 17(5): 703-8.*

[4] NUTTALL D, HAINES JF, TRAIL II. A study of the microenvironment of pegged and keeled glenoid components compared using radiosterometric analysis. *J Shoulder Elbow Surg 2007; 16(3 Suppl): S65-S70.*

[5] RAHME H, MATTSON P, WIKBLAD L, NOWAK J, LARSSON S. Stability of cemented in-line pegged glenoid compared with keeled glenoid components in total shoulder arthroplasty. *J Bone Joint Surg 2009; 91A(8): 1965-72.*

[6] LECROIX D, MURPHY LA, PRENDERGAST PJ. Three-dimensional finite element analysis of glenoid replacement prostheses : A comparison of keeled and pegged anchorage systems. *J Biomech Eng 2000; 122(4): 430-6.*

[7] ROCHE C, ANGIBAUD L, FLURIN PH, WRIGHT T, ZUCKERMAN J. Glenoid loosening in response to dynamic multi-axis eccentric loading: A comparison between keeled and pegged designs with an equivalent radial mismatch. *Bulletin of the Hospital for Joint Diseases 2006; 63(3-4): 88-92.*

[8] FOX TJ, CIL A, SPERLING JW, SANCHEZ-SOTELO J, SCHLECK CD, COFIELD RH. Survival of the glenoid component in shoulder arthroplasty. *J Shoulder Elbow Surg 2009; 18: 859-63.*

[9] THROCKMORTON TW, ZARKADAS PC, SPERLING JW, COFIELD RH. Pegged versus keeled glenoid components in total shoulder arthroplasty. *J Shoulder Elbow Surg 2010 Feb; 9 (Epub ahead of print).*

[10] SPERLING JW, COFIELD RH, SCHLECK CD, HARMSEN WS. Total shoulder arthroplasty versus hemiarthroplasty for rheumatoid arthritis. Results of 303 consecutive cases. *J Shoulder Elbow Surg 2007; 16(6): 683-90.*

[11] WALCH G, BADET R, BOULAHIA A, KHOURY A. Morphologic study of the glenoid in primary glenohumeral osteoarthritis. *J Arthroplasty 1999; 14(6): 756-60.*

CLINICAL AND RADIOGRAPHIC ANALYSIS OF A PARTIALLY CEMENTED GLENOID IMPLANT- 5 YEAR MINIMUM FOLLOW-UP

R.S. CHURCHILL, C. ZELLMER, H.J. ZIMMERS, R. RUGGERO

ABSTRACT

Background

The purpose of this study is to review clinical and radiographic findings on a consecutive group of 20 shoulders that underwent total shoulder arthroplasty with a partially cemented glenoid component at a minimum of five years follow-up.

Methods

Twenty patients that received a partially cemented polyethylene glenoid were evaluated with Simple Shoulder Tests (SST), Constant scores, and radiographs. Five year post-op radiographs were compared with respective six week post-op radiographs. Independent evaluation assigned every glenoid a lucency grade from 0 (no lucency) to 5 (gross lucency) and assessed the central peg for bone presence between the radial fins.

Results

Mean SST and Constant scores were 11.1 and 82.4, respectively. Mean lucency scores increased from 0.1 to 0.3 from six weeks to five year follow-up ($p=0.05$). 15/20 patients had similar or increased bone presence between the central peg fins at five year follow-up, none of which had a worsening lucency score at five years. The 5/20 patients which had decreased or absent bone presence at five years had worsening lucency scores from a mean of 0.2 to 1.0 at five years ($p=0.05$). There was no difference in SST score ($p=0.54$) or Constant score ($p=0.37$) between the two groups.

Conclusions

This partially cemented glenoid component had low rates of lucencies at five year minimum follow-up. Similar or increased bone growth between the radial fins of the central peg at five years was associated with no progression of glenoid lucencies. Decreased or absent bone presence between the radial fins at follow-up correlated with slight advancement of glenoid lucent lines over five years.

INTRODUCTION

Glenoid loosening is a commonly encountered problem in total shoulder arthroplasty [9, 10, 19, 20]. Currently most glenoid designs are of two varieties, pegged or keeled. Several studies have shown a reduced incidence of lucent lines on immediate post operative and follow-up radiographs for pegged glenoid designs [2, 4, 8]. Modern cementing techniques have helped reduce the incidence of lucent lines on initial post operative radiographs for keeled radiographs [12, 17, 18]. However, despite this improvement, in a recent randomized clinical trial by Edwards *et al.*, pegged implants were shown to be superior to keeled implants in the reduction of lucent line formation at two year minimum follow-up [4].

In 2001, Wirth reported on a novel, partially cemented, pegged glenoid implant trialed in a canine model [19]. This study found the partially cemented pegged implant superior to a keeled implant design. This new implant design had three cemented peripheral pegs and an uncemented central peg. The uncemented central peg was larger and had four sequentially spaced radial fins at its distal tip. This space between adjacent fins allowed for possible bone growth incorporation to improve long term fixation. In 2001, the minimally cemented pegged glenoid implant became available for clinical use in total shoulder arthroplasty. Despite over eight years of widespread clinical use, no long term data on the implant exists.

The purpose of this study was to determine the midterm results of this novel, partially cemented, pegged glenoid implant design. With its unique central peg radial fin design, our hypothesis was that bone growth between the fins would occur resulting in improved glenoid fixation and reduced lucent line formation.

MATERIALS AND METHODS

This retrospective study was approved by our institutional review board. Between October 2002 and May 2004 a total of 33 total shoulder arthroplasties were performed on 32 patients with the diagnosis of primary glenohumeral osteoarthritis. All patients were operated on by a single, fellowship trained, shoulder reconstruction specialist. Patients were contacted between February 2009 and May 2009 for review. Of the original 32 patients, nine were deceased, three had moved out of state and could not be located, and one had just undergone open heart surgery and was unavailable for review. Thus 20 shoulders were available for review.

All patients underwent a standard total shoulder arthroplasty with implantation of the Global Advantage humeral prosthesis and the Anchor Peg glenoid prosthesis (DePuy, Warsaw, IN) (fig. 1). The Anchor Peg glenoid was available in six

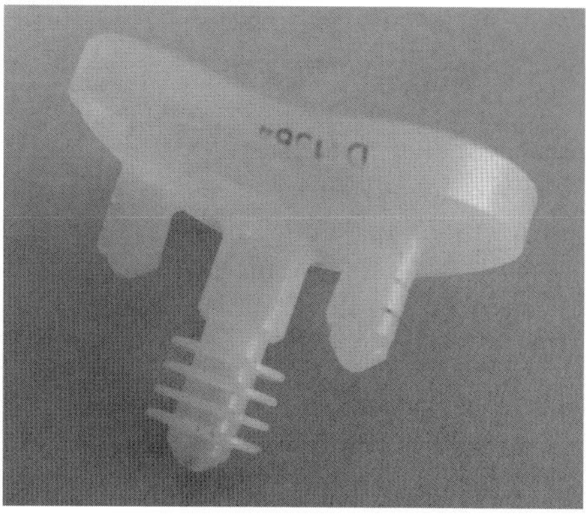

Fig. 1: DePuy Anchor peg glenoid.

sizes, [40, 44, 48, 52, 56, and 56XL]. It was made of ultra high molecular weight polyethylene which was gamma sterilized in a nitrogen vapor barrier package. The three peripheral peg diameters were 4.7 mm, the central peg minimum diameter was 5.4 mm, and fin diameter was 9.4 mm. A standard deltopectoral approach was utilized in all patients. The subscapularis was taken down leaving a 1cm stump on the lesser tuberosity. The humeral head was dislocated and the rotator cuff was inspected to verify there was no evidence of a rotator cuff tear. A standard 135° humeral head cut was made in anatomic retroversion and remaining humeral osteophytes removed. The humeral shaft was reamed and broached to the appropriate size. The glenoid was exposed in standard fashion with anterior and inferior capsular releases. The glenoid center point was drilled and glenoid reaming was performed when necessary to obtain a concentric fit with the glenoid implant. The center hole was then overdrilled to accept the Anchor Peg center post. The three hole peripheral drill guide was inserted and the three peripheral holes were drilled into the glenoid. The glenoid trial was then inserted to ensure proper fitting. Copious irrigation was then performed and the glenoid bone dried with suction. Final preparation of the three peripheral holes was completed with a CO_2 irrigation system to dry the holes prior to cementing. Cement was placed in the three peripheral holes under pressure by way of a 2oz syringe. No cement was placed in the center hole. The Anchor Peg glenoid was impacted and held with manual pressure in position for 15 minutes while the cement hardened. Humeral head trialing was then completed and the final Global Advantage humeral stem and head were impacted on the back table and then implanted. The subscapularis was then repaired back to its 1cm stump on the lesser tuberosity.

Post-operatively patients were started on a passive shoulder elevation and external rotation program the day of surgery. Patients were limited to 140° of forward elevation and 40° of external rotation. A sling was employed for the surgical day only. The following day the dressing and drain were removed and the sling discontinued. Stretching continued for two weeks on a self-directed basis. At two weeks, internal rotation up the back and cross body adduction were added under the instruction of a physical therapist. The limit of 140° forward elevation was discontinued at this time. At six weeks, standard AP, Grashey, and axillary lateral radiographs of the shoulder were obtained. At this time patients were offered a physical therapy strengthening program if desired.

Patients were contacted for follow-up between February 2009 and May 2009. SST, Constant scores and fluoroscopically aligned Grashey view radiographs were obtained at minimum five year follow-up. The fluoroscopic alignment was performed to ensure the x-ray beam was parallel to the glenoid bone-implant interface [11]. The radiographs were evaluated independently by three musculoskeletal radiologists. Radiographic lucency around the pegs of the glenoid implant were graded according to a modification of the Lazarus method [15] as well as assessing for the presence of bone within the fins of the central glenoid peg. The Lazarus grading system was originally described for a five peg, fully cemented, glenoid implant. The current glenoid implant under evaluation was cemented only for the three peripheral pegs. The center, larger peg, which has four distal radial fins for bone incorporation was uncemented. The three peripheral pegs were scored in accordance with the Lazarus method (table I). The grading of the central peg was performed separately as a modification to the Lazarus grading system. Since the central peg is cementless, no bone cement interface is present, therefore the central peg grading was completed by way of measuring the lucency of the bone in the region of the central peg (table II). The presence of bone between the fins of the central peg was evaluated as present or absent. The five year minimum follow-up films were then assessed for any change in the central peg bone presence and were graded as increased, decreased, absent, or similar to the initial six week post operative radiographs. The final peripheral peg and central peg lucency grades were the grade assigned by at least two of the three radiologists. In no case did all three radiologists disagree on the lucency grade. Weighted kappa analysis [14] (table III) was used to calculate the reliability of intra-observer and inter-observer agreement for the peripheral peg lucency grades and the central peg lucency grades. CT scan imaging of the glenoid was performed on two randomly selected patents based upon their five year follow-up X-rays. One patient was selected from the group with radiographic evidence of bone present between the central peg fins, and one patient was selected from the group without radiographic evidence of central peg bone presence.

Statistical analysis was completed by standard *t*-test with significance set at p=0.05. The peripheral peg and central peg lucency scores were calculated independently.

Table I: Grading system for pegged glenoid components

0	No radiolucency
1	Incomplete radiolucency around one or two pegs
2	Complete radiolucency (≤ 2mm wide) around one peg only, with or without incomplete radiolucency around one other peg
3	Complete radiolucency (≤ 2mm wide) around two or more pegs
4	Complete radiolucency (> 2mm wide) around two or more pegs
5	Gross loosening

Table II: Grading system for glenoid components with cementless center peg

0	Center lucency diameter < or = 9mm
1	Center lucency diameter 10-13mm partial length
2	Center lucency diameter 10-13mm complete length
3	Center lucency diameter > 13mm partial length
4	Center lucency diameter > 13mm complete length
5	Gross loosening

Table III: Interpretation of Kappa Values

Kappa	Agreement
< 0	Less than chance agreement
0.0-0.20	Slight agreement
0.21-0.40	Fair agreement
0.41-0.60	Moderate agreement
0.61-0.80	Substantial agreement
0.81-0.99	Almost perfect agreement

RESULTS

Patient demographics are listed in table IV. Initial six week post operative radiographs demonstrated 18 shoulders with no detectable peripheral peg lucency

(Lazarus grade 0), and two shoulders with Lazarus grade 1 lucency. Thus the group Lazarus lucency score at six weeks was 0.1 (range 0-1). 18 shoulders had a grade 0 central peg lucency score (no detectable lucency) and two shoulders with grade 1 lucency. Thus, 10% of the six week post operative films had evidence of glenoid lucent lines. Central peg bone incorporation was present in 18 shoulders and absent in two shoulders.

Table IV: Patient demographic data.

Number shoulders	20
Male	10
Female	10
Follow Up Data	
Mean age	74.6 years (range 62-90)
Mean FU	67.3 months (range 60-76)
SST	11.1 (range 9-12)
Constant Score	82.4 (range 71-94)

At five year follow-up, 75% of the shoulders had no evidence of glenoid lucency. Fifteen shoulders had no detectable peripheral peg lucency, four shoulders with Lazarus *grade 1* lucency, and one shoulder with Lazarus *grade 2* lucency, for a group Lazarus lucency score of 0.3 at five year minimum follow-up. Central peg lucency scores were grade 0 in 17 shoulders (no detectable lucency), one shoulder with *grade 1* lucency, and two shoulders with *grade 3* lucency for a group central peg lucency score of 0.3 at five year minimum follow-up. Central peg bone incorporation was present in 17 shoulders and absent in three shoulders (fig. 2, 3). Central peg bone presence, when compared to the respective six week post operative films, was similar or increased in 15 shoulders and decreased or absent in five shoulders.

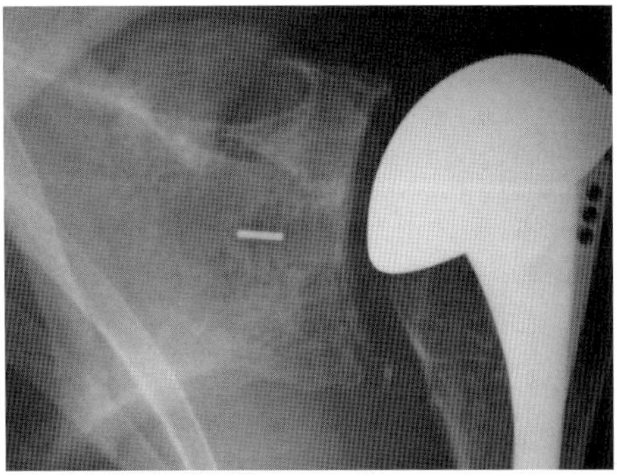

Fig. 2: 5 year follow up radiograph with bone presence between the central peg radial fins.

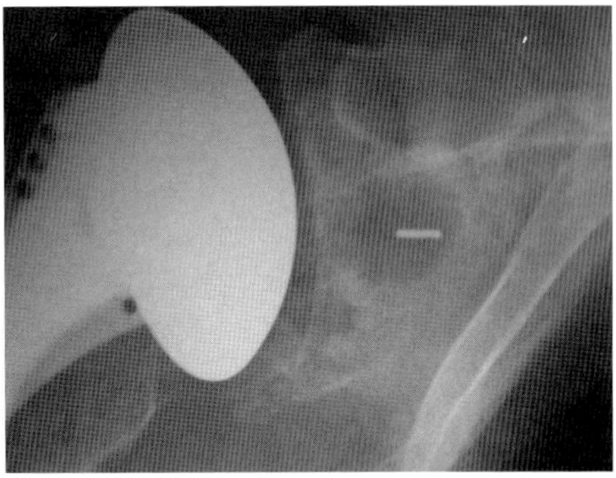

Fig. 3: 5 year follow up radiograph showing no central peg bone presence and evidence of lucency surrounding the central peg.

The group Lazarus lucency score increased from 0.1 at six weeks to 0.3 at minimum five year follow-up ($p=0.05$). The group central peg lucency score also showed advancement from 0.1 to 0.3, ($p=0.05$). Of the 15 shoulders with similar or increased central peg bone presence, no shoulder showed an increase in peripheral peg Lazarus lucency score, one had central peg lucency advancement from grade 0 to grade 1, and one had improvement in central peg lucency from grade 1 to 0. The five shoulders with decreased or absent central peg bone presence accounted for all of the peripheral peg lucency advancement (table V). This group of five shoulders had a six-week peripheral peg Lazarus score of 0.2 which advanced to 1.0 at five year follow-up (p=0.05). The central peg lucency score in these five patients increased from 0.2 to 1.2 (range 0-3) but did not achieve statistical significance (p=0.09). There was no difference in age (p=0.64), SST score (p=0.54), or Constant score (p=0.37) between the two groups (table VI).

Table V: Individual lucency scores and central fin bone presence grades.

Peripheral Peg		Central Peg		Fin Bone Presence		
6 week	5-7 yr	6 week	5-7 yr	6 week	5-7yr	Inrc/Similar/Decr
0	0	0	0	Y	Y	I
0	0	0	0	Y	Y	I
0	0	0	0	Y	Y	I
0	0	0	0	Y	Y	I
0	0	1	0	Y	Y	I
0	0	0	0	Y	Y	I
0	0	0	0	N	Y	I
1	1	0	0	Y	Y	I
0	0	0	0	Y	Y	S
0	0	0	0	Y	Y	S
0	0	0	0	Y	Y	S
0	0	0	0	Y	Y	S
0	0	0	1	Y	Y	S
0	0	0	0	Y	Y	S
0	0	0	0	Y	Y	S
1	1	0	0	Y	N	D
0	1	0	0	Y	Y	D
0	2	0	3	N	N	D
0	0	0	0	Y	Y	D
0	1	1	3	Y	N	D

Table VI : Patient data based upon central peg bone presence at five year follow up.

	Decreased/Absent Bone	Increased/Similar Bone	p-Value
Male/Female	2/3	8/7	
Mean age	76.0	74.1	p=0.64
SST	10.8	11.2	p=0.54
Constant Score	79.6	82.9	p=0.37

Preoperative glenoid posterior erosion was present in five shoulders, posterior humeral subluxation of 25% or more occurred in four shoulders, and 17 of the shoulders required glenoid reaming to achieve concentric fit with the glenoid implant. There was no correlation between these preoperative glenoid findings and the development of glenoid lucent line formation.

Weighted kappa values for the intra-observer agreement of the radiologic lucency scoring were fair (kappa 0.27) for the peripheral pegs and moderate (kappa 0.46) for the central pegs. The inter-observer agreement kappa values were also fair (kappa 0.31) for the peripheral pegs and moderate (kappa 0.52) for the central pegs.

The CT scan of the patient randomly selected from the group with similar or increased central peg bone presence is shown in figure 4 with their corresponding radiograph in figure 5. This clearly demonstrates the bone presence between three of the radial fins. Figure 6 is the CT scan image of the patient randomly selected from the decreased or absent central peg bone group. Their corresponding radiograph is shown in figure 3. The lucency surrounding the central peg and lack of radial fin bone presence, identified on the standard radiograph, are well demonstrated on the CT scan.

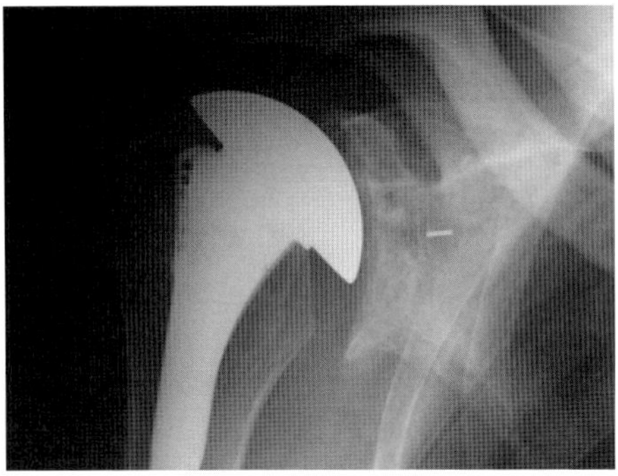

Fig. 5: Corresponding 5 year follow up X-ray image of patient in figure 4, also depicting bone presence between three of the central peg radial fins.

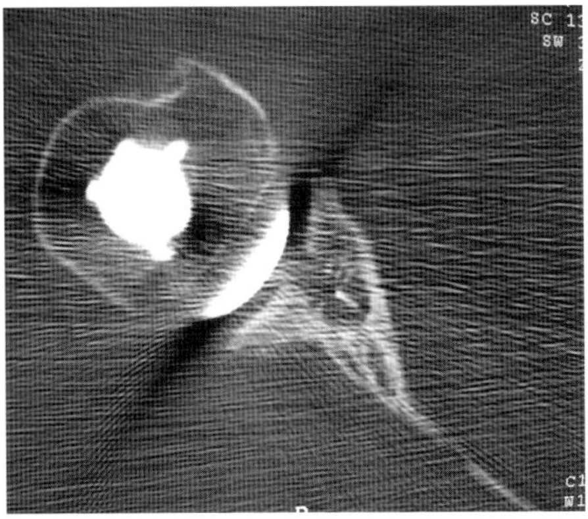

Fig. 4: 5-year follow up CT scan image of a patient with bone presence between the central peg radial fins.

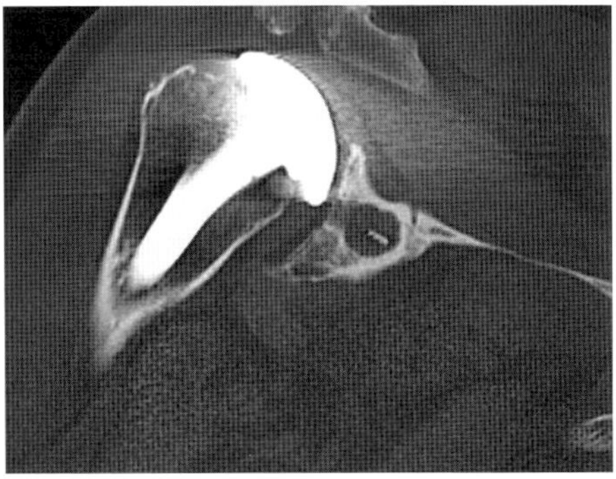

Fig. 6: 5-year follow up CT scan image of patient in figure 3. Note no indication of bone presence between the central peg radial fins and evidence of generalized lucency surrounding the central peg.

DISCUSSION

This study focuses on the immediate and midterm results of a novel, partially cemented, pegged glenoid design. These results support our hypothesis regarding improved longevity and reduced lucency formation with central peg bone incorporation.

Glenoid component loosening continues to be a common mode of failure in total shoulder arthroplasty [7, 10, 19, 20]. Loosening has been associated with the progression of glenoid lucent lines [1, 3, 16]. Multiple glenoid designs exist, including, screw fixation, metal backed, bone ingrowth, and all-polyethylene. Studies report superior results with cemented all-polyethylene implants [2, 6]. Polyethylene implants are available in several designs, including keeled, pegged, inline pegged, and partially cemented pegged.

Gartsman in 2005 reported initial post operative glenoid lucent lines present in 39% of keeled and 5% of pegged glenoid designs [8]. Edwards found similar results with 41% of keeled implants demonstrating lucent lines on initial post operative radiographs [5]. Bone preparation techniques such as compaction have shown a reduction in immediate post operative lucent line presence for keeled implants. Szabo reported 11% immediate lucent line presence advancing to 17% at two years using the compaction method with keeled implants [18]. One other recent report utilizing the compaction method identified 15% of keeled implants with immediate post operative lucent lines increasing to 46% at minimum two year follow-up [4]. Mileti reported 14% of keeled implants had immediate lucent line presence advancing to 95% at average 3.9 year follow-up [16]. Numerous studies have shown superiority of pegged over keeled implants [12, 13, 15, 19]. Pegged implant studies range from 0-10% lucent line presence on initial post operative radiographs and 15% at minimum two year follow-up [2, 4, 8].

Our study utilizes a partially cemented pegged design which has an uncemented central peg with radial fins allowing for bone incorporation. This design was proven superior to a keeled design in initial canine evaluation [19]. Currently no short or midterm reports exist for this implant. Our six-week post operative radiograph evaluation detected two shoulders with evidence of lucent lines. This 10% lucency rate correlates well with other fully cemented pegged designs [2, 4, 8]. At minimum five year follow-up our patient population had advancement to 25% lucent line presence. The presence of bone incorporation around the central peg fins was present in 85% of the glenoids at minimum five-year follow-up. This bone incorporation was graded as increased or similar in 15/20 shoulders and decreased or absent in 5/20 shoulders compared to their respective six week post operative films. None of the patients with increased or similar bone presence at five years had advancement in glenoid lucency. This group had only a single shoulder with peripheral peg grade 1 lucency at six weeks. This did not progress beyond grade 1 and remained the only shoulder in that group with peripheral peg lucency at five-year follow-up. In patients where the central peg bone incorporation was decreased or absent, mean peripheral peg lucency scores increased from 0.2 to 1.0 ($p=0.05$) and accounted for all of the worsening lucency grades at minimum five-year follow-up. These patients were also noted to have increased central peg lucency with modified Lazarus scores increasing from a group mean of 0.2 to 1.2, ($p=0.09$).

The two CT scans obtained correlated well with their respective X-ray findings. The patient with bone presence between three of the radial fins on xray had CT images which also identified bone present between the radial fins. The patient with five year follow-up radiographs which lacked radial fin bone presence and demonstrated lucency surrounding the central peg, had identical findings clearly depicted on their CT images. While CT scanning was completed in just two patients, in these two patients the X-ray and CT images demonstrated excellent correlation.

Despite the small numbers available, central peg bone incorporation does appear to virtually eliminate the development and progression of lucent line formation. Comparison of patients with similar or increased central peg bone to those with decreased or absent bone noted no difference in age, gender, preoperative glenoid erosion, or preoperative posterior humeral head subluxation. Reaming and soft tissue tensioning techniques were similar in all cases. The five patients with decreased or absent central peg bone incorporation have no identifiable reasons for this occurrence. While these five patients did have slight, but statistically significant advancement in glenoid lucent line formation, no patient in the study had clinical findings associated with the presence of glenoid lucent lines. These minor glenoid lucencies will likely progress, and at some point may become symptomatic, but at the present time they are radiologic findings that lack clinical significance.

This study has several limitations. First, the study size of 20 patients is small. However, despite this constraint, significance was reached in group glenoid lucency progression, as well as peripheral peg lucency progression in patients with decreased or absent bone presence between the central peg radial fins. Second, the six-week post-operative radiographs were not fluoroscopically aligned to insure a perfectly orthogonal view of the glenoid implant. While the six-week post-operative radiographic images remain good quality, a minor misalignment may underestimate the amount of bone presence between the radial fins, or potentially obscure lucent lines surrounding the peripheral pegs. Thirdly, no established grading system exists for this partially cemented glenoid implant. As such, a modification of the Lazarus grading system is presented for characterization of the uncemented central peg.

Future large scale, long-term, studies are indicated to evaluate the ultimate benefits of bone incorporation between the central peg radial fins and how this may reduce the formation of lucent lines and glenoid failure. Additional data regarding the proposed modification of the Lazarus grading system for the uncemented central peg will determine the relevance of this proposed grading system in determining the progression of glenoid lucency.

CONCLUSIONS

This partially cemented glenoid component had low rates of lucencies at five year minimum follow-up. These rates correspond favorably to those reported in the literature. The majority of patients had bone presence between the central peg radial fins at follow-up. When compared to respective six-week post-operative films, similar or increased bone growth between the radial fins of the central peg was associated with no progression of glenoid lucencies at five-year follow-up. Further, large scale, long-term studies are indicated to determine the clinical significance of these findings.

REFERENCES

[1] BARRETT WP, FRANKLIN JL, JACKINS SE, WYSS CR, Matsen III FA. Total shoulder arthroplasty. *J Bone Joint Surg 1987; 69A: 865-72.*

[2] BARWOOD S, SETTER KJ, BLAINE TA, BIGLIANI LU. The incidence of early radiolucencies about a pegged glenoid component using cement pressurization. *J Shoulder Elbow Surg 2008 Sep-Oct;17(5): 703-8.*

[3] BOILEAU P, AVIDOR C, KRISHNAN SG, WALCH G, KEMPF J, MOLE D. Cemented polyethylene versus uncemented metal-backed glenoid components in total shoulder arthroplasty: A prospective, double-blind, randomized study. *J Shoulder Elbow Surg 2002; 11:351-9.*

[4] EDWARDS TB, LABRIOLA JE, STANLEY RJ, O'CONNOR DP, ELKOUSY HA, GARTSMAN GM. Radiographic Comparison of Pegged and Keeled Glenoid Components Using Modern Cementing Techniques: A Prospective Randomized Study. *ASES Specialty Day Presentation, Las Vegas, NV, Feb 28, 2009.*

[5] EDWARDS TB, SABONGHY EP, ELKOUSY H, WARNOCK KM, Hammerman SM, O'Connor DP, et al. Glenoid component insertion in total shoulder arthroplasty: comparison of three techniques for drying the glenoid before cementation. *J Shoulder Elbow Surg 2007; 16(3 Suppl): S107-110.*

[6] FOX TJ, CIL A, SPERLING JW, SANCHEZ-SOTELO J, SCHLECK CD, COFIELD RH. Survival of the glenoid component in shoulder arthroplasty. *J Shoulder Elbow Surg 2009; Mar 16 [Epub].*

[7] FRANKLIN JL, BARRETT WP, JACKINS SE, MATSEN III FA. Glenid loosening in total shoulder arthroplasty. Association with rotator cuff deficiency. *J Arthoplasty 1988; 3: 39-46.*

[8] GARTSMAN GM, ELKOUSY HA, WARNOCK KM, EDWARDS TB, O'CONNOR DP. Radiographic comparison of pegged and keeled glenoid components. *J Shoulder Elbow Surg 2005; 14: 252-7.*

[9] HASAN SS, LEITH JM, CAMPBELL B, KAPIL R, SMITH KL, MATSEN FA, 3rd. Characteristics of unsatisfactory shoulder arthroplasties. *J Shoulder Elbow Surg 2002; 11: 431-41.*

[10] IBARRA C, DINES DM, McLAUGHLIN JA. Glenod replacement in total shoulder arthroplasty. *Orhop Clin North Am 1998; 29:403-13.*

[11] KELLEHER IM, COFIELD RH, BECKER DA, BEABOUT JW. Fluoroscopically positioned radiographs of total shoulder arthroplasty. *J Shoulder Elbow Surg 1992; 1: 306-11.*

[12] KLEPPS S, CHIANG AS, MILLER S, JIANG CY, HAZRATI Y, FLATOW EL. Incidence of Early Radiolucent Glenoid Lines in Patients Having Total Shoulder Replacements. *Clin Orthop 2005; 435: 118-25.*

[13] LACROIX D, MURPHY LA, PRENDERGAST PJ. Three-dimensional finite element analysis of glenoid replacement prostheses: a comparison of keeled and pegged anchorage systems. *J Biomech Eng 2000; 122: 430-6.*

[14] LANDIS JR, KOCH GG. The measurement of observer agreement for categorical data. *Biometrics 1977;33: 159-74.*

[15] LAZARUS MD, JENSEN KL, SOUTHWORTH C, MATSEN FA, 3rd. The radiographic evaluation of keeled and pegged glenoid component insertion. *J Bone Joint Surg Am 2002; 84-A: 1174-82.*

[16] MILETI J, BOARDMAN ND 3rd, SPERLING JW, COFIELD RH, TORCHIA ME, O'DRISCOLL SW *et al.* Radiographic analysis of polyethylene glenoid components using modern cementing techniques. *J Shoulder Elbow Surg 2004 Sep-Oct;13(5): 492-8.*

[17] NORRIS BL, LACHIEWICZ PF. Modern cement technique and the survivorship of total shoulder arthroplasty. *Clin Orhop 1996; 328: 76-85.*

[18] SZABO I, BUSCAYRET F, EDWARDS TB, NEMOZ C, O'CONNOR DP, BOILEAU P *et al.* Radiographic comparison of two glenoid preparation techniques in total shoulder arthroplasty. *Clin Orthop Relat Res 2005 Feb;(431): 104-10.*

[19] WIRTH MA, KORVICK DL, BASAMANIA CJ, TORO F, AUFDEMORTE TB, ROCKWOOD CA Jr Radiologic, mechanical, and histologic evaluation of 2 glenoid prosthesis designs in a canine model. *J Shoulder Elbow Surg 2001; 10: 140-8.*

[20] WIRTH MA, ROCKWOOD CA Jr Complications of total shoulder-replacement arthroplasty. *J Bone Joint Surg Am 1996; 78:603-16.*

HYBRID GLENOID RESURFACING: EXPERIENCE AND RESULTS

S.M. LAMBERT

DEFINITION

Hybrid glenoid resurfacing (HGR) combines two different physical mechanisms of implant fixation to obtain an optimal transference of joint-reaction force into the supporting cortical structure of the scapula (the lateral column, the base of the coracoid, and the spine of the scapula) through the vault of the glenoid.

The vault of the glenoid is supported between two buttresses, cranially (the supraglenoid tubercle region), and caudally (the infraglenoid tubercle region and lateral column of the scapula). Anteriorly and posteriorly the vault is bounded by walls of thin cortical bone of varying morphology, but at its medial (apical) extent the apex is again thick cortical bone. Implants which distribute load effectively and efficiently into the cranial and caudal buttresses are likely to survive better over the longer term. Thus implants which achieve fixation medially in juxtaposition with or into these buttresses may achieve improved long term durability. The cement mantle around a hip implant deforms by flow under hysteresis allowing implants to "bed in" over time. These mechanical conditions do not apply in the shoulder: the in vivo behaviour of a glenoid implant cement mantle depends on the distribution of force into the asymmetric vault of the glenoid, the strength of the supporting cancellous bone mantle, and the effectiveness of load-transfer into the cortical walls of the glenoid. The variation in width and zonal distribution of lucent lines around cemented glenoid implants, whether keeled or pegged, suggests that the evolution of lucencies in different zones of the implant-bone interface is caused through different zone-specific physical mechanisms. The more contact surface area (CSA) between implant and bone the better for fixation. However a greater CSA results in greater bone displacement and loss, particularly on retrieval during revision surgery, requiring sophisticated augmentation techniques particularly for non-contained defects of the glenoid vault. The geometric shape with the greatest surface area of contact with the least volume of displaced material is a cylinder or rod: a large core dia-

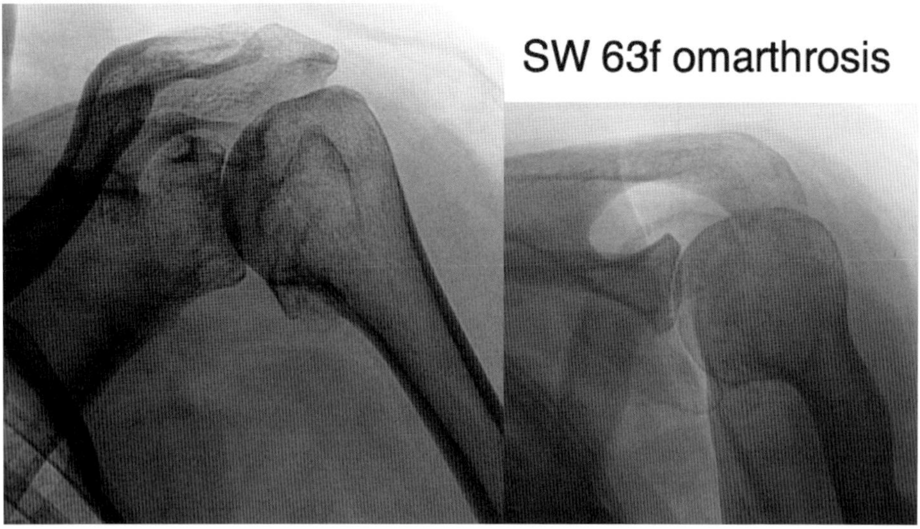

Fig. 1:
a) Omarthrosis: concentric, congruent, good bone quality of glenoids vault.
b) Short glenoid shell screws: note parallelism and positioning of the screws. The small horizontal line within each of the shell screws is the radiological marker within the pegs of the glenoid component.

meter hollow screw produces radial preload on bone into which it is introduced, suggesting a potential osteoprotective or osteoregenerative advantage over time for implantation into bone of poor quality. A cement interface permits primary fixation in bone with a relatively elastic load-transfer, but a potentially negative effect on bone quality in the longer term. Thus an implant which combines the advantages of primary fixation in bone and a positive time-dependant influence on bone health with the relatively elastic, hence more effective, load-shedding characteristics of a cement interface might demonstrate better longevity than either the traditional pure cement or mechanical (uncemented) interfaces (fig. 1).

PROBLEMS WITH CURRENT GLENOID COMPONENT FIXATION

Cemented fixation

A well-integrated and contiguous cement mantle can, and often does, give excellent durable fixation of a glenoid component over time, and modern polymer technology ensures a low rate of primary component wear provided the joint reaction force remains directed into the glenoid vault. Polymer wear currently appears to be a minor cause of aseptic glenoid component loosening: granuloma disease is not a common feature of glenoid component failure. The integrity of the rotator cuff is the major factor in determining the centralisation force acting on the glenoid: the normal evolution of cuff degeneration may be different in patients with osteoarthritis but is certainly a major concern in the inflammatory arthropathies. Cranial humeral head migration, particularly during initiation of abduction, will occur if the supra-equatorial rotator cuff is insufficient, creating abnormal resultant joint reaction forces on the glenoid. If this causes deformation of the polymer-cement interface and abnormal cancellous bone loading profiles leading to stress concentration and stress-shielding within the vault, then loosening, particularly in poor quality bone, will eventually occur. Ultimately, the fate of the glenoid component appears more dependant on the fate of the rotator cuff than on the properties of the component itself.

It follows that the younger the patient, the more likely that rotator cuff dysfunction will be a survival-determining factor for the glenoid component, and revision will be a necessary consideration at the outset.

Failure leading to revision of cemented components is characterised by loss of cancellous bone material from the vault, creating either contained or non-contained cavities. Contained cavities are relatively easy to deal with using fixation of a revision prosthesis which bypasses the cavity to gain primary fixation, but which provides loading conditions on the graft used to fill the cavity to enhance secondary osseo-integrative fixation. Non-contained cavities are more difficult to deal with requiring structural augmentation of bone and polyaxial fixation into the scapula, while again enhancing secondary osseo-integrative fixation. If the problem of cavitation could be avoided in the first instance then the problem of revision would be simplified.

The hollow screws used in HGR displace less bone, provide a compressive radial preloading on bone and, in whichever direction the glenoid reaction force is applied through the possible 360 degree range, there is a zone of the surface of the screw which resists deformation or displacement. Removal of screws from cancellous bone leaves a track determined by the core diameter of the screw, without more bone being lost than the volume of the cylinder of the screw. This permits non-augmented (hence simpler) revision replacement of the glenoid component.

Cementless fixation

A flat-backed metal base-plate loads the glenoid vault through contact with the cortical rim of the prepared glenoid. Incomplete contact will lead to stress-shielding and so progressive bone lysis at the zone of incomplete contact, including within the glenoid vault. This can be anticipated and minimised by extra screw fixation, permitting load-sharing/distribution into the cortical bone struts of the scapula. Most base-plates are flat: radial preload of the glenoid vault would be improved by a convex back surface to the component. If asymmetric primary screw fixation is achieved then it is a matter of time before there is motion between the components of the base-plate system, metallosis, and loosening.

The hollow screws used in HGR obtain cancellous bone fixation and, if necessary, primary cortical fixation using longer screws into the vault of the osteoporotic glenoid or into a medialised vault. The convex back of the glenoid resurfacing prosthesis generates radial distribution of force into the glenoid vault consistent with the natural trabecular pattern of the metaphyseal bone. The cemented interface between the hollow screws and the polyethylene glenoid component permits non-destructive micromotion of the glenoid component so distributing load into the screws: no failure of the pegs of the glenoid component has been noted to date.

ADVANTAGES OF HGR

HGR provides adaptability to challenging glenoid conditions and to the changing rotator cuff environment.

GLENOID FOSSA DEFORMITY

1) Screw fixation into the glenoid permits a greater part of the spectrum of degenerative glenoid morphologies to be treated by simple total shoulder replacement without augmentation or compromise of the position, alignment, or fixation of the glenoid component. The medialised glenoid fossa (the deepest part of the floor of the glenoid is medialised to the level of the base of the coracoid) can accommodate short hollow screws with cortical fixation and permit protection of the "at-risk" glenoid especially in the inflammatory arthritides where a hemi-arthroplasty solution might otherwise be selected (giving poorer outcomes for pain and further glenoid erosion) (fig. 2).

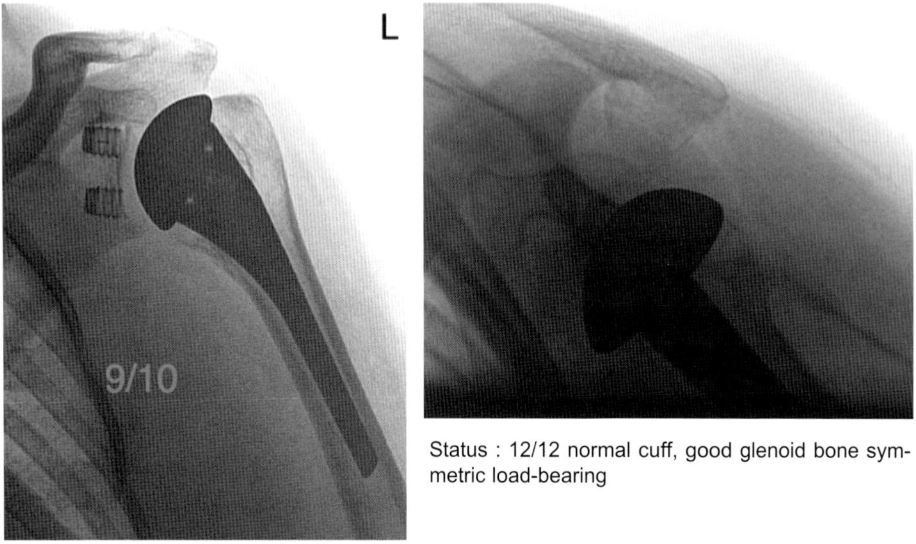

Status : 12/12 normal cuff, good glenoid bone symmetric load-bearing

Fig. 2: In situations where the glenoid neck is short, shell screws can still provide a durable basis for glenoid fixation where a keeled or pegged cemented implant would have been potentially difficult to implant successfully.

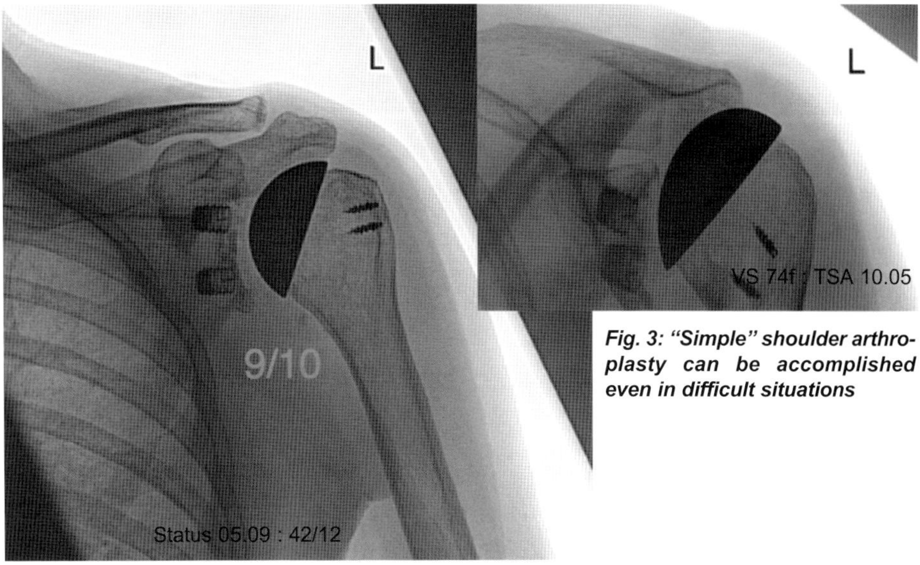

Fig. 3: "Simple" shoulder arthroplasty can be accomplished even in difficult situations

2) If the glenoid and scapular metaphysis are deformed by fracture with malunion complicated by post-traumatic arthritis, then the hollow screws can be sited to accommodate existing fracture fixation implants, and still permit glenoid protection (fig. 3).

GLENOID FOSSA DYSPLASIA

3) Retroversion, partial or complex hypoplasia of the glenoid with arthritis can be corrected with the hollow screw fixation of the glenoid component in HGR. The rationale for not correcting retroversion of the glenoid for total shoulder replacement does, in part, reflect the difficulty of gaining secure primary implantation of the glenoid component if standard cemented or non-cemented fixation is used: if the glenoid vault is reamed to neutral version insufficient bone will sometimes be left for fixation of the glenoid component. Short hollow screws can be used to gain secure primary fixation in very shallow fossae after correcting for congenital (or degenerative) retroversion.

REVISIBILITY

As noted, removal of the hollow screws of HGR leaves a greater volume of glenoid vault bone stock for immediate non-augmented revision replacement: this gives the operating surgeon more options for revision particularly if the rotator cuff condition is favourable (when it would be undesirable to proceed to excision hemiarthroplasty, or reversed polarity replacement).

SURGICAL TECHNIQUE IN HGR: PITFALLS

To gain maximum advantage from the HGR method the accuracy of implantation of the hollow screws is paramount, but difficult.

Parallelism

Parallelism of the screws for optimal cementation of the polyethylene glenoid component is not always easy to achieve particularly in bone of varying quality: the softer bone of osteoporosis can allow the screw to be placed helically rather than axially and so offset or non-parallelism can be created.

Positioning

The hollow screws should be placed close to the robust bone of the tubercular regions of the glenoid: the caudal screw is usually placed first (the range of possible positions is least), and this determines the position of the cranial screw, which is placed as close to the supraglenoid region as permitted, anterior to the dorsal concavity of the scapular neck at this point so that the screw does not penetrate the dorsal scapular cortex. Should the cranial screw penetrate at this point the suprascapular nerve is within range of injury.

Penetration

Longer screws are used in osteoporotic bone (fig. 4) and in dysmorphic glenoid conditions but in general the shorter screws are used in glenoids with normal bone quality. Penetration of the glenoid vault anteriorly or posteriorly is not necessarily a problem provided good cortical contact is gained and the two screws are parallel: should there be divergence or convergence of the screws then further medial displacement of the screws is possible on implantation of the glenoid component.

RESULTS OF HGR

In 2008, Hertel presented the 2 to 8 year review of HGR using the Epoca *(Synthes, Dubendorf, Switzerland)* shell-screw system. This was a single-surgeon, prospective, non-randomised cohort study conducted from 1999 to 2006 of 70 glenoids in 63 patients. Nine patients had inadequate radiographs, leaving 61 glenoids in 54 patients with sufficient information for the study. At a mean follow-up of 54 months (range 24 to 97 months) lucent lines were noted in 8 glenoids (13%), which, in one case, were greater than 2 mm in at least one zone. No clinically relevant loosening was noted. No revision surgery was indicated. The mean Constant Score at the latest review was 63 (range 19-84). The mean Oxford Shoulder Score was 17 (range 12-44).

Lucent lines were seen in cases in which cement had extruded from the hollow screws under the glenoid component. It is assumed that motion of the glenoid component under load caused the cement to fragment so creating the rare condition of cement-related bone lysis. This author has not noted a similar complication in over 60 similar cases even with cement extrusion.

The author has revised three glenoid components in which hollow screws had been used, two for haematogenous infection and one during revision for early massive rotator cuff failure. The screws were readily removed in the first two cases, but bone stock was preserved and interval revision arthroplasty was possible using another large-pitch screw fixed-fulcrum device with adequate primary fixation. The screws were much better integrated in the third case but again readily removed, once the cement had been retrieved from the cavity of the screws using a mechanical cement-removal instrument. Revision was completed as in the first cases.

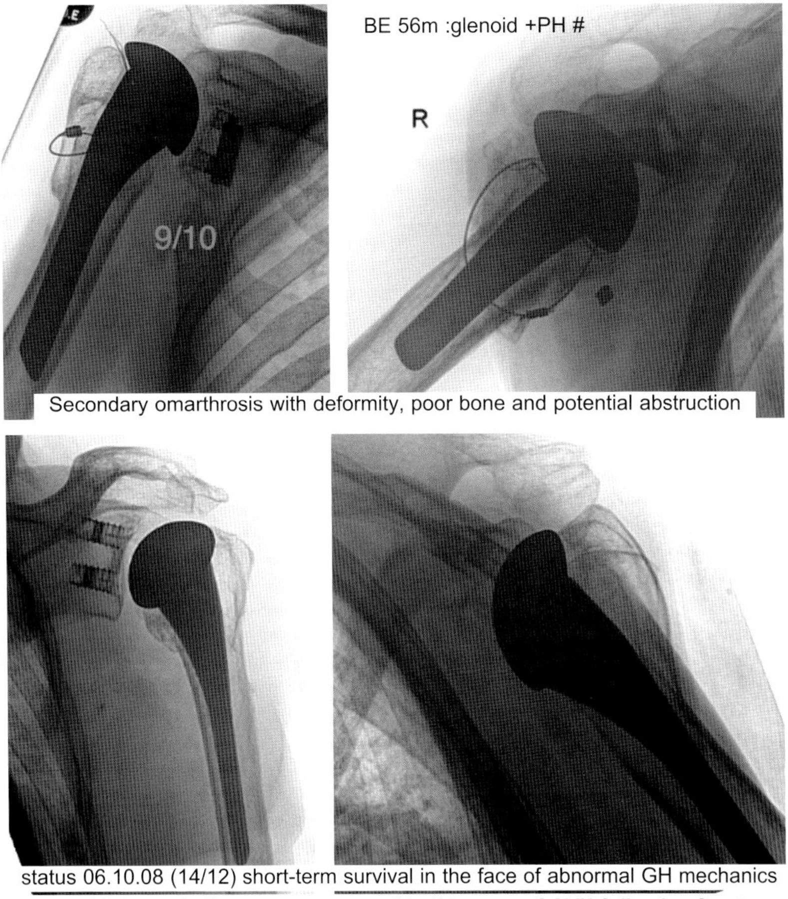

Fig. 4: 76f: long shell screws were used in this case of AVN following fracture of the proximal humerus in which the glenoid vault was osteopaenic

CONCLUSION

HGR appears to be a reliable and durable method in the short to medium term, and, importantly, preserves the volume and quality of glenoid vault bone stock. Aseptic glenoid wear is rare and loosening is not usually symptomatic or progressive enough to require revision. It appears that the extrusion of cement from the screws under the glenoid component might be implicated in the low incidence of lucent lines around this prosthesis.

CLINICAL AND RADIOLOGICAL FOLLOW-UP OF THE AEQUALIS THIRD-GENERATION CEMENTED TOTAL SHOULDER REPLACEMENT

A MINIMUM TEN-YEAR STUDY

A. KHAN, T.D. BUNKER, J.B. KITSON

There are no long-term published results on the survival of a third-generation cemented total shoulder replacement. We describe a clinical and radiological study of the Aequalis total shoulder replacement for a minimum of ten years. Between September 1996 and May 1998, 39 consecutive patients underwent a primary cemented total shoulder replacement using this prosthesis. Data were collected prospectively on all patients each year, for a minimum of ten years, or until death or failure of the prosthesis. At a follow-up of at least ten years, 12 patients had died with the prosthesis intact and two had emigrated, leaving 25 available for clinical review. Of these, 13 had rheumatoid arthritis and 12 osteoarthritis. One refused radiological review leaving 24 with fresh radiographs.

Survivorship at ten years was 100% for the humeral component and 92% for the glenoid element. The incidence of lucent lines was low. No humeral component was thought to be at risk and only two of the glenoid. The osteoarthritic group gained a mean 65° in forward flexion and their Constant score improved by a mean 41.4 points. The rheumatoid group gained a mean of 24° in flexion and their Constant score improved by 29.4 points. This difference may have been due to failure of the rotator cuff in 75% of the patients with rheumatoid arthritis. This a third generation total shoulder replacement gives an excellent result in patients with osteoarthritis and an intact rotator cuff.

Patients with rheumatoid arthritis have a 75% risk of failure of the rotator cuff at ten years.

Fixation of the glenoid component is one of the limiting factors in both first- and second-generation total shoulder replacement (TSR) [1-4]. The rate of loosening seen with the second-generation Neer II modular TSR in long-term studies was 24% at 9.5 years [5] and 40% at 7.7 years [6] which was of considerable concern. This has led to the cautious use of a glenoid component even when the evidence points to the functional superiority of TSR over hemiarthroplasty in the short- and medium-term [7].

The Aequalis TSR (Tornier Inc, St Ismier, France) is an unconstrained third-generation prosthesis with variable medial and posterior offset which replicates the complex shape of the proximal humerus. The non-conforming anatomically pear-shaped glenoid component, should, in theory, improve glenohumeral kinematics by restoring the mechanical lever arm of the abductors, thereby reducing excessive translation of the humeral head, eccentric loading and loosening [8].

This study describes a third-generation modular posterior offset TSR performed using a contemporary cementing technique.

PATIENTS AND METHODS

In September 1996 we began to use a third-generation prosthesis, the Aequalis (Tornier Inc). In 2008 we obtained approval of the Ethics Committee to review patients in whom this prosthesis had been implanted for more than ten years. Between September 1996 and May 1998, 30 consecutive Aequalis TSRs were implanted in 36 women and three men. Data were collected prospectively on all patients on an annual basis, for a minimum of ten years, or until death or failure of the prosthesis. During this period 12 patients died from unrelated causes at a mean of 5.75 years (2.0 to 10.0) from the initial operation. Two emigrated and were eventually lost to follow-up after one and six years, respectively. None of these patients showed signs of radiological loosening at the time of their last follow-up. The remaining 25 patients were reviewed by one of the authors (AK) who had not been involved in the original surgery. The mean time to follow-up was 10.6 years (10.0 to 12.0). Obtaining 100% follow-up was difficult since many patients were in their ninth decade of life, and some had moved to live with younger relatives. For two of these, review was by telephone. One had radiography at his local hospital and the other refused to attend for this examination. Radiological data were therefore available for 24 patients and clinical information for all 25.

The pre-operative diagnosis of the 25 surviving patients was rheumatoid arthritis (RA) in 13 (52%) and osteoarthritis (OA) in 12 (48%). Two had a small tear of the rotator cuff seen at operation. There were 24 women and one man with a mean age of 78.6 years (38 to 84). The glenoid bone stock was assessed pre-operatively on anteroposterior (AP) and axial radiographs and again at operation. Of the 13 patients with RA, two had severe erosion of the glenoid, one extending to the base of the coracoid and the other causing severe retroversion. Of the 12 patients with OA, six had erosions. According to the classification of Walch *et al* [9] four were A1, one was A2 and the other B1. The state of the rotator cuff was assessed clinically before surgery and by direct inspection and palpation operatively.

Operative technique

The senior author (TDB) carried out all the operations using the same surgical approach and cementing technique. Each patient had a scalene block and general anaesthesia. An extended deltopectoral approach was used. The quadrilateral space was carefully dissected and the posterior circumflex humeral vessels and axillary nerve identified and marked with a silastic sling. This protected the neurovascular bundle during the release of the inferior capsule, which was believed to be the key to a good exposure of the glenoid and allowed the shoulder to move freely post-operatively. The superior capsule, including the coracohumeral and superior glenohumeral ligaments, was divided thereby allowing complete exposure of the margins of the glenoid. A biceps tenodesis to pectoralis major was performed in all cases.

A small tear of the rotator cuff was identified but not repaired in two patients with OA. All the others had an intact cuff, although this was attenuated in five of the 13 with RA. In the rheumatoid patient whose glenoid had been eroded to the base of the coracoid, osteotomy of the coracoid was needed to expose the margins of the glenoid. An allograft from a femoral head was screwed to the native glenoid before the implantation of a cemented glenoid component. In the other rheumatoid patient with a severely retroverted glenoid and posterior subluxation of the head of the humerus, the glenoid was reamed in an attempt to correct the retroversion before implanting the glenoid component. No bone graft was used. In the osteoarthritic patients, the glenoid was reamed according to the manufacturer's recommendations.

A standard cementing technique was used in each patient. The glenoid was irrigated using the Exeter lavage system (Howmedica International Ltd, London, United Kingdom) and the slot in the glenoid for the keel of the implant was dried with an adrenaline (1:200,000)-soaked swab. Palacos R bone cement with gentamicin (Schering-Plough Ltd, Welwyn Garden City, United Kingdom) was packed into the prepared, washed and dried bone and pressurised with the glenoid component. On the humeral side, an appropriately-sized Exeter cement restrictor (Howmedica International Ltd) was inserted. The bone surface was washed using the Exeter lavage system (Howmedica), dried with suction and swabs, and Palacos cement with gentamicin was inserted down the intramedullary canal with digital pressure.

Implants

A keeled ultra-high-molecular-weight all-polyethylene flat-backed glenoid component was used in all cases. In 22 patients small components were used and in the other three, a medium-sized implant. In 13 patients a neck-stem angle of 130° (125° to 140°) was used and in 15 a head of 46 mm × 17 mm (39 to 50). We used 9 mm femoral components in 22 patients and of 6.5 mm in the other three. These were implanted with 30° of retroversion in each case. Posterior offset was reproduced by rotation of the component of the humeral head to the appropriate position.

Rehabilitation

A sling was used for 48 hours for comfort and to allow recovery from the scalene block. At this stage, patients were given gentle pendulum exercises. For the first six weeks the emphasis was on passive and then active forward elevation and abduction to 90° and external rotation to neutral. Free movements were allowed after six weeks.

All the patients were assessed pre-operatively using the American Shoulder and Elbow Surgeons Score (ASES) [10] and that of Constant and Murley [11]. Follow-up assessment was performed by one of the authors (AK) who had not been involved in the surgery and using the ASES, the Constant and the Oxford shoulder score (OSS) [12]. The range of post-operative movement in each direction was measured using a goniometer (Baseline, Chattanooga Group, Chattanooga, Tennessee). Strength was assessed with the arm at 90° of abduction in the plane of the scapula using the mean of three measurements with resistance against a calibrated 30 1b spring balance (Reuben Heaton Ltd, Warwickshire, United Kingdom) maintained for three seconds. This was recorded on the Constant score forms.

Radiological assessment

Standardised AP radiographs in the plane of the scapula and axillary views at a tangent to the glenoid, were taken throughout the study. At follow- up these were assessed for radiolucent lines by two authors not involved in the original surgery (AK, JBK). The glenoid was assessed according to the method of Lazarus *et al* [13] as follows: grade 0, no lucent lines; grade 1, a lucent line under the base plate, but not affecting the keel; grade 2, an incomplete lucent line around the keel; grade 3, a complete lucent line around the keel which was non-progressive and less than 2 mm wide; grade 4, a complete lucent line around the keel greater than 2 mm wide; and grade 5, movement of the glenoid component relative to the native scapula and therefore considered to be loose. Glenoid components graded as 4 and 5 were deemed to be 'at risk'.

The humerus was assessed by the method of Sperling *et al* [14]. The stem was divided into thirds. Zones 1 to 3 referred to the cement-bone interface adjacent to the lateral three thirds, and zones 5 to 7 the interfaces adjacent to the medial three thirds. Zone 4 represented the tip of the stem and zone 8 the undersurface of the head. A radiolucent line > 2 mm wide in three or more zones or gross loosening indicated that the humeral component was at risk. Superior migration was recorded as movement of the centre of the humeral head with respect to the centre of the glenoid as described by Deutsch *et al.* [15] An excursion of 5 mm or more was taken to represent failure of the cuff [5, 15-17].

Statistical analysis

Kaplan-Meier [18] survival curves were constructed using loosening of the component and revision for any cause as end-points. Pre- and post-operative measurements of active movement, pain and the Constant score were compared using the Friedman test. An unpaired *t*-test was used to compare the post-operative scores of groups of patients with intact and impaired rotator cuffs. A p-value ≤ 0.05 was considered to be significant.

RESULTS

Clinical

There was significant improvement in the Constant score in each group after ten years. Pain, function and activity were all significantly better ($p < 0.001$, table I).

Patients with OA had the best results at follow-up. In this group the mean pain score on the visual analogue scale (VAS) improved markedly from 6.0 to 1.0. The mean flexion increased from 65° to 130° and the adjusted Constant score improved from 26.0% to 92.8%. By contrast, the two patients who had small tears at the initial operation had developed massive tears of the cuff with pseudoparalytic shoulders at follow-up. Their flexion was worse than before surgery, but the adjusted Constant score was better, 22.0% to 50.0%, because their pain was negligible. The VAS was reduced from 7.0 to 4.0. Despite the massive tears their glenoid components did not loosen.

Table I: Pre- and post-operative clinical details (mean) of the patients

Pre-operative		Post-operative*	
OA†			
Constant Pain score	2.1	Constant Pain score	14.4
CS‡ (% adjusted)	18.0 (*26.0*)	CS (% adjusted)	59.4 (*92.8*)
Pain VAS§	6.8	Pain VAS	1.0
ASES¶ score	24.3	ASES score	74.9
		Oxford score	20.3
Range of movement (°)			
Flexion	65	Flexion	130
Abduction	55	Abduction	121
External rotation	9	External rotation	48.8
Internal rotation	Buttock	Internal rotation	T8
OA with cuff tear			
Constant pain score	2.5	Constant pain score	7.5
CS (% adjusted)	14.2 (*22.0*)	CS (% adjusted)	26.0 (*50.0*)
Pain VAS	7.0	Pain VAS	4.0
ASES score	35	ASES score	38.8
		Oxford score	38.5
Range of movement (°)			
Flexion	50	Flexion	45
Abduction	37	Abduction	8
External rotation	20	External rotation	20
Internal rotation	Buttock	Internal rotation	LSJ
Rheumatoid arthritis			
Constant Pain score	3.1	Constant pain score	10.5
CS (% adjusted)	14.0 (*20.0*)	CS (% adjusted)	43.4 (*62.8*)
Pain VAS	7.7	Pain VAS	1.2
ASES score	14.8	ASES score	59.5
		Oxford score	33
Range of movement* (°)			
Flexion	61	Flexion	84.6
Abduction	33	Abduction	43
External rotation	8	External rotation	41.2
Internal rotation	Thigh/buttock	Internal rotation	GT

* data exclude the two revision cases, one with rheumatoid arthritis and one with OA
† OA, osteoarthritis
‡ CS, Constant score
§ VAS, visual analogue scale
¶ ASES, American shoulder and elbow surgeons

The patients with RA also improved considerably. Their mean pain score (VAS) decreased from 7.7 to 1.2 at ten years. Flexion improved from a mean of 61° to 135° two years after surgery, but because of the deficiency in the cuff in nine of 12 of these patients, the mean flexion was only 84.6° at ten years. This was reflected in the adjusted Constant score which improved from a mean of 14.0 to 67.2 at two years, but decreased to 43.4 at ten years (Table I).

RADIOLUCENT LINES AND OSTEOLYSIS

Humerus

The radiographs of 24 patients were reviewed. After ten years, radiolucent lines were present in a single zone around 12 humeral components and in two humeral zones in four radiographs. In each case, they were less than 2 mm wide. There were no cases of revision for loosening of a 'humerus at risk' (table II).

Glenoid

There were two revisions for glenoid loosening (Table II). Both patients had an unusual indication for TSR. The first had suffered a thalamic stroke which caused athetosis of her left arm and severe arthrosis. The athetoid movement could not be controlled by medication either pre- or post-operatively. She developed lucent lines around the glenoid keel and eventually displaced the glenoid component. This was removed eight years after the initial operation, leaving her with a hemiarthroplasty. The second patient had RA with a severely retroverted glenoid fossa and pre-operative posterior subluxation. The glenoid was not grafted and the socket remained retroverted. She continued to have episodes of posterior subluxation and dislocation and the glenoid component eventually loosened. It was removed four years after the initial operation and a posterior bone block from the iliac crest was inserted in an attempt to keep her hemiarthroplasty located. In each of these cases, we assume that the cuff had failed since there was proximal migration of the humeral component of more than 5 mm.

Table II: The radiological review of 24 patients at ten years

Parameter	Number	OA*	OA with cuff	RA†
No glenoid radiolucent lines	11	6	1	2
Grade 1, 2 or 3 radiolucent lines	11	3	1	7
Glenoid at risk	2	0	0	2
Revision of glenoid	2	1	0	1
No humeral radiolucent lines	10	4	1	4
Humeral lucency < 2 mm	16	6	1	8
Humerus at risk	0	0	0	0
Superior migration of humeral head	14	2	2	9

* OA, osteoarthritis
† RA, rheumatoid arthritis

At radiological review, two glenoids were thought to be loose (Table II). Both patients had severe RA and were satisfied with their TSRs ten and 12 years after the initial operation despite complete lucent lines (grade-4 lucency) around the keel of their prosthesis and obvious failure of the rotator cuff, with gross upward migration of the humeral head. One patient had a femoral head allograft screwed to her native scapula for gross medialisation. When followed up at 12 years she had severe failure of the cuff with erosion of the acromion and distal clavicle by the superiorly displaced humeral component. Despite the use of allograft we included her in our final analyses. Both patients felt that they were better than before surgery and did not need revision.

Incomplete radiolucent lines were seen around a further 11 glenoid components of which two were around the keel. All were less than 2 mm in width. These results are summarised in Table II.

Integrity of the rotator cuff

The rotator cuff was intact in 36 patients at the time of surgery. Of the three patients with a tear in the cuff, two had a small full-thickness tear with a cuff of poor quality, and one had a massive tear with arthropathy. She died six years after her operation. In each case the tears progressed with superior migration of the humeral component of more than 5 mm (Table II).

Of the 24 patients reviewed radiologically at least ten years post-operatively, nine of 12 with RA had clinical and radiological evidence of failure of the cuff. If the patient with the revision is excluded, they had a mean Constant score of 43.4 points (adjusted Constant score 62.8%); Table I). Two osteoarthritic patients, who had an intact cuff at surgery, developed a deficiency of the cuff after ten years. Overall, there was a rate of cuff failure of 54.2% (13 of 24) at a minimum of ten years. The groups were further subdivided according to the state of the cuff at ten years. Those with an intact cuff achieved a better Constant score (table III). This difference did not, however, reach statistical significance (p = 0.052) because of the small number of patients in the study.

A presumption of failure of the cuff was made if the patient was pseudoparalytic, or had a grossly positive Jobe and

Table III. Mean shoulder scores at ten years or more comparing the effect of cuff failure*

				Active range of movement (°)†					
Pathology	**Number of patients**	**Pain (VAS)**	**Constant pain score**	**Flexion (°)**	**External rotation (°)**	**Internal rotation (°)**	**Abduction (°)**	**Constant score (% adjusted)‡**	**OSS§**
Osteoarthritis with intact cuff	8	0.25	14.38	140	54.3	T7	126	60.43 (*94.4*)	19.88
Osteoarthritis with cuff failure‡	3	3	10	90	30	LSJ	53	34.7 (*54.1*)	33.67
Rheumatoid arthritis with intact cuff	3	3.3	8.3	93	38	T12	60	42.0 (*60.9*)	40
Rheumatoid arthritis with cuff failure	8	0.375	11.25	85	43	Thigh	34	43.9 (*63.6*)	29.63

* data exclude the two revisions with failure of the cuff (one RA and one OA patient) and an RA patient who declined a radiograph

† excludes two patients from telephone review (one RA and one OA). Mode values given for internal rotation

‡ includes one patient with OA who developed failure of the cuff and two with tears of the cuff at the initial operation

§ OSS, Oxford shoulder score

Moyners test [19], weakness of external rotation and marked weakness on strength testing for the Constant score at 90° of abduction, elevation of the humeral head on resisted cuff action and a radiograph which showed increased upward migration of at least 5 mm. Since advanced imaging modalities such as ultrasonography were not used there may be a degree of inaccuracy in our diagnosis.

Complications

There were only two revisions, both for aseptic loosening of the glenoid component, one of which was secondary to recurrent posterior dislocation. There were no other dislocations. This gave a revision rate of 8% from all causes. There were no peri-operative deaths. The mean age of the patients who died was 79.3 years (59 to 91). The 59-year-old patient died from chronic obstructive pulmonary disease and complications of a rheumatoid cervical spine seven years after her initial operation. All 12 deaths were from unrelated causes. There were no cases of infection, neurovascular complications, thromboembolic event or peri-prosthetic fracture.

Survivorship

Survival of the humeral component for revision for any cause as an endpoint was 100%, with survival for aseptic or septic loosening of 100%. Survivorship curves of the glenoid with revision for any cause as an endpoint were constructed and survival of the glenoid at a minimum of ten years with revision for any cause as the end point was 92% (95% confidence interval (CI) 85.7 to 100). Using survival analysis, the probability of the glenoid loosening radiologically at 12 years was 85.2% (95% CI 71.9 to 98.5. In the worst-case analysis, in which the two shoulders lost to follow-up were regarded as failures, survival was 86.2% (95% CI 72 to 99) at 12 years.

DISCUSSION

Loosening of the glenoid is one of the commonest complications of TSR [1-4, 20]. In earlier studies the incidence of radiolucent lines at the glenoid cement-bone interface has ranged from 55% to 80% [21]. This has improved with modern cementing techniques [13, 21, 22] Sperling, Cofield and Rowland [23] showed an estimated glenoid survival of 97% at ten years using the Neer II prosthesis. However, Stewart and Kelly [5] had a revision rate of 8.1% and a radiological loosening rate of 27% at 9.5 years and Sojbjerg *et al* [6] showed loosening in 40% of their patients at 7.7 years.

Several studies [24, 25] have shown anatomical variability in the proximal humerus, particularly in the diameter of the head and in the medial and posterior offset from its centre in relation to the longitudinal axis of the humerus. This resulted in a more anatomical third generation of shoulder prostheses with variable head size and offset such as the Tornier Aequalis. Roentgenographic stereometric analysis has shown that by translating and rotating less, offset humeral heads produce less eccentric loading of the glenoid than standard heads thereby potentially reducing the risk of loosening of the glenoid component [26]. Our study assesses the survival of such a third-generation prosthesis at a minimum of ten years. Our results are encouraging as far as survival is concerned but devastating in terms of failure of the rotator cuff in the rheumatoid patient. The 100% survival of the cemented humeral component, with none at risk, is a considerable improvement on the results of the uncemented Neer II implant which had rates of loosening of 40% and 24% at 7.7 and 9.5 years, respectively [5, 6]. Our study suggests that a surgeon can be confident that a third-generation humeral component will survive for at least ten years.

Survival of 93% after ten years for the glenoid component is also reassuring. This is a better result than historical studies would have predicted. In retrospect, the two revisions in our study were as much a failure of indication as of technique. One glenoid component failed after being implanted into an athetoid patient and the other when severe retroversion of a posteriorly subluxed shoulder was not corrected at the time of the initial surgery. However, both patients would probably have suffered from marked erosion and pain in the glenoid had they been given a hemiarthroplasty.

Lucent lines around the glenoid component have been a concern in the past [21, 23] In our study there were only two glenoids at risk and in both of these patients there was severe failure of the rotator cuff. One had a femoral head allograft between the glenoid component and the native scapula which had survived for 12 years. The relative paucity of glenoid lucent lines in the other patients at ten years is in sharp contrast to the high incidence of loosening seen in other series because of the 'rockinghorse effect' [27] not least considering that 53.8% of the patients showed radiological and clinical evidence of failure of the rotator cuff. These results are better than the medium-term multicentre results from the originators of the Aequalis prosthesis [28]. This study reassures us that it is appropriate to replace the glenoid.

There are several potential weaknesses in our study. One was the relatively small number of patients available for review. However, these numbers were similar to those in the long-term studies of Sneppen *et al* [29] and of Stewart and Kelly [5] and to the mid-term studies of Raiss *et al.* [8] We failed to follow-up the two patients who had emigrated, but achieved complete clinical follow-up of those remaining in the country despite many being in their ninth decade of life. We used proximal migration of the humeral component as evidence of failure of the rotator cuff. Although an indirect parameter, its accuracy has been validated by numerous studies [30-32] including its use in evaluating TSR [5, 15-17].

The radiographs were not set up with image-intensifier control, but they were standardised and were performed by a dedicated musculoskeletal radiographer for all except one patient. Only films which were perpendicular to the glenoid were accepted.

The principal strength of our study was that it reviewed the survival of a third-generation TSR with a minimum follow-up of ten years performed by a single surgeon, using the same prosthesis and technique at the same hospital.

Our study highlights a problem which we had not anticipated, that of failure of the cuff in 75% of the rheumatoid patients ten years after TSR. Paradoxically, this did not adversely affect the mean shoulder scores. Patients with an intact cuff had a mean Constant score of 42 whereas those with a tear scored 43.9. This was because one rheumatoid patient with an intact cuff scored poorly for function and had a VAS of 9. If she is excluded from the analysis, the mean Constant score for those with an intact cuff rises to 59. In the osteoarthritic group those with an intact cuff had a Constant score of 60, whereas those with failure had a score of 34.7. None of the osteoarthritic group had radiological evidence of loosening of the glenoid.

Our study has shown that deficiency of the rotator cuff rather than loosening of the glenoid is the most common long-term complication of a third-generation TSR. Two other studies confirm this. Sojbjerg *et al* [6] showed failure of the cuff in 43% of their 69 rheumatoid patients with a mean follow-up of 7.7 years and Stewart and Kelly [5] found superior subluxation in 57% of 58 consecutive TSRs performed for RA.

Our study found a survival of 100% for the humeral stem and of 93% for the socket at a minimum follow-up of ten years.

The incidence of lucent lines and sockets at risk is much less than reported in previous studies, but failure of the rotator cuff occured in 75% of rheumatoid patients by ten years.

The authors *wish to thank Dr R. Powell, Clinical Research Advisor, Clinical Governance and Research Department, Royal Devon & Exeter Hospital & Peninsula Medical School for his help with this study.*
No benefits *in any form have been received or will be received from a commercial party related directly or indirectly to the subject of this article.*

REFERENCES

[1] WIRTH MA, ROCKWOOD CA. Complications of total shoulder replacement arthroplasty. *J Bone Joint Surg [Am] 1996; 78-A:603-16.*

[2] BARRETT WP, FRANKLIN JL, JACKINS SE, WYSS CR, MATSEN FA 3rd Total shoulder arthroplasty. *J Bone Joint Surg [Am] 1987; 69-A:865-72.*

[3] HASAN SS, LEITH JM, CAMPBELL B, *et al.* Characteristics of unsatisfactory shoulder arthroplasties. *J Shoulder Elbow Surg 2002; 11: 431-41.*

[4] BOHSALI KI, WIRTH MA, ROCKWOOD CA. Complications of total shoulder arthroplasty. *J Bone Joint Surg [Am] 2006; 88-A: 2279-92.*

[5] STEWART MPM, KELLY IG, Total shoulder replacement in rheumatoid disease: 7- to 13-year follow-up of 37 joints. *J Bone Joint Surg [Br] 1997; 79-B:68-72.*

[6] SØJBJERG JO, FRICH LH, JOHANNSEN HV, SNEPPEN O. Late results of total shoulder replacement in patients with rheumatoid arthritis. *Clin Orthop 1999; 366: 39-45.*

[7] RADNAY CS, SETTER KJ, CHAMBERS L, *et al.* Total shoulder replacement compared with humeral head replacement for the treatment of primary glenohumeral osteoarthritis: a systematic review. *J Shoulder Elbow Surg 2007; 16: 396-402.*

[8] RAISS P, ALDINGER PR, KATSEN P, RICKERT M, LOEW M. Total shoulder replacement in young and middle-aged patients with glenohumeral osteoarthritis. *J Bone Joint Surg [Br] 2008; 90- B: 764-9.*

[9] WALCH G, BADET R, BOULAHIA A, KHOURY A. Morphologic study of the glenoid in primary glenohumeral osteoarthritis. *J Arthroplasty 1999; 14: 756-60.*

[10] RICHARDS RR, AN KN, BIGLIANI LU, *et al.* A standardized method for the assessment of shoulder function. *J Shoulder Elbow Surg 1994; 3: 347-52.*

[11] CONSTANT CR, MURLEY AH. A clinical method of functional assessment of the shoulder. *Clin Orthop 1987; 214: 160-4.*

[12] DAWSON J, FITZPATRICK R, CARR A. Questionnaire on the perceptions of patients about shoulder surgery. *J Bone Joint Surg [Br] 1996;78-B: 593-600.*

[13] LAZARUS MD, JENSEN KL, SOUTHWORTH C, MATSEN FA 3rd The radiographic evaluation of keeled and pegged glenoid component insertion. *J Bone Joint Surg [Am] 2002; 84-A: 1174-82.*

[14] SPERLING JW, COFIELD RH, DRISCOLL SW, TORCHIA ME, ROWLAND CM. Radiographic assessment of ingrowth total shoulder arthroplasty. *J Shoulder Elbow Surg 2000; 9: 507-13.*

[15] DEUTSCH A, ALTCHEK DW, SCHWARTZ E, OTIS J, WARREN RF. Radiologic measurement of superior displacement of the humeral head in the impingement syndrome. *J Shoulder Elbow Surg 1996; 5: 186-93.*

[16] HAINES JF, TRAIL IA, NUTTALL D, BIRCH A, BARROW A. The results of arthroplasty in osteoarthritis of the shoulder. *J Bone Joint Surg [Br] 2006; 88-B: 496-501.*

[17] TRAIL IA, NUTTALL D. The results of shoulder arthroplasty in patients with rheumatoid arthritis. *J Bone Joint Surg [Br] 2002; 84-B: 1121-5.*

[18] KAPLAN EL, MEIER P. Nonparametric estimation from incomplete observations. *J Am Stat Assoc 1958; 53: 457-81.*

[19] JOBE FW, MOYNES DR. Delineation of diagnostic criteria and a rehabilitation program for rotator cuff injuries. *Am J Sports Med 1982; 10: 336-9.*

[20] MATSEN FA 3rd, CLINTON J, LYNCH J, BERTELSEN A, RICHARDSON ML. Glenoid component failure in total shoulder arthroplasty. *J Bone Joint Surg [Am] 2008; 90-A: 885-96.*

[21] BREMS J. The glenoid component in total shoulder arthroplasty. *J Shoulder Elbow Surg 1993; 2: 47-54.*

[22] NORRIS BL, LACHIEWICZ PF. Modern cement technique and survivorship of total shoulder arthroplasty. *Clin Orthop 1996; 328: 76-85.*

[23] SPERLING JW, COFIELD RH, ROWLAND CM. Neer hemiarthroplasty and Neer total shoulder arthroplasty in patients fifity years old or less: long-term results. *J Bone Joint Surg [Am] 1998;80-A: 464-73.*

[24] BOILEAU P, WALCH G. The three dimensional geometry of the proximal humerus: implications for surgical technique and prosthetic design. *J Bone Joint Surg [Br] 1997; 79-B: 857-65.*

[25] ROBERTS SN, FOLEY AP, SWALLOW HM, WALLACE WA, COUGHLAN DP. The geometry of the humeral head and the design of the prosthesis. *J Bone Joint Surg [Br] 1992; 73-B: 647-50.*

[26] NUTTAL D, HAINES JF, TRAIL IA. The micromotion of pegged glenoid components in total shoulder replacements. *J Bone Joint Surg [Br] 2008; 90-B(Suppl II): 350.*

[27] BARRETT WP, FRANKLIN JL, JACKINS SE, WYSS CR, MATSEN FA 3rd Total shoulder arthroplasty. *J Bone Joint Surg [Am] 1987; 69-A: 865-72.*

[28] EDWARDS TB, KADAKIA NR, BOULAHIA A, *et al.* A comparison of hemiarthroplasty and total shoulder arthroplasty in the treatment of primary glenohumeral osteoarthritis: results of a multicenter study. *J Shoulder Elbow Surg 2003; 12: 207-13.*

[29] SNEPPEN O, FRUENSGUARD S, JOHANNSEN HV, *et al.* Total shoulder replacement in rheumatoid arthritis: proximal migration and loosening. *J Shoulder Elbow Surg 1996; 5: 47-52.*

[30] WEINER DS, MACNAB I. Superior migration of the humeral head: a radiological aid in the diagnosis of tears of the rotator cuff. *J Bone Joint Surg [Am] 1970; 52-A: 524-7.*

[31] LEHTINEN JT, BELT EA, LYBACK CO, *et al.* Subacromial space in the rheumatoid shoulder: a radiographic 15 year follow-up study of 148 shoulders. *J Shoulder Elbow Surg 2000; 9:183-7.*

[32] VAN DE SAND MHJ, ROZING PM. Proximal migration can be measured accurately on standardised anteroposterior shoulder radiographs. *Clin Orthop 2006; 443: 260-5.*

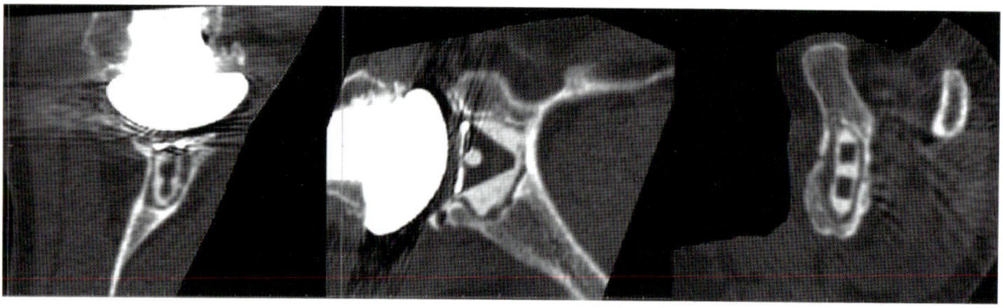

Fig. 1

processing software to generate 3-D reconstructions of each CT-scan. This software benefits from extremely fast OpenGL standard 3-1 D graphic capabilities, which are optimized for exploiting any available hardware graphic accelerator boards. The 3-D surface reconstructions were created using the surface rendering function in OsiriX with software settings optimized for metal (pixel value, 2000; high resolution, 0.50; smooth iterations, 80). To avoid measurement errors, all image reconstructions were made using the native section scans of 0.625 mm thickness.

The scapulae were reconstructed in 3D and digitalised reference (ROI) points were plotted along the lateral border of the scapula and the deepest part of the supraspinous fossa in order to determine the plane of the scapular blade. The metallic marker of the glenoid implant was used to evaluate the positioning of the glenoid relative to the plane of the scapula. This was staple-shaped in the Neer II prosthesis (fig. 2).

The ROI points were then transferred to a second programme: 3D-RESHAPER®. This software permitted calculation of the best

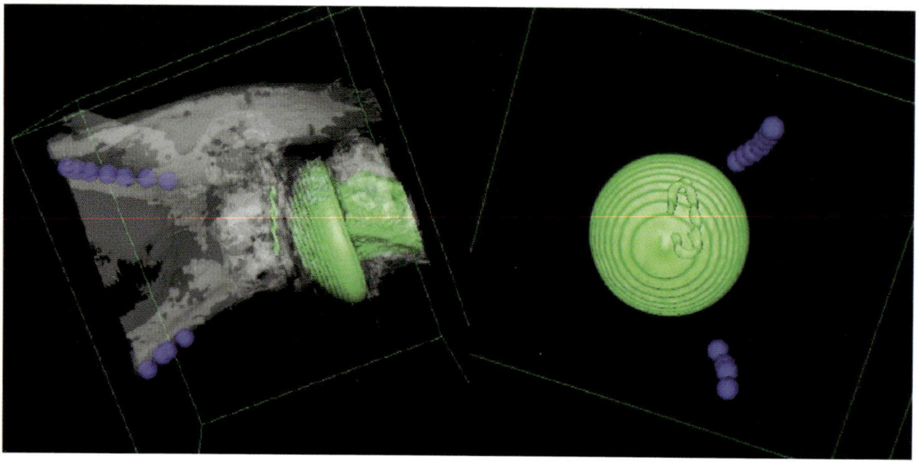

Fig. 2

plane of the scapula and the best plane of the glenoid according to the previously digitalised ROI points and measured the relationship of the planes relative to one another.

Four parameters of glenoid positioning were studied: glenoid version, glenoid inclination, glenoid rotation and the antero-posterior offset distance of the glenoid relative to the scapular plane.

The version was calculated by measuring the angle between the plane of the glenoid and the plane of the scapula. The inclination was calculated by measuring the angle between a line drawn perpendicularly from the centre of the glenoid in the scapular plane, and a line drawn along the floor of the supraspinous fossa. Rotation was calculated by measuring the angle between the supero-inferior axis of the glenoid and the scapular plane. The offset was measured as the shortest distance between the centre of the glenoid metallic marker and the scapular plane.

Using a standardised protocol, both a senior consultant shoulder surgeon and a musculoskeletal radiologist reviewed the CT scans looking for the presence of radiolucent lines and/or osteolysis. The radiolucent lines were ranked according to the Molé scoring system [5]. A four-point scale was chosen to rank osteolysis: no osteolysis, osteolysis restricted to one or more of the glenoid fixation areas, major osteolysis involving the whole glenoid fixation without cortical disruption, and major osteolysis involving the whole glenoid fixation with cortical disruption.

To determine the patterns of polyethylene wear, we used a recently published and validated technique, which employed three-dimensional (3-D) computed tomography to determine acetabular wear in total hip arthroplasty. The technique has a reported accuracy of 0.08 mm and a reproducibility of 0.04 mm [6].

For each of the 3-D image reconstructions, the humeral head was digitized with an average of 33 points (SD, 9; from 13 to 64) evenly dispersed on the spherical portion. The glenoid component was digitized using an average of 9 points (SD, 0.8; from 8 to 12) dispersed on the staple shaped metallic marker of the glenoid. The humeral head is therefore represented by a cloud of points that lie on a unique sphere and the glenoid component by a succession of points that lie on a unique staple shaped area in space. While digitalizing a point on a metallic component, OsiriX placed the point precisely on the metal surface in the 3-D view with a spatial accuracy of 0.001 mm.

The coordinates of digitized points were exported from OsiriX to a file as comma separated variables (CSV). Geometric analysis software, 3D Reshaper® *(Technodigit, Gleizé, France)*, was used to deduce the coordinates of the articular head center by fitting a sphere to its point cloud, and the center of the glenoid component by fitting a circle to its point array, in both cases using the method of least squares (fig. 3). The point coordinates were further manipulated in spreadsheets

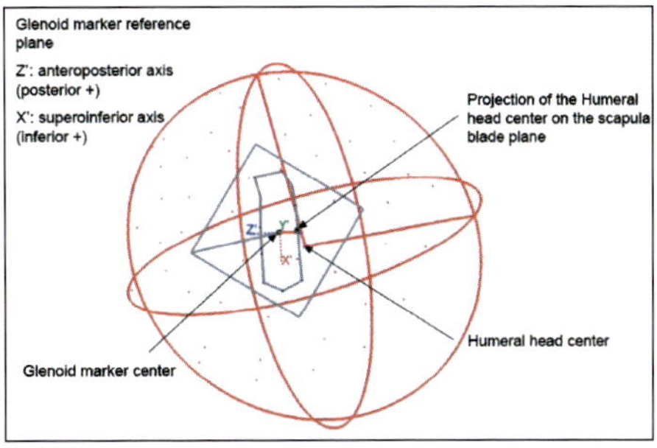

Fig. 3

using Microsoft EXCEL® (Microsoft Corp, Redmond, WA) to deduce the head-glenoid eccentricity vector in the reference plane of the scapular shape marker (wear vector), and to calculate the amount of glenoid polyethylene (PE) wear.

Statistical evaluation

Nonparametric statistical analysis was performed with use of SPSS 10.0 for (SPSS, Chicago, Illinois) to determine relationships between variables. Significance was set at $p < 0.05$.

RESULTS

Clinical outcome

On examination at latest follow up, the active forward flexion was on average 131° (SD 31°; range 40° to 170°) and the active abduction was on average 128° (SD 35°; range 25° to 170°). The average Constant score was 78 points (SD 25; range 7 to 90).

Radiological outcome

The mean Molé score for radiolucent lines was 9 points (SD 4; range 1 to 15). The lucency score on computed tomography correlated significantly with patient follow up ($p<0.001$). Four patients had no osteolysis around the glenoid; 12 had osteolysis restricted to one or more of the glenoid fixation areas; 10 had major osteolysis involving the whole glenoid fixation without cortical disruption; and 5 had major osteolysis involving the whole glenoid fixation with cortical disruption.

Glenoid positioning parameters

The results of the four glenoid positioning parameters are reported in Table 1. These parameters were scored so that retroversion was positive and anteversion negative; superior inclination was positive and inferior inclination negative; clockwise rotation was positive for a right shoulder and anticlockwise rotation was positive for a left shoulder. The average version was 5.53° but with a standard deviation of 12.22° (from -19 to +29°), implying a large variation in the implant positioning. Equivalent results were reported for the other three positioning parameters.

Table 1: Results of the glenoid implant postional parameters

	Average	SD	Min	Max
Retroversion (°)	5,53	12,22	-19	+29
Superior inclination (°)	14,28	18,91	-16	+60
Rotation (°)	3,54	13,28	-25	+33
Off-set distance (mm)	5,81	3,16	0	+13,6

Glenoid wear pattern

The results of the wear pattern are reported in Table 2. The wear pattern was scored so that posterior wear was positive and anterior wear negative; inferior wear was positive and superior negative. The absolute offset distance between the centre of the glenoid marker and the projection of the humeral head centre on the glenoid marker plane (wear vector) was on average 2.790 mm (SD, 1.703; from 0.631 to 6.516). The offset distance along the antero-posterior axis of the glenoid marker correlated significantly with glenoid version ($R2=0.425$; $p<0.01$). The offset distance along the supero-inferior

Table 2: Glenoid wear pattern

	Average	SD	Min	Max
Absolute offset distance (Wear vector) (mm)	2,79	1,704	0,632	6,516
Offset distance along the antero-posterior axis (mm)	0,701	2,687	-5,478	+6,206
Offset distance along the supero-inferior axis (mm)	-0,653	1,677	-3,948	+4,287
Amount of PE worn (mm)	0,208	1,508	0,007	0,834

axis of the glenoid marker correlated significantly with glenoid inclination. The wear vector correlated significantly with duration of follow-up ($R2=0.267$; $p=0.024$) and with the Molé score ($R2=0.141$, $p=0.114$). The amount of PE wear also correlated significantly with duration of follow-up ($R2=0.25$; $p=0.016$) and Molé score ($R2=0.176$, $p=0.176$).

DISCUSSION

Glenoid failure: Material or Surgical Failure? This series demonstrates that the glenoid component positioning significantly affects PE wear, the orientation of wear (wear vector) and the occurrence of radiolucent lines. Accurate glenoid component positioning is therefore the prerequisite for preserving the PE (Material) from early failure.

This study used CT-scans to calculate the humeral head penetration in glenoid PE and the glenoid wear patterns. This has been made possible by the advent of novel computer data processing techniques, which are both accurate and reproducible. The 3-D CT technique used in this study has been recently published and validated in the determination of acetabular wear patterns in total hip arthroplasties, with an accuracy of 0.08 mm and a reproducibility of 0.04 mm [6]. Our study is the first attempt to assess the in situ wear in TSA. The CT technique addresses the shortcomings of cadaveric and retrieval studies [2, 3]: a greater number of prostheses can be analyzed and early patterns of wear can be measured. The direction of wear in relation to the position and orientation of the glenoid prosthesis can be assessed.

In this study, the wear vectors along the supero-inferior axis and antero-posterior axis were significantly correlated with the version and inclination of the glenoid respectively. Neutral glenoid version and neutral or slight inferior inclination resulted in central loading of the glenoid, minimising wear.

These results are in keeping with previous Finite Element Analysis studies: Hopkins *et al.* [7], Oosterom *et al.* [8] and Nyffeler *et al.* [9] performed in-vitro experiments analysing the effects of the glenoid version and inclination on glenoid implant fixation. They all concluded that variation in version and inclination lead to eccentric loading of the implant. This eccentric loading of the glenoid component (so-called "Rocking Horse Effect") is associated with component failure. In our study, both the wear vector and amount of PE wear were significantly associated with the occurrence of radiolucent lines (and osteolysis) around the implant. These results confirm that eccentric loading leads to greater wear and component failure.

CONCLUSION

This in vivo computed tomographic study successfully demonstrates a direct relationship between wear patterns and the position of the glenoid component in TSA. With regard to loosening of the glenoid component in TSA, we conclude that the surgical failure induces the material failure.

REFERENCES

[1] BOHSALI KI, WIRTH MA, ROCKWOOD CA Jr Complications of total shoulder arthroplasty. *J Bone Joint Surg Am 2006; 88-10: 2279-92.*

[2] SCARLAT MM, MATSEN FA, 3rd Observations on retrieved polyethylene glenoid components. *J Arthroplasty 2001; 16-6: 795-801.*

[3] WIRTH MA, AGRAWAL CM, MABREY JD, DEAN DD, BLANCHARD CR, MILLER MA, ROCKWOOD CA, Jr Isolation and characterization of polyethylene wear debris associated with osteolysis following total shoulder arthroplasty. *J Bone Joint Surg Am 1999; 81-1: 29-37.*

[4] GREGORY T, TAILLIEU F, BARING T, VANDENBUSSCHE E, HANSEN UN, MÜTSCHLER C, AMIS AA, EMERY R, AUGEREAU B. A new CT-scan protocol for the in-vivo analysis of glenoid failure after total shoulder arthroplasty. *10th International Congress on Shoulder Surgery Salvador, Bahia, Brasil, 2007.*

[5] MOLE D RO, RIAND N, LEVIGNE C, WALCH G. Cemented glenoid components: results in osteoarthritis and rheumatoid arthritis. In: Walch G BP, *ed. Shoulder arthroplasty. Berlin: Springer, 1999: 163-71.*

[6] VANDENBUSSCHE E, SAFFARINI M, HANSEN UN, TAILLIEU F, MUTSCHLER C, AUGEREAU B, GREGORY TM. Measurement of Femoral Head Penetration in Polyethylene using a 3-Dimensional Ct-scan technique. *Acta Orthopaedica 2010.*

[7] HOPKINS AR, HANSEN UN, AMIS AA, KNIGHT L, TAYLOR M, LEVY O, COPELAND SA. Wear in the prosthetic shoulder: association with design parameters. *J Biomech Eng 2007;129-2: 223-30.*

[8] OOSTEROM R, ROZING PM, BERSEE HE. Effect of glenoid component inclination on its fixation and humeral head subluxation in total shoulder arthroplasty. *Clin Biomech (Bristol, Avon) 2004; 19-10: 1000-8.*

[9] NYFFELER RW, SHEIKH R, ATKINSON TS, JACOB HA, FAVRE P, GERBER C. Effects of glenoid component version on humeral head displacement and joint reaction forces: an experimental study. *J Shoulder Elbow Surg 2006; 15-5: 625-9.*

RECENTERING THE HUMERAL HEAD IN THE HORIZONTAL PLANE IN TSA

P. HABERMEYER

INTRODUCTION

Neer *et al.* [15, 17] observed that substantial posterior glenoid wear caused static posterior subluxation of the humeral head in patients with primary osteoarthritis (OA). To study its natural course and discriminate retroversion from posterior erosion and dysplasia, Walch *et al* [21] classified glenoid morphology in the transaxial plane in primary OA (fig. 1).

Reasons for decentering of the humeral head in primary arthritis are not fully understood. Apart form a contracture or insufficiency of the active stabilizers (the rotator cuff and joint capsule), changes in the passive stabilizers (an increased glenoid version or humeral head version) are likely causes of decentralization of the humeral head in OA [14, 17, 21].

Humeral-head decentering in the transverse plane is defined as deviation of the center of rotation of the humeral head from the glenoid center-line [11]. In a total shoulder arthroplasty (TSA), it is important to detect and correct decentering of the humeral head to avoid early polyethylene wear and loosening of the glenoid component caused by an eccentric posterior rim loading [4, 11, 13].

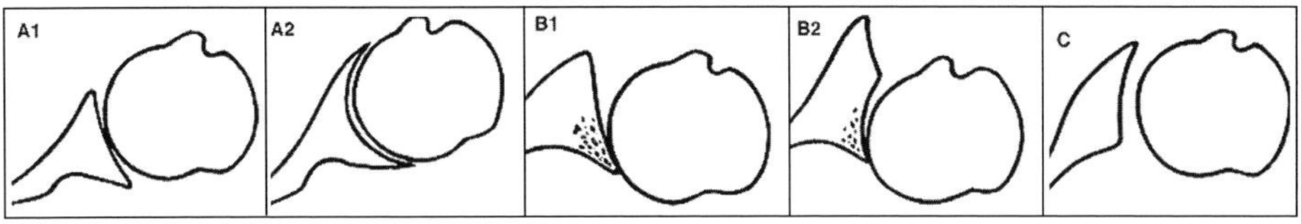

Fig. 1. The three classifications of glenoid morphology as described by Walch et al. [21] are shown. Type A was characterized by an equal balance of forces acting on the glenoid and a centralized head. Glenoid wear was minor (Type A1) or major with substantial central wear causing a glenoid cup (Type A2). Type B had asymmetric force distribution on the glenoid leading to either a loss of joint space (predominantly posterior), subchondral sclerosis (more marked on the posterior edge of the glenoid), and/or multiple posterior geodes (Type B1) or by a posterior cup which gave the appearance of a double concavity on the glenoid surface (Type B2). Type C was arbitrarily defined as glenoid retroversion greater than 25° and represents glenoid dysplasia.

Moskal *et al.* [13] compared 80 successful TSAs with 53 failed TSAs. Forty-six percent of glenoid components in the failed group were malverted (angled > 0° anterior or > 20° posterior to the plane of the scapula) compared with none in the successful group. Of the failed TSAs, glenoid components had lucent lines in 76% of patients, were loose in 66%, and migrated in 26% compared with 29%, 0%, and 0%, respectively, in patients with successful TSAs. There was a correlation between posterior glenohumeral instability and posterior glenoid component malversion. In addition, Nyffeler and Gerber showed [18] that version of the glenoid component and direction of the force vectors of the rotator cuff muscles influence the position of the humeral head. If the glenoid is inserted in retroversion, the center of the humeral component is displaced posteriorly by 0.5 mm per degree of version, leading to posterior loading and tilting, resulting in glenoid component loosening. Boulahia and Kempf [3] reported a series of 481 TSAs in patients with primary OA in relation to the glenoid morphology with a mean followup of 45 months. There was a higher complication rate after TSA for Type B2 glenoids. In this study 30% of the patients who received a bone graft for correction of the glenoid retroversion experienced failure of graft incorporation. Posterior subluxation of the humeral head occurred in 85% of patients with uncorrected glenoid retroversion greater than 20°. Iannotti and Norris [10] examined 128 patients treated with TSAs for primary OA after a mean followup of 46 months. They found significantly better functional results after TSAs in patients with severe or moderate eccentric glenoid erosion than for hemiarthroplasty. In patients with postoperative posterior subluxation, hemiarthroplasties and TSAs achieved lower final scores and were more painful than in patients with a centered humeral head. Ten of the 12 patients with glenoid loosening and posterior subluxation had moderate to severe glenoid erosion or subluxation of the humeral head preoperatively. Based on this experience, Iannotti and Norris stated that glenoid erosion should be corrected by reaming the high side, performed in combination with glenoid component implantation in order to recenter the humeral head. They also stated that humeral head subluxation is associated with a less favorable result regardless of the type of shoulder arthroplasty and must be considered in the preoperative planning.

In patients undergoing total shoulder arthroplasty we sought to evaluate if static posterior decentering of the humeral head one to OA could be recentered by surgical glenoid alignment in the transverse plane along with soft tissue balancing. We also wished to determine how pre-operative glenoid deformity affects the ability to recenter the humeral head with total shoulder arthroplasty. We investigated whether the preoperative humeral head position and glenoid morphology influences postoperative functional results as measured by the Constant and Murley Score.

MATERIALS AND METHODS

Seventy-seven consecutive patients (45 women, 30 men) with OA of the shoulder were treated by TSA using one type of shoulder prosthesis (Arthrex, Karlsfeld, Germany). All patients were prospectively enrolled in this study. Patients with etiologies of glenohumeral arthritis other than idiopathic OA were excluded. The average age of the patients was 67.6 years (range, 47-85 years) at the time of surgery. All patients were clinically and radiographically followed up for a mean of 2 years (range, 1-7 years) by one observer (PM).

During the TSA we did not correct the glenoid anatomy in Type A glenoids. In Type B glenoids (41 patients) (fig. 2), deformities of the high anterior side were lowered by eccentric reaming. In eight patients, bone grafting was performed after reaming the high side. Indications for bone grafting were massive excentric glenoid deformity in which reaming the anterior high side would lead to weakening of the anterior scapular neck. The bone graft was sized to fit between the metal back of the glenoid component and the bony surface. Seventy-five patients received a cementless metal-backed glenoid component and two patients received a cemented glenoid component.

The surgical technique consisted of a release of the pectoralis major tendon in cases with massive contraction of the pectoralis major muscle, the mobilization of the postero-superiore rotator cuff, the release of the coracohumeral ligament, the release of the subscapularis tendon described by Matsen [11], as well as a capular release using the technique of bi-focal capsulotomy. The bi-focal capsulotomy starts with the preliminary ligation of anterior humeral circumflex artery and vein, followed by the horizontal incision of the rotator interval to the base of the coracoid. The subscapularis tendon is completely vertically incised adjacent to the bicipital groove downwards to the latissimus dorsi tendon (Hockey-cut). Then the subscapularis tendon is completely subperiosteally detached from the humeral shaft together with the inferior capsule from anterior to posterior around the humeral neck ("humeral capsulotomy"). The coracohumeral ligament is released around the base of the coracoid. Subsequently a juxtaglenoidal semicircular incision of the capsule is performed,

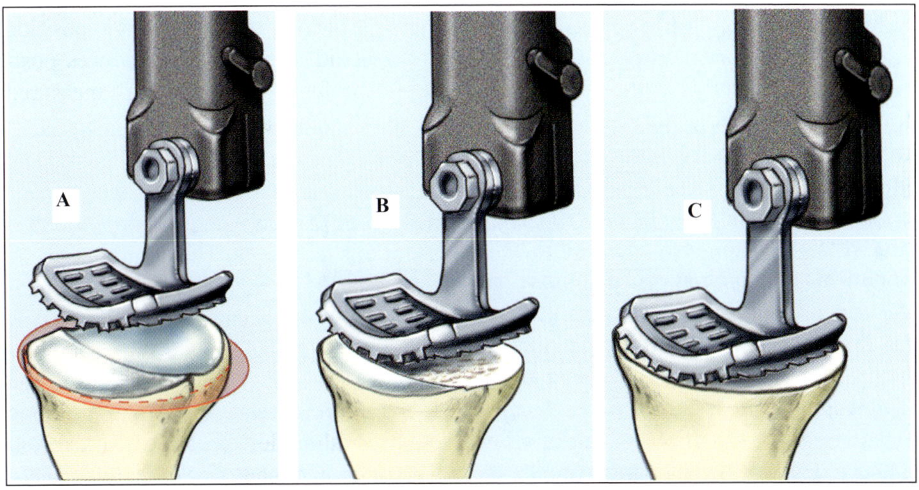

Fig. 2A-C. (A) The illustration shows anterior glenoid reaming. The glenoid must be reamed up to the plane indicated by the lightly shaded area (extending from the dashed lines outward to the solid dark line) by lowering the high side. (B) This illustration shows anterior glenoid reaming. The anterior high side was partially reamed. (C) This illustration shows a completely reamed glenoid with a concentric bony surface.

starting below the base of the coracoid in the area of the anterior scapular neck extending along the glenoid rim up the the 7 o'clock position posteriorly ("rim side capuslotomy"). Then the long head of the biceps tendon is partially tenotomized and the subscapularis muscle is subfascial mobilized in the subscapular fossa.

Functional results were documented using the adjusted Constant and Murley score [5, 8] to exclude a potential impact of age and gender on shoulder function. This evaluation was performed preoperatively and at 3 months, 6 months, and then annually during the postoperative period. The patients had standardized radiographic examinations in three planes (true AP in neutral rotation, axillary and y views) preoperatively, and at 6 weeks, 3 months, 6 months, and then annually after surgery.

The true AP view was taken standing. The X-ray cassette is positioned in the plane of the scapula behind the patient with the arm positioned in neutral rotation at the side. The beam passes in an anterior-to-posterior direction 10° tilted perpendicular to the scapula. The axillary radiograph was taken with the upright patient sitting adjacent to the X-ray table and positioning the arm in 70° to 90° abduction and 90° flexion of the elbow on the xray table. The X-ray cassette was placed on the table directly beneath the shoulder, and the X-ray machine was situated directly over the shoulder so that the beam passed in a superior-to-inferior direction through the shoulder (fig. 3).

Glenoid wear in the transversal plane was assessed in the axillary view using the classification of glenoid morphology according to Walch *et al.* [21] Decentralization of the humeral head also was documented using the technique described below on the axillary radiograph. Glenoid morphology also was assessed intraoperatively by the surgeon.

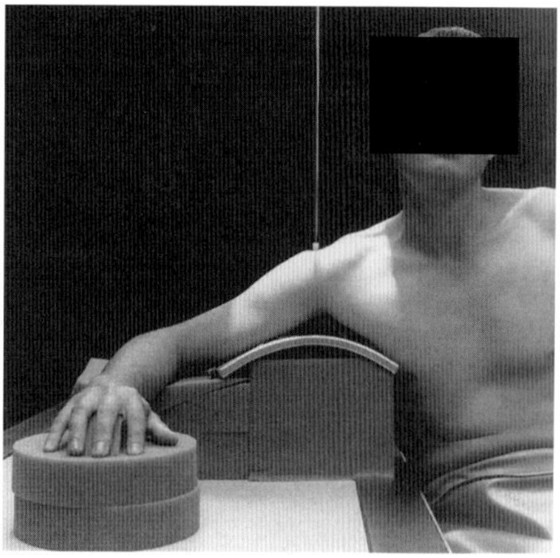

Fig. 3. A photograph shows the technique for taking an axillary view radiograph.

We defined decentering of the humeral head as a deviation of the center of the humeral head in the transverse plane of ± 5 mm in relation to the glenoid center line (fig. 4). The glenoid center line is defined as the plane of the scapula passing through the center of the glenoid [11]. Measurement of decentering was performed preoperative and postoperatively using this technique. The condition of the rotator cuff also was assessed intraoperatively. The rotator cuff was categorized as being intact, or having a deep partial tear or complete tear. Univariate analyses of an association between the glenoid morphology in the transverse plane classified according to Walch *et al.* [21] the decentralization of the humeral head, and the intraoperative state of the rotator cuff were done using Pearson's chi square test for categorical data.

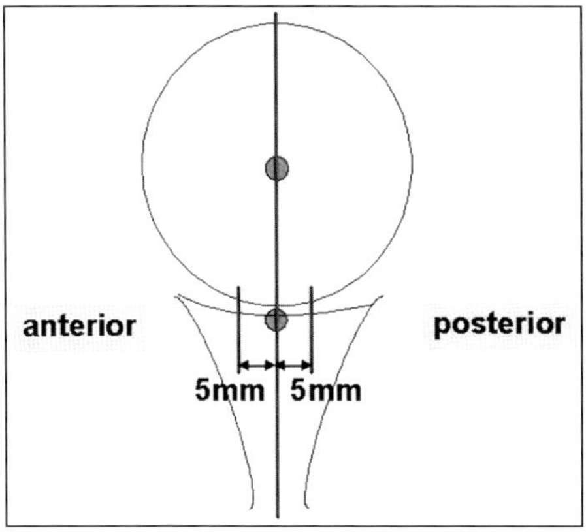

Fig. 4. A diagram shows the method for assessing decentering of the humeral head in the transversal plane. Decentering of the humeral head was defined as a deviation of the center of the humeral head greater than 5 mm anteriorly and posteriorly respectively from the center of the glenoid.

We performed Wilcoxon signed rank tests for differences in distribution of preoperative and postoperative centering of the humeral head. The Mann-Whitney U test was used to assess for differences in distribution of age, length of followup, and preoperative and postoperative Constant and Murley score as a function of the different types of glenoid wear. Constant and Murley score improvements were determined using the Wilcoxon test. Significance was set at $p < 0.05$.

All statistical analyses were performed using SPSS version 11.0 for Windows (SPSS Inc, Chicago, IL).

RESULTS

Radiographically, preoperative posterior glenoid wear was observed in 63.7% (49 patients) of the patient series and concentric glenoid wear was documented in 36.4% (28 patients) (Table 1). There was no association between glenoid wear and state of the rotator cuff. There was also no relationship between the state of the rotator cuff and the type of glenoid wear or preoperative position of the humeral head (Table 2).

Table 1: Intraoperative state of rotator cuff in relation to the glenoid wear

	Total	Concentric Glenoid wear	Eccentric glenoid wear	Type A1 glenoid	Type A2 glenoid	Type B1 glenoid	Type B2 glenoid
RC intact	58 (75.3%)	19 (67.9%)	39 (79.6%)	8 (80%)	11 (61.1%)	21 (84%)	18 (75%)
Deep partial tear of SSP	17 (22.1%)	8 (28.6%)	9 (18.4%)	1 (10%)	7 (38.9%)	3 (12%)	6 (25%)
Complete SSP tear	2 (2.6%)	1 (3.6%)	1 (2%)	1 (10%)	0	1 (4%)	0

Table 2: Intraoperative state of rotator cuff related to the position of the humeral head preoperatively

	Humeral head centered pre-OP	Humeral head decentered anteriorely pre-OP	Humeral head decentered posteriorely pre-OP
RC intact	33 (70.2%)	5 (83.3%)	20 (83.3%)
Deep partial tear of SSP	12 (25.5%)	1 (16.7%)	4 (16.7%)
Complete SSP tear	2 (4.3%)	0	0

In all patients the postoperative centering of the humeral head in the transversal plane was improved ($p < 0.0001$). A preoperatively, posteriorly, decentered humeral head position was corrected in all patients (fig. 5). Two of the six patients with anterior decentering preoperatively had anterior decentering postoperatively. The other four patients had recentering of the humeral head as a result of the surgery. Anterior decentering occurred in 15 patients postoperatively. Preoperatively, eight of these patients had centered humeral heads, five had posteriorly decentered humeral heads, and two had anteriorly decentered humeral heads (Table 3).

At follow-up there was no difference in the distribution of humeral head position regardless of the preoperative state of glenoid wear. In the 28 patients with concentric glenoid wear (Type A glenoid), no surgical correction of the glenoid anatomy was performed. Of these 28 patients, 22 (79%) had a centered and two (7.1%) had a posterior decentered humeral head preoperatively. Postoperatively, two (9%) of these patients had anterior decentering. No posterior decentering was observed in this group at followup.

In the 49 patients with an eccentric glenoid wear (Type B glenoid), surgical correction of the glenoid deformity was performed. Preoperatively, only 25 of these patients (51%) had a centered humeral head and 22 patients (44.9%) had posterior decentering of the humeral head. No posterior decentering was observed in any of these patients postoperatively, and in 42 patients (86%) the humeral head was centered.

Overall, there was significant improvement ($p < 0.05$) in the Constant and Murley score from preoperative to postoperative. There were no differences in the preoperative and postoperative Constant and Murley scores between patients with preoperatively centered and posteriorly decentered shoulders (Table 4). Futhermore, the preoperative Constant and Murley score was not correlated with the type of glenoid wear. The

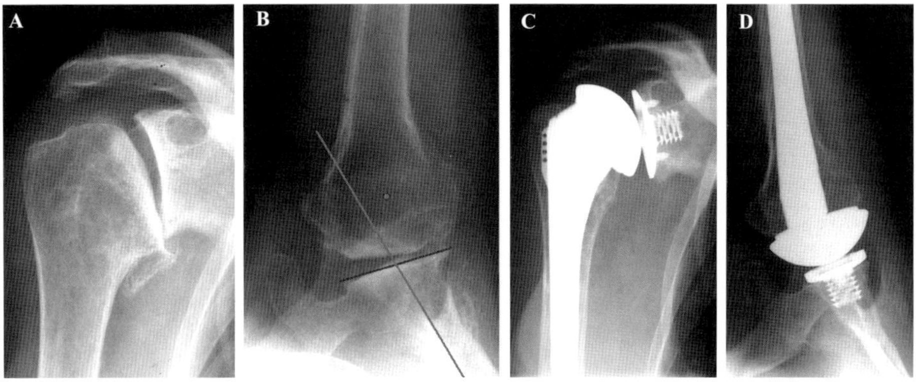

Fig. 5A-D. (A) A true AP radiograph shows a patient with severe OA. (B) The axillary view shows posterior glenoid wear and posterior decentering of the humeral head. (C) The true AP radiograph control taken 2 years postoperatively shows a centered humeral head in the coronal plane. (D) The axillary radiograph control taken 2 years postoperatively shows a recentered humeral component.

Table 3: Distribution of glenoid wear related to the decentering of the humeral head

Humeral Head position	Total (%)		Concentric glenoid wear (%)		Eccentric glenoid wear (%)		Type A1 Glenoid (%)		Type A2 Glenoid (%)		Type B1 Glenoid (%)		Type B2 Glenoid (%)	
	Pre-op	Post-op	Pre-op	Post-op	Pre-op	Post-op	Pre-op	Post-op	Pre-op	Post-op	Pre-op	Post-op	Pre-op	Post-op
centered	47 (61)	62* (80.5)	22 (78.6)	20 (71.4)	25 (51)	42* (85.7)	8 (80)	8 (80)	14 (77.8)	12 (66.7)	20 (80)	22 (88)	5 (20.8)	20* (83.3)
anterior	6 (7.8)	15* (19.5)	4 (14.3)	8 (28.6)	2 (4.1)	7* (14.3)	2 (20)	2 (20)	2 (11.1)	6 (33.3)	2 (8)	3 (12)	0	4* (16.7)
posterior	24 (31.2)	0*	2 (7.1)	0	22 (44.9)	0*	0	0	2 (11.1)	0	3 (12)	0	19 (79.2)	0*

* significant difference in distribution of humeral head position preoperatively versus postoperatively

Table 4: Constant score related to the different types of glenohumeral decentering

	Centred glenohumeral joint (pre-OP)		Posterior decentred glenohumeral joint (pre-OP)		Anterior decentered glenohumeral joint (pre-OP)	
	Pre-OP	Post-OP	Pre-OP	Post-OP	Pre-OP	Post-OP
Relative Constant score (%)	51.6	102*	47.6	90*	25.6	94.9*
Pain (pts)	5.4	13.8*	6.4	12.7*	4.2	14*
Activity of daily living (pts)	8	18.1*	8.2	15.8*	5.8	17.7*
Range of motion (pts)	19.8	33.5*	16.7	29.9*	13.6	30.3
Strength (pts)	4.7	8.3*	4.3	7.6*	0.4	7.2

* significant difference between pre- and post-op data.

overall Constant and Murley score as well as the subcategories for pain, activities of daily living, total range of motion, and strength improved ($p < 0.05$) postoperatively regardless of the types of pre-operative glenoid wear (Table 5).

Postoperatively, patients with eccentric glenoid wear had a lower ($p = 0.008$) overall Constant and Murley score as well as in the subcategories of activities of daily living ($p = 0.013$) and range of motion ($p = 0.013$). There was no difference in the subscore for pain and strength. Postoperatively, patients with a Type A2 glenoid achieved better Constant and Murley scores than patients with a Type B1 glenoid ($p = 0.012$) or Type B2 glenoid ($p = 0.007$). Patients with a Type A2 glenoid had better ($p = 0.006$) pain relief compared with patients who had a Type A1 glenoid. There was no difference in postoperative shoulder function in patients with a Type B1 glenoid compared with patients who had a Type B2 glenoid.

There were complications (2.6%) from the implantation technique. Bone-graft resorption occurred in one of eight patients followed by glenoid loosening requiring revision surgery 32 months postoperatively. In another patient, incongruence of the bony surface of the glenoid and the metal back of the glenoid component led to loosening with breakage of a fixation screw requiring revision 20 months postoperatively. In both cases the cementless glenoid component were replaced using a cemented glenoid component. No radiolucencies around the glenoid or humeral components were observed on any of the postoperative radiographs.

Table 5: Pre- and postoperative Constant score in relation to glenoid wear

	Total		Concentric glenoid wear		Eccentric glenoid wear		Type A1 glenoid		Type A2 glenoid		Type B1 glenoid		Type B2 glenoid	
	Pre-OP	**Post-OP**	**Pre-OP**	**Post-OP**	**Pre-OP**	**Post-OP**	**Pre-OP**	**Post-OP**	**Pre-OP**	**Post-OP**	**Pre-OP**	**Post-OP**	**Pre-OP**	**Post-OP**
Relative Constant score (%)	49.4	97.5*	49.6	106.2*	48.7	92.1*	47.5	100*	50.8	110.6*	48.3	95.6*	49.2	89.1*
Pain (pts)	5.7	13.5*	5.4	14.3*	5.8	13*	4.6	13.5*	5.9	14.9*	5.4	13.1*	6.2	12.8
Acitivity of daily living (pts)	7.9	17.3*	8.8	18.7*	7.3	16.5*	9.4	18*	8.4	13.31*	6.7	17.1*	8	15.9*
Range of motion (pts)	18.4	32*	17.8	34.8	18.7	30.4*	18.4	33*	17.5	35.9*	19.2	31.3*	18.1	29.6*
Strength (pts)	4.4	8	4.6	8.1	4.1	7.9*	4.6	9.6*	4.6	6.8	3.9	8.7*	4.3	7.1*

* significant difference between pre- and post-op data.

DISCUSSION

We evaluated whether static posterior decentering of the humeral head in patients with glenohumeral OA and posterior glenoid wear could be recentered during TSA.

As all 77 patients underwent soft tissue balancing during shoulder arthroplasty and due to the fact that we found no difference in the distribution of the position of the humeral head at follow-up between patients with pre-operative concentric wear and those with eccentric glenoid wear, we suggest that correction of the glenoid deformity by reaming seems possible in TSA.

Our two-year results showing recentering of the glenohumeral joint, especially in patients with posterior decentering preoperatively, were confirmed by Gerber [22] and seem to be stable for at least four years. Gerber [22] examined 23 patients who had received a total shoulder arthroplasty due to an osteoarthritis with posterior decentering of the humeral head after an average of 42 months. In twenty-one out of the twenty-three patients the posterior decentering was reversed.

Assessing the centering of the shoulder using an axillary X-ray instead of an axillary CT-scan is a potential weakness of our study. However, during CT scanning the patient must lie in a supine position with the arm internally rotated relaxing the anterior capsule and permitting artifactual posterior subluxation of the humeral head simulating posterior decentering of the humeral head. As the assessment of glenoid morphology according to Walch *et al.* [21] was performed using the axillary view, and assessed intraoperatively by the surgeon. CT scanning was not necessary.

There are studies of the anatomy and degenerative changes of the glenoid in the transverse plane in OA [6, 21]. Posterior glenoid wear and its surgical management are well-described [17, 19, 21]. Glenoid version can be correlated to the severity of osteoarthritic changes. Posterior humeral head subluxation is commonly associated with posterior glenoid erosion [2]. Radiographic studies of osteoarthritic shoulders show that posterior subluxation of the humeral head is not correlated with the presence of glenoid retroversion [1, 21] but to the morphologic type of glenoid wear [21]. These findings are corroborated by our study. We found a positive correlation between posterior decentralization of the humeral head and glenoid morphology as described by Walch *et al.* [21].

Rotator cuff disease is uncommon in patients with primary OA, occurring in 10% to 23% of patients [1, 7]. In our study, a supraspinatus tendon tear was seem intraoperatively in 24.7% (19 patients) of patients. Only two of these patients had a complete supraspinatus tendon tear. There was no association between the state of the rotator cuff and centering of glenohumeral joint or glenoid deficiency.

Previous studies have described reconstruction of glenoid bone stock using bone grafting and screw fixation, reporting the postoperative functional results, rates of radiolucency, and complications [9, 19]. However, we found no studies describing recentering of the glenohumeral joint after correction of glenoid alignment during TSA. Neer and Morrison [16] were the first to report on bone grafting for severe glenoid deficiency. In their series of 463 consecutive TSAs only 4.3% of their patients required glenoid bone grafting. After a mean follow-up of 4.4 years they reported that approximately 15% of patients (three patients) had complications. In two patients the fixation screws broke, and in another patient the fixation screw was worn as a result of contact with the humeral component. Eighty-five percent of their patients achieved satisfactory and excellent functional results. In a series of 953 TSAs reported by Steinmann and Cofield [19], 28 patients (3.2%) required glenoid bone grafting. After a mean follow-up of 5.3 years three loose glenoids components were observed (10.7%). Nonetheless, 82% of their patients achieved excellent and satisfactory functional results. They concluded that the clinical and radiographic results are similar to those for TSA overall. Hill and Norris [9] performed bone grafting for glenoid deficiency in 16% (21 patients) of their TSAs. Seventeen patients were followed up after a mean 70 months. The graft failed in 18% (three patients) because of nonunion or migration of the graft. Five (29%) of these failures required glenoid revision and 47% had unsatisfactory functional results. In our series, bone grafting was performed for severe glenoid deficiency in eight or 10.4% of TSAs. Failure occured in one patient because of nonunion of the bone graft and jurhe surgery was required. With a mean follow-up of 39 months in the patients who required bone grafting, an adjusted Constant and Murley score of 95.6% was achieved which is comparable to the Constant and Murley score of our patients with concentric glenoid wear.

Miller *et al.* examined 41 patients who had TSAs at a mean clinical follow-up of 1.9 years. They found a positive lift-off test in 67% and a positive belly-press test in 66.6% of cases [12], indicating an insufficiency of the subscapularis muscle. Postoperative anterior and anterosuperior decentering of the humeral component can be caused by subscapularis deficiency. Therefore, the influence of surgical glenoid alignment for patients with postoperative anterior or anterosuperior decentering is unclear.

Our midterm results suggest a that decentered humeral head caused by glenoid deficiency in the transversal plane can be recentered by lowering the high side, and in severe glenoid deficiency by bone grafting with soft tissue balancing. Because of the recentering, the preoperative posterior humeral head position does not influence the postoperative functional result. The complication rate with this technique is low in our study and complications were observed only in patients who had eccentric glenoid wear preoperatively. We recommend normalizing posterior glenoid wear during glenoid preparation during TSA to avoid early glenoid loosening.

REFERENCES

[1] BADET R, BOILEAU P NOEL E, WALCH G. Arthrography and computed arthrotomography study of seventy patients with primary glenohumeral osteoarthritis. *Rev Reum Engl Ed. 1995; 62: 555-62.*

[2] BELL RH, NOBLE JS. The management of significant glenoid deficiency in total shoulder arthroplasty. *J Shoulder Elbow Surg. 2000;9: 248-56.*

[3] BOULAHIA A, KEMPF JF. Influence de la morphologie de la glène sur les résultats cliniques des arthroplasties de l'épaule dans l'omarthrose primitive : etude multicentrique de 481 cas. In: Walch G, Boileau P, Molé D, eds. 2000 Prothèses d'Epaule : recul de 2 à 10 ans [2000 shoulder prostheses : two to ten year folow-up]. *Montpellier, France: Sauramps Medical; 2001:87-94.*

[4] COLLINS D, TENCER A, SIDLES J, MATSEN F. Edge displacement and deformation of glenoid components in response to eccentric loading. *J Bone Joint Surg Am. 1992; 74: 501-7.*

[5] CONSTANT CR, MURLEY AH A clinical method of functional assessment of the shoulder. *Clin Orthop Relat Res. 1987; 214:160-64.*

[6] DE WILDE FL, BERGHS BM, VANDEVYVER F, SCHEBENS A, VERDONK R. Glenohumeral relationship in the transverse plane of the body. *J Shoulder Elbow Surg. 2003; 12: 260-67.*

[7] EDWARDS TB, BOULAHIA A, KEMPF JF, BOILEAU P, NÉMOZ C, WALCH G. The influence of rotator cuff disease on the results of shoulder arthroplasty for primary osteoarthritis. *J Bone Joint Surg Am. 2002;84: 2240-48.*

[8] GERBER C. Integrated scoring systems for the functional assessment of the shoulder. In: Matsen FA, Fu FH, Hawkins RJ, eds. The Shoulder: A Balance of Mobility and Stability. *Rosemont, IL: The American Academy of Orthopaedic Surgeons; 1992: 531-50.*

[9] HILL JM, NORRIS TR. Long-term results of total shoulder arthroplasty following bone-grafting of the glenoid. *J Bone Joint Surg Am. 2001;83: 877-83.*

[10] IANNOTTI JP, NORRIS TR. Influence of preoperative factors on outcome of shoulder arthroplasty for glenohumeral osteoarthritis. *J Bone Joint Surg Am. 2003; 85: 251-58.*

[11] MATSEN FA, LIPPITT SB, SIDLES JA, HARRYMAN DT. Practical Evaluation and Management of the Shoulder. *Philadelphia, PA: WB Saunders Company; 1994: 151-220.*

[12] MILLER SL, HAZRATI Y, KLEPPS S, CHIANG A, FLATOW EL. Loss of subscapularis function after total shoulder replacement: a seldom recognized problem. *J Shoulder Elbow Surg. 2003; 12: 29-34.*

[13] MOSKAL MJ, CAMPBELL B, SMITH KL, MATSEN FA. The position of prosthetic components in failed and successful shoulder arthroplasties. *Orthopaedic Research Report. 1999: 59-61.*

[14] MULLAJI AB, BEDDOW FH, LAMB GH. CT measurement of glenoid erosion in arthritis. *J Bone Joint Surg Br. 1994; 76: 384-88.*

[15] NEER C 2nd Replacement arthroplasty for glenohumeral osteoarthritis. *J Bone Joint Surg Am. 1974; 56: 1-13.*

[16] NEER CS 2nd, MORRISION D. Glenoid bone grafting in total shoulder arthroplasty. *J Bone Joint Surg Am. 1988;70: 1154-62.*

[17] NEER CS 2nd, WATSON KC, STANTON FJ. Recent experience in total shoulder replacement. *J Bone Joint Surg Am. 1982; 64: 319-37.*

[18] NYFFELER RW, GERBER C. The relevance of anatomical reconstruction. In: Walch G, Boileau P, Molé D, eds. 2000 Prothèses d'Epaule : recul de 2 à 10 ans. [2000 shoulder prostheses : two to ten year follow-up]. *Montpellier, France : Sauramps medical; 2001:57-59.*

[19] STEINMANN SP, COFIELD RH. Bone grafting for glenoid deficiency in total shoulder replacement. *J Shoulder Elbow Surg 2000;9: 361-67.*

[20] VON EISENHART-ROTHE R, KROETZ M, WIEDEMANN E, ENGLMEIER KH, GRAICHEN H. Fixed and functional decentering of the head of the humerus in patients with omarthrosis. *Unfallchirurg. 2002; 105: 517-22.*

[21] WALCH G, BADET R, BOULAHIA A, KHOURY A. Morphologic study of the glenoid in primary glenohumeral osteoarthritis. *J Arthroplasty. 1999;14: 756-60.*

[22] GERBER C, COSTOUROS JG, SUKTHANKAR A, FECENTESE SF. Static posterior humeral head subluxation and total shoulder arthroplasty. *J Shoulder Elbow Surg 2009: 18: 505-10.*

NEW METHODS OF PRE OPERATIVE PLANNING FOR MANAGEMENT OF GLENOID BONE LOSS

J.P. IANNOTTI

Glenoid deformity and bone loss are characteristic of arthritic and post traumatic conditions and present specific challenges for prosthetic reconstruction. Correction of pathologic version is important when placing a glenoid component [1-4]. Traditional methods for pre operative planning included the use of plain radiographs and CT scanning. Both plain radiographs and 2D scanning have been shown to subject to errors resulting from variations in the plane of imaging in relation to the plane of the scapula [5]. The use of 3D imaging has improved the ability to define glenoid anatomy but currently available methods lack the ability to quantify the amount or location of bone loss or define patient specific glenoid version. This is particularly true when there is both central as well as eccentric bone deformity. Anatomic studies define a 20 degree variation in natural glenoid version [6, 7]. Ideally, correction of pathologic version to the patient's native version and would be preferable than to correct version perpendicular to the plane of the scapula or some other arbitrary selected value. Determining patient specific version, bone loss and the location of the native glenoid fossa joint line would require new methods of imaging and a normal scapula on the opposite side. If a normal scapula were available a 3D reconstruction of the scapula could be obtained and superimposed upon the abnormal scapula [7-10]. In the absence of a normal opposite scapula and an imaging method to allow for analysis of the two scapulae other methods would be required.

Our research and development team has over the last several years defined and validated a novel concept and method to determine normal anatomy from the pathologic anatomy (Fig. 1). For the shoulder we defined the shape of the interior of the normal glenoid vault and define this shape to be essentially the same between individuals. From this we developed a consistent method of placing the vault sample within the 3D space of the pathologic glenoid using developed software that utilizes 3D CT scans [7-10] (Fig. 2-8). We have compared the vault method with other methods of measuring glenoid version [11, 12]. We have validated the reproducibility and accuracy of the vault method in the shoulder [8-10] and have applied this to other joints that have complex boney anatomy [13]. Further development of the software has given us a joint and implant specific pre operative surgical simulator allowing the surgeon to perform patient specific pre operative planning (Fig. 9-12). Future development of these tools will be commercially available and should allow the surgeon to more precisely plan the surgical procedure to define the best method for preparation of the bone, placement of the implant and selection of the implant best suited to manage the patient's condition. We have linked the information obtained from the imaging tools to allow for the design and fabrication of patient specific bone preparation tools that will assist the surgeon to more accurately execute the pre operative plan and place the implant in the desired location (Fig. 13-17).

New Methods of Measuring Bone Loss:
Hypothesis

- A standardized anatomic implant shape in the correct sizes for an individual patient can be used as a tool to measure bone loss.
- Pre operative planning tool to facilitate decision making and link to new instrumentation to facilitate the surgical procedure

Fig. 1

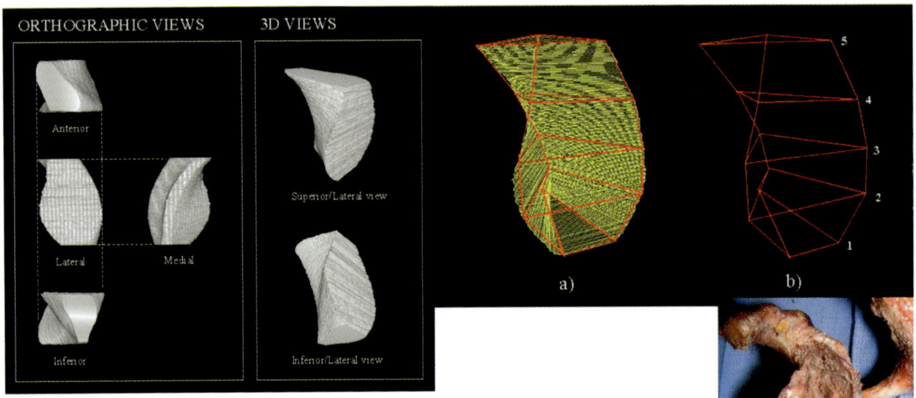

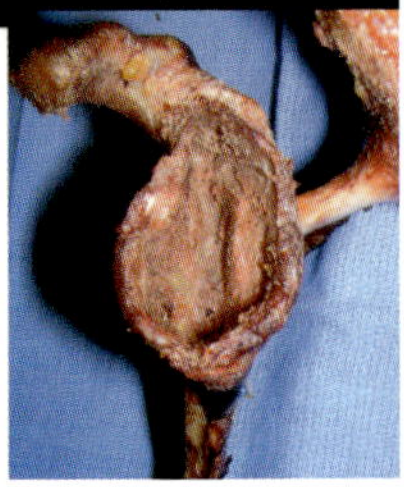

Fig. 2 : The Glenoid Vault Defined: Solid Computer Models of the Shape

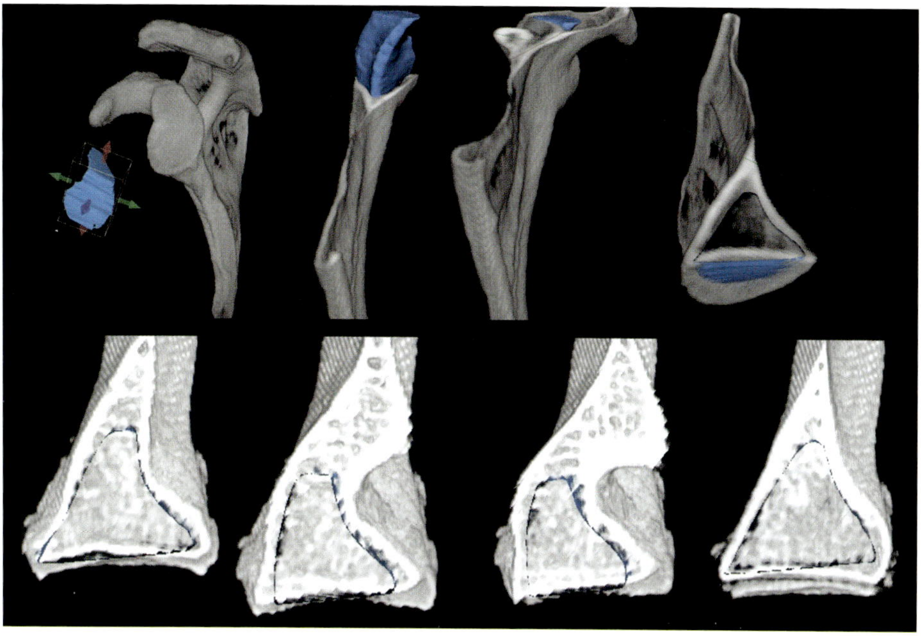

Fig. 3: Computer Surgery in 11 Cadaver Scapula
With five sized vaulted glenoid models all fit with less than 2mm difference between the endosteal wall and outer dimension of the component

Predicting Version and Bone Loss from Pathologic Glenoid

- 12 patients with unilateral OA.
- Bilateral CT scans of scapulae.
- Processed with Volsuite.
- Register scapulae to same coordinates in space.
- Use normal side as patient-specific glenoid template.
- Compare glenoid bone volume changes:
  - Abnormal side to normal side
  - Abnormal side to vault implant

Fig. 4

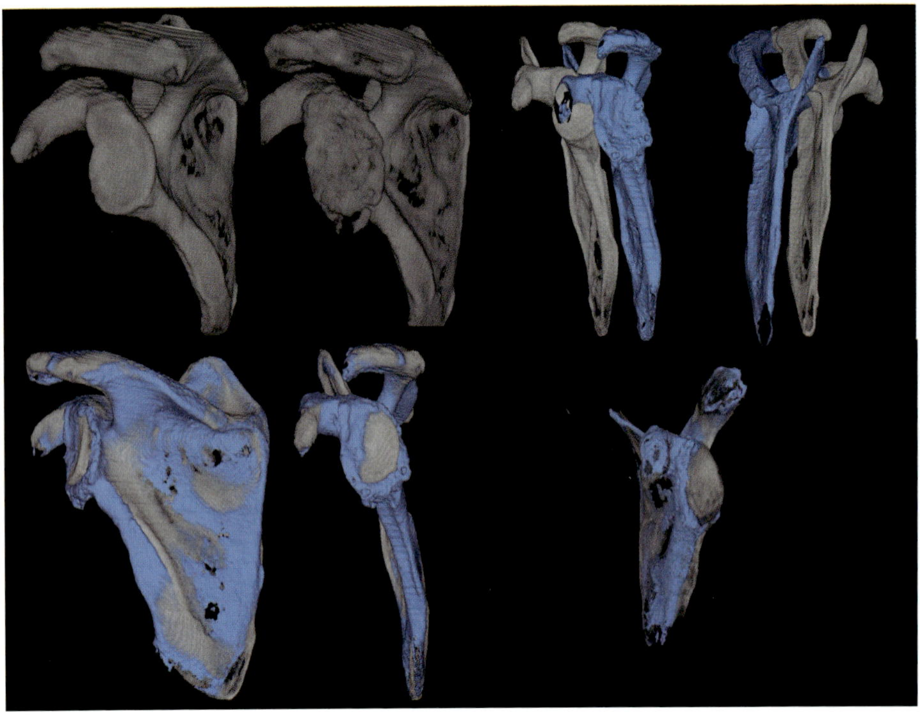

Fig. 5

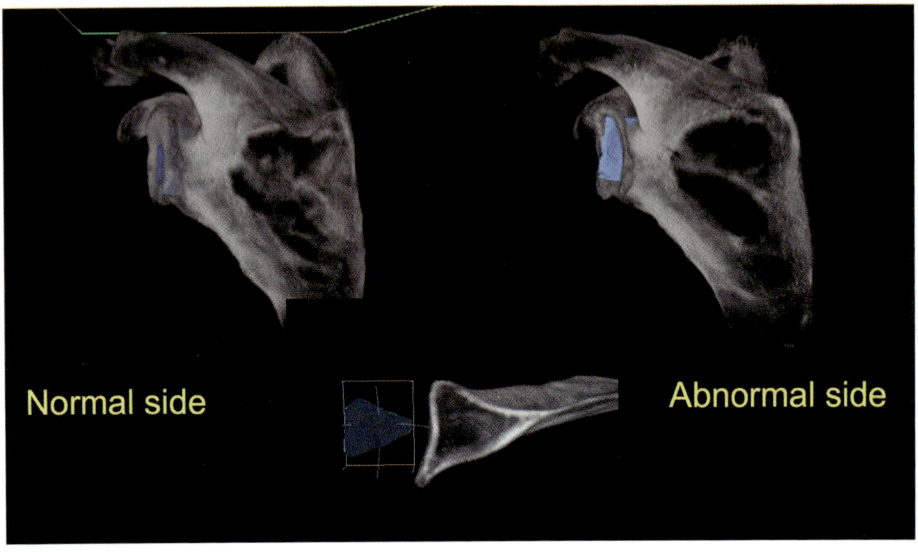

Fig. 6: Use of the standard glenoid "implant" model. Surrogate to using the opposite normal shoulder (12 samples less than 1% difference in calculated bone loss and 3 degrees of version between the two methods, kappa value 0.75)

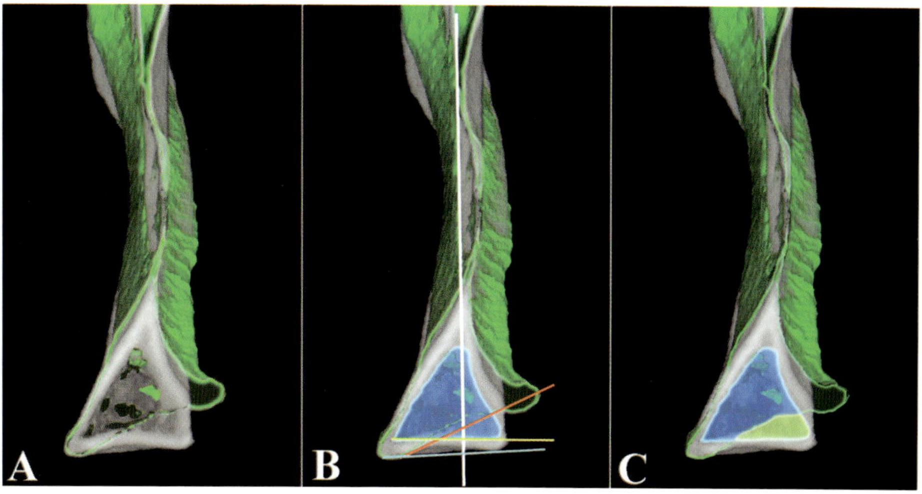

Fig. 7: Use of the vault model to define glenoid bone loss and glenoid version
A: Grey is normal and green abnormal scapula: B: blue is vault model, red line is abnormal version, blue normal version on normal scaplua and yellow is predicted normal version from vault model

Results

- Virtual vault implant accurately estimated bone loss of abnormal side (0.8 +/- 1.5%)
- Correlation coefficient = 0.99
- Assessment of correct glenoid retroversion within 3 degrees of opposite shoulder.
- In all paired scapulae, this represented a highly consistent method of estimating bone loss due to osteoarthritis.

Fig. 8

Pre – Operative Planning Tool

- Using these techniques can we define for a given patient the consequences of surgical management of glenoid bone loss that are patient and implant specific?
- Can we use that information to perform the surgery with greater accuracy?

Patents pending

Fig 9

Pre – Operative Surgical Simulator

- Functional capabilities
  - Import patient's CT scan
  - Fast (< 5 minutes) user-guided preprocessing
  - Quantify distances and angles between surgical landmarks
  - Virtually drill and ream surgical surfaces
  - Test location and size of bone grafts
  - Interactively place vault model to quantify bone loss
  - Interactively place implant models in both scapula and humerus; verify size and fit

Fig 10

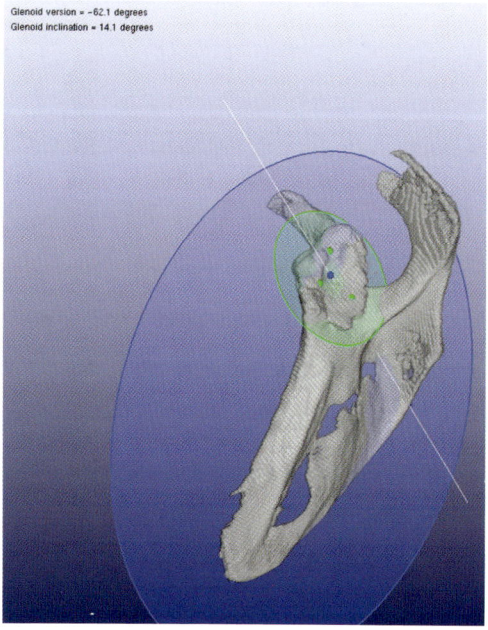

***Fig. 11:* Blue represents plane of the scapula and green plane of the glenoid fossa: Retroversion 62 degrees and inclination angle 14 degrees**

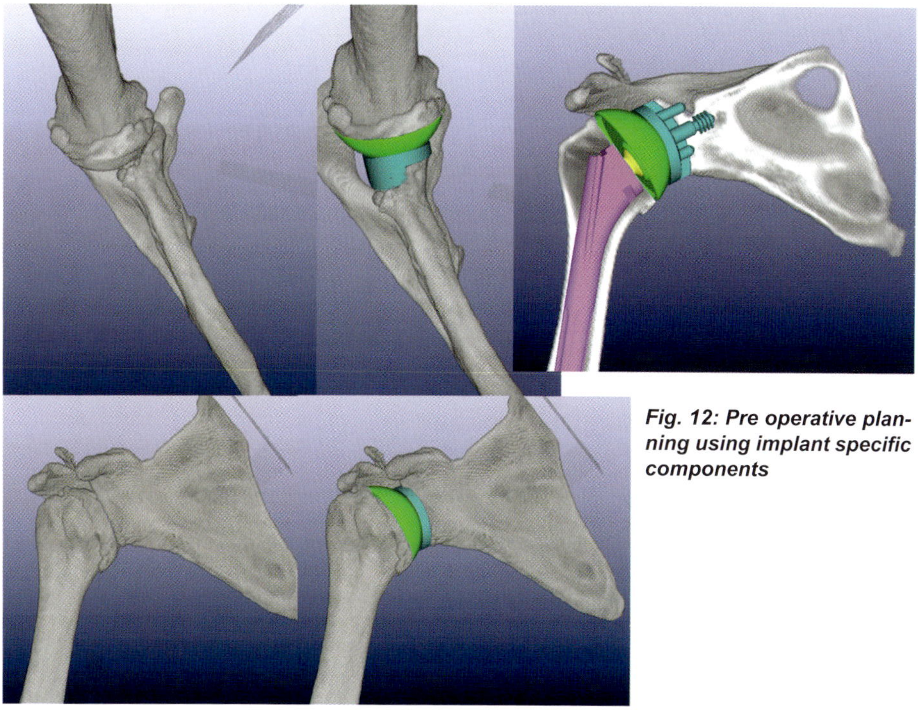

***Fig. 12:* Pre operative planning using implant specific components**

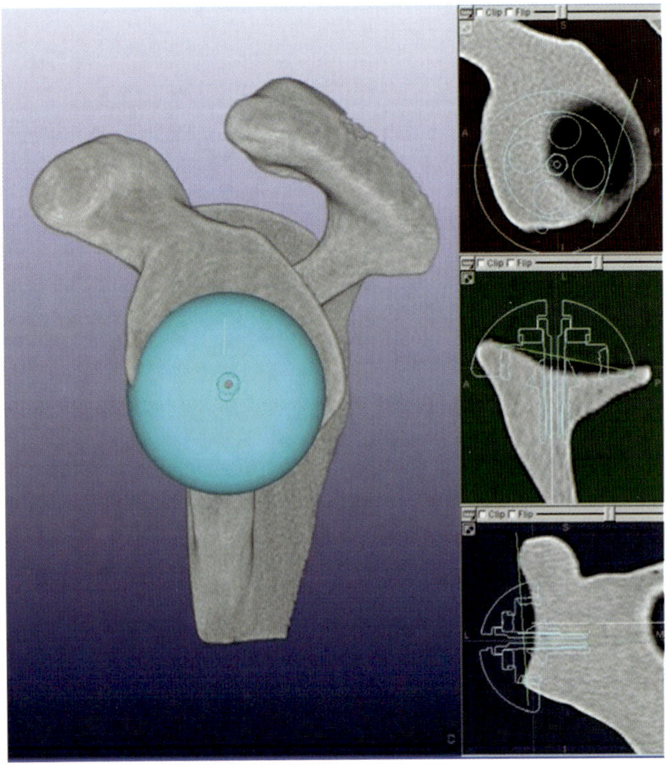

Fig. 13: Pre clinical testing of Simulator and the Glenoid Positioning System: Glenosphere and screw position

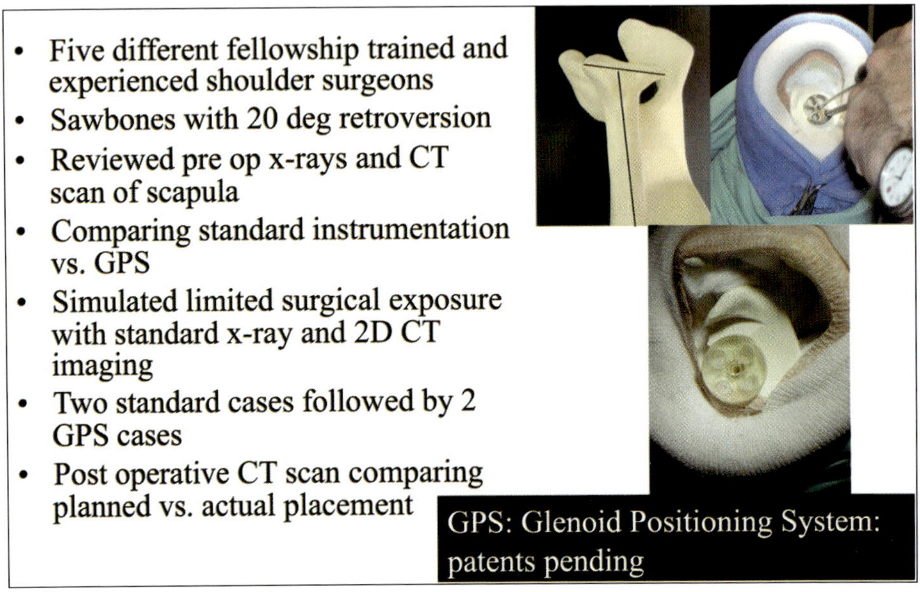

Fig. 14: Pre-Clinical Trial Glenoid Positioning System: Saw-Bones

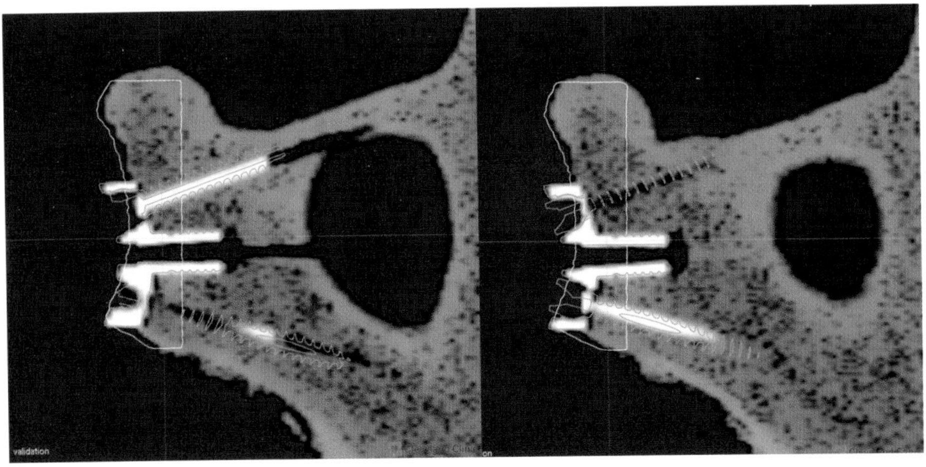

Fig. 15: Patient Specific Instruments: Pre Clinical Trial: Sawbones Example
Pre operative planning (blue lines) vs. post operative CT of the actual metaglene and screw placement using GPS system (sous les images) Pre operative planning (blue lines) vs. post operative CT of the actual metaglene and screw placement using GPS system

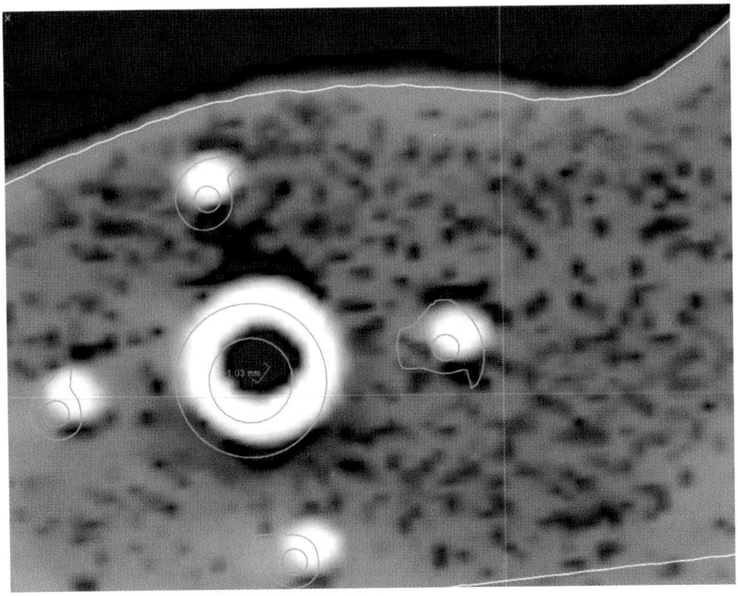

Fig. 16: Pre Clinical Trial: Sawbones
Pre operative planning (blue lines) vs. post operative CT of the actual metaglene and screw placement using GPS system

Metaglene Position	GPS Method (n = 10) Mean difference (+/- SD) Range	STD Method (n = 10) Mean difference (+/- SD) Range
Superior - Inferior	0 mm (0.5 mm) Range 1 mm	1 mm (3.0 mm) Range 8 mm
Anterior – posterior	0 (0.5 mm) Range 1 mm	1 (3.0 mm) Range 8 mm
Version	2 degrees (1 deg) Range 2 degrees	-12 degrees (10 deg) Range 20 degrees

Fig. 17: Metaglene position: Planned vs. Actual GPS vs. Standard Surgical Technique

REFERENCES

[1] FARRON A, TERRIER A, BUCHLER P. Risks of loosening of a prosthetic glenoid implanted in retroversion. *J Shoulder Elbow Surg 2006; 15: 521-26.*

[2] FAVRE P, MOOR B, SNEDEKER JG, GERBER C. Influence of component positioning on impingement in conventional total shoulder arthroplasty.

[3] IANNOTTI JP, SPENCER EE, WINTER U, DEFFENBAUGH D, WILLIAMS GR. Prosthetic positioning in total shoulder arthroplasty. *J Shoulder Elbow Surg 2005; 14: 111S-121S.*

[4] SPENCER EE

[5] BOKOR DJ, O'SULLIVAN MD, HAZAN GJ. Variability of measurement of glenoid version on computed tomography scan. *J Shoulder Elbow Surg 1999; 8: 595-8.*

[6] CHURCHILL RS, BREMS JJ, KOTSCHI H. Glenoid size, inclination, and version: An anatomic study. *J Shoulder Elbow Surg 2001; 10: 327-32.*

[7] KWON YW, POWELL KA, YUM JK, BREMS JJ, IANNOTTI JP. Use of three-dimensional computed-tomography for the analysis of the glenoid anatomy. *J Shoulder Elbow Surg 2005; 14: 85-90.*

[8] CODSI MJ, BENNETTS C, GORDIEV K, BOECK DM, KWON YW, BREMS JJ *et al.* Normal glenoid vault anatomy and validation of a novel glenoid implant shape. *J Shoulder Elbow Surg 2008; 17: 471-8.*

[9] SCALISE JJ, BRYAN J, POLSTER J, BREMS JJ, IANNOTTI JP. Quantitative analysis of glenoid bone loss in osteoarthritis using three-dimensional computed tomography scans. *J Shoulder Elbow Surg 2008; 17: 328-35.*

[10] SCALISE JJ, CODSI MJ, BRYAN J, IANNOTTI JP. The three-dimensional glenoid vault model can estimate glenoid version in osteoarthritis. *J Shoulder Elbow Surg 2008; 17: 487-91.*

[11] DE WILDE LF, BERGHS BA, VANDWYVER F, SCHEPENS A, VERDONK RC. Glenohumeral relationship in the transverse plane of the body. *J Shoulder Elbow Surg 2003; 12: 260-7.*

[12] GATHANAPI A, McCARRON J, IANNOTTI JP Accuracy of Different Methods to Predict Normal Glenoid Version in Pathologic *J. Shoulder and Elbow Surgery in review 2010*

[13] BARSOUM abstract AAOS 2010.

HORIZONTAL GLENOID DEFICIENCY (B2 & C) RESULTS OF GLENOID BONE GRAFT IN PRIMARY TSA

C. LÉVIGNE, J. GARRET, P. BOILEAU, C. MORAGA, G. WALCH

Horizontal posterior glenoid deficiency is not rare in primary osteoarthritis and may be a challenging problem for indication and surgical technique in shoulder arthroplasty.

Walch in 1999 proposed a classification of horizontal glenoid morphology based on 113 cases of primary osteoarthritis analyzed by computed tomography scans [1]. Both types B2 and type C are characterized by an increase of glenoid retroversion corresponding to a posterior bone deficiency. Independently of the unknown mechanism, the main difference between type B2 and type C is that B2 has a biconcave aspect and is associated with posterior subluxation of the humeral head whereas in type C, the head remains relatively centered and glenoid wear is uniformly distributed (Fig. 1).

Combination of bone graft reconstruction and non-constrained total shoulder arthroplasty is one of the methods proposed for surgical management of these posterior defects. The goal of this study was to analyze the results.

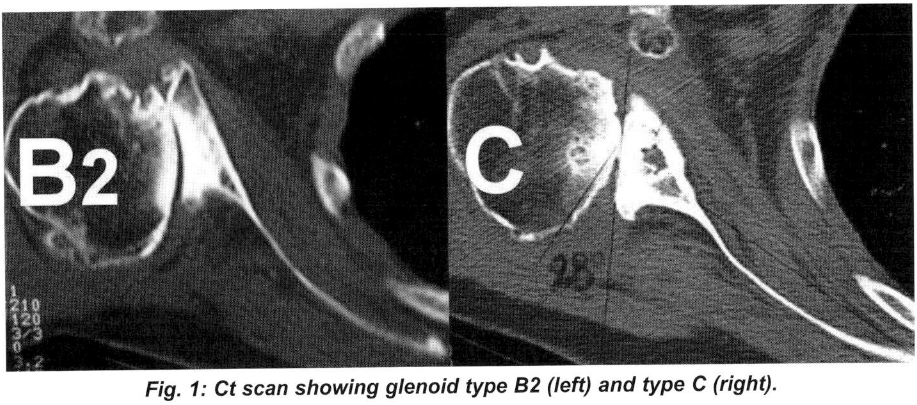

***Fig. 1:** Ct scan showing glenoid type B2 (left) and type C (right).*

MATERIAL AND METHODS

This is a retrospective multicenter study of 9 cases of total shoulder arthroplasty implanted between 1997 and 2004 in osteoarthritis with static posterior instability. Out of these, seven cases have been operated between 1997 and 1999 and only two cases have been operated since 2000. Eight cases were type B2 glenoid and one case was type C in the Walch classification on the CT scan [1]. There were 6 women and 5 men with a mean age of 69 years (range, 56-84 years) at the time of the procedure.

Preoperative constant score was 29 pts (range, 11-61 pts). Active anterior elevation averaged 99° (range, 60-150.). Active external rotation arm at the side was 16° (range, 0-30.) Three grades of defect were definited according drawn distance between the vertical line flush to the most medial point of the spinoglenoid notch, radiographic landmark that we found to be most reproducible regardless of beam orientation (Fig. 2) : Grade1 (minor) if glenoid wear extends less than 1/3 of the distance between the original joint line and the vertical lime at the spinoglenoid notch, grade 2 (moderate) if glenoid wear extends 1/3 and 2/3 of this distance and grade 3 (severe) if it reaches beyoud 2/3 third of this distance. Using this classification, the glenoid defect was defined grade 1 in 1 case, grade 2 in 5 cases and grade 3 in 3 cases.

Surgical procedure included in all cases structural corticocancellous autograft harvested from resected humeral head. In 8 cases the graft was first secured by independent cortical screws (2 screws 4.5 in 5 cases, three screws 3.5 in 2 cases, and 4 screws 2 mm in one case), and cemented keeled polyethylene glenoid (Tornier) was implanted. The ninth case corresponds to the type C glenoid who received an uncemented glenoid with a graft secured by the metal-back and one additional screw. Six patients had an additional posterior capsular plication. Postoperatively, 4 patients were immobilized in neutral rotation for six weeks, the others in a regular sling. Passive rehabilitation began the next day after surgery in all cases.

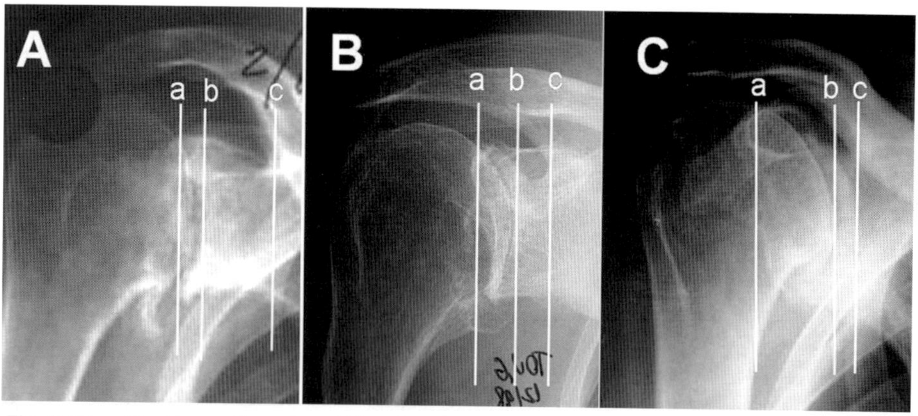

Fig. 2: Classification in 3 grades of the glenoid defect on AP view: (a) is the vertical line figuring the original joint line, (b) is the vertical line flushing with the most medial point of the defect and (c) is the vertical line flushing with the most medial point of the spinoglenoid notch. A- grade1: ab < 1/3 ac B- grade 2 : ab= 1/3-2/3 ac C- grade 3 : ab > 2/3.

RESULTS

One patient was revised 12 months after the index procedure for posterior dislocation and subsequent migration of the glenoid implant. The glenoid was removed and converted into hemiarthroplasty. We included in the results her status before revision because the other cases of glenoid migration have not been reoperated and thus remain included, and also because we consider glenoid migration was a graft-related complication. The other patients have been reviewed with a minimum of two years follow-up. Average follow-up was 90 months (range, 12-145 months).

At the last follow-up, the mean Constant score was 52 points (range, 20-83 pts). The functional result was rated excellent in 2 cases (score >70 pts), good in 3 cases (score 50-70 pts), fair in 2 cases (score 30-50 pts) and poor in 2 cases (score <30 pts). Active anterior elevation (AEE) reached in average 111° (range, 70-160°), active external rotation (AER) arm at the side was 37° in average (range 10-80°).

Radiographic evaluation concerns the 9 cases of the series. We observed 5 cases of glenoid migration associated with graft failure (56%): one concerns the metal-back glenoid with medial migration (Fig. 3), one presented posterior dislocation before glenoid migration and the three others showed a collapse of the graft and a subsequent glenoid migration before two years of follow-up (Fig. 4). Graft healing has been observed in 4 cases. We did not observe partial resorption.

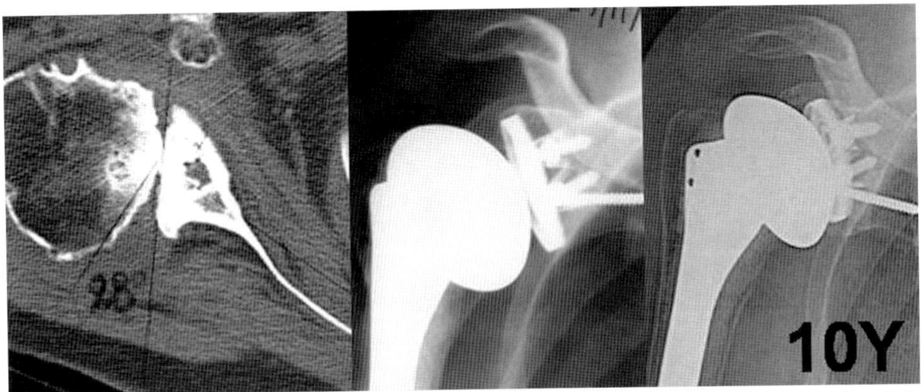

Fig. 3: Case of glenoid type C treated by glenoid metalback combined with graft (center). After 10 years there is graft resorption and medial migration of glenoid component (right).

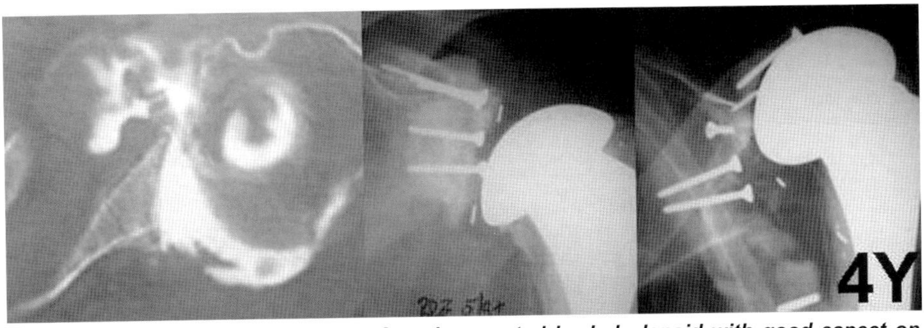

Fig. 4: Combination of posterior graft and cemented keeled glenoid with good aspect on postoperative view (center). After 4 years, collapse of the graft and glenoid migration.

There was a good concordance between radiological evolution and clinical results. Graft healing was always associated with a good clinical result: mean values of Constant score, AAE and AER were respectively 68 pts, 135° and 33°. The case of metal-back glenoid medial migration did relatively well with a Constant score of 57 pts at 12 years of follow-up. The four glenoid migrations were associated with the four worse clinical results: mean values of Constant score, AAE and AER were respectively 35 pts, 85° and 48°.

Posterior dislocation in one case and collapse of the graft prior to glenoid migration in three cases occurred into the two first postoperative years. There was no influence of follow-up on the result.

Additional capsular plication did not improve the clinical results and did not prevent posterior dislocation nor glenoid migration in this series. Similarly postoperative immobilisation in neutral rotation was done in 4 out of the 5 cases who had glenoid failures.

Results according to the grade of the defect show that grade 3 defects are associated with worse clinical results (worse constant score and active elevation) and increase of glenoid failures (Table 1).

DISCUSSION

Preoperative planning is essential in osteoarthritis because posterior defect is frequent and needs specific surgical management. The defect is not correctly analyzed with radiographs and needs transversal analysis by CT-scan or at least by MRI. This permits to distinguish type B from type C, to measure the retroversion angle and to evaluate the residual glenoid bone (glenoid depth, antero-posterior glenoid diameter). In our view, radiographic AP view remains useful to appreciate and to classify the grade of the defect which seems to have an incidence on the result. In this study, we attempted to quantify the defect using a classification that we have used previously for rheumatoid arthritis [2], whereby glenoid wear is measured relative to the projection of the base of the coracoid process. This appeared to be an imprecise method, possibly due to the variability of the orientation of the radiologic beam. We observed that the projection of the spinoglenoid notch was clearer, more accurate and reproducible regardless of the beam orientation. While this new classification requires validation, it proved to be helpful and relevant in this study (Fig. 2).

Table 1

	N	Constant score (pts)	AAE(°)	AER(°)	XR migration (nb)
Grade 1	1	57	120	10	1
Grade 2	5	55	128	28	1 (20%)
Grade 3	3	40	80	60	3 (100%)

Surgical management of glenoid deficiency has been the purpose of many reports and different methods have been proposed in the literature. Trying to compensate the excessive glenoid retroversion by changing the humeral version has been proven to be ineffective [3]. Filling the defect with cement leads to early glenoid loosening and cannot be recommended. Some authors prefer the option of hemiarthroplasty, considering the high failure risk in combining reconstruction and cemented glenoid component, but also accepting persisting posterior subluxation and a limited functional result [4]. In the "pitonnage" technique, there is no bone graft, but head screws may serve as solid support for the posterior part of the glenoid; we did not find any series reporting the results of this method.

Neer and Morrison reported on 19 cases with excellent results with a combination of bone grafting and four different glenoid components. They did not have any glenoid loosening or graft subsidence at an average of 4 years follow-up [5]. Steinman and Cofield reported good results in 23 of 28 patients who underwent bone grafting for glenoid deficiency [6]. As an alternative treatment, Rice and Cofield noted satisfactory mid-term pain relief and improvement in function in patients with an asymmetric glenoid component; however, instability was not always corrected with these implants [7]. Norris reported in a first study no evidence of loosening in 9 corticocancellous bone grafts performed for peripheral glenoid deficiency [8]. He was less optimistic in a second series with 4 failures out of 12 cases of posterior defect [9].

The results of our series are not convincing with 56% graft subsidence and glenoid migration (5 cases). One of these concerns the only type C of the series complicated by glenoid osteolysis and medial migration of the metal-back glenoid. Considering the high prevalence of this complication with this glenoid design, we cannot conclude that it was a graft related complication [10]. The four other cases were type B2, one grade 2 and three grades 3, treated by graft combined with cemented keeled polyethylene glenoid, who failed by glenoid loosening and graft subsidence. The persisting posterior static instability participates in the failure at least in two cases, with one fixed dislocation occurring 3 months after the operation and one recurrent subluxation followed by glenoid migration after one year. It is possible that graft collapse preceded the recurrence of subluxation in the two other cases based on the observation of the radiographic evolution. In these four cases posterior capsular plication was combined and did not prevent the failure. Moreover three out of four were immobilized in neutral rotation during 6 weeks. Even if this protection has not been efficient in this series, we think however it is important, the most difficult part of this management being the capacity tolerate the device and ability to avoid wrong mobilisation during this period, especially for body care.

It is interesting to note that 4/8 grafts healed without recurrence of posterior ubluxation in similar anatomic conditions (Fig. 5). We believe that surgical details are important to enhance healing: micro perforations of glenoid sclerotic bone, solid graft fixation with at least 2 screws perpendicular to the contact area and, of course, out of the way of glenoid keel or pegs. We agree with other authors that an additional posterior transdeltoid small approach may be very useful to achieve a correct direction of the screws in these posterior defects. The technique of fixation of the graft is not standardized: we try to sculpture and match the humeral graft to the glenoid with minimal abrasion. Others prefer ingeniously to reshape the glenoid to receive a geometric graft [11]: it is probably better for the stability of graft fixation but, in our view, detrimental for an already reduced bone stock.

In this series only humeral head autograft has been used. In rare cases of osteopenic bone, corticocancellous iliac graft may be used. We did not find any author recommending allogenic graft in primary arthropathies.

In clinical practice our indications are based on the preoperative CT-scan:

- *For type B*, we select the mid-axial transversal cut and we draw the line from the posterior glenoid rim correcting glenoid retroversion to 10°. If the residual depth of the glenoid medial to the line measure more than 15 mm and antero-posterior glenoid diameter more than 20 mm, our option will be to ream more anteriorly. Beyond these limits, we consider that residual bone is no longer sufficient to admit a new cemented glenoid and the joint line would be excessively medialised. A combination of cemented glenoid and bone graft was our prior option but this choice is really challenging and the results are not convincing. It is the main reason that there are only 2 cases out of nine in this multicenter series between 2000 and 2007… In our indications, we have a place for hemi in limited goal situations but mostly for reversed arthroplasty which is more relevant in combination with structural graft [12]. It is interesting to note that 4 cases of B2 glenoid were successfully treated by reverse arthroplasty and bone graft during the same period in this multicenter study.

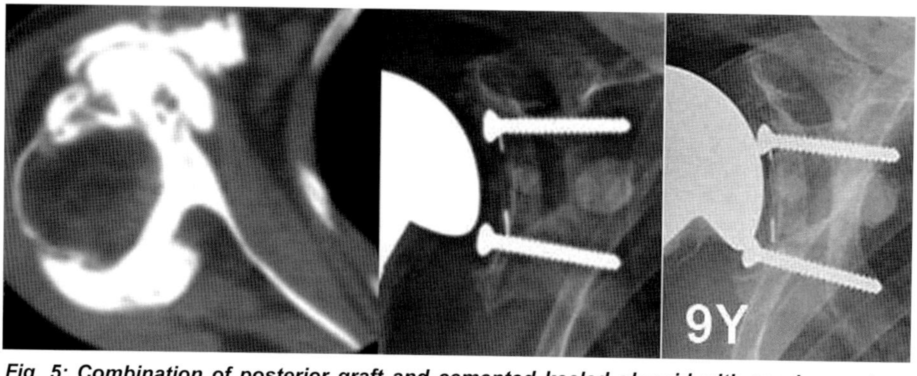

Fig. 5: Combination of posterior graft and cemented keeled glenoid with good aspect on postoperative view (center). After 9 years, graft is healed and there is no glenoid loosening.

- *For glenoid type C*, indications are controversial as well: Sperling reported bad results of hemiarthroplasty in this particular pattern and suggest addressing the defect by bone graft or glenoid osteotomy or an augmented component [13]. We prefer to implant the glenoid component without any procedure to reorientate the glenoid because of the absence of posterior subluxation [14].

In conclusion, bone-grafting for posterior glenoid deficiency in primary total shoulder replacement is a technically demanding procedure and is associated with a high rate of failure. Static posterior instability is not always reduced by correction of glenoid retroversion and is likely to be an important factor of failure. In our practice, this procedure has now very limited indications and reverse total arthroplasty is getting now more indications in this challenging pattern. For the rare residual indications, this study shows that graft healing may be obtained in combination with cemented glenoid but attention to detail and meticulous surgical technique is required.

REFERENCES

[1] WALCH G, BADET R, BOULAHIA A, KHOURY A. Morphologic study of the glenoid in primary glenohumeral osteoarthritis. *J Arthroplasty 1999;14: 756-60.*

[2] LÉVIGNE C, FRANCESCHI JP. Rheumatoid arthritis of the shoulder. Radiologic presentation and results of arthroplasty. In: G Walch and P Boileau, Editors, Shoulder Arthroplasty, *Springer, Berlin 1999: 221-32.*

[3] SPENCER EE, VALDEVIT A, KAMBIC H, *et al.* The effect of humeral component anteversion on shoulder stability with glenoid component retroversion. *J Bone Joint Surg Am 2005; 87 (4):808-14.*

[4] NEER CS, MORRISON DS Glenoid Bone-Grafting in Total Shoulder Arthroplasty. *J Bone Joint Surg 1988; 70(8):1154-62*

[5] NEER CS, MORRISON DS Glenoid Bone-Grafting in Total Shoulder Arthroplasty. *J Bone Joint Surg 1988; 70(8): 1154-62.*

[6] STEINMANN SP, COFIELD RH Bone grafting for glenoid deficiency in total shoulder replacement. *J Shoulder Elbow Surg 2000; 9(5): 361-7.*

[7] RICE RS, SPERLING JW, MILETTI J, SCHLECK C, COFIELD RH Augmented Glenoid Component for Bone Deficiency in Shoulder Arthroplasty. *Clin Orthop Relat Res 2008; 466; 579-83.*

[8] NORRIS TR Bone graft for glenoid deficiency in total shoulder replacement. Proceedings of the Third International Conference on Surgery of the Shoulder. *Tokyo: Professional Postgraduate Services; 1987. P 373-6.*

[9] HILL JM, NORRIS TR Long-Term Results of Total Shoulder Arthroplasty Following Bone-Grafting of the Glenoid. *J Bone Joint Surg 2001; 83(6): 877-83.*

[10] BOILEAU P, AVIDOR C, KRISHNAN S, WALCH G, KEMPF JF, MOLE D. Cemented polyethylene versus uncemented metal-backed glenoid components in total shoulder arthroplasty: A prospective, double-blind, randomized study. *J Shoulder Elbow Surg 2002;11(4): 351-59.*

[11] SCALISE J. Management of Glenoid Bone Deficiency in Total Shoulder Arthroplasty for Osteoarthritis. *Tech Shoulder Elbow Surgery 2008; 9(4): 208-15.*

[12] NEYTON L, BOILEAU P, NOVÉ-JOSSERANT L, EDWARDS TB, WALCH G. Glenoid bone grafting with a reverse design prosthesis. *J Shoulder Elbow Surg 2007; 16(3S): 71-8.*

[13] SPERLING JW, COFIELD RH, STEINMANN SP Shoulder Arthroplasty for Osteoarthritis Secondary to Glenoid Dysplasia. *J Bone Joint Surg 2002; 84(4): 541-6*

[14] EDWARDS, TB, BOULAHIA A, KEMPF JF, BOILEAU P, NEMOZ C, WALCH G. Shoulder arthroplasty in patients with osteoarthritis and dysplastic glenoid morphology. *J Shoulder Elbow Surg 2004; 13(1):1-4.*

AUGMENTED GLENOID COMPONENT FOR BONE DEFICIENCY

R.H. COFIELD, R.S. RICE

RECONSTRUCTIVE OPTIONS

When addressing with bone loss or alteration of bone shape in reconstructive surgery, one has in general three choices: selective bone preparation, bone grafting, use of an augmented or custom component – or some combination thereof. Selective reaming of the high side has been used in shoulder arthroplasty to prepare glenoids with irregular glenoid wear and has been effective when the amount of bone loss is not too extreme. Segmental bone grafting of the glenoid is not commonly necessary but can be done efficiently should grafting the glenoid be needed [1]. As published in 1982, Neer suggested the possibility of an asymmetrically thick polyethylene glenoid component, but this implant was seldom used [2].

We over time have developed a number of special glenoid components including those having an angled keel, those that were 2 mm thicker than usual to account for central bone loss and restore the joint line, an augmented metal-backed ingrowth component with screws, and a posteriorly augmented all-polyethylene glenoid component for treatment of the typical patient with a biconcave glenoid related to osteoarthritis and segmental wear.

Very recently there has been a biomechanical study performed on a custom posterior-step glenoid, this idea being presented as a poster at the 2010 AAOS Annual Meeting. On mechanical testing, there was essentially no difference when implanting this component in a cadaver when compared with a more standard glenoid component [3].

CASE SERIES

This report focuses on the use of an augmented all-polyethylene glenoid component for bone deficiency in shoulder arthroplasty. The material forming the basis of this report was published in 2008 by Rice and co-authors [4]. In constructing the implant the keel was perpendicular to the surface of the component resting against the bone and the articulating surface was prepared such that the posterior portion of the component was thicker by 0.44, 0.51, or 0.58 inches depending upon the size of the component. This change corrected the slope of the glenoid by approximately 4 degrees.

Between January 1, 1995, and December 31, 1999, this implant was placed in 13 patients with 14 operated shoulders. All had osteoarthritis. The average patient age was 66 years (range, 52 to 78 years). There were 12 men with 13 operated shoulders and one woman. Clinical follow-up averaged 5 years (range, 2.1 to 8 years). X-ray follow-up was available for 12 shoulders and averaged 3.9 years (1 to 8 years). The surgical technique was modified. The centering hole for the glenoid was moved 2 to 3 mm posteriorly depending on the size of the patient. The glenoid surface was reamed with approximately 5 degrees of posterior inclination using a bullet-tipped reamer. The glenoid component was then cemented in place with the thicker portion posteriorly, using the standard technique for cementing glenoid components. Importantly for stability, it was necessary to adjust the humeral head size. A system was used that included 26 sizes of humeral head components. The anterior capsule was released from the subscapularis preserving the anterior band of the inferior glenohumeral ligament with its attachments to the glenoid and to the inferior aspect of the humeral neck. The subscapularis was lengthened by freeing it from the anterior capsule and often by shifting the attachment site on its humerus medially by 1 cm. Occasionally the posterior capsule was plicated using longitudinal sutures placed from within the joint.

Clinical results were, in general, quite favorable. Pain on a 1 to 5 scale was reduced from 4.3 to 2.1 ($P = 0.0001$). Two shoulders postoperatively maintained a grade 4 score. Satisfaction as expressed by the patients was much better in 4, better in 7, the same in 2, and worse in 1. Active elevation improved on average from 99 degrees to 160 degrees ($P = 0.0001$). External rotation improved from 35 degrees to 56 degrees ($P = 0.057$). Internal rotation improved from the thumb being able to touch the sacrum to L3 ($P = 0.12$). The Neer rating was 5 excellent, 7 satisfactory, and 2 unsatisfactory. The latter related to residual pain.

The only complications were clinically apparent subluxation. This was moderate in the posterior direction in 3 shoulders, and severe in the anterior direction in 1 shoulder. This last patient had Parkinsonism and dislocated postoperatively; closed reduction and external support were applied. No reoperations were necessary in this patient group.

The radiographic results were available postoperatively for 12 of the 14 shoulders. Preoperative posterior subluxation was present in 11 of the 12 shoulders with postoperative follow-up. Postoperatively, there was posterior subluxation in 3 shoulders. One glenoid had a complete 2 mm lucent line and a shift in component position. This glenoid was considered as loose. In this patient there was also moderate posterior humeral subluxation postoperatively. No other glenoid components or humeral components had significant lucent lines. They either had no lucent lines or incomplete 1 mm lucent lines.

In discussing this material, one can see this is a small number of patients and the follow-up is mid-term at best.

We would conclude from this study that no unanticipated problems developed when using this augmented glenoid. However, it did not always control posterior subluxation. Therefore, it seemed marginally effective. Of note, considering the method of construction of this implant, the implant offset the central point of contact toward the thicker area, such that the central point of contact no longer rested over the center of the keel portion of the component but slightly posterior to it.

We feel that this design because of its marginal effectiveness has limited usefulness. We would consider new designs, and these would include both all-polyethylene and metal-backed ingrowth components, the latter supplemented by screw fixation. The articular surface of the component should be perpendicular to the keel or pegs. The thicker aspect of the component would have two configurations: a slope posteriorly of 2.5 degrees, 5 degrees, and 7.5 degrees and a set of stepped components with steps 2 mm, 4 mm, or 6 mm in thickness. This variety of augmented components should be useful in compensating for bone loss related to arthritic wear. To apply these newer components, one would need modified instrumentation including guides, a special reamer, and a set of rasps.

REFERENCES

[1] STEINMANN SP, COFIELD RH Bone grafting for glenoid deficiency in total shoulder arthroplasty. *J Shoulder Elbow Surg 9:361-367, 2000.*

[2] NEER CS, WATSON KC, STANTON FJ Recent experience in total shoulder replacement. *J Bone Joint Surg 64A: 319-337, 1982.*

[3] KIRANE YM, LEWIS GS, SHARKEY NA, ARMSTRONG AD Custom posterior-step glenoid prostheses for treating biconcave osteoarthritic glenoid defects. *Poster Presentation, N° P293 at the Annual Meeting, American Academy of Orthopaedic Surgeons, New Orleans LA, March 9-13, 2010.*

[4] RICE RS, SPERLING JW, MILETTI J, SCHLECK C, COFIELD RH Augmented glenoid component for bone deficiency in shoulder arthroplasty. *Clin Orthop 466: 579-583, 2008.*

REVISION OF HUMERAL HEAD REPLACEMENT TO TOTAL SHOULDER ARTHROPLASTY FOR GLENOID EROSION:
OUTCOMES OF THE ANATOMIC VERSUS THE REVERSE GLENOID

F. SIRVEAUX, F. WEIN, J. ARMENGOL, J. PORCELLINI

INTRODUCTION

The development of glenoid osteoarthritis (OA) is a concern after humeral replacement whatever the etiology of the arthroplasty. Sperling *et al.* [1] reported 72% of glenoid erosion at more than 10 years of follow-up. Parsons *et al.* [2] showed that glenoid cartilage erosion affected the functional results particularly for less than 1 mm of residual joint space. However, the rate of humeral head replacement (HHR) revision for glenoid erosion remains low – 15% according to Sperling *et al.* [3] and 8,1% according to Radnay *et al.* [4] in a systematic review. The literature on the results of revision to TSA for failed HHA is very poor. Hattrup [5] reported 17 cases with 30% of unsatisfactory results, Caroll *et al.* [6] reported 16 cases with 47% of unsatisfactory results, and Sperling and Cofield [7] reported 18 cases with 38% of unsatisfactory results. In the series of Dines *et al.* [8], the results were more encouraging, with 11 good results of 16 cases. Ravenscroft *et al.* [9] (17 cases) concluded that revision for failed HHR improves pain but not function. Overall, results are less impressive than those of primary TSA.

The results of TSA after failure of HHR could be compromised by asymmetric erosion, soft tissue imbalance, humeral malposition, and secondary cuff deficiency [6]. Levy *et al.* demonstrated that pain and function can be improved by using reverse shoulder arthroplasty (RSA) for HHR failure related to glenohumeral arthritis and cuff deficiency despite a high rate of complications –mainly related to the prosthesis and to bone loss [10]. Thus, there are two options for failed HHR revision: conversion to TSA or RSA. The goal of this study was to analyze the indications for conversion of HHA to TSA and RSA and then compare the results of both.

PATIENTS & METHODS

Patients

This retrospective, international, multicenter study collected cases of revision of HHR with glenoid erosion to either TSA or RSA. The exclusion criteria were: revision of HHR without glenoid erosion, revision of HHR without glenoid component implantation, tumors, absence of radiographs prior to the revision. The number of patient included in each center is reported in Table 1. For the clinical and radiographic analysis, we excluded cases with less than 18 months of follow-up.

Table 1: Number of cases included

Center	N
Lyon	48
Nice	19
Nancy	14
U.S.A.	27
Italy	9
Tours	7
Spain	7

We were able to include 131 cases. They included 93 females and 38 males. The etiologies leading to the initial HHR, gender distribution, and mean age are reported in Table 2. The mean age at the time of revision surgery for the entire series was 65 years (range, 31 to 85; median, 66).

The initial HHR was monoblock in 12 cases, modular in 74 cases, bipolar in 11 cases, and unknown in 34 cases. The mean interval from the time of HHR to revision was 42.7 months (range, 2 to 255 months; median, 24.5 months). The functional evaluation before revision is reported in Table 3.

Preoperative antero-posterior (AP) radiographs were available in 126 cases. In all cases, we found a preoperative narrowing of the glenohumeral joint with significant glenoid erosion. In the remaining cases the glenoid erosion had been noted in the operative report. In 35 out of the 50 cases of HHR for fracture (70%), the glenoid erosion was associated with tuberosity migration or malunion. Three patients had had a history of infection after the primary HHR.

Table 2: Distribution of etiology for primary HHR implantation, gender, and mean age.

Etiology leading to initial HHR	No. of cases	Gender		Mean age
		Female	male	
Acute fracture	50	39	11	64.7
Osteoarthritis	17	14	3	63.5
Cuff tear arthropathy	8	4	4	71.0
Rheumatoid arthritis	3	3	0	56.0
Fracture sequelae	31	21	10	56.4
Osteonecrosis	2	1	1	37.5
Miscellaneous	3	2	1	51.0
Unknown	17	10	7	63.5
Total	**131**	**93**	**38**	**61.7**

Table 3: Clinical evaluation before revision (AAE, active anterior elevation)

	Pain	Activity	Mobility	Strength	Constant score	Adjusted Constant score	AAE
Mean	4.1	5.3	8.2	1.9	19.3	24.9	57.9
Min-max	0-15	0-14	0-28	0-15	0-58	0-79	0-130
Median	5	6	8	0	19	23	60

We classified the glenoid erosion using the classification of Favard in the frontal plane [11]. We found 27 cases of glenoid erosion type E0, 30 of E1, 39 of E2, 25 of E3, and 4 of E4. Only 42 had axillary radiographs. Among those according to the Walch classification [12], we found 14 cases of type A1, 14 of type A2, 1 of type B1, 11 of type B2 and 2 of type C.

Operative technique

In 74% of the cases, the revision procedure was performed by a surgeon different from the one who performed the HHR. The deltopectoral approach was used in 118 cases and the anterosuperior approach was used in 8 cases (leaving 5 unknown cases).

The stem of the HHR was removed in 119 cases and left in place in 12 cases. A longitudinal humerotomy was performed in 25 cases and a diaphyseal window in 5 cases. In 35 cases (26.7%) a proximal humeral bone defect was noted after removing the stem. An intraoperative humeral fracture occurred in 12 cases (9.1%).

The HHR was revised to a RSA in 99 cases (fig. 1). In 2 cases, the HHR was converted to a RSA with the same stem left in place. In the other 97 cases, the stem needed to be removed. In 32 cases, the HHR was converted to a TSA (fig. 2). Among this group, the stem was removed in 22 cases and left in place in 10 cases. A long stem (150 or 180 mm) was used in 55 RSAs and in 3 TSAs.

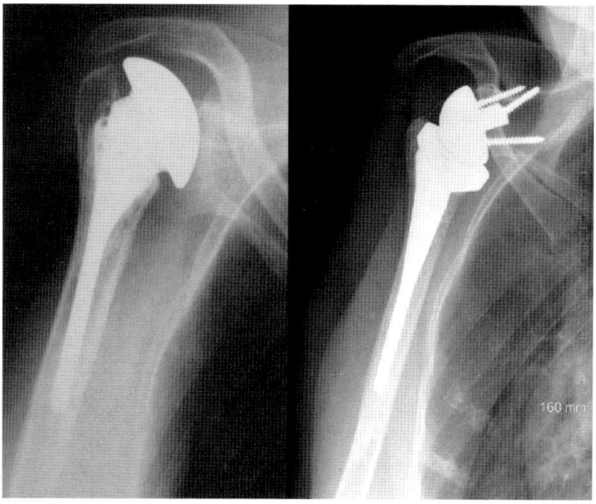

Fig. 1: Radiograph in 2003 of HHR performed for 71-year-old woman for primary OA in 2001, showing glenoid erosion (type-E2) with upward migration; AP view after revision to RSA in 2009.

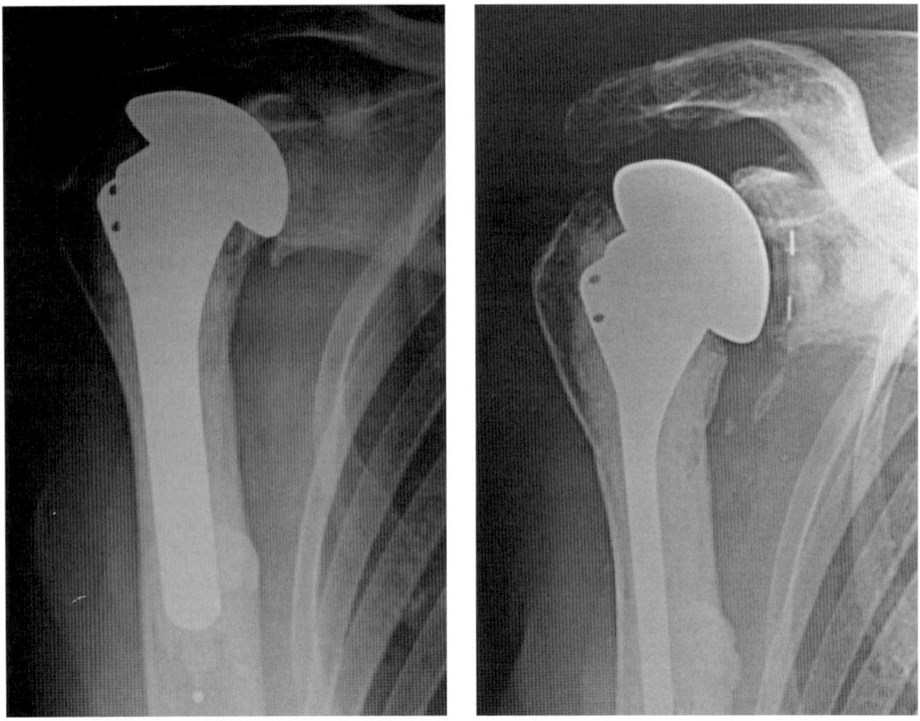

Fig. 2: Radiograph in 2007 of HHR performed for 58-year-old woman for primary OA in 2003; revision to TSA performed in 2009 due to painful glenoid.

On the glenoid side, there was no bone defect in 38 cases (29%). The defect was considered minimal and central in 38 cases (29%). A large central defect was noted in 18 cases (13%). A cortical defect was noted in 20 cases (15%). Before implanting the glenoid component, morcellized graft was used in 2 cases and a structural graft was used in 10 cases. The status of the cuff was evaluated during the procedure. For TSA, the glenoid component was cemented in all but 4 cases (metal-back glenoid). For RSA, an uncemented, long-pegged base plate was used in 4 cases and a standard-pegged base plate was used in the other cases.

Data Analysis Methods

For evaluation of the preoperative data, intraoperative data, and complications, we used the entire series. The patients with less than 24 months of follow-up were excluded from the clinical evaluation at last follow-up. For ordinal and continuous measurements, a paired *t*-test was performed to detect differences between preoperative and postoperative values. The ANOVA, Pearson, and Chi2 tests were used to compare RSA to TSA. A p value <0.05 was considered statistically significant.

RESULTS

Complications

In the TSA group, there were no early post-operative complications. One patient suffered a traumatic diaphyseal fracture with humeral and glenoid loosening. This patient was revised to a long stem HHR in another institution. One patient had a secondary rotator cuff tear and was not revised. Two patients underwent reoperation (revision rate, 6.2%); one was the patient with the humeral fracture, another was a patient with a TSA was revised again to a RSA for recurrent glenoid loosening.

In the RSA group, 12 patients suffered complications (complication rate 12%). There were 2 dislocations, 6 infections, 1 humeral dissociation, one hematoma, one bone resorption behind the glenoid base plate, and one iliac crest fracture. Ten patients had reoperations (revision rate, 10%). One dislocation was reoperated on for replacement of the polyethylene insert. Another dislocation was treated with revision of the humeral stem. Neither dislocation recurred. Five out of 6 infected prostheses were reoperated on: 1 debridement and 4 one-stage prosthesis revisions. One patient was reoperated on for debridement of a post-operative hematoma. The patient with glenoid base plate bone erosion was reoperated on for glenoid component revision. One patient had an open arthrolysis for stiffness.

Both the complication rate and the reoperation rate were significantly higher in the RSA group.

Overall results

We included patients with more than 2 years of follow-up. Six patients were deceased before 2 years of follow-up, 3 were lost and one has less than 2 years of follow-up. This leaves 121 patients included for functional evaluation. The mean follow-up was 59 months (range, 24 to 203; median, 45). All parameters of functional evaluation were significantly improved (Table 4). Removing the stem or leaving it in place did not influence the results or the complication rate.

Table 4: Functional results for 121 included cases, * $p<0.001$ (paired T test).

	Before revision	Last follow-up
Pain	4.1	11*
Activity	5.3	12.2*
Mobility	8.1	18.7*
Strength	1.9	6.6*
Constant score	19.4	48.3*
Adjusted Constant score	26%	67%*
Active anterior elevation	58	111*
Active external rotation	4.5	12.3*

Concerning the subjective results, 83% patients were very satisfied or satisfied with their operation, and 17% were disappointed or unsatisfied. We did not find any statistical influence of age, etiology, or glenoid morphology in the frontal or the sagittal plane.

RSA versus TSA

Patients revised with a RSA were significantly older than those revised with a TSA (67 versus 59 years old, $p=0.001$). The distribution of the etiology of the primary HHR was significantly different. Reverse shoulder arthroplasty was more frequently used for revision of HHR done for acute fractures and fracture sequelae. Eighty-three percent of the monoblock HHRs and 100% of the bipolar HHR were revised with a RSA.

The choice between TSA and RSA was strongly influenced by the status of the rotator cuff at time of revision ($p<0.001$) as reported in Table 6.

On the preoperative radiographs, the distribution of glenoid morphology according to Favard was different between the two groups (fig. 3).

Analysis of the pre-revision functional status demonstrated that the preoperative status was different between TSA and

Table 5: Primary indication for HHR (CTA, cuff tear arthropathy; MT, massive tear; OA, osteoarthritis; RA, rheumatoid arthritis; misc., miscellaneous).

	CTA-MT	Acute fracture	Fracture sequelae	Osteo-necrosis	OA	RA	Misc.
RSA	8	45	22	0	10	3	11
TSA	0	5	9	2	7	0	9
Mean age at revision	73.6	68.1	60.3	41.5	69.3	50.3	63.0

Table 6: Status of rotator cuff at time of revision of HHR.

	Subscapularis		Supraspinatus		Infraspinatus		Teres minor	
	Normal	Torn	Normal	Torn	Normal	Torn	Normal	Torn
RSA	26	54	11	73	17	53	49	19
TSA	23	3	22	2	23	1	23	0

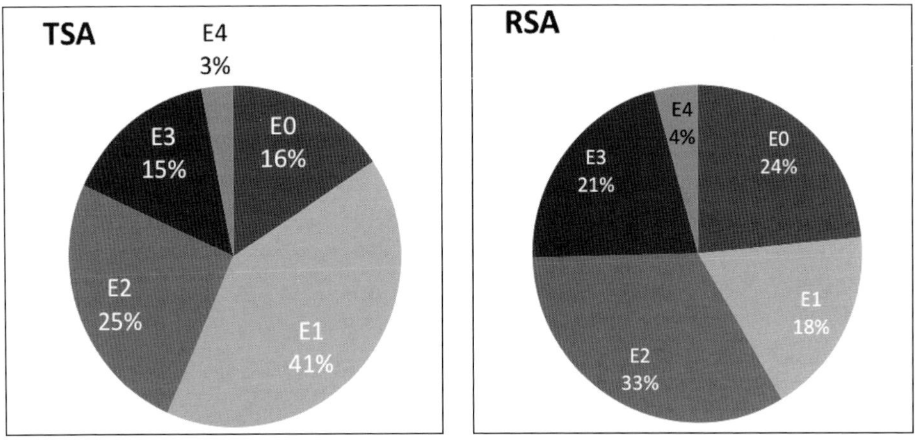

Fig. 3: Distribution of glenoid morphology in frontal plane before revision.

RSA conversion. As reported in Table 7, patients who had received a RSA were significantly older than those who received a TSA: a mean age at revision of 66.9 years versus 59 years, respectively. Furthermore, the mobility was significantly lower and the loss of strength was greater in the RSA group.

Table 7: Preoperative Constant score according to the type of revision prosthesis for 131 cases (AAE, active anterior elevation; AER, active external rotation), * p<0.05.

	RSA	TSA
N	99	32
Age	66.9	59*
Pain	3.9	4.8
Activity	5	6.1
Mobility	7.4	10.5*
Strength	1.3	3.7*
Constant score	17.5	24.8*
AAE	53	70*
AER	1.9	11.3*

Considering the cases with more than 2 years of follow-up, 91 RSAs and 30 TSAs were included. The Constant score was not statistically different between the two groups at final follow up. The Constant score averaged 47.3 points in the RSA group and 51.6 points in the TSA group. For all the components of the Constant score, the degree of improvement was not significantly different. Because the active external rotation was higher in the TSA group before revision, the TSA obtained a better range of motion in active external rotation at final follow-up: 25.3° versus 8.4° ($p<0.005$). Subjectively, 19.6% of the patients in the RSA group were unsatisfied or disappointed versus 6.6% in the TSA group.

The radiographs at final follow revealed 45% incidence of scapular notching in the RSA group. Regarding notch size, there were 28 patients in grade 1, 7 in grade 2, 2 in grade 3 and 8 in grade 4. Thirty-nine percent of the patients developed an inferior glenoid spur [13]. There were 9 cases with a radiolucent line around the central peg of the prosthesis but no base plate migration or loosening. We did not find any relationship between scapular notching and Constant score. The size of the notch was significantly influenced by the length of follow up (fig. 4).

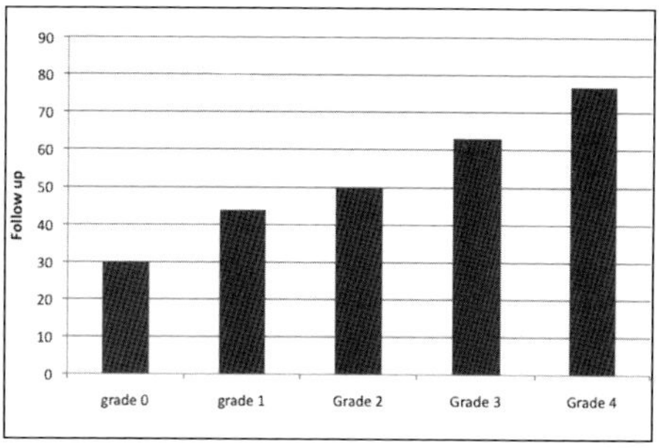

Fig. 4: Influence of follow-up on scapular notch size in RSA.

In the TSA group, radiographic evaluation at final follow up revealed a 46% incidence of glenoid radiolucent lines and 2 glenoid component migrations (one cemented, and one metal-back). Around the humerus, 25% had radiolucent lines but no humeral stems migrated.

DISCUSSION

This study demonstrates that revision of HHR for glenoid erosion improves the shoulder in terms of pain and function. The choice between TSA or RSA is above all dependent on the status of the rotator cuff. TSA and RSA allow similar functional results but the rate of complications of RSA is higher. Overall results reported in this study are better than those previously published in the literature [5-7, 9]. However, this study has several limitations. It is a retrospective and multi-center study. Several data are missing, especially concerning the description of the patients' status before HHR and details of the HHR implants. Radiographs were not taken in a standardized manner. The indications for revision were not uniform. The decision to revise could have been influenced by such factors as rotator cuff deficiency, tuberosities nonunion, asymmetrical glenoid erosion. Analysis of the preoperative data demonstrates that the TSA and RSA groups were definitely different. The accuracy of the comparison between the two groups is therefore debatable. Further prospective studies are needed to validate these results.

Nevertheless, this is the largest reported series of HHR revision and the only one comparing TSA and RSA in that context. Although this study includes patients with different diagnoses, they all reached the common end-point of glenoid arthrosis after a HHR.

Most of the previous series reporting revision of HHR reported poor functional results because the authors had used Neer's criteria [5-7]. Caroll *et al.* [6] reported an unsatisfactory outcome in 47% despite 50° of improvement in active forward elevation and 73% patients being subjectively satisfied. As in previous reported series [8], our study demonstrated a significant improvement in pain after both TSA and RSA. Yet, our results are in contradiction with those reported by Ravenscroft *et al.* [9], who did not find any functional improvement. Our gain in active forward elevation was similar to the series of Sperling and Cofield [7], Caroll *et al.* [6] and Dines *et al.* [8].

Our study highlights the importance of patient selection before revising a HHR. The history and physical exam, and the assessment of the rotator cuff and bone stock is mandatory. As noted by Hattrup [5], removal of the humeral stem is often necessary because of poor stem position or to improve exposure. The potential advantage of using a modular implant was not confirmed by our study. In the study by Carroll *et al.* [6], 50% of the HHR modular stems had to be removed. In the 17-case series reported by Ravenscroft *et al.* [9], all the stems were left in place, but overall functional results remained poor. The surgeon must prepare for the possible need for stem removal instruments as well as a long-stemmed implant prior to the procedure.

Revision of HHR remains a challenging procedure and the results never reach the results of the primary shoulder arthroplasty. The surgeon is confronted with scar tissue, rotator cuff deficiency, asymmetrical glenoid wear and substantial bone loss. That is why Levy *et al.* reported on the conversion to RSA in cases of rotator cuff-related or tuberosity-related failure [10, 14]. In our series, the patients with cuff deficiency were likely to be treated with a RSA. These patients were older than those treated with TSA, they had a poorer range of motion before revision and a higher rate of eccentric glenoid erosion, all of which made them poor candidate for conversion to TSA. The possibility of patient selection for conversion to TSA allowed us to improve the results of that group in our series and to decrease its rate of complications.

Reverse shoulder arthroplasty gave similar results even with the poorer preoperative condition of its patients. Still, the higher risk of complications with RSA must be kept in mind. The same findings were reported by Levy *et al.* in their series [14]. These authors concluded that complications were mainly related to bone loss. In our series, around 20% of patients revised with a RSA obtained unsatisfactory subjective results. Finally, the surgeon must considerer that the long-term results of RSA are less favorable after revision surgery [15].

CONCLUSION

Revision of HHR for painful glenoid OA improves pain and function of the shoulder. When possible, conversion to a TSA should be considered, and the necessary preparations should always be taken for a potential stem removal. A conversion to a reverse is proposed for cases of rotator cuff deficiency, soft-tissue imbalance, and asymmetric glenoid erosion. The preoperative assessment should always include an evaluation of the available bone stock, and the patient should always be informed of the generally high risk of postoperative complications.

REFERENCES

[1] SPERLING JW, COFIELD RH, ROWLAND CM. Neer hemiarthroplasty and Neer total shoulder arthroplasty in patients fifty years old or less. Long-term results. *J Bone Joint Surg Am 1998; 80: 464-73.*

[2] PARSONS IMT, MILLETT PJ, WARNER JJ. Glenoid wear after shoulder hemiarthroplasty: quantitative radiographic analysis. *Clin Orthop Relat Res 2004, 120-5.*

[3] SPERLING JW, COFIELD RH, ROWLAND CM. Minimum fifteen-year follow-up of Neer hemiarthroplasty and total shoulder arthroplasty in patients aged fifty years or younger. *J Shoulder Elbow Surg 2004; 13: 604-13.*

[4] RADNAY C, SETTER K, CHAMBERS L, LEVINE W, BIGLIANI LU, AHMAD CS. Total shoulder replacement compared with humeral head replacement for the treatment of primary glenohumeral osteoarthritis: a systematic review. *J Shoulder Elbow Surg 2007; 16: 396-402.*

[5] HATTRUP S. Revision total shoulder arthroplasty for painful humeral head replacement with glenoid arthrosis. *J Shoulder Elbow Surg 2009; 18: 220-24.*

[6] CARROLL R, IZQUIERDO R, VASQUEZ M, BLAINE T, LEVINE WN, BIGLIANI LU. Conversion of painfull hemiarthroplasty to total shoulder arthroplasty: long term results. *J Shoulder Elbow Surg 2004; 13: 599-603.*

[7] SPERLING JW, COFIELD RH. Revision total shoulder arthroplasty for the treatment of glenoid arthrosis. *J Bone Joint Surg [Am] 1998; 80: 860-67.*

[8] DINES J, FEALY S, STRAUSS EJ, ALLEN SH, CRAIG E, WARREN RF, DINES D. Outcomes analysis of revision total shoulder replacement. *J Bone Joint Surg [Am] 2006; 88: 1494-1500.*

[9] RAVENSCROFT M, CHARALAMBOUS C, HAINES J, TRAIL I. Outcome of stemmed shoulder hemiarthroplasty revision. *Arch Orthop Trauma Surg 2009; 129: 797-99.*

[10] LEVY J, FRANKLE M, MIGHELL M, PUPELLO D. The use of the reverse shoulder prosthesis for the treatment of failed hemiarthroplasty for proximal humeral fracture. *J Bone Joint Surg Am 2007; 89: 292-300.*

[11] FAVARD L, LAUTMAN S, SIRVEAUX F, OUDET D, KERJEAN Y, HUGUET D.

Hemiarthroplasty versus reverse arthroplasty in the treatment of osteoarthritis with massive rotator cuff tear. In: Walch G, Boileau P and Mole D, eds. 2000 shoulder prosthesis... Two to ten year follow-up. *Montpellier: Sauramps Medical; 2001. p. 261-8.*

[12] WALCH G, BADET R, BOULAHIA A, KHOURY A. Morphologic study of the glenoid in primary glenohumeral osteoarthritis. *J Arthroplasty 1999; 14: 756-60.*

[13] SIRVEAUX F, FAVARD L, OUDET D, HUQUET D, WALCH G, MOLE D. Grammont inverted total shoulder arthroplasty in the treatment of glenohumeral osteoarthritis with massive rupture of the cuff. Results of a multicentre study of 80 shoulders. *J Bone Joint Surg Br 2004; 86: 388-95.*

[14] LEVY JC, VIRANI N, PUPELLO D, FRANKLE M. Use of the reverse shoulder prosthesis for the treatment of failed hemiarthroplasty in patients with glenohumeral arthritis and rotator cuff deficiency. *J Bone Joint Surg Br 2007; 89: 189-95.*

[15] GUERY J, FAVARD L, SIRVEAUX, F, OUDET D, MOLE D, WALCH G. Reverse total shoulder arthroplasty. Survivorship analysis of eighty replacements followed for five to ten years. *J Bone Joint Surg Am 2006; 88: 1742-47.*

LESSONS LEARNED FROM THE HYLAMER EXPERIENCE & TECHNICAL SALVAGE FOR GLENOID RECONSTRUCTION

T.R. NORRIS, S. ABDUS-SALAAM

INTRODUCTION

Neer was an early pioneer in shoulder arthroplasty for proximal humeral fracture treatment [1, 2].

He reported on total shoulder arthroplasty for arthritis in 1974 and 1982 [3, 4].

Indications for shoulder arthroplasty have expanded to include treatment for primary and secondary shoulders pathology with the rotator cuff intact, and more recently for those with cuff deficits. As more surgeons gain experience with the shoulder, the use of shoulder arthroplasty increases annually. According to the U.S. Department of Health and Human Services the number of total shoulder arthroplasties increased 145% between 1997 and 2005 [5]. The number of patients of all ages who underwent total shoulder arthroplasty in 2004, 2005 and 2006 was 15,400, 16,500 and 18,300, respectively [6]. As demonstrated in the hip and knee arthroplasty literature [7], the revision burden of shoulder arthroplasty will increase with the aging of the United States population and with the increase in the number of procedures performed.

Salvaging a failed shoulder arthroplasty is technically challenging [8-17]. Whereas the greater tuberosity healing is the main challenge obtaining a satisfactory result in prosthetic fracture treatment, in degenerative arthritis, the glenoid has been the weak link in arthroplasty. Whereas glenoid arthritis is the most common reason to revise a humeral head arthroplasty [18], glenoid component loosening has been the most common cause for revision total shoulders [19].

Glenoid component failure is a result of wear, fragmentation, shift or loosening. Polyethylene debris and osteolysis can lead to a spectrum from minor to severe glenoid bone loss [20].

The problem became more rapidly apparent in the 1990s when DuPont/DePuy introduced highly cross-linked polyethylene sterilized by gamma irradiation in air. Unfortunately, this combination of polyethylene and sterilization method dramatically shortened the time in which the polyethylene would wear, fragment, shift, or loosen [21, 22]. In turn, many more cases presented in a short time period for glenoid component revision in 3 to 5 years rather than 10 to 15 years [19].

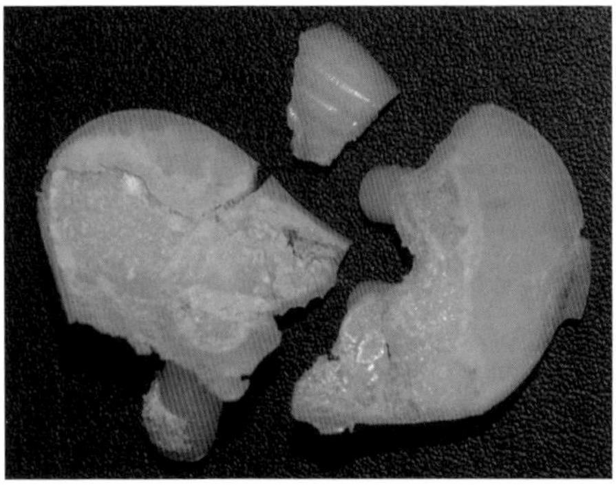

With component loosening, there can be significant glenoid bone loss [15, 20, 23, 24]. This includes, at minimum, the space occupied by the component and methyl methacrylate. These mechanical factors of loosening plus the reaction to the polyethylene debris with osteolysis leads to a spectrum from minor to severe glenoid bone loss.

Traditionally, approaches to address the bone deficits have met with only moderate success. Additional scar and an increase chance of infection may adversely affect the outcome with each additional surgery.

Removal of the glenoid component alone, either open or arthroscopically invariably results in medial humeral head migration with progressive glenoid bone loss. Revisions, when necessary become more difficult. A primary glenoid exchange has a high loosening and failure rate in the face of a large glenoid defect, particularly if the glenoid rim is compromised.

The shoulders fare better with grafting the glenoid defect when converting to a humeral head replacement, total shoulder or reverse shoulder arthroplasty. Many grafting and prosthetic techniques have been described, but grafting and obtaining sufficient strong bone to incorporate and support a new glenoid component is challenging.

Impaction grafting with allograft of the defect when converting a failed total shoulder for glenoid loosening to a humeral head arthroplasty at the time of component removal similarly results in graft resorption in 50 per cent at an average of 33 months [26].

Alternatively, the allograft chips can be impacted in a 2-stage procedure with reimplantation of a cemented glenoid component with only fair outcome [20, 27, 28]. Reimplantation of a glenoid component when possible has better outcomes than converting to a humeral head replacement alone [20].

Similarly, autogenous iliac bone grafts to address glenoid defects without reimplantation of a cemented glenoid has been tried when the total shoulder is revised to a humeral head arthroplasty. If the patient has pain after the graft has incorporated in 6 months, then the humeral head arthroplasty can be revised to an anatomic or reverse shoulder arthroplasty [14, 28, 29].

Alternatively, a two-stage procedure has been employed to reimplant the glenoid after graft consolidation, but this does require the second procedure [27-29].

Assuming the rotator cuff is functional and sufficient, an anatomic total shoulder replacement has been preferred in the one or two stage reconstructions. In cases with absence of the subscapularis or superior cuff deficiency, the reverse shoulder more recently has been a better option [30].

Managing large glenoid defects are particularly problematic. Antuna classified glenoid bone deficiencies into central, peripheral, or combined. Each of these are subdivided as mild, moderate, and severe [20].

Williams and Iannotti have a very comprehensive classification that would cover all deficits encountered, but may not be a clinically useful as one which concentrates on the three types seen for our patient population needing structural bone grafts [23].

The categories seen in our cases with glenoid component loosening all have defects begin in the central cavity where the component is first placed. Humeral head arthroplasty alone in these revisions have given less predictable pain relief and function and there is a high incidence of painful glenoid arthrosis [26]. Reimplantation of a cemented anatomic glenoid component into a large defect in one stage without grafting leads to high loosening rate and frequently need revision [31].

Converting the failed total shoulder to a humeral head replacement with allograft impaction is one alternative in an effort to avoid the iliac donor site discomfort with autogenous grafting. Unfortunately, multiple studies demonstrate problematic subsidence of cancellous allograft into the glenoid deficits. This results in a painful arthrokatadysis of the humeral head into the scapula with little bone for later glenoid reconstruction [20, 26, 27, 32].

A single stage revision with a large iliac crest bone graft and an anatomic cemented glenoid component raises concerns in that the polymethylmethacrylate (PMMA) may impede graft healing in anatomic total shoulder arthroplasty.

Neyton and Walch described implanted a tricortical iliac crest bone graft into the glenoid defect with an interval of 6 months between stages to permit bone incorporation. These structural autografts do not have the subsidence associated with cancellous allograft and autografts [33, 34]. Unfortunately, with each additional surgery, functional recovery is delayed, the quality of the tissues likely decreases while the incidence of sepsis increases.

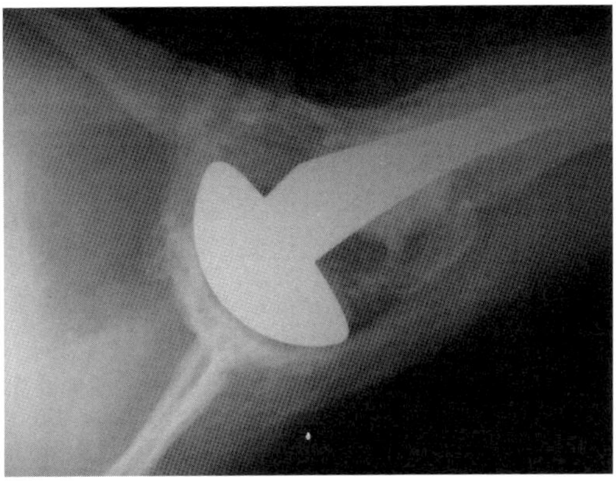

Conversion TSA to HHA with cancellous allograft subsidence

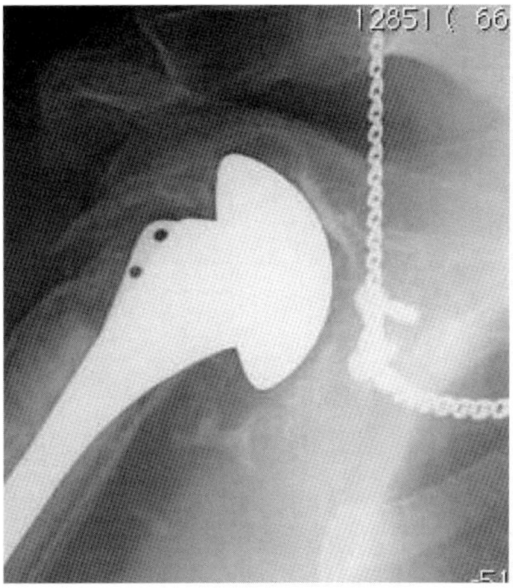

As in primary shoulder arthroplasty, better function and pain relief with longevity are obtained with resurfacing both the humeral head and the glenoid [35].

It is not a surprise that experience to date favors bone grafting the glenoid defect in a primary conversion to a humeral head arthroplasty. The cancellous allografts and autografts lack the structure to effective resist the humeral head loads. They have a high subsidence and failure rate. Structural iliac crest autografts with the crest facing the humeral head described by Neyton and coauthors have the best incorporation rate with the least subsidence. It leaves the choices open for performing an anatomic total or reverse shoulder arthroplasty in the future if necessary. Its disadvantage is that is requires two operations. Loss of adequate rotator cuff function favors the reverse arthroplasty at the time of revision. In our experience, many of our patients have already had multiple procedures and compromised rotator cuff for function.

In this article, we report our preliminary results of a one-stage glenoid reconstruction using tricortical iliac crest bone graft with a reverse shoulder arthroplasty to salvage failed anatomic and reverse shoulder arthroplasties with a large glenoid defects [36, 37].

The rationale is the glenoid baseplate can compress the bone graft and protect it sufficiently to allow healing while still observing the principles of glenosphere positioning [38-40].

MATERIALS AND METHODS

Between 2004 and 2009, 52 patients underwent revision shoulder arthroplasty with tricortical iliac crest bone graft (TICBG) at our institution. Twenty-nine shoulders in 28 patients are included in the study. The inclusion criteria include a complete preoperative evaluation, operative reports and one-year postoperative clinical and radiographic evaluations. Sixteen patients had incomplete medical records and 8 had radiographic follow-up less than one year. The mean age was 63.1years. The sex distribution was 15 men and 13 women. The reasons for revision were failed total shoulder arthroplasty (TSA) in 26 patients, failed reverse shoulder arthroplasty (RSA) in 2 patients and one failed humeral head replacement (HHR) with severe glenoid erosion. In the failed total shoulder arthroplasty group, the causes for revision were aseptic glenoid loosening in 17/26 (65.4%), sepsis in 6/26 (23.1%), instability in 2/26 (7.7%), chronic dislocation in 1/26 (3.8%) and in 1/26 (3.8%) aseptic glenoid loosening and instability occurred concomitantly. In the failed reverse shoulder arthroplasty group, the causes of revision were aseptic glenosphere loosening in 2/2 (100%). The failed humeral head replacement had a fixed dislocation with erosion of 60% of the glenoid.

Post-operative radiographs were reviewed for evidence of graft healing. We determined the graft to be healed if a bone block was present under the glenoid baseplate without lucent lines and if no change in component position was noted on immediate post-operative and follow-up radiographs. Minimum follow-up was one year or until revision. The junior and senior authors independently reviewed all radiographs. Anterior-posterior (AP) and lateral scapular radiographs were taken at the first follow-up visit. Subsequently, AP in internal and external rotation, axillary lateral and scapular Y views were taken routinely at 2, 6, and 12 weeks, 6 months and then annually. Patient demographics are reported in Table 1.

Table 1: Demographic data: N=29 TICBG

Shoulder	Revision Indication	Cause of Rev.	# Prior Procedures	XR F/U (mo.'s)	Age (years)	Sex	Prior Sepsis
1	Failed RSA	aGSL	3	36	58	F	no
2	Failed TSA	sepsis	7	32	51	M	yes
3*	Failed TSA	sepsis	9	19	43	F	yes
4	Failed HHR	Glen oa	1	25	54	M	no
5*	Failed TSA	aGL	6	3	75	F	no
6*	Failed TSA	Chr dis	12	6	54	F	no
7	Failed RSA	aGSL	4	12	71	F	no
8*	Failed TSA	aGL	20	38	71	M	no
9	Failed TSA	aGL	2	57	59	F	no
10	Failed TSA	Instab, aGL	7	29	52	M	no
11	Failed TSA	aGL	1	12	74	M	no
12	Failed TSA	Instab.	10	23	37	M	no
13*	Failed TSA	sepsis	13	9	47	F	yes
14	Failed TSA	aGL	5	22	51	M	no
15	Failed TSA	aGL	1	15	79	F	no
16	Failed TSA	aGL	1	22	60	M	no
17*	Failed TSA	aGL	2	21	60	M	no
18	Failed TSA	aGL	4	27	57	F	no
19	Failed TSA	aGL	2	14	58	F	no
20	Failed TSA	sepsis	5	12	66	M	yes
21	Failed TSA	sepsis	3	14	72	M	yes
22*	Failed TSA	aGL+H	1	35	67	M	no
23	Failed TSA	aGL	6	29	59	M	no
24	Failed TSA	sepsis	3	12	74	M	yes
25	Failed TSA	Instab	2	17	69	F	no
26	Failed TSA	aGL	8	13	68	M	no
27*	Failed TSA	aGL	3	5	60	M	no
28	Failed TSA	aGL	1	30	62	F	no
29	Failed TSA	aGL	1	59	59	F	no

TECHNIQUE

The surgical technique consisted of glenoid exposure and debridement of prosthetic fragments and any fibrous or necrotic debris. Tissue cultures were sent and held for 14 days. Antibiotics were started after harvesting deep cultures.

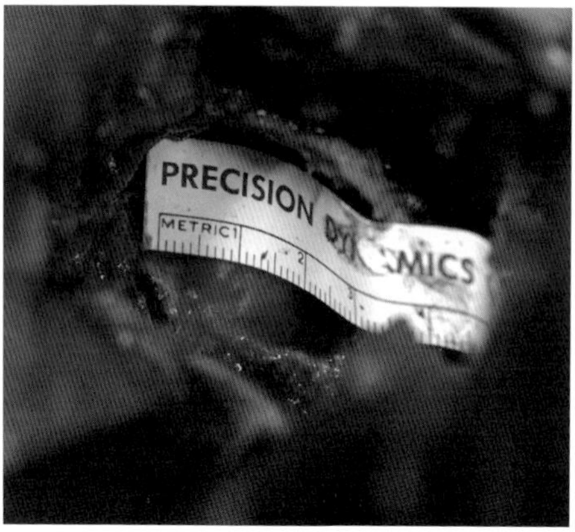

Measure and size defect

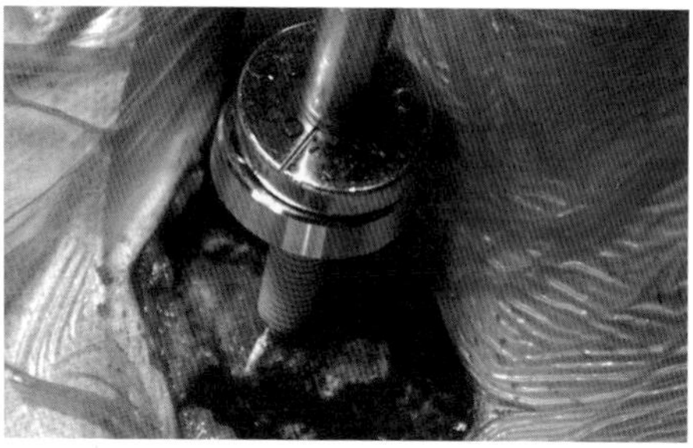

Harvest graft on iliac crest with baseplate attached

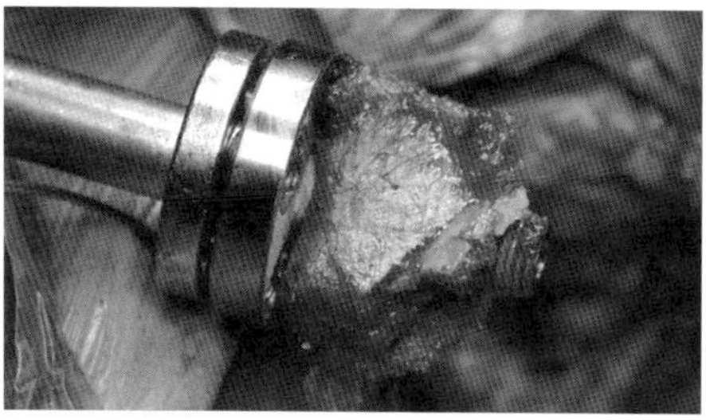

Remove graft and trim to fit glenoid defect

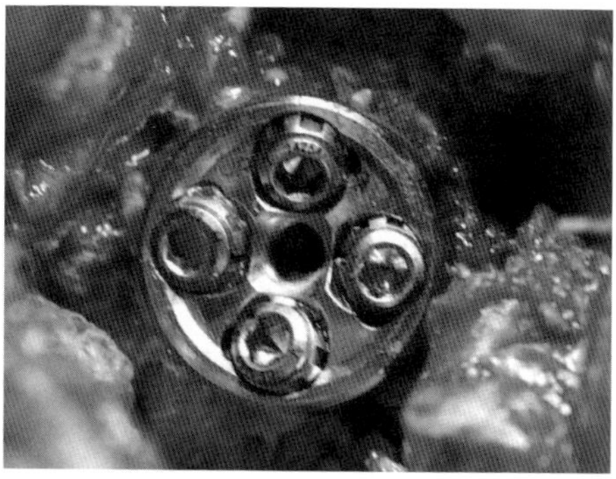

Secure graft and baseplate to native glenoid

The technique may be viewed as a video supplement at http//www.vumedi.com/node/54195 for the detailed surgical technique. The Aequalis Reversed Shoulder Prosthesis (Tornier, Inc., Edina, MN) was used in all revisions. In the post-operative period, an abduction pillow and sling is used for 5 weeks. Patients were instructed in hospital by physical and occupational therapist on active ROM exercises for hand, wrist and elbow and sling care on post-operative day 1. Instructions for shoulder pendulums were also given but were began on post-operative day 21. Patients were allowed to begin passive forward elevation in plane of scapula at 3 weeks and active ROM with forward flexion stretching exercises at home or with a therapist at 6 weeks. Strengthening began at 12 weeks.

RESULTS

Twenty-eight patients and 29 shoulders were included in this series (see Table 2). Average follow-up was 23.2 months (12-57 months). Twenty-six failed TSA, 2 failed RSA and one failed HHR were salvaged using one stage TICBG and RSA.

Table 2: Results

Shoulder	Graft healed	Revision indication	# Prior proc.'s	Cause of Failure	Prior sepsis	Age (yrs)	Final result
1	yes	Failed RSA	3	NA	no	58	-
2	yes	Failed TSA	7	NA	yes	51	-
4	yes	Failed HHR	1	NA	no	54	-
7	yes	Failed RSA	4	NA	no	71	-
9	yes	Failed TSA	2	NA	no	59	-
10	yes	Failed RSA	7	NA	no	52	-
11	yes	Failed TSA	1	NA	no	74	-
12	yes	Failed TSA	10	pain/stiff	no	37	fusion
14	yes	Failed TSA	5	NA	no	51	-
15	yes	Failed TSA	1	NA	no	79	-
16	yes	Failed TSA	1	NA	no	60	-
18	yes	Failed TSA	4	NA	no	57	-
19	yes	Failed TSA	2	NA	no	58	-
20	yes	Failed TSA	5	NA	yes	66	-
21	yes	Failed TSA	3	NA	yes	72	-
23	yes	Failed TSA	6	NA	no	59	-
24	yes	Failed TSA	3	NA	yes	74	-
25	yes	Failed TSA	2	NA	no	69	-
26	yes	Failed TSA	8	NA	no	68	-
28	yes	Failed TSA	1	NA	no	62	-
29	yes	Failed TSA	1	NA	no	59	-
3	no	Failed TSA	9	sepsis	yes	43	Healed/ TICBG x2
5	no	Failed TSA	6	sepsis	no	75	Healed 3-stage revision
6	no	Failed TSA	12	aGSL	no	54	Pending revision
8	no	Failed TSA	20	aGSL	no	71	Rev to LP RSA, healed
13	no	Failed TSA	13	sepsis	yes	47	resection
17	no	Failed TSA	2	aGSL	no	60	Healed TICBG
22	no	Failed TSA	1	aGSL	no	67	Rev to LP RSA, healed
27	no	Failed TSA	3	aGSL	no	60	Rev to LP RSA, healed

Twenty-one of 29 (72.4%) bone grafts healed with one procedure. With additional surgery 28 of 29 (96.6%) of the grafts healed. Eight of 29 (27.6%) of the bone grafts failed the first attempted TICBG. Three failures were due to sepsis and 5 from aseptic loosening. One of three (33%) of the septic failures had prior sepsis. All but one septic failure was successfully revised in two stages using a RSA and a second TICBG. The other septic failure ultimately required resection arthroplasty after failing the 2-stage reconstruction due to repeat sepsis. Three of five (60%) of the aseptic glenosphere failures were initially fixed with a short post (15mm) baseplate in which the baseplate post did not engage the native scapula. One of five had a long post (25 mm) and superior tilt on initial postoperative radiograph. All 5 of these were successful revised with a TICBG in an additional procedure with a long post baseplate in which the post was fixed in the native scapula. The number of prior procedures was statistically significant between the failed (n=8.5) and the healed (n=3.7) grafts, p=0.011. The group with failure to heal the graft were slightly younger (59.6 to 61.4 years) but this was not significant, p=0.478. Two patients had additional subsequent surgeries for periprosthetic humeral shaft fractures without disturbing the healed TICBG.

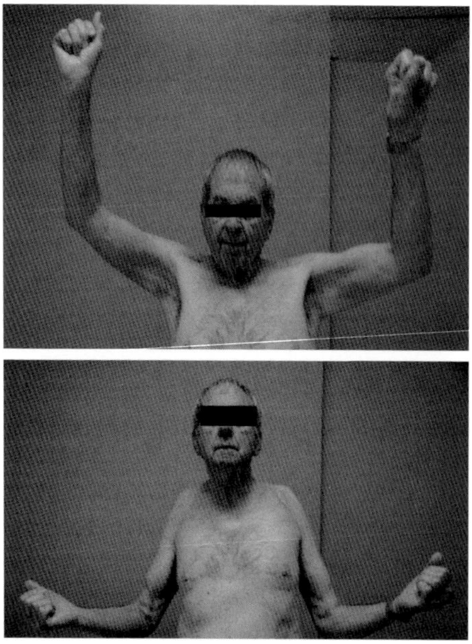

Example of post-op elevation and rotation after bilateral TICBGs in revision TSA with glenoid loosening to a RSA

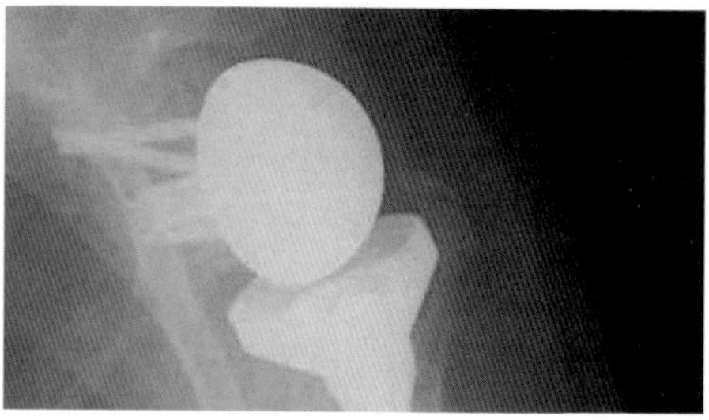

Post-operative healed graft and secure baseplate

DISCUSSION

Salvaging a failed shoulder arthroplasty is technically challenging. Complications related to the glenoid are a leading cause of revision shoulder arthroplasty [8-17]. Glenoid component failure is a result of wear, fragmentation, shift or loosening. Polyethylene debris and osteolysis lead to a spectrum from minor to severe bone loss. The one-stage reconstruction of glenoid defects with a tricortical structural iliac crest has several advantages over a two-stage procedure. With one-stage, there will be less scarring in patients who often present after multiple shoulder procedures. In our study, the mean number of procedures was 5.1 (range 1-20) overall, 3.7 in the successful TICBG group and 8.5 in the failed TICBG group. Additional surgical insult to an already traumatized soft tissue envelope can be minimized with a one-stage procedure. Second, each surgical procedure increases the chance of sepsis. Even with good initial graft fixation, sepsis will ultimately lead to failure and require additional procedures to obtain the final outcome. Three of our eight TICBG failures occurred due to sepsis.

Our results also highlight three technical points necessary for successful one stage glenoid reconstruction with TICBG. Initially, reconstructions were using the standard baseplates with a 15mm central post. The short post did not provide fixation in the native scapula; the four peripheral screws were not reliable for fixation alone. In our series three of the five aseptic failures occurred with implants with short post baseplates. At the senior author's request, the Tornier engineers Yves-Alain Raton and Laurent Comtat developed the longer 25mm and 30 mm baseplate posts to insure post would engage the patient's scapula with the additional graft. The 25 mm long post baseplate is now FDA approved and is used in all of these cases with bone grafts. The rationale for successful TICBG healing is the glenoid baseplate can compress the bone graft and protect it during healing. For these reasons, two compression screws and two locking screws for our peripheral screws are now preferred in accord with the designers' original intention. On several occasions 4 peripheral locking screws were used. The one aseptic glenosphere failure did have 4 peripheral locking screws glenosphere with a cephalad tilt for its original fixation. This went on to loosen and required a second procedure to obtain healing. At revision there was partial resorption of the TICBG under the baseplate. In addition to surgeon error in not tilting the baseplate inferiorly, there was concern with the resorption under the baseplate. The locking screws without compression might have contributed to the failure.

The in-situ technique to ream the iliac graft and seat the baseplate while on the iliac crest simplifies the carpentry of harvesting the necessary size and shape of the graft. The baseplate and graft can then be contoured to fit the glenoid defect. It would be more challenging to ream, shape the graft and implant the post thru the free graft if the graft was harvested first.

A simplified classification is proposed to address the defects encountered in this cohort of patients. With glenoid loosening sufficient to require an iliac graft, there are no mild defects or only peripheral defects as described by Antuna [20]. All defects from glenoid loosening begin as central cavitary defects. The average length of a central polyethylene peg or keel is 15 mm. Add to this the volume of the PMMA and additional bone loss from polyethylene induced osteolysis, there is even less bone available to hold a new component without grafting. Whether it is loosening by mechanical, chemical (polyethylene-mediated osteolysis) or by sepsis, the glenoid defect usually involves a majority of the central cavity.
Although pegged glenoid components are thought to be more bone conserving, the intercalary cancellous bone is replaced with rubbery fibrous tissue between the pegs. The resultant defect is frequently as large or larger than found with keeled glenoid components.

Antuna's peripheral bone loss classification alone is not encountered in revision arthroplasty for glenoid loosening. It is applicable to shoulder instability, fixed dislocations, and osteoarthritic wear patterns. Only one patient in our series had a severe peripheral wear pattern cause by a chronically subluxed humeral head replacement that involved 50% of the glenoid. In this instance, no glenoid had previously been implanted. This was the one exception to the wear pattern reported for the remaining patients. This was managed by asymmetrically shaping the TICBG to fit the posterior glenoid deformity, but differs from the pattern seen during revision for glenoid loosening. The

TICBG is an effective technique for some moderate and all severe central and combined defects. Milder central defects are more appropriately local bone grafts such as the distal clavicle if available.

The modification of Antuna's classification offered by Williams and Iannotti [23] subdivides the glenoid into subchondral bone, the glenoid rim and vault regions. It is more comprehensive and descriptive for the 8 potential defects seen in revision arthroplasty.

A more simplified classification of glenoid bone loss encountered during revision arthroplasty for glenoid loosening is proposed. Smaller defects, other bone graft sources such as the distal clavicle may be sufficient and are not considered in this review.

Classification of Glenoid Bone Loss Encountered During Revision for Glenoid Loosening In TSA

Type 1-central cavitary defect
Type 2-central bone loss and one scapular wall
- 2A-anterior wall
- 2B-posterior wall

Type 3-central bone loss with absence of anterior and posterior scapular walls

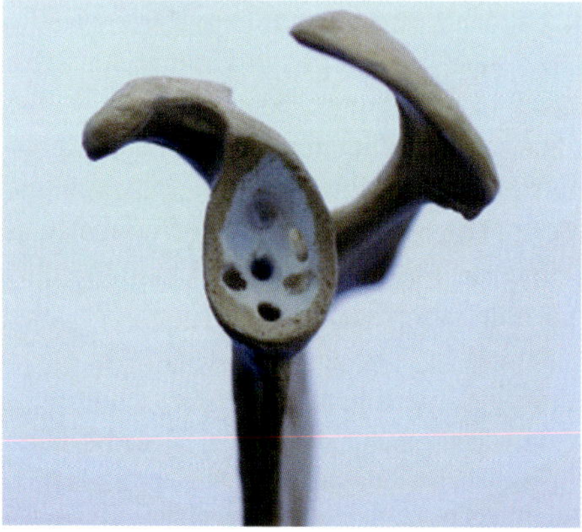

Type 1: cavitary central bone loss, rim and walls intact

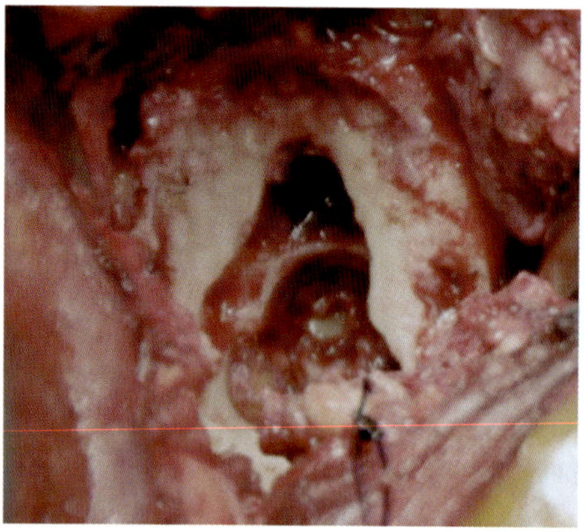

Type 1 cavitary bone loss

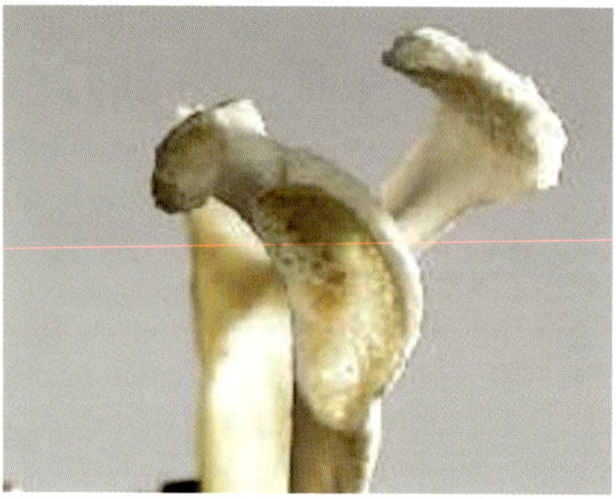

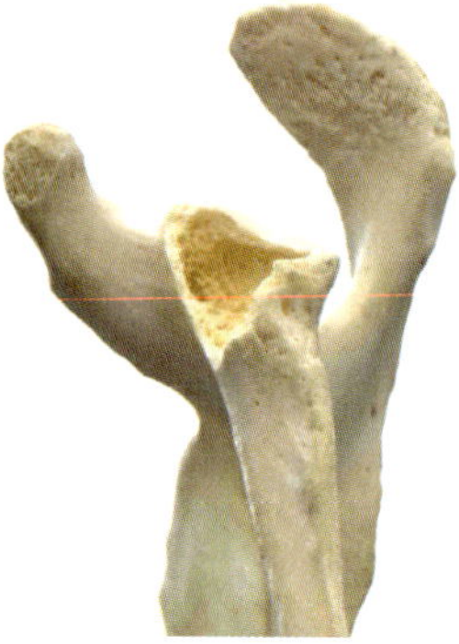

Type 2A: cavitary + anterior loss of glenoid rim and scapular vault.

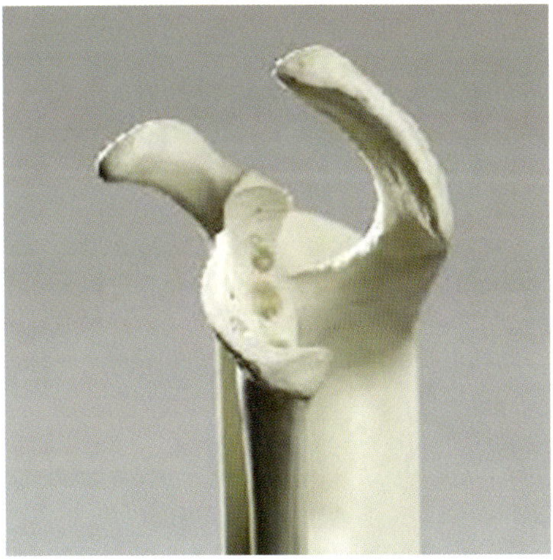

Type 2B: Cavitary + posterior glenoid rim and wall

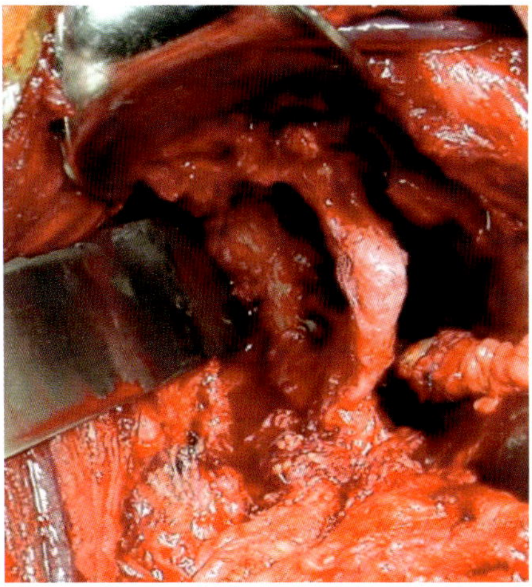

Type 2B-cavitary central and posterior peripheral glenoid defect

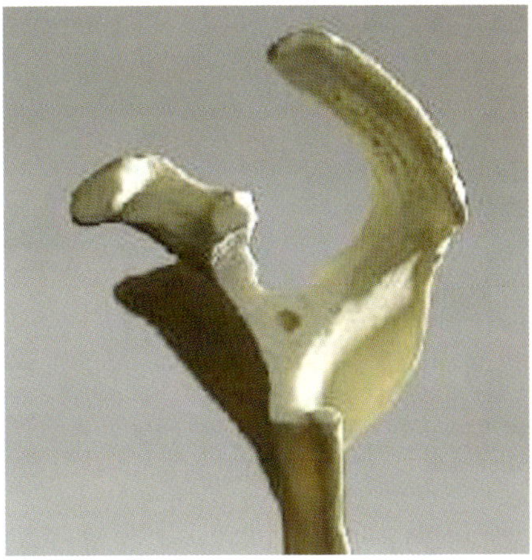

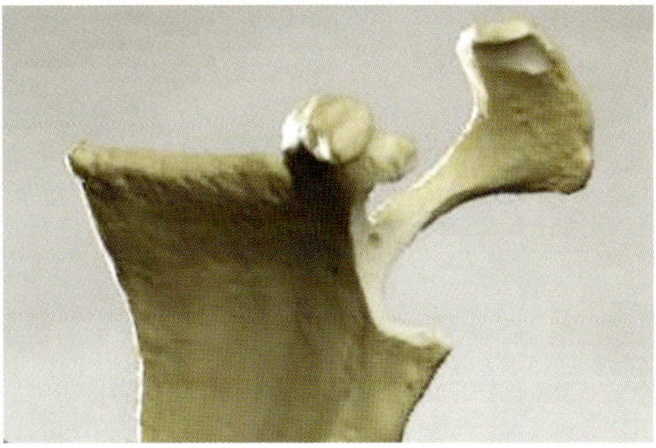

Type 3: Cavitary + loss of anterior and posterior rim and wall

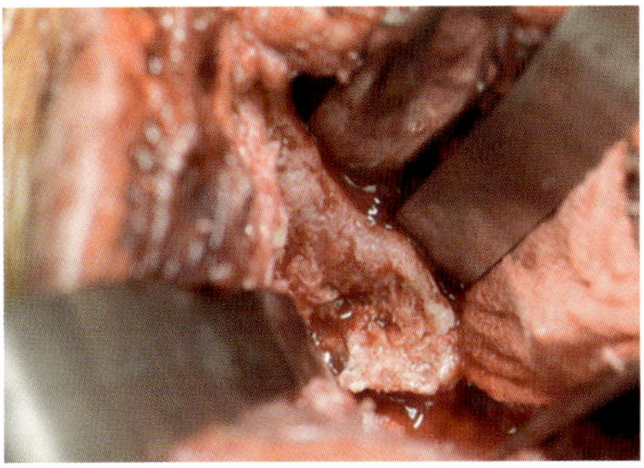

The more severe Type 3 defects have the cavitary central defect with loss of both the anterior and posterior walls. The pillar of the scapula and the base of the coracoid are frequently preserved and project laterally, while the bone in between is absent. The three categories reflect what is seen clinically in these patients.

The purpose of the review is to determine whether or not the one-stage iliac crest bone graft offers a reasonable option to address these glenoid reconstructions. As many patients had multiple prior procedures with or without prior sepsis, the standard functional scores did not seem to be relevant for determining success or failure of the procedure. The goal was to obtain graft healing and a stable baseplate-glenosphere construct for the reverse shoulder arthroplasty. The technique of one-stage glenoid reconstruction with TICBG is feasible with a successful outcome if the graft heals.

The classification for glenoid bone loss captures the defects seen and has implications for the graft size and shape needed, as well as what scapular bone remains for the fixation.

In conclusion, one-stage glenoid reconstruction with TICBG is reasonable option with a good chance of success in these complicated cases. Twenty-one of twenty-nine shoulders had successful healing of the graft in the one-stage. Seven of the remaining eight shoulders required additional surgery to gain healing; one went on to a resection arthroplasty for recurrent sepsis. She has not had a recurrence of her infection since the resection.

In this early experience, there was a learning curve. The standard 15 mm post is the same length of the keel or central peg in the standard glenoid component. Engaging the native scapula with a longer baseplate post give better fixation into the scapula as it was soon discovered. In-situ preparation of the TICBG and baseplate prior to transfer into the glenoid simplifies the procedure.

REFERENCES

[1] NEER CS II, BROWN TH J^r, MCLAUGHLIN HL Fracture of the Neck of the Humerus with Dislocation of the Head Fragment. *Am J Surg, 85: 252-8. 1953.*

[2] NEER CS II. Articular Replacement for the Humeral Head, *J. Bone Joint Surg Am, Apr 1955; 37: 215-228.*

[3] NEER CS II. Replacement Arthroplasty for Glenohumeral Osteoarthritis. *J. Bone and Joint Surg, 56-A: 1-13, Jan. 1974.*

[4] NEER CS, WATSON KC, STANTON FJ. Recent experience in total shoulder replacement. *J Bone Joint Surg Am 1982; 64: 319-37.*

[5] U.S. Department of Health and Human Services

[6] U.S. Department of Health and Human Services

[7] KURTZ S, ONG K, LAU E, MOWAT F, HALPERN M, Projections of Primary and Revision Hip and Knee Arthroplasty in the United States from 2005 to 2030, *J Bone Joint Surg Am, Apr 2007; 89: 780-85.*

[8] MATSEN FA III, BICKNELL RT, LIPPITT SB Shoulder arthroplasty: the socket perspective. *J Shoulder Elbow Surg, Sep 2007; 16(5 Suppl): S241-7.*

[9] BOHSALI KI, WIRTH MA, ROCKWOOD CA J^r. Complications of Total Shoulder Arthroplasty, *J. Bone Joint Surg Am, Oct 2006; 88: 2279-92.*

[10] DINES JS, FEALY S, STRAUSS E J, ALLEN A, CRAIG EV, WARREN RF, DINES DM Outcomes Analysis of Revision Total Shoulder Replacement, *J Bone Joint Surg Am, Jul 2006; 88: 1494-1500.*

[11] WIRTH MA, ROCKWOOD CA J^r Current concepts review. Complications of Total Shoulder-Replacement Arthroplasty, *J Bone Joint Surg Am, Apr 1996; 78: 603-16.*

[12] WIRTH MA, ROCKWOOD CA J^r Complications of shoulder arthroplasty. *Clin Orthop, 307: 47-69, 1994.*

[13] WIRTH MA, SELTZER DG, SENES HR, PANNONE A, LEE J, ROCKWOOD CA J^r An

analysis of failed humeral head and total shoulder arthroplasty. *Orthop Trans, 18: 977-978, 1994-5.*

[14] HASAN SS, LEITH JM, CAMPBELL B, KAPIL R, SMITH KL, MATSEN FA III, Characteristics of unsatisfactory shoulder arthroplasties. *J Shoulder Elbow Surg, 2002; 11(5): 431-41.*

[15] DEUTSCH A, ABBOUD JA, KELLY J, MODY M, NORRIS T, RAMSEY ML *et al.* Clinical results of revision shoulder arthroplasty for glenoid component loosening. *J Shoulder Elbow Surg 2007;16: 706-16.*

[16] PEARL ML, ROMEO A, WIRTH MA, YAMAGUCHI K, NICHOLSON GP, CREIGHTON RA, Decision making in contemporary shoulder arthroplasty. *Instr Course Lect, Jan 2005; 54: 69-85.*

[17] FRANTA K, LENTERS TR, MOUNCE D, NERADILEK B, MATSEN FA III, The complex characteristics of 282 unsatisfactory shoulder arthroplasties. *J Shoulder Elbow Surg, Sep 2007; 16(5): 555-62.*

[18] SPERLING JW, COfiELD RH. Revision total shoulder arthroplasty for treatment of glenoid arthrosis. *J Bone Joint Surg Am 1998; 80:860-7.*

[19] SPERLING JW, COfiELD RH, ROWLAND CM. Minimum fifteen-year follow-up of Neer hemiarthroplasty and total shoulder arthroplasty in patients aged fifty years or younger. *J Shoulder Elbow Surg 2004;13: 604-1325.*

[20] ANTUNA SA, SPERLING JW, COFIELD RH, AND ROWLAND CM, Glenoid revision surgery after total shoulder arthroplasty. *J Shoulder Elbow Surg, May 2001; 10(3): 217-24.*

[21] ROCKWOOD CA Jr, WIRTH MA. Observation on retrieved Hylamer glenoids in shoulder arthroplasty: Problems associated with sterilization by gamma irradiation in air. *J Shoulder Elbow Surg: March/April 2000,191-7.*

[22] WIRTH MA, AGRAWAL CM, MABREY JD, DEAN DD, BLANCHARD CR, MILLER MA, ROCKWOOD CA Jr Isolation and Characterization of Polyethylene Wear Debris Associated with Osteolysis Following Total Shoulder Arthroplasty. *J Bone Joint Surg Am. 1999; 81:29-37.*

[23] WILLIAMS GW, IANNOTTI JP Options for glenoid bone loss: composites of prosthetics and biologics. *J Shoulder Elbow Surg:6 (5S), 267S-272S.*

[24] DEUTSCH A, ABBOUD JA, KELLY J, MODY M, NORRIS T, RAMSEY ML *et al.* Clinical results of revision shoulder arthroplasty for glenoid component loosening. *J Shoulder Elbow Surg 2007;16: 706-16.*

[25] RM CARROLL, R IZQUIERDO, M VAZQUEZ, TA BLAINE, WN LEVINE, LU BIGLIANI Conversion of painful hemiarthroplasty to total shoulder arthroplasty: long-term results. *J Shoulder Elbow Surg, Nov 2004; 13(6): 599-603.*

[26] PHIPATANAKUL WP, NORRIS TR. Treatment of glenoid loosening and bone loss due to osteolysis with glenoid bone grafting. *J Shoulder Elbow Surg, 2006:15 (1) 84-7.*

[27] ANTUNA S, SPERLING JW, COfiELD RH. Reimplantation of a glenoid component after component removal and allograft bone grafting: a report of 3 cases. *J Shoulder Elbow Surg 2002;11: 637-41.*

[28] CHEUNG EV, SPERLING JW, COFIELD RH, Reimplantation of a Glenoid Component Following Component Removal and Allogenic Bone-Grafting. *J Bone Joint Surg Am, Aug 2007; 89: 1777-83.*

[29] NEYTON L, BOILEAU P, NOVE-JOSSERAND L, EDWARDS TB, WALCH G Glenoid bone grafting with a reverse design prosthesis. *J Shoulder Elbow Surg, May 2007; 16(3 Suppl): S71-8.*

[30] MATSEN, FA III, BOILEAU P, WALCH G, GERBER C, BICKNELL RT. The Reverse Total Shoulder Arthroplasty. *J Bone Joint Surg Am, Mar 2007; 89: 660-7.*

[31] HILL JM, NORRIS TR. Long-term results of total shoulder arthroplasty following bone-grafting of the glenoid. *J Bone Joint Surg Am 2001;83: 877-83.*

[32] COFIELD RH Bone grafting for glenoid bone deficiencies in shoulder arthritis: a review. *J Shoulder Elbow Surg, Sep 2007; 16(5 Suppl): S273-81.*

[33] NEYTON L, WALCH G, NOVE-JOSSERAND L, EDWARDS TB Glenoid corticocancellous bone grafting after glenoid component removal in the treatment of glenoid loosening. *J Shoulder Elbow Surg 2006;15(2): 173-9.*

[34] NEYTON L, WALCH G, NOVE-JOSSERAND L, EDWARDS TB Glenoid corticocancellous bone grafting after glenoid component removal in the treatment of glenoid loosening. *J Shoulder Elbow Surg 2006; 15(2):173-9.*

[35] GARTSMAN GM, RODDEY TS, HAMMERMAN SM. Shoulder arthroplasty with or without resurfacing of the glenoid in patients who have osteoarthritis. *J Bone Joint Surg Am 2000;82: 26-34.*

[36] NORRIS TR, KELLY JD, HUMPHREY CS. Management of Glenoid Bone Defects in Revision Shoulder Arthroplasty: A New Application of the Reverse Total Shoulder Prosthesis. *Techniques Shoulder Elbow Surgery. 2007. 8(1): 37-46.*

[37] NORRIS TR Reconstruction of Glenoid Bone Loss in Total Shoulder Arthroplasty. In Shoulder Concepts 2008-Arthroscopy and Arthroplasty. *Ed: Pascal Boileau, Sauramps Medical. ISBN: 978-2-84023-5729. 2008. 397-404.*

[38] NYFFELER RW, WERNER CM, GERBER C Biomechanical relevance of glenoid component positioning in the reverse Delta III total shoulder prosthesis. *J Shoulder Elbow Surg. 2005; 14(5) 524-8.*

[39] KELLY JD, HUMPHREY CS, NORRIS TR Optimizing glenosphere position and fixation in reverse shoulder arthroplasty. Part One. The twelve-mm rule. *JSES 2008, vol. 17(4) 589-94.*

[40] HUMPHREY CS, KELLY JD, NORRIS TR Optimizing glenosphere position and fixation in reverse shoulder arthroplasty, Part Two: The three-column concept. *JSES: 2008, 17(4), 595-601.*

GLENOID REMOVAL OR GLENOID BONE GRAFTING?

L. NEYTON, B. MELIS, N. BONNEVIALLE, P. BOILEAU

INTRODUCTION

While total shoulder arthroplasty has proven effective in pain relief and improvement of function, there are concerns regarding the occurrence of loosening of the glenoid component over the long term. When the glenoid component fails and loosens, small to large cavitary lesions are created in anatomically small bone volumes. When combined with defects of the thin cortical vault walls, implantation of a new glenoid component may not be possible. To date, defects are either neglected or managed with reconstruction techniques. Simple removal of the loose glenoid component has been proposed as a non reconstructive option. Bone grafting the glenoid defect without new glenoid component implantation combined with hemiarthroplasty is a reconstructive option.

The current retrospective study was designed to answer the hypothesis that patients who have undergone glenoid component removal, either isolated or associated to a bone graft, could get acceptable functional results at mid-term follow-up.

MATERIALS AND METHODS

Inclusion criteria were: revision total shoulder arthroplasty (TSA) because of aseptic glenoid loosening or glenoid component failure; glenoid component removal, either isolated or associated to a bone graft; a minimum of two years follow-up after revision; clinical and radiographical evaluation pre-operatively and at last follow-up. Clinical evaluation used the Constant-Murley score.

Preoperative, postoperative, and most recent radiographs of the shoulder were analyzed. These included an AP view and a lateral view. Periprosthetic glenoid lucency was recorded according to Molé [1]. Medial migration of the humeral head after glenoid component removal was recorded as moderate (<10 mm), or severe (≥ 10 mm). Inclusion with follow-up less than 2 years could be accepted in case of re-implantation. Glenoid loosening because of infection and revision glenoid component were excluded.

Between 1991 and 2007, 154 shoulders underwent revision shoulder arthroplasty for glenoid loosening or failure and were included in the retrospective, multicenter Glenoid Day database. Among these, 50 shoulders underwent glenoid removal. During surgery, 1 of 2 revision methods were used - either simple removal of the loose glenoid implant or removal of the implant with bone grafting. One patient was lost to follow-up. Thus, 49 shoulders in 49 patients were included in the present study.

Of the 49 procedures, 26 were performed in men and 23 in women. The mean age was 69.3 years (range, 42 to 91 years). Thirty-six procedures were on the dominant extremity. The primary diagnosis for the 49 shoulder arthroplasties was primary osteoarthritis in 24, rheumatoid arthritis in 6, fracture sequelae in 6, avascular osteonecrosis in 2, instability osteoarthrtis in 1. Of the primary arthroplasties, 10 primary diagnoses were not known.

The glenoid component for the primary arthroplasty were all-polyethylene cemented in 37, metal-back bone ingrowth in 12. All the all-polyethylene glenoid components were loose according to the Molé classification. Metal-back components revealed 6 loosenings and 6 failures because of dissociation of the polyethylene in 3 cases and polyethylene wear in 3. The mean time-interval from the primary TSA to revision was 5.7 years (range, 0.5 to 13 years). It was 3.6 years (range, 0.8 to 10 years) for Group I (simple glenoid removal group) and 6.2 years (range, 0.5 to 13 years) in Group II (glenoid removal and bone grafting group). The mean time from revision to most recent follow-up or before re-operation was 4.8 years (range, 1 to 10 years). It was 6.2 years (range, 3 to 14 years) for Group I and 4.4 years (range, 1 to 10 years) for Group II. There were 5 patients with less than 2 years follow-up as a result of re-revision during the follow-up period.

Glenoid bone loss was graded intraoperatively based on location as cavitary or combined defects. The glenoid component and surrounding bone cement (if present) were removed in all cases. Eleven shoulders had simple glenoid component removal (*Group I*). Removal of the loose glenoid component was performed under arthroscopic control in three cases and in open surgery in eight cases. Glenoid bone loss was graded as cavitary in 9 and combined in 2.

After component and cement removal, the defect was grafted with autologous bone from the ipsilateral iliac crest to the involved shoulder in 38 cases (*Group II*). The defect was grafted with morcellized cancellous bone chips in 7 cases. Glenoid bone loss was graded as cavitary in six cases. In one case, the defect was graded as combined because of anterior perforation, but the vault was considered to be continent enough to support filling with the graft. The defect was grafted with iliac crest tricortical autologous graft in 31 cases. Glenoid bone loss was graded as cavitary in 22 and combined in 9. The graft was impacted into the defect and was considered to have sufficient primary stability in 27 cases. The graft had to be fixed with screws in 4 cases.

Mean preoperative pain in Group I was 4.3 (range, 0 to 8), and that in Group II was 5.1 (range 0 to 15). The mean preoperative range of motion for group I was 59° (range, 20 to 90) for active elevation,

10° (range, -50° to 80) for external rotation and reached the buttock (range, thigh to T7) for internal rotation. The mean preoperative range of motion for group II was 98° (range, 30 to 180) for active elevation, 24° (range, -10 to 60) for external rotation and sacrum (range, thigh to T7) for internal rotation. The mean preoperative Constant and adjusted score in Group I were 15.4 (range, 5 to 26) and 19 (range, 7 to 37), respectively. The mean preoperative Constant and adjusted score in Group II were 37 (range, 11 to 84) and 46 (range, 15 to 103), respectively.

RESULTS

Complications and Re-operations

Thirteen complications (26.5%) and 10 (20%) re-operations were recorded. These events are summarized in Table I.

Group I Glenoid Removal (n=11)

In Group I, one shoulder had a reimplantation. This patient had painful severe glenoid wear and rotator cuff tear three years postoperatively and underwent reverse shoulder arthroplasty without glenoid bone grafting.

There was an overall improvement in pain rating from 4.3 to 8 (p=0.004) with simple glenoid removal. Active elevation improved from a mean of 59° to 93° (p=0.04) and external rotation from a mean of 10° to 12.5° (p=0.86). Internal rotation improved from buttock level to sacrum (p=0.18). Constant score and adjusted Constant score improved from a mean 15.4 to 37 (p=0.0012) and 19 to 51 (p=0.0002), respectively (Table II).

At most recent follow-up or before re-operation, the SSV was available for seven patients who rated their shoulder at

Table I. Complications and Re-operations

Complication		Treatment	
Infection P.Acnes	1	Resection Arthroplasty	1
Graft Migration	2	None	
Painful Glenoid Erosion	5	New Glenoid Implant	5
Painful Glenoid Erosion and RC Tear	3	Reverse Shoulder Arthroplasty	3
Contact Head/Screws	1	Screw Removal	1
Iliac Crest Fracture	1	None	
Total	13 (26.5%)		10 (20%)

Table II. Glenoid Removal Results

n=11	Pre revision	FU (75 months)	*p*
Age		63	69
Pain	4	8	0.004
Constant score	15	37	0.0012
Adj Constant score	19	51	0.0002
AAE	59	93	0.04
IR	BUTTOCK	SACRUM	NS
ER	10	12	NS

a mean 40% (range, 5 to 70%) of a normal shoulder. Six patients were satisfied or very satisfied with their result and five were disappointed or unhappy.

All eleven shoulders had complete sets of preoperative and postoperative radiographs. Postoperatively, medial shifting of the humeral head component into the glenoid after glenoid component removal was moderate in 6 (mean follow-up 73.6 months) and severe in 5 (mean follow-up 76.6 months). Periprosthetic humeral lucency was present in 1 shoulder (incomplete and <1 mm) and was asymptomatic.

Group II Glenoid removal and bone grafting (n=38)

Seven shoulders have had reimplantation because of continuing pain at a mean 21.5 months (range, 11 to 37); five had implantation of a new glenoid component and two were converted to a reverse shoulder arthroplasty.

At the most recent follow-up or before re-revision, the mean pain score improved from 5.1 to 8.6 ($p<0.0001$). Mean active elevation improved from a mean of 98° to 113.6° ($p=0.006$) and external rotation from a mean of 24° to 26° ($p=0.65$). Internal rotation did not change (sacrum). Constant score and adjusted Constant score improved from a mean 37 to 49.2 ($p=0.004$) and 46 to 64.7 ($p<0.0001$), respectively (Table III).

At most recent follow-up evaluation or before re-operation, the SSV was available for eleven patients who rated their shoulder at a mean 53% (range, 10 to 85%) of a normal shoulder. Nineteen patients were satisfied or very satisfied with their result and ten were disappointed or unhappy. The information was not available in 9 patients.

Thirty-eight shoulders had complete sets of preoperative and postoperative radiographs. Postoperatively, medial shifting of the humeral head component into the bone graft was moderate in 24 (mean follow-up 45 months) and severe in 14 (mean follow-up 61 months).

Group Comparisons

Glenoid Removal vs Glenoid Bone Grafting (Results are listed in Table IV)

There was a trend towards better pain, Constant and adjusted Constant score, active anterior elevation in the glenoid bone grafting group, but this difference was not statistically significant.

Table III. Glenoid removal and bone grafting results

n=38	Pre revision	FU (53 months)	*p*
Age	64	68	
Pain	5	8.6	<0.0001
Constant score	37	49	0.004
Adj Constant score	46	65	<0.0001
AAE	98	113	NS
IR	SACRUM	SACRUM	NS
ER	24	26	NS

Table IV. Glenoid Removal vs Glenoid Bone Grafting

	Removal n=11	Glenoid Bone Graft n=38	p
Pain	8	8.6	NS
Constant score	37	49	NS
Adjusted Constant score	51	65	NS
Active anterior elevation	93	113.6	NS
MM≥10 mm	6 (54.5%)	14 (37%)	–
SSV	40	53	–

The rate of severe medial migration of the humeral head into the glenoid was lower in the glenoid bone graft group.

Cancellous Bone Grafting vs Tricortical Bulk Grafting

Seven shoulders had cancellous bone grafting and 31 had tricortical bone grafting. With the numbers available, there was no statistically significant difference between the groups (Table V).

Medial Migration: Moderate vs Severe

Nineteen cases (38.8%) demonstrated severe medial migration into the glenoid at a mean follow-up of 63 months. Medial shifting of the humeral head component into the glenoid was severe in 5 cases out eleven cases in the removal group. Medial shifting of the humeral head component into the bone graft was severe in 3 cases out of seven with morcellized cancellous bone grafting compared to eleven cases out of 31 with bulk tricortical bone grafting.

Thirty cases (61.2%) demonstrated moderate medial migration: 6 in the removal group, 4 in the morcellized cancellous bone grafting group and 20 in the bulk tricortical bone grafting group.

There was a trend toward better pain, Constant and adjusted Constant score, active anterior elevation, but this difference was not statistically significant in the moderate medial migration group.

Table V. Cancellous Bone Grafting versus Tricortical Bulk Grafting

	Cancellous n=7	Tricortical n=31	p
Pain	8.4	8.6	NS
Constant score	50	49	NS
Adjusted Constant score	68	64	NS
Active anterior elevation	110	114	NS
MM≥10mm	3	11	–
SSV	43	59	–

Table IV: Medial Migration: Moderate vs Severe

	Moderate Medial Migration n=30	Severe Medial n=19	*p*
Pain	8.2	8.8	NS
Constant score	48.9	43.1	NS
Adjusted Constant score	63	59.6	NS
Active anterior elevation	111.6	104.7	NS

DISCUSSION

Isolated removal of the loose glenoid implant is a simple procedure avoiding the problem of reconstruction of glenoid bone stock. The removal of the loose glenoid implant is performed through a revision deltopectoral approach and through the rotator interval avoiding subscapularis re-violation. The procedure can also be performed arthroscopically [2]. This procedure provides acceptable results in regard to pain, but low mobility and function because medialization of the humeral head and wear of the remaining glenoid bone reduces the rotator cuff and deltoid moment arms [3, 4]. Absence of glenoid reconstruction precludes, *a priori*, further glenoid re-implantation. In the present study, re-implantation of a non-cemented metal-back glenoid component of a reverse shoulder arthroplasty was performed in one case despite severe medialization. At the time of this study, the follow-up following the re-implantation procedure was too short to allow clinical and radiographic evaluation. We have adopted a cautious approach to simple glenoid removal, reserving this for frail or non motivated patients, and perform it arthroscopically.

The goal of glenoid reconstruction is to provide a solid area and a fulcrum point for the prosthetic head. Therefore, an ideal reconstruction technique should offer sufficient primary resistance, healing to the native glenoid, avoid secondary subsidence, and resist humeral head medialization. Moreover, glenoid reconstruction should allow component reimplantation at the same time or in a staged procedure if needed. In the present study, among the seven shoulders with initial glenoid bone grafting that required re-revision, six shoulders had had glenoid reconstruction with bulk tricortical graft and did not require additional glenoid bone grafting by the time of re-revision. One shoulder had had cancellous bone grafting and required re-grafting at the time of re-revision because of insufficient bone stock.

Morcellized cancellous graft is used to fill central cavitary contained defects i.e glenoid vaults that are intact or near intact. Cheung and Cofield impacted morcellized cancellous allogenic bone grafts (CanPac, AlloSource) into the glenoid defect and noted subsequent mean medialization of the humeral head in relation to the glenoid of 7.5 mm [5]. Despite this medialization, second-stage glenoid component implantation was possible and the results of seven cases were evaluated at an average follow-up of seventy-nine months. Pain scores significantly improved, but range of motion did not, with an average anterior elevation of 88°. Similar subsidence was observed by Scalise and Iannotti with a mean 7 mm medialization [6]. In this study, we used autologous cancellous chips from the ipsilateral iliac crest to fill cavitary defects and found similar clinical and radiographic results. Based on our previous experience [7], our preferred technique for glenoid bone loss management is tricortical (iliac crest) structural reconstruction. We use a bulk autograft in central cavitary defects as well as in peripheral defects. In cases with intact glenoid vaults, the graft is contoured with a burr or a rongeur and impacted in the central defect. Additional cancellous bone chips harvested at the same time are used to complete the reconstruction. Impaction into a contained defect provides, as a general rule, sufficient primary stability to the graft. However, careful attention should be paid to the primary stability of the graft and additional fixation should be performed if the stability is not sufficient to avoid graft migration, as we observed in two cases in the present study.

In case of central and peripheral combined defects, the graft is secured to the remaining glenoid with screws. Use of metallic screw fixation risks contact with the humeral head resulting in metallosis and possible need for re-revision and screw removal. If deemed necessary, bioabsorbable screws should be used.

The purpose of this study is to report the outcomes of two treatment methods for managing symptomatic failed glenoid components. The present study has a number of shortcomings, as the sample size in the two treatment groups was small, the length of follow-up varied and the treatment selection was not randomized. There was little difference in the outcome between the 2 groups. The only difference was a better trend to resist medial migration in the glenoid bone grafting group. With the numbers available we could not detect any statistically significant difference between morcellized cancellous bone grafting and bulk tricortical bone grafting. However, there was a trend to better resistance to medial migration with bulk tricortical bone grafting. Additionally, there is a trend to better functional results when medial migration is moderate.

Isolated removal of a loose cemented glenoid component is a less invasive option that can be indicated in frail or non motivated patients. Bone grafting of glenoid deficiency is important to restore the joint-line for improvement of joint kinematics and to offer the possibility of later reimplantation if pain relief is not achieved. This proved to be necessary for 7 patients of the 38 so treated. As such, these results suggest acceptable functional results at mid-term follow-up with glenoid removal and a benefit of glenoid bone grafting compared to simple removal.

REFERENCES

[1] MOLÉ D, ROCHE O, RIAND N, LEVIGNE C, WALCH G. Cemented glenoid component: results in osteoarthritis and rheumatoid arthritis. In: Walch G, Boileau P (eds): Shoulder arthroplasty, *Springer Verlag, Berlin, 1999, 163-71.*

[2] O'DRISCOLL SW, PETRIE RS, TORCHIA ME. Arthroscopic removal of the glenoid component for failed total shoulder arthroplasty: a report of five cases. *J Bone Joint Surg Am 2005; 87: 858-63.*

[3] HAWKINS RJ, GREIS PE, BONUTTI PM. Treatment of symptomatic glenoid loosening following unconstrained shoulder arthroplasty. *Orthopedics. 1999; 22: 229-34.*

[4] NEYTON L, SIRVEAUX F, ROCHE O, MOLÉ D, BOILEAU P, WALCH G. Results of revision surgery for glenoid loosening: a multicenter series of 37 shoulder prosthesis. *Rev Chir Orthop Reparatrice Appar Mot. 2004;90: 111-21.*

[5] CHEUNG EV, SPERLING JW, COFIELD RH. Reimplantation of a glenoid component following component removal and allogenic bone-grafting. *J Bone Joint Surg Am 2007; 89: 1777-83.*

[6] SCALISE JJ, IANNOTTI JP. Bone grafting severe glenoid defects in revision shoulder arthroplasty. *Clin Orthop Relat Res. 2008; 466: 139-145.*

[7] NEYTON L, WALCH G, NOVÉ-JOSSERAND L, EDWARDS TB. Glenoid corticocancellous bone grafting after glenoid component removal in the treatment of glenoid loosening. *J Shoulder Elbow Surg. 2006;15: 173-9.*

ASEPTIC GLENOID LOOSENING OR FAILURE IN TOTAL SHOULDER ARTHROPLASTY: RESULTS OF REVISION WITH GLENOID REIMPLANTATION

N. BONNEVIALLE, B. MELIS, L. NEYTON, C. TROJANI, P. BOILEAU

ABSTRACT

Background

Re-implantation and cementation of a new all-polyethylene glenoid component in cases of symptomatic glenoid failure or loosening is a well established surgical strategy. However, the results of this intervention have not been clearly evaluated. Our purpose was to investigate whether such a procedure solves the problem of glenoid loosening and restores painless shoulder function.

Material and methods

Retrospective multicenter cohort study of 42 consecutive anatomical total shoulder arthroplasties (TSA) with symptomatic failed glenoid components revised by re-implantation of a new all PE, cemented glenoid component. Revision surgery was performed by a senior shoulder surgeon in all cases. The mean patient age was 60 years at the first TSA and 67 years at the time of revision. The indication for TSA was primary osteoarthritis in the majority of cases. All patients were reviewed clinically and radiologically; the mean follow-up following revision surgery was 74 months (24 to 138).

Results

The failed initial glenoid component was metal-backed in 32 cases and all-polyethylene cemented in 10 cases. The main cause of glenoid failure was component loosening in 19 patients (45%) and polyethylene wear or dissociation in 23 (54%). Associated rotator cuff complications were observed in 45% of cases (19/42) consisting of rotator cuff tears in 2 cases and subscapularis insufficiency in 17. The prosthesis was unstable in 19% of cases (8/42). At last follow-up, 7 patients (17%) had already been re-revised as a result of symptomatic recurrent glenoid implant loosening. Conversion to a hemiarthroplasty was performed in 3 cases, a reverse arthroplasty in 3 cases and one resection arthroplasty was performed for infection. The overall rate of recurrent glenoid loosening (re-revision + Molé score ≥12) was 67%. Soft tissue problems and prosthetic instability were significantly associated with recurrent loosening. Of the 10 associated bone grafts performed during the revision procedure, 4 were partially and 6 were totally lysed. For the 35 patients who still had their glenoid prostheses in place at last review, the mean Constant score was 57 points (+16 points); the mean active anterior elevation 125° (+19°) and the mean pain score 11 points (+5 points).

Conclusion

Revision of an anatomical TSA by re-implantation and cementation of a new all-polyethylene glenoid component does not solve the problem of glenoid loosening or failure; the functional benefit for the patient is modest. Soft tissue imbalance and instability are underestimated preoperatively and explain in part, the high rate of recurrent glenoid loosening. Patients with severe glenoid bone defects, soft tissue problems and/or prosthetic instability represent clear contraindications to re-implantation with an all PE cemented glenoid component.

INTRODUCTION

The number of Total Shoulder Arthroplasties (TSA) implanted for degenerative pathologies affecting the shoulder joint has increased dramatically during the last decades. The glenoid component remains the “weak link” in the survival of TSA [1, 10]. The main complication of cemented all-polyethylene glenoid components at long-term follow-up is aseptic loosening. The use of metal-back uncemented components has been associated with other modes of failure such as polyethylene liner wear and dissociation [3, 5, 8, 9, 13].

Glenoid component re-implantation is one potential therapeutic option that can be employed when revising TSA for symptomatic glenoid loosening or failure. Little is reported in the literature concerning the functional and radiological outcomes following this procedure. The outcome of revision shoulder arthroplasty seems to be poorer than that following a primary arthroplasty. It also appears to be associated with higher rates of failure of re-implanted glenoid components [2, 4, 6, 7, 12].

We hypothesized that, in cases of glenoid loosening or failure, revision of TSA by re-implantation of a new cemented glenoid component would be a reliable therapeutic option.

MATERIAL AND METHODS

Inclusion and exclusion criteria

A retrospective multicenter study was performed with the participation of 8 different centers specialising in shoulder surgery.

The inclusion criteria were: *1)* revision of a TSA performed between 1991 and 2006, *2)* for an aseptic glenoid failure, *3)* with glenoid reimplantation; and *4)* a minimum radiological and clinical follow-up of 2 years. Excluded were revisions using others therapeutic options such as *1)* glenoid removal without re-implantation, *2)* isolated glenoid bone grafting, *3)* reverse shoulder arthroplasty, or *4)* resection arthroplasty.

In a series of 137 TSA revised for an aseptic glenoid failure, 48 had glenoid components re-implanted. Three patients were lost to follow-up and 3 patients died before the minimum 2 year follow-up.

Thus, 42 arthroplasties (41 patients) were included in this study.

Patients

The procedure was performed in 15 men and 26 women with an average age of 60.5 years (35-77) at the time of primary TSA and 67 years (40-84) at revision surgery. The right shoulder was operated upon in 26 cases, the left in16 and the dominant side in 26 cases.

The indication for TSA was primary osteoarthritis in 33 cases, rheumatoid arthritis in four cases, post-instability arthropathy in three cases, sequela of fracture in one case and avascular necrosis in one case. Pre-operative CT-scans were available in 33 cases. The glenoid morphology according to the Walch classification was type A1 in 17 cases, type A2 in six cases, type B1 in four cases, and type B2 in six cases [14].

Surgical technique and implants

All procedures were performed by a senior surgeon specialising in shoulder surgery. The mean interval between primary TSA and revision was 64 months (4-131). Four patients were operated upon for glenoid loosening or failure before the end of the first post-operative year. In these four cases there was no objective evidence of occult deep prosthetic infection that may have contributed to such an early failure.

All revision prostheses were implanted via a delto-pectoral approach. The status of the rotator cuff tendons were verified and any partial or full-thickness lesions were systematically repaired following prosthetic implantation. The humeral stem was removed in 19 shoulders to assist in glenoid exposure. A humerotomy was required in 3 cases.

The glenoid component was removed and the presence and extent of glenoid bone loss was evaluated. A defect was present in 37 shoulders (86%): 25 were classified as central and 12 were combined (central and peripheral). The new glenoid component was all-polyethylene and cemented in all cases. The backside geometry was flat in 26 shoulders and convex in 16.

In 10 cases, a supplemental bone grafting procedure was performed in order to improve component stability and fill encountered osseous defects (25%). Seven structural iliac crest bone grafts (three for central and four for peripheral defects), two allografts (one for a central and one for a peripheral defect) and one cancellous impacted graft (central defect) were utilised. Revision was carried out as a one-stage procedure in all cases except for one where there was a delay of six months between grafting and glenoid reimplantation. In five cases, the graft was stabilized with screws and in the remainder impaction was sufficient to achieve primary graft stability.

Clinical and radiological evaluation

All patients were reviewed clinically and radiologically with a mean follow-up of 74 months (24-138).

The pre- and post-operative clinical evaluation consisted of measurement of active shoulder mobility and the Constant score, which was then adjusted for age and gender. At last follow-up, subjective satisfaction was assessed by asking the patients if they were very satisfied, satisfied, disappointed or unhappy with the outcome following the intervention.

Subscapularis function was specifically evaluated as part of the pre- and post-operative clinical examination using the lift-off test, belly press test and observing for increased external rotation with the arm by the side. The degree of subscapularis muscle fatty infiltration was assessed on the pre-operative CT-scans, when available.

The radiographic analysis consisted of antero-posterior views in neutral rotation and an axillary view. Glenoid periprosthetic radiolucencies were scored according to the classification of Molé [11]. Clear migration of the component or a score above 12 points was considered indicative of glenoid loosening. Loosening was not registered as a complication unless its presence had resulted in a revision procedure being performed.

Statistical methods

Descriptive statistics of the clinical data were performed. For quantitative variables, the t-test and Mann-Whitney test were used to determine significance. For qualitative variables, a $\chi 2$ test or Fisher's exact test was used. The significance level was set at 0.05. Statistical analysis was performed using Medical 8.0 software.

RESULTS

Causes of revision of primary TSA

The revised glenoid component was metal-backed (MB) in 32 cases, all-polyethylene cemented (PE) flat in 8 and convex in 2. Nineteen (45%) glenoid failures were due to component loosening and 23 (54%) occurred as a result of polyethylene wear or dissociation, principally from a metal back baseplate.

In addition to glenoid loosening or failure of the primary TSA, additional complications were frequently observed. Rotator cuff problems consisted of two postero-superior rotator cuff tears (one infra-spinatus and one supra-spinatus) and 17 (40%) cases of subscapularis insufficiency (proven clinically and/or on CT-scan in six cases and detected intraoperatively in eleven cases). In eight (19%) cases, there was evidence of prosthetic instability. This occurred in an anterior direction in three cases. Posterior humeral prosthetic subluxation was identified in five cases.

Post-revision complications

The overall complication rate was 45% (19/42). Complications were classified as either affecting the implant or the periarticular soft tissues. When both occurred in combination, the complication related to the implant was presented. The complication data is summarized in Table I.

Nine shoulders (21%) underwent further surgical treatment. In seven cases (17%), a revision of the glenoid implant was necessary because of poor post-operative clinical outcomes, which were unacceptable to the patient. Conversion to a RSA was performed in three cases; to a hemiarthroplasty in three cases and one resection arthroplasty was performed deep infection. The remaining two cases consisted of an open arthrolysis and an arthroscopic debridement of intra-articular cement loose bodies.

Table I: Postoperative complications and reoperations. (Cs, total Constant score; Fu, follow-up; pts, points).

Complications n=19 (45%)	Reoperations n=9 (21%)	Comments
Implant		
Glenoid loosening n=7	Conversion in RSA (n=3)	Cs 30 pts at Fu
	Conversion in HA (n=3)	Cs 23 pts at Fu
	Resection arthroplasty	Late deep infection
Soft tissue disorders		
Stiffness n=1	Open arthrolysis	History of instability arthropathy for index TSA. Cs 55 pts at Fu
Subscapularis tear (anterior subluxations) n=3	None	Cs 48 pts at Fu
Infraspinatus tear (upward migration) n=5	None	Upward migration of the prosthesis. No revision because a low functional demand (Cs 23 pts at Fu)
Posterior subluxation n=2	None	Cs 34 pts at Fu
Loose bodies n=1	Arthroscopic debridment	Loose bodies of cement with a glenoid component still in place.

Functional results

The functional results were evaluated in the 35 shoulders with the glenoid implant still in place and are summarized Table II. The mean follow-up post revision surgery was 74 months (24-138).

All domains of the Constant score and all ranges of shoulder mobility increased at follow-up. However, significant improvements were only achieved for the pain and activity domains, absolute Constant score, adjusted Constant score and the active anterior elevation.

In terms of the subjective evaluation, the outcome was considered to be very satisfactory in 18 cases and satisfactory in 10. Nine patients were disappointed and four were unhappy with the result. Of those patients with glenoid loosening at last follow-up, 12 (43%) remained satisfied or very satisfied with the outcome following surgery.

Table II: Functional results according to the Constant score and active mobility.

	Preoperative	Review	Gain	P-value
Constant score				
Pain (/15 points)	**6.2**±3 [0 ;15]	**11.2**±3.6 [3 ;15]	**5**±4 [-4 ;11]	<0.0001 *(t-test)*
Activity (/20 points)	**9.3**±4,6 [0 ;20]	**14.4**±5 [4 ;20]	**5.1**±6.5 [-6 ;20]	<0.0001 *(t-test)*
Mobility (/40 points)	**21.9**±11 [4 ;40]	**25.7**±10.7 [0 ;38]	**3.8**±12.3 [-22 ;34]	0.2 *(t-test)*
Strength (/25 points)	**3.8**±3.7 [11 ;83]	**5**±3.2 [0 ;15]	**1.3**±4.5 [-8 ;10]	0.0056 *(Mann-Whitney test)*
Absolute Constant score (/100 points)	**41.3**±19.9 [0 ;16]	**56.7**±19.09 [18 ;85]	**15.4**±22.7 [-32 ;67]	0.0003 *(t-test)*
Adjusted Constant score (%)	**54.2**±25.4 [14 ;119]	**79.3**±29.7 [26 ;127]	**23.7**±33.5 [-47 ;107]	<0.001 *(t-test)*
Active Mobility				
Anterior Elevation (degrees)	**106.1**±41 [30 ;180]	**125.4**±35.9 [60;180]	**19.3**±42.8 [-90 ;140]	0.04 *(t-test)*
External Rotation at side (degrees)	**28.7**±21.3 [0 ;80]	**29.7**±19.6 [-20 ;60]	**1**±22.1 [-50 ;50]	0.8 *(t-test)*
Internal Rotation (points)	**4.7**±2.9 [0;10]	**5.2**±2.4 [0 ;10]	**0.5**±2.6 [-6 ;8]	0.43 *(t-test)*

Overall radiological results

The radiological results were analysed in the cases where the glenoid component had been retained at last follow up. A radiolucent line around the glenoid implant was identified in 34 (97%) shoulders. The Molé score was higher or equal to 12 points in 21 (50%) cases. As previously reported, seven (17%) TSAs required further revision for poor clinical outcome. Thus, the overall rate of glenoid loosening was 67% (28/42) for the entire series at last follow-up (Fig. 1).

No humeral stem met the radiographic criteria for being loose although proximal radiolucent lines were observed in 19 cases (50%) at last follow-up.

Bone Graft Evolution

Specifically analysing the 10 cases in whom glenoid reimplantation had been performed in combination with a glenoid bone graft, there were no instances where the bone graft could be considered as well healed. Partial resorption had occurred in six cases while in four cases the bone grafts has resorbed completely. At last follow-up, the glenoid component was loose in six cases (60%) and further surgery had been performed in three cases as previously reported: Two patients with symptomatic glenoid loosening were revised to a reverse prosthesis (fig. 2). One patient developed a late deep infection necessitating resection arthroplasty with insertion of an antibiotic impregnated cement spacer.

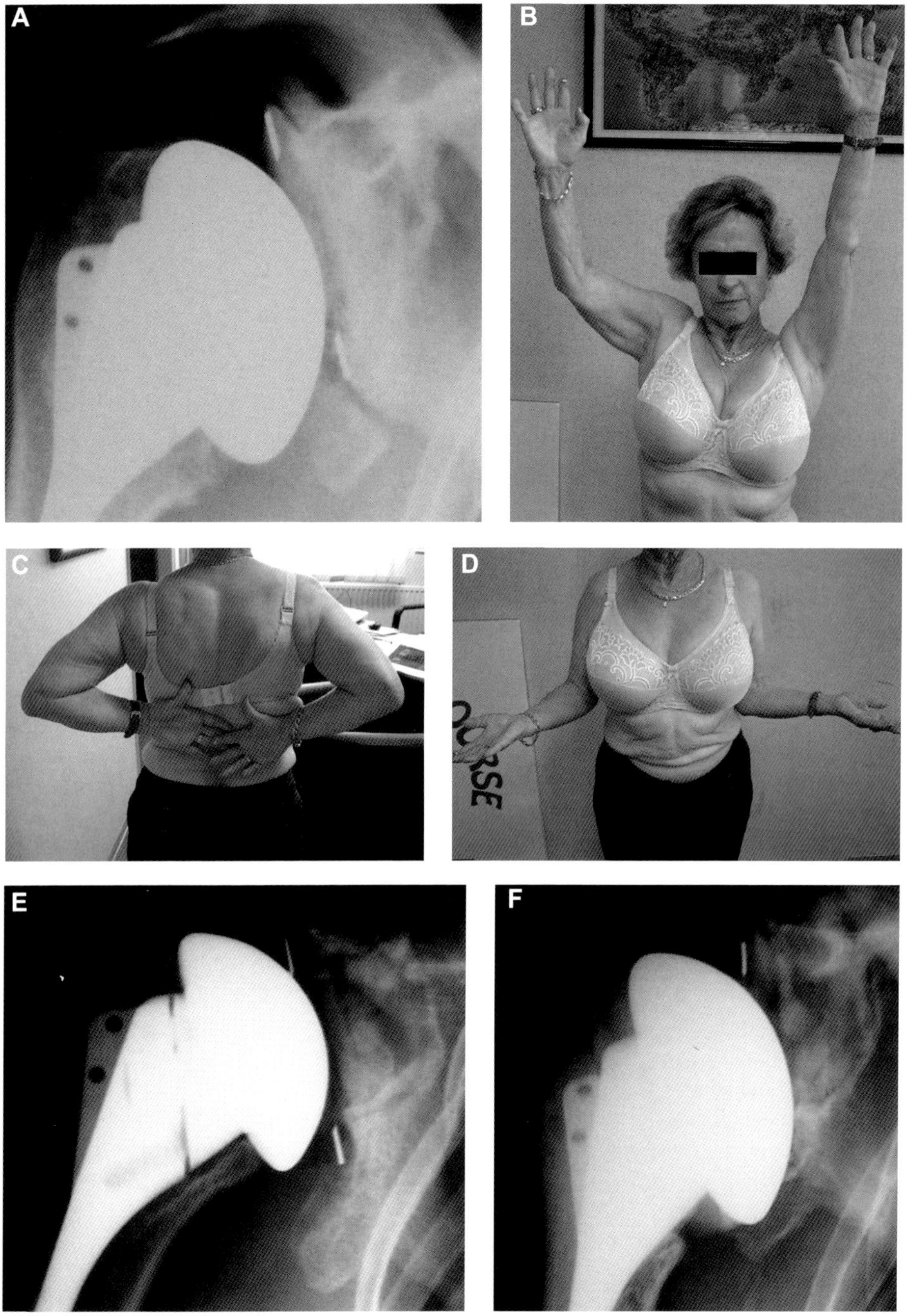

Fig. 1: A 76 years old woman, in whom a TSA was revised for glenoid loosening 12 years ago (A). At the follow-up, the Constant score is 77 points without pain: score of 15/15 (B,C,D). On plain radiograph, the glenoid component was clearly loose as soon as 4 years of follow-up (E) but did not require a new revision surgery. At the last follow-up, osteolysis increased, the prosthesis is anterior subluxated and the glenoid component migrated (F).

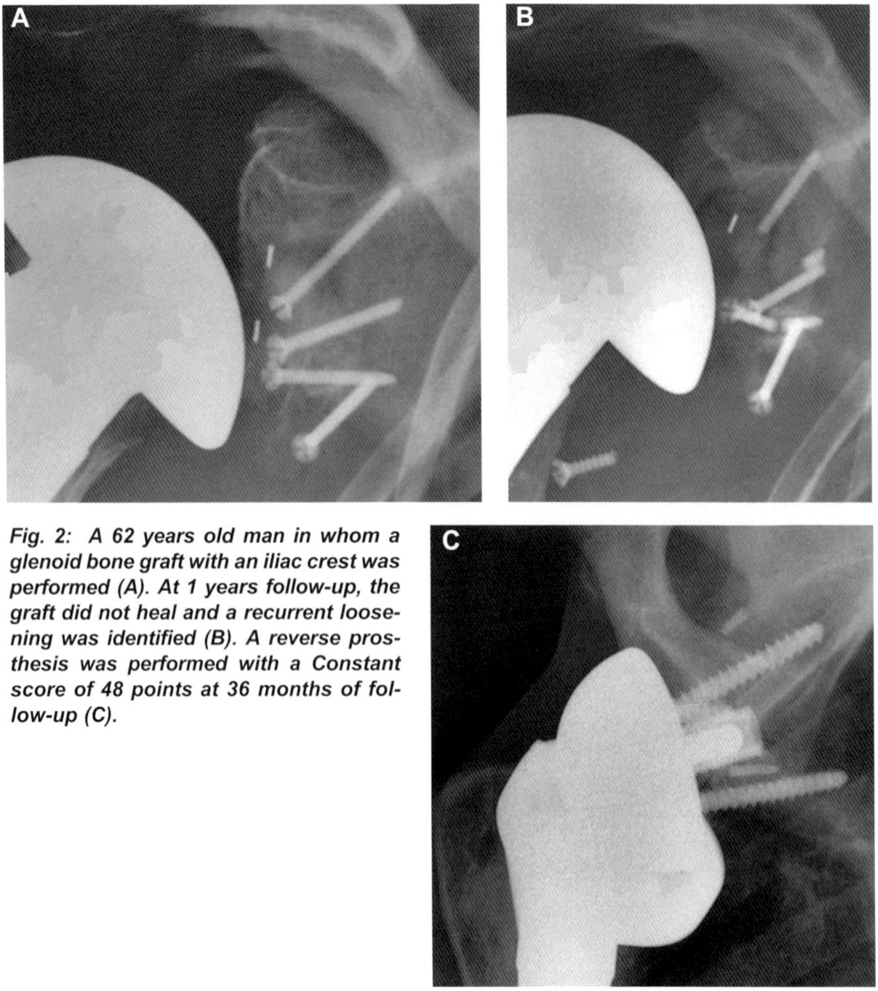

Fig. 2: A 62 years old man in whom a glenoid bone graft with an iliac crest was performed (A). At 1 years follow-up, the graft did not heal and a recurrent loosening was identified (B). A reverse prosthesis was performed with a Constant score of 48 points at 36 months of follow-up (C).

Correlations between glenoid loosening and functional results at follow-up

Clinically, glenoid loosening was responsible for a significant decrease in the pain score (mean reduction 3.3 points). However, there was no statistically significant difference in the absolute Constant score. (52 vs 63 points) (Table III).

Correlations between glenoid loosening and soft tissue problems at follow-up

Soft tissue problems (rotator cuff tear, prosthesis instability) were recorded in two different groups: group I (n=28) with glenoid loosening (revised or with a Molé score $\geq$12) and group II (n=14) without glenoid loosening. Soft tissue problems

Table III: Correlations between radiological glenoid loosening and the Constant score. (n=35, FU=74 months).

	n=35		
	Radiological glenoid loosening	Absence of radiological loosening	P value
Pain (points)	**10**±3.8 [3;15]	**13.3**±1.9 [10 ;15]	0.007 *(t-test)*
Mobility (points)	**22.4**±12.1 [0 ;38]	**26.6**±11.2 [0 ;38]	0.28 *(t-test)*
Activity (points)	**13.2**±5.3 [4 ;20]	**15.6**±4.2 [8;20]	0.16 *(t-test)*
Strength (points)	**4.4**±3.8 [0 ;15]	**6**±1.5 [4 ;8]	0.14 *(t-test)*
Cs score (points)	**52.1**±21.7 [18;85]	**63.7**±14.3 [41 ;81]	0.09 *(t-test)*
Adjusted Cs score (%)	**72.4**±29.8 [26 ;123]	**89.6**±25.6 [53;127]	0.08 *(t-test)*

were significantly more frequently observed in group I (57%) than in group II (14%) (p=0.02).

Others correlations

No correlation were found between glenoid loosening and age, gender, arm dominance, native glenoid morphology (Walch classification), or type of implant.

DISCUSSION

The optimal management of the loose or failed glenoid component in TSA remains unclear. Our study does not confirm our hypothesis as revision of an anatomical TSA by reimplantation of a new glenoid component does not solve the problem of glenoid loosening or failure. In the present series, the overall rate of recurrent glenoid loosening or failure after reimplantation of a new glenoid implant was 67% (28/42) at a mean follow-up of 74 months. A radiolucent line was present in 97% of cases (34/35) and seven patients (17%) had to be re-revised for recurrent glenoid loosening or failure. Glenoid bone defects were present in 37 (86%) shoulders in our series. In 10 cases, glenoid bone grafting was performed in combination with glenoid reimplantation, mainly using iliac crest graft performed synchronously. The results of bone grafting were unsatisfactory as a high rate of graft lysis was encountered and recurrent glenoid loosening occurred in six (60%) cases.

Recurrent glenoid loosening or failure after reimplantation of a new glenoid component is multifactorial. Associated complications (such as rotator cuff insufficiency or prosthetic instability) are frequently underestimated and therefore, not treated (or poorly treated) at the time of revision surgery. In our study, we found that soft tissue failures were often evident pre-operatively: 40% of cases of subscapularis insufficiency and 19% of antero-posterior prosthetic subluxations were diagnosed before revision surgery.

Postoperatively, there was a significant correlation between glenoid loosening and the presence of soft tissue disorders. Even if the clinical diagnosis is difficult to formulate in patients with painful shoulders, every effort should be made to identify soft tissue imbalance as it clearly compromises re-implantation of a new glenoid component. We concur with Deutsch *et al.* [6], who compared clinical outcomes of revision TSA in groups with and without preoperative prosthetic antero-posterior instability, that soft tissue instability is predictive of post-operative outcome.

In our study, 21% of already revised patients required further surgery, mainly for recurrent glenoid failure. This is comparable to the figures of between 10 and 80% reported elsewhere in the literature. [2, 4, 5, 6, 7, 12]. However, the rate remains low in comparison to the rate of radiological loosening identified (67%). One potential explanation for this is that as the age of the patient increases with follow-up, the functional demands decrease correspondingly.

The main weakness of our study is that it is a multicenter study, incorporating the results of many different surgeons. Although a mean follow-up of 74 months may not be sufficient to fully evaluate prosthetic outcome, our series represents the longest follow-up reported in the literature to date, as well as the largest series of cases.

CONCLUSION

Revision of an anatomical TSA by re-implantation of a cemented all-polyethylene glenoid component does not solve the problem of glenoid loosening or failure; the functional benefit for the patient is modest. Soft tissue imbalance and instability are preoperatively underestimated and partly explain the high rates of recurrent glenoid loosening. Patients with severe glenoid bone defects, soft tissue problems and/or prosthetic instability are clear contraindications to re-implantation of an all PE cemented glenoid implant.

REFERENCES

[1] ADAMS JE, SPERLING JW, HOSKIN TL, MELTON LJ 3rd, COFIELD RH. Shoulder arthroplasty in Olmsted County, Minnesota, 1976-2000: a population-based study. *J Shoulder Elbow Surg. 2006;15: 50-5.*

[2] ANTUNA SA, SPERLING JW, COFIELD RH, ROWLAND CM. Glenoid revision surgery after total shoulder arthroplasty. *J Shoulder Elbow Surg. 2001 May-Jun; 10(3): 217-24.*

[3] BOILEAU P, AVIDOR C, KRISHNAN SG, *et al.* Cemented polyethylene versus uncemented metal-backed glenoid components in total shoulder arthroplasty: a prospective, double-blind, randomized study. *J Shoulder Elbow Surg 2002; 11: 351-9.*

[4] CHEUNG EV, SPERLING JW, COFIELD RH. Revision shoulder arthroplasty for glenoid component loosening. *J Shoulder Elbow Surg. 2008 May-Jun; 17(3): 371-5.*

[5] COFIELD RH. Uncemented total shoulder arthroplasty: a review. *Clin Orthop 1994; 304:86-93.*

[6] DEUTSCH A, ABBOUD JA, KELLY J, MODY M, NORRIS T, RAMSEY ML, IANNOTTI JP, WILLIAMS GR. Clinical results of revision shoulder arthroplasty for glenoid component loosening. *J Shoulder Elbow Surg. 2007 Nov-Dec;16(6): 706-16.*

[7] DINES JS, FEALY S, STRAUSS EJ, ALLEN A, CRAIG EV, WARREN RF, DINES DM. Outcomes analysis of revision total shoulder replacement. *J Bone Joint Surg Am. 2006 Jul; 88(7): 1494-500.*

[8] FOX TJ, CIL A, SPERLING JW, SANCHEZ-SOTELO J, SCHLECK CD, COFIELD RH. Survival of the glenoid component in shoulder arthroplasty. *J Shoulder Elbow Surg 2009;17: 859-63.*

[9] KASTEN P, PAPE G, RAISS P, BRUCKNER T, RICKERT M, ZEIFANG F, LOEW M. Mid-term survivorship analysis of a shoulder replacement with a keeled glenoid and a modern cementing technique. *J Bone Joint Surg Br. 2010 Mar; 92(3): 387-92.*

[10] KOZAK LJ, DEFRANCES CJ, HALL MJ. National Hospital Discharge Survey: 2004 annual summary with detailed diagnosis and procedure data. National Center for Health Statistics. *Vital Health Stat 13(162). 2006.*

[11] MOLE D, ROCHE O, RIAND N. Cemented glenoid component. In:Walch G, Boileau P, Molé D, eds. *Shoulder arthroplasty. Berlin: Springer; 1999.P. 163-71.*

[12] SAJADI KR, KWON YW, ZUCKERMAN JD. Revision shoulder arthroplasty: an analysis of indications and outcomes. *J Shoulder Elbow Surg. 2010 Mar; 19(2): 308-13.*

[13] TAUNTON MJ, MCINTOSH AL, SPERLING JW, COFIELD RH. Total shoulder arthroplasty with a metal-backed, bone-ingrowth glenoid component. Medium to long-term results. *J Bone Joint Surg Am. 2008 Oct; 90(10): 2180-8.*

[14] WALCH G, BADET R, BOULAHIA A, KHOURY A. Morphologic study of the glenoid in primary glenohumeral osteoarthritis. *J Arthroplasty 1999 Sep; 14(6): 756-60.*

ASEPTIC GLENOID LOOSENING OR FAILURE IN TOTAL SHOULDER ARTHROPLASTY:
RESULTS OF REVISION WITH REVERSE SHOULDER ARTHROPLASTY

B. MELIS, N. BONNEVIALLE, L. NEYTON, G. WALCH, P. BOILEAU

Background

Glenoid failure or loosening in total shoulder arthroplasty (TSA) is often associated with other major complications such as glenohumeral instability and rotator cuff tears. Revision surgery is frequently complicated by deficient glenoid bone stock and the multi-factorial aetiology of glenoid component failure. Reverse shoulder arthroplasty has been proposed as a potential surgical strategy in the management of such cases. Our purpose was to evaluate if the reverse shoulder arthroplasty (RSA) is a reliable therapeutic option in cases of glenoid failure or loosening associated with bone loss and/or cuff tear or instability.

Material and methods

Retrospective multicenter cohort study of 37 consecutive anatomical TSA with symptomatic failed glenoid components revised by RSA. Revision surgery was performed by a senior shoulder surgeon in all cases. The mean patient age was 64 years at the first TSA and 71 years at the time of revision. The indication for TSA was primary osteoarthritis in the majority of cases. All patients were reviewed clinically and radiologically. The mean follow-up after revision surgery was 46.6 months (24 to 104).

Results

The initial failed glenoid component was metal-backed in 19 cases and cemented all-polyethylene in 18. The main cause of glenoid failure was component loosening in 25 patients (67%) and polyethylene wear or dissociation in 12 (33%). Associated rotator cuff tears occurred in 24 cases (65%); subscapularis insufficiency was present in 29 cases (78%) and prosthetic instability was present in 13 cases (35%). Glenoid bone loss was observed in all cases. At the last follow-up, 8 patients (22%) had already been re-revised because of symptomatic recurrent glenoid implant loosening (3), prosthetic anterior instability (3) or humeral subsidence (2). The RSA had been converted to a hemiarthroplasty (HA) in 1 case and a resection arthroplasty was performed in one other. Of the 29 (78%) associated bone grafts performed, 6 (21%) were partially and 1 (3%) was completely lysed. Of the 35 patients with their RSA still in place at last review, the mean Constant score was 55.2 points (+31 points), the mean anterior active elevation 121° (+53°) and the mean pain score 11.5 points (+7.5 points)

Conclusion

RSA solves the issues of glenoid loosening or failure and of bone graft incorporation. Significant improvements in functional results were observed. However, TSA revision with RSA is risky surgery and is associated with both significant complication rates and probability of re-revision. Extreme care must be taken to prevent complications and to ensure proper initial positioning of the implant.

INTRODUCTION

Loosening is the most common reason for revision of uncontrained total shoulder arthroplasties (TSA). Loosening rates have been reported at between 0 and 20% at medium term follow-up [2, 4, 6, 11, 12]. At long-term follow up, loosening rates of 50% and a 5% rate of revision surgery have been described [19, 21]. Several factors such as cuff tears, component malpositioning, tuberosity malunion and glenohumeral instability can contribute to glenoid component failure. A minority of revisions are performed for glenoid loosening in isolation [7]. The multifactorial nature of the associated problems encountered in glenoid component failure further complicate revision TSA, already itself a technically demanding procedure. Several studies have reported greater symptomatic and functional improvement in patients with glenoid component reimplantation compared to those treated with removal and bone grafting [1, 5, 8]. The feasibility of glenoid resurfacing depends largely on the status of glenoid bone stock. Persistent glenohumeral instability, rotator cuff tears and malunion of the greater tuberosity are all risk factors for poor outcome following glenoid revision with an anatomical TSA [8]. RSA has been suggested as a viable surgical option to treat glenoid loosening associated with these major complications [14, 15, 17]. The purpose of this study was to evaluate the results of RSA for the treatment of glenoid failure or loosening. We hypothesised that, in the case of glenoid failure or loosening associated with bone loss and/or cuff tear or instability, revision by RSA would be a reliable therapeutic option.

MATERIAL AND METHODS

Inclusion and exclusion criteria

A retrospective multicenter cohort study was carried out. The inclusion criteria were TSA revised by RSA for aseptic glenoid loosening or failure with a minimum clinical and radiological follow-up of 2 years. The exclusion criteria were other therapeutic options such as glenoid removal (isolated or associated with glenoid bone grafting), glenoid reimplantation and resection arthroplasty.

Between 1991 and 2006, in 7 centers specialising in shoulder surgery, 40 TSA were revised using RSA for aseptic glenoid loosening or failure. One patient was lost to follow-up and two patients died during the minimum 2 years follow-up period that represents the basis of this study. Thus, the study group included 37 revisions performed in 37 patients. Of the 37 procedures, 16 were performed in men (43%) and 21 in women (57%). The dominant side was involved in 26 cases (70%). The mean age at index TSA was 64.4 years (range, 44 to 79) and 71.0 years (range, 52 to 82) at revision. The indication for TSA was primary osteoarthritis in 22 cases (59%), post-instability osteoarthritis in 3 (8%), sequela of fracture in 3 (8%), rheumatoid arthritis in 2 (5%) and miscellaneous in 7 cases (20%). In 22 cases (59%) the primary TSA had been implanted in other institutions. The mean interval between primary TSA and revision was 75.3 months (range, 0.1 to 168). The mean interval between revision and most recent follow up was 46.6 months (range, 24 to 104).

Clinical evaluation

Demographic data, dates and details of procedures performed, preoperative and postoperative history, physical examination, radiographic findings and complications were recorded for each patient on a standard shoulder form. Constant scores and subjective results were calculated. The results were evaluated as excellent for adjusted Constant scores ≥100%, good if between 85% and 99%, fair if between 65% and 84% and poor if <65%. Active forward elevation and external rotation were recorded in degrees; internal rotation as the highest posterior spinal vertebra reached by the thumb. Eight patients, unable to return for follow-up visit, answered a validated shoulder questionnaire, which record pain, function, activities of daily living, range of motion and satisfaction.

Radiological evaluation

A radiographic analysis was performed for each patient. For each failed TSA, the presence of anterior or posterior instability, superior humeral head migration, humeral component subsidence, humeral radiolucent lines (RLL) according to Cofield's classification [20], glenoid loosening according to Molé's [13] classification, glenoid component migration, glenoid polyethylene wear or dissociation and glenoid bone loss were analyzed. Glenoid bone defects were classified as cavitary or combined as recorded on the operation note. Rotator cuff tears were analyzed in pre-revision CT scans or MRI's and confirmed intra-operatively. Anterior or posterior subluxation of the prosthesis, humeral subsidence, humeral RLL according to Gruen's [10] classification, scapular notch according to Sirveaux's [18] classification, glenoid bone spurs, RLL around screws and the central peg, glenoid component loosening and healing of glenoid bone grafts were analyzed for the RSAs at latest follow-up.

Surgical technique

Revision was performed through a deltopectoral approach in 35 cases (95%) and through a supero-lateral approach in 2 cases (5%). The humeral stem was removed in 34 cases (92%). Humerotomy was performed before stem removal in 5 cases (13.5%). A humeral fracture occurred in 4 cases (11%) (diaphyseal in 3 cases and of the greater tuberosity in 1 case) during humeral stem extraction, each requiring fixation. One of these patients underwent subsequent hardware removal. In 2 cases (5%) a cortical breach occurred during humeral preparation or stem implantation.

In 3 cases (8%), the stem was retained and an adaptator was applied (Fig. 1). An Aequalis (Tornier) reverse prosthesis was implanted in 25 cases (67%) and a Delta reverse (Depuy) in 12 (33%). The stem was cemented in 33 cases (89%). A metallic spacer was added in 2 cases (5%). Bone grafting was performed in 29 cases (78%) consisting of a structural iliac crest bone graft in 21 cases, autologous cancellous bone graft in 5 and allograft in 3 cases. A long peg glenoid was used in 8 cases (22%). The diameter of the glenosphere was 36 mm in 35 cases (95%) and 42 mm in 2 cases (5%). The revision was performed as a two-stage procedure in 3 cases (8%). Before the long peg glenoid component became available, the choice to perform a staged procedure was at the discretion of the surgeon depending on the degree of bone loss encountered. In the first stage a short peg glenoid with bone graft was implanted without inserting a humeral component in order to avoid early shearing forces on the bone graft. The second stage of humeral component implantation was performed six months later (Fig. 2).

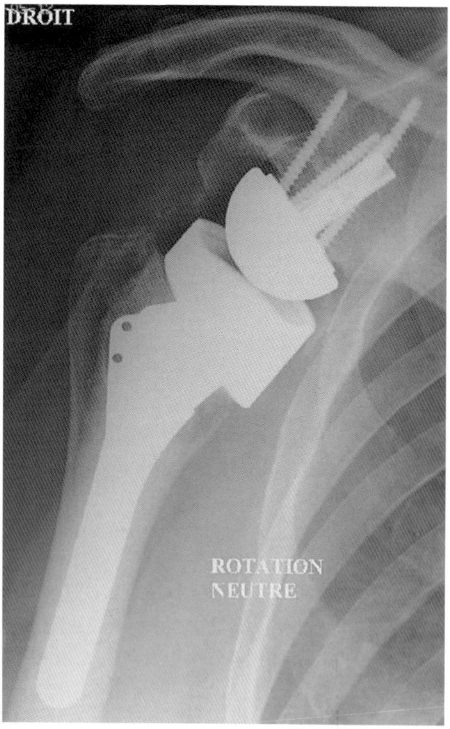

Fig. 1. Adaptator used to avoid humeral stem removal.

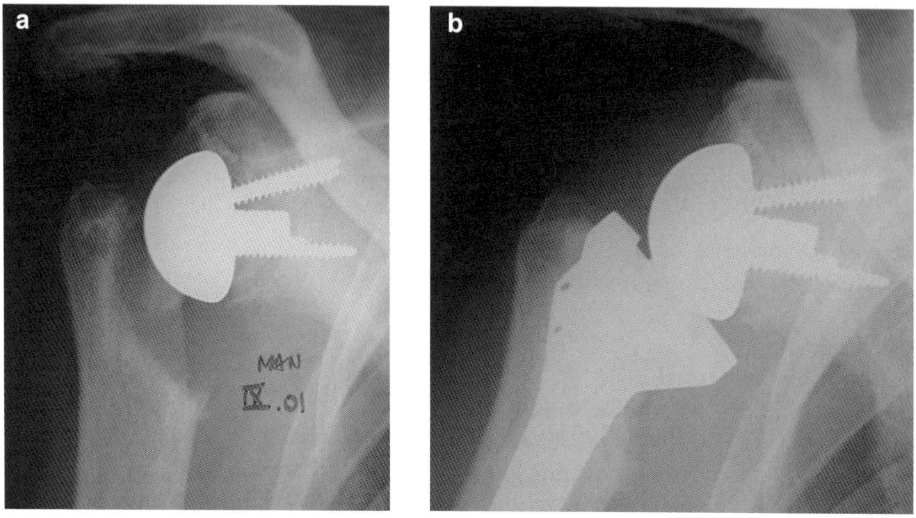

Fig. 2. Glenoid revision in a two stage procedure. First stage procedure (a): glenoid and bone graft implantation; Second stage procedure (b): humeral implantation 6 months after.

Statistical methods

Descriptive statistics of the clinical data were performed. For quantitative variables, the *t*-test and Mann-Whitney test were used to determine significance. For qualitative variables, a $\chi 2$ test or Fisher's exact test was used. The significance level was set at 0.05. Statistical analysis was performed using Medical 8.0 software.

RESULTS

Patients/Causes of revision

The TSA glenoid component was all-polyethylene cemented in 18 (4 flat, 14 convex) (49%) and metal-backed in 19 cases (51%). The humeral component was cemented in 28 cases (76%) and press-fit in 9 (24%). The cause of the revision was glenoid loosening (Molé score ≥12 and ≥10 respectively for polyethylene and metal back components) in 25 cases (67%) (Fig. 3 and 4) and polyethylene wear or dissociation in 12 (33%) (Fig. 5). Glenoid loosening occurred early (<2 years) in 5 cases (20%) and late (>2 years) in 20 cases (80%). Of the 25 loose glenoid components, implant migration was observed in 12 cases (48%) (medialized 4, inferior tilt 3, superior tilt 1, anterior tilt 1, associated 2, dislocated 1). The additional complications that

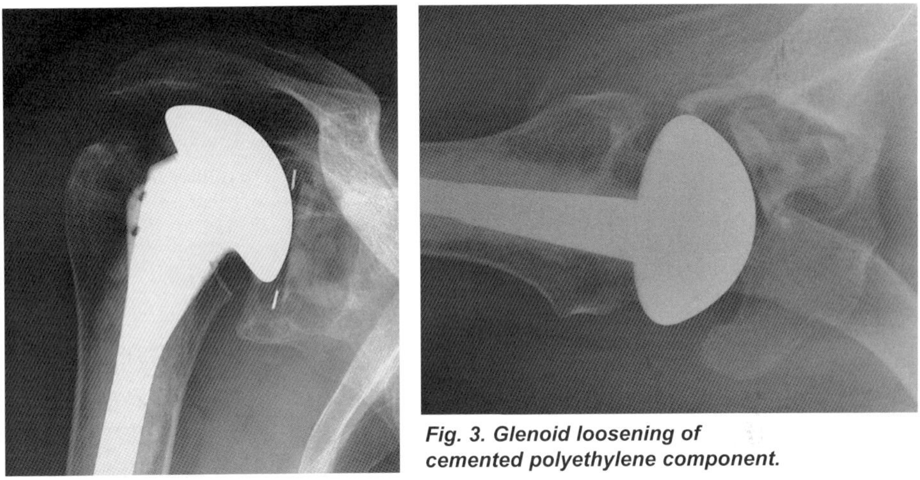

Fig. 3. Glenoid loosening of cemented polyethylene component.

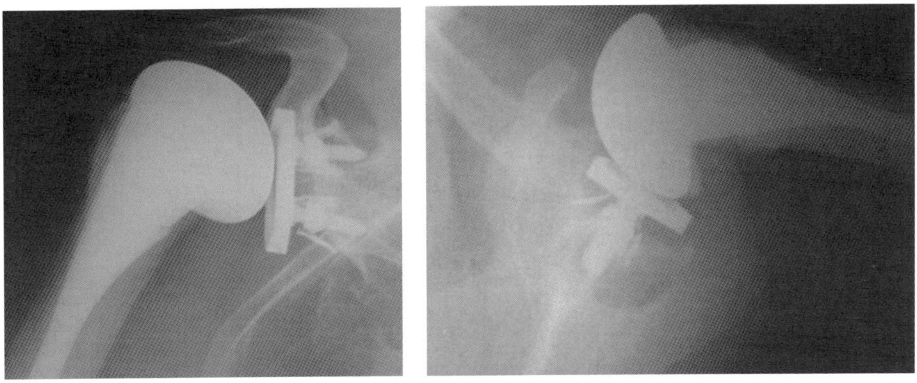

Fig. 4. Glenoid loosening of metal back component.

occurred in association with glenoid failure are shown in table I. A rotator cuff tear was present in 24 cases (65%) involving the supraspinatus tendon in 21 cases (57%), the infraspinatus in 13 (35%) and the subscapularis in 20 cases (54%) (Fig. 6).

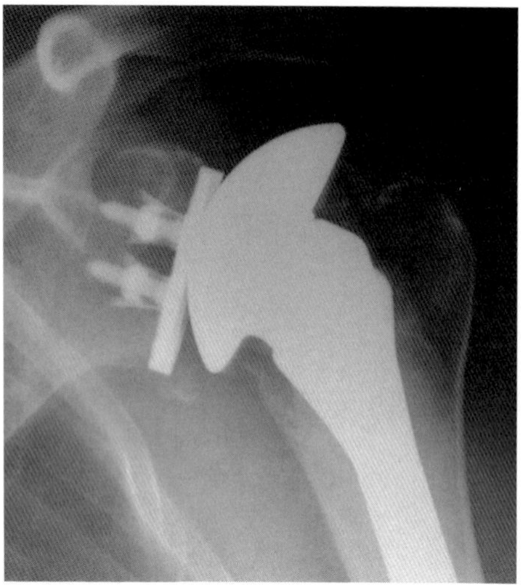

Fig. 5. Polyethylene wear without glenoid loosening.

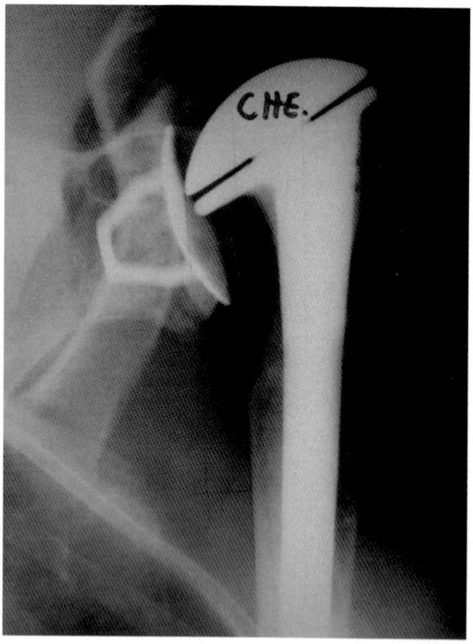

Fig. 6. Glenoid loosening associated with cuff tear.

Table I. Pre-operative associated complications with glenoid loosening or failure

	Rotator Cuff Tear n=24					Instability n=13		Glenoid Bone Loss n=37	
	Isolated Ssp n=2	Isolated Ssc n=3	Ssp+ Ssc n=6	Ssp+ Isp n=2	Ssp+Isp+ Sscap n=11	Ant n=7	Post n=6	Cavitary n=27	Combined n=10
Glenoid loosening n=25	1	1	3	1	9	4	3	19	6
Polyethylene wear or dissociation n=12	1	2	3	1	2	3	3	8	4

Ssp = supraspinatus; **Ssc**=subscapularis; **Isp**=infraspinatus; **Ant**=anterior; **Post**=posterior

Clinical or radiological insufficiency of the subscapularis musculo-tendinous unit was found in a further 9 patients. Prosthetic instability existed in 13 cases (35%) (anterior in 7 cases and posterior in 6) (Fig. 7 and 8). Anterior instability was significantly correlated with early glenoid loosening (p=0,007). Clinical subscapularis insufficiency (positive belly press, lift off test and increased external rotation) was evident in all cases of anterior instability. Cavitary bone loss (Fig. 9) was pre-

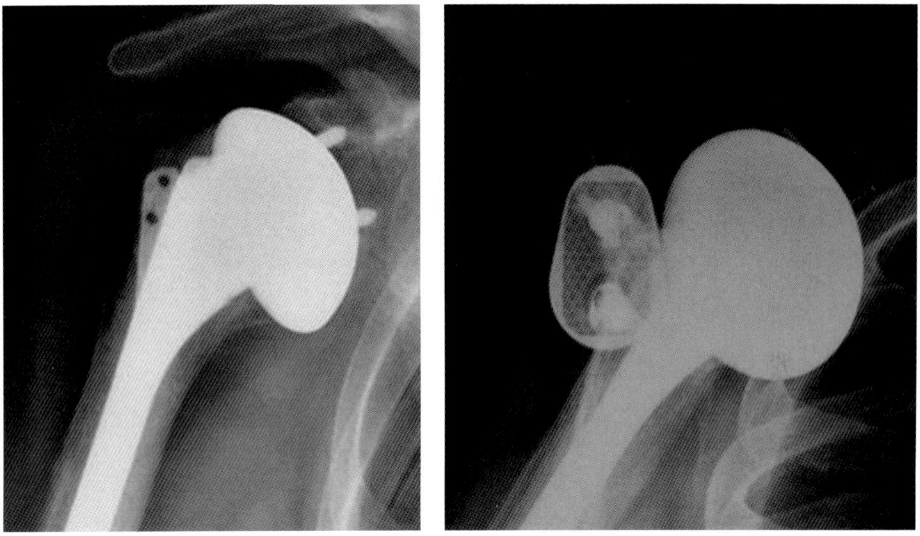

Fig. 7. Anterior prosthetic instability.

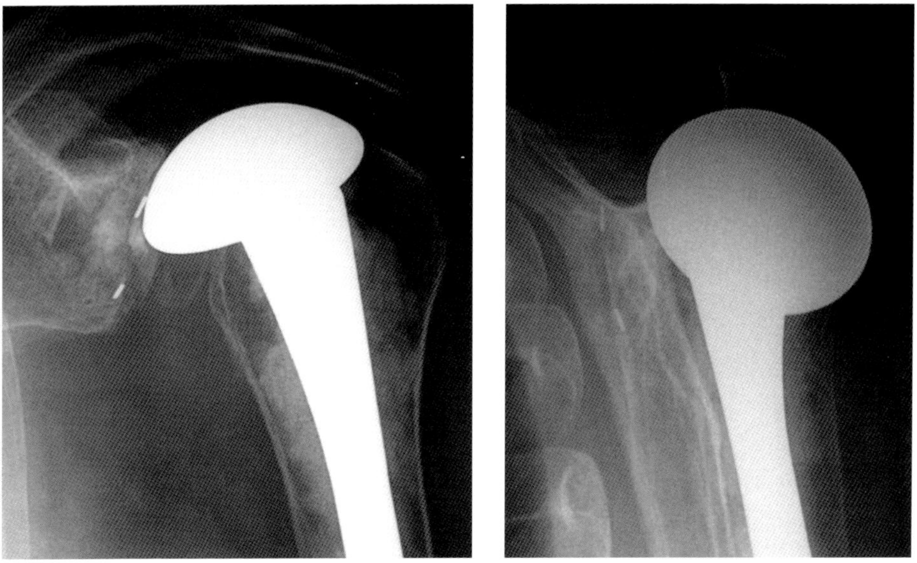

Fig. 8. Posterior prosthetic instability.

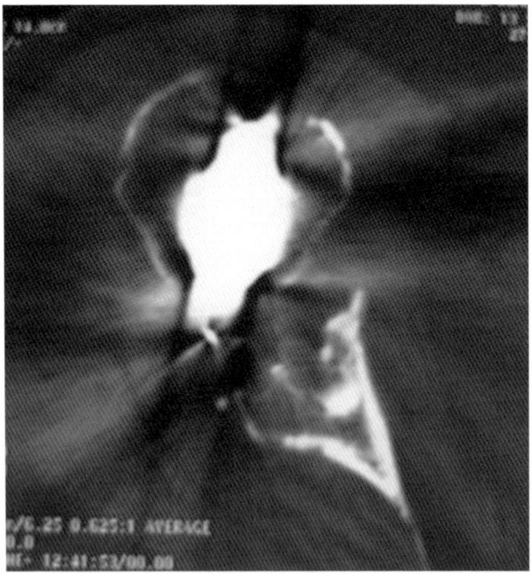

Fig. 9. Cavitary bone loss.

sent in 27 cases (73%) while combined bone loss was encountered in 10 cases (27%) (Fig. 10). Combined bone loss was more frequent after removal of metal back (8 cases) than cemented polyethylene components (2 cases).

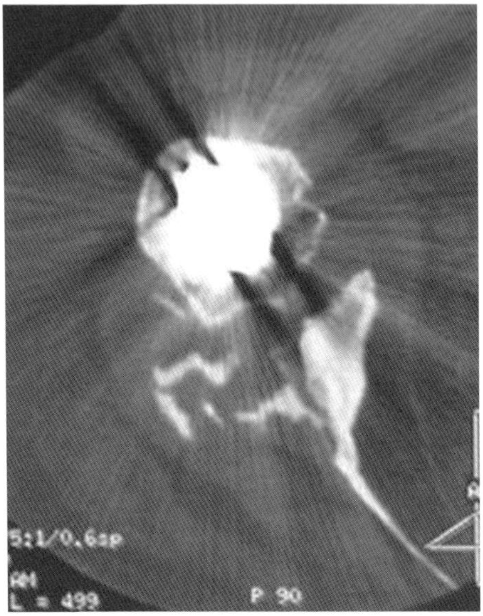

Fig. 10. Combined bone loss.

Complications and Re-revisions

A postoperative complication occurred in 11 patients (30%) and re-revision was required in 8 of these (22%). The analysis of postoperative complications and re-revisions is presented in table II. Glenoid loosening and instability were the most common complications observed. Recurrent glenoid loosening occurred: 5 years after revision, due to bone graft resorption, in one patient in whom a custom designed glenosphere with an "acromion plate" had been implanted; 10 months after revision in one patient where an adaptator had been implanted without stem removal over-tensioning the bone graft and glenoid component; and three years after revision in one patient where, even if the procedure had been performed in two stages, the peg of the baseplate did not extended beyond the bone graft into the native glenoid (Fig. 11). Glenosphere and adaptator removal with conversion to hemiarthroplasty was performed in one case and a reimplantation of a glenosphere with a long peg extending through the bone graft into the native glenoid bone was performed in the other two cases. In these two cases, at last follow-up the graft had healed and no signs of loosening were observed.

Table II. Post-operative Complications and Re-revisions

Complication n=11 (30%)	**Re-revision n=8 (22%)**
Glenoid loosening (n=3)	Conversion to HA (1) Glenoid revision (graft+ long peg) (2)
Anterior instability (n=3)	Metallic spacer (2) Closed reduction (1)
Humeral problem (subsidence/fracture) (n=2)	Stem replacement (1) Prosthesis removal (1)
Infection (n=2)	-
Haematoma (n=1)	-

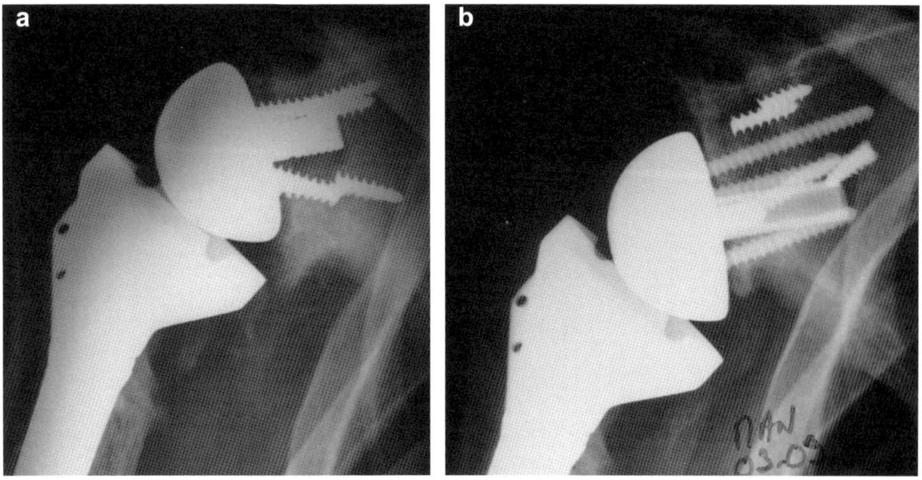

Fig. 11. Recurrent glenoid loosening (a) and re-revision with bone graft and long peg glenoid implanted in the native bone (b).

Instability due to humeral shortening occurred in two cases, immediately postoperatively in one and at one month following surgery in the other. An additional humeral metallic spacer was implanted to address the issue of shortening in each case. In one of these patients a fracture of the greater tuberosity had also occurred at the time of reverse prosthesis implantation. In a third case, instability occurred three months after surgery requiring closed reduction and immobilization. A 36 mm glenosphere had been used in all cases. No recurrence of instability was observed in any case at latest follow-up (Fig. 12).

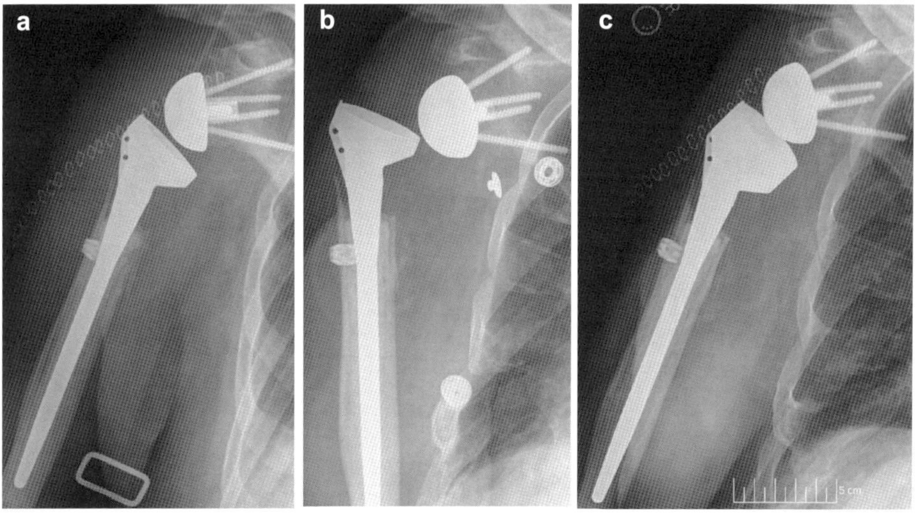

Fig. 12. RSA instability appeared 1 month after revision (b) and re-revision was performed with additional metallic spacer (c).

Subsidence of the humeral stem was observed in 2 cases. In the first case, a cortical breach had occurred at the time of RSA humeral component implantation. Ablation of the cemented stem was required and an uncemented stem was implanted. It was not possible to achieve complete axial stability with the uncemented stem and a tendency towards subsidence persisted. This RSA has since been removed in another institution. Further clinical and radiologic information was not recorded.

In the second case, subsidence occurred in a cemented stem three years after surgery leading to a humeral stress fracture. In this case, stem subsidence had already occurred in the primary TSA prior to RSA revision. No evidence of peri-prosthetic infection was identified. A further stem revision was performed.

One patient had a postoperative haematoma that spontaneously resorbed and did not require further surgery.

Two cases of infection were observed: both patients were painfree with a mean Constant score respectively of 71 and 54. Radiolucencies around the glenoid baseplate without migration of the implant were observed in both cases. In one case, bone graft lysis had occurred (Fig. 13). At last follow-up, neither patient had been re-revised. Both remain under surveillance for possible future glenoid loosening.

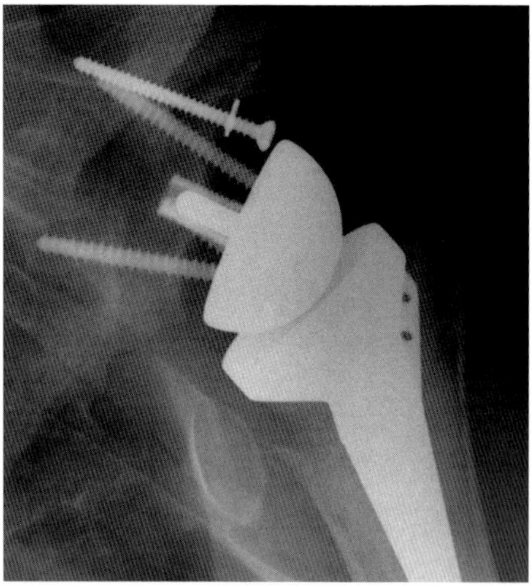

Fig. 13. Lysis of bone graft in one patient with low grade infection.

Functional results

The functional results are summarized in Table III. These results have been evaluated in the 35 patients who retained their

Table III. Functional Results according to the Contant scoring system and Mobility [n=35; FU=46.6 m (24 to 104)]

	Pre-revision	Last FU	p value
Pain	4.0 ± 2.6	11.5 ± 2.8	P<0.0001
Activity	6.1 ± 2.9	14.5 ± 4.1	P<0.0001
Mobility	11.7 ± 7.4	22.1 ± 8.5	P<0.0001
Strength	2.5 ± 3.5	7.1 ± 5.4	P=0.0001
Total CS	24.3 ± 12.5	55.2 ± 17.1	P<0.0001
Adj CS	31.6 ± 16.5	75.6 ± 21.5	P<0.0001
EAA	68° ± 38.9	121° ± 31.6	P<0.0001
ER1	16° ± 18.9	17° ± 16.1	n.s.
IR	3.2(S1) ± 2.7	3.8(S3) ± 2.5	n.s.

prostheses at latest follow-up. All parameters of the Constant Score were significantly improved as well as the active anterior elevation (AAE). However, the mobility in internal and external rotation did not change following surgery. According to the adjusted Constant score the results were excellent in 14% of cases, good in 26%, fair in 23% and poor in 37%. Despite these results, 32 of 37 patients (86%) were satisfied or very satisfied at last follow-up. The five dissatisfied patients consisted of two patients in whom the reverse prosthesis had been removed, two patients with persistent pain and one patient with a poor functional result.

Radiological results

Glenoid notching was classified as grade 0 in 16 cases (46%), grade 1 in 15 (43%) and grade 2 in 4 cases (11%). A glenoid bone scapular spur was observed in 15 cases (43%). Glenoid RLLs around the screws and/or around the central peg were present in 3 cases (9%). In 2 of these 3 cases, a low-grade infection was identified. The bone graft healed in 22 out of 29 cases (76%) (Fig. 14). Partial graft resorption was observed in 6 cases (21%). The only case of bone graft lysis (3%) was observed in the setting of a low-grade infection.

Correlations

No significant statistical correlations were found between the Constant score and primary diagnosis, cause of the revision (glenoid loosening/polyethylene wear), type of glenoid component revised and associated complications (cuff and subscapularis status, instability, bone loss). Although the mean Constant score was slightly better in patients in whom bone grafts had been performed (mean 57 pts) than those without bone grafting (mean 50 pts), the difference was not significant with the numbers available (p=0.3). The mean Constant score in patients with intra or post-operative complications not re-operated upon was lower (mean 48 pts) than in patients not experiencing complications (mean 58 pts) but the difference was not significant (p=0.1).

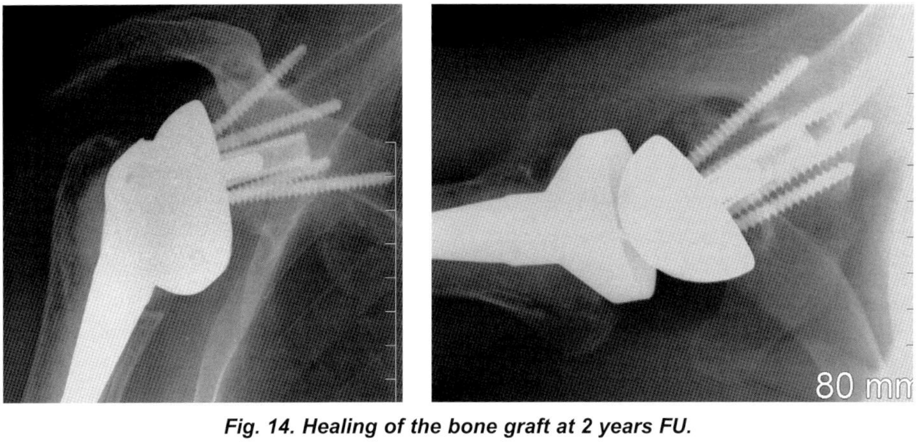

Fig. 14. Healing of the bone graft at 2 years FU.

DISCUSSION

Our study confirms our hypothesis: revision of glenoid loosening or failure with a RSA is a reliable therapeutic option, specifically in cases of severe glenoid bone loss and associated complications such as rotator cuff tear or instability. Of the 37 patients, revised with a RSA for glenoid loosening or failure in the present study, 24 (65%) had an associated rotator cuff tear and 13 (35%) had prosthetic instability. Glenoid bone loss was present in all 37 patients, cavitary in nature in 27 and combined in 10. Although revision with RSA permits the solution of multiple problems simultaneously, it is risky surgery: postoperative complications occurred in 11 patients (30%) and re-revision was required in 8 of them (22%). Global functional results were good, particularly in relation to the gains achieved in AAE and pain. The main advantage of RSA is that it permits reconstruction of glenoid bone loss, due to implant fixation of the bone graft with the metallic baseplate.

Different therapeutic options have been proposed for patients presenting with glenoid loosening or failure. Modest functional improvements and humeral head medialization/protrusion have been reported following glenoid removal and corticocancellous grafting without glenoid prosthetic reimplantation [1, 16]. Better functional results, pain relief and a higher degree of satisfaction have been reported in cases of glenoid reimplantation [1, 8]. In general, revision with prosthetic components provide the best outcomes, whereas soft-tissue reconstructions can be expected to yield poorer results [9]. Addressing instability is essential when revising the glenoid component for loosening [1]. The combination of glenoid bone loss, instability and rotator cuff deficiency appears to be a common constellation of findings in cases requiring revision for glenoid failure. RSA would seem to represent the ideal solution in addressing this complex problem. Norris [17] has pioneered a technique for the management of failed total shoulder arthroplasties with glenoid deficiency and/or rotator rotator cuff dysfunction creating instability. Using this technique good preliminary results for RSA performed in combination with tricortical autologous iliac bone grafting were reported. Neyton [14, 15] found encouraging clinical and radiographical results at short term follow-up in a small series of TSA revised with RSA and bone grafting; in this series no radiographic evidence of bone graft lysis or compression was observed at follow up. Our outcomes are comparable to those of Neyton [15] for pain improvement. Although better range of motion and function was observed in our series, a lower rate of bone graft healing and more frequent recurrent glenoid loosening was identified, possibly accounted for by the longer duration of follow-up. Although similar to those previously published for RSA implanted in the setting of revision surgery [3], the complication and re-revision rates observed in this series remain high [22]. Recurrent glenoid loosening, recurrent instability and infection are among the main complications that may be anticipated.

The present study had several limitations. It is retrospective, multicenter and represents the results of different surgeons. The minimum follow-up of two years is too short to judge the final results following revision arthroplasty. Nevertheless, our study represents the largest series of TSA revised with RSA for aseptic glenoid loosening or failure. The reported results encourage us to continue to perform this procedure for specific indications. Selective use of the reverse prosthesis may be the key to reducing the high rate of complications encountered, in general. One stage implantation of with inferiorly tilted long peg glenoid baseplates engaging the native glenoid bone is mandatory in order to avoid recurrent glenoid loosening. Restoration of humeral length, use of large diameter glenospheres and lateralisation are needed to prevent instability. In cases of metal back glenoid component failure without loosening, a specially adapted glenosphere can be implanted onto the metal back glenoid implant, obviating the need to remove the baseplate, with obvious benefits in terms of preservation of glenoid bone stock.

CONCLUSION

RSA solves the issues of glenoid loosening or failure occurring in association with other major complications such as severe glenoid bone loss, rotator cuff tears and/or prosthetic instability. The problem of glenoid bone graft incorporation is addressed with the use of long peg baseplates which achieve stable fixation in the native glenoid bone. In this study, 76% of bone grafts healed and 86% of patients were satisfied or very satisfied with the outcome following surgery. However, TSA revision with RSA is risky surgery. The complication and re-revision rates are high. Extreme care must be taken to prevent complications and to ensure proper initial positioning of the implant.

REFERENCES

[1] ANTUNA SA, SPERLING JW, COFIELD RH, ROWLAND CM Glenoid revision surgery after total shoulder artrhoplasty. *J Shoulder Elbow Surg. 2001; 10: 217-24.*

[2] BARRETT WP, FRANKLIN JL, JACKINS SE, WYSS CR, MATSEN FA III. Total shoulder arthroplasty. *J Bone Joint Surg (Am) 1987; 69: 865-72.*

[3] BOILEAU P, WATKINSON D, HATZIDAKIS A.M, HOVORKA I. Neer Award 2005: The Grammont reverse shoulder prosthesis: Results in cuff tear arthritis, fracture sequelae, and revision arthroplasty. *J Shoulder Elbow Surg 2006; 15: 527-40.*

[4] BRENNER BC, FERLIC DC, CLAYTON ML, DENNIS DA Survivorship of unconstrained total shoulder arthroplasty. *J Bone Joint Surg (Am)1989; 71: 1289-96.*

[5] CHEUNG EV, SPERLING JW, COFIELD RH Revision shoulder arthroplasty for glenoid component loosening. *J Shoulder Elbow Surg. 2008; 17(3): 371-5.*

[6] COFIELD RH Total shoulder arthroplasty with the Neer prosthesis. *J Bone Joint Surg (Am) 1984; 66: 899-906.*

[7] COFIELD RH, EDGERTON BC. Total shoulder arthroplasty: complications and revision surgery. *Instr Course Lect 1990; 39: 449-62.*

[8] DEUTSCH A, ABBOUD JA, KELLY J, MODY M, NORRIS T, RAMSEY ML, IANNOTTI JP, WILLIAMS GR. Clinical results of revision shoulder arthroplasty for glenoid component loosening. *J Shoulder Elbow Surg. 2007;16(6): 706-16.*

[9] DINES JS, FEALY S, STRAUSS EJ, ALLEN A, CRAIG EV, WARREN RF, DINES DM. Outcomes analysis of revision total shoulder replacement. *J Bone Joint Surg Am. 2006; 88(7): 1494-500.*

[10] GRUEN TA, McNEICE GM, AMSTUTZ HC. “Modes of failure” of cemented stem-type femoral components: a radiographic analysis of loosening. *Clin Orthop 1979; 141: 17-27.*

[11] HAWKINS RJ, BELL RH, JALLAY B Total shoulder arthroplasty. *Clin Orthop 1989; 242: 188-94.*

[12] KELLY IG, FOSTER RS, FISHER WD Neer total shoulder replacement in rheumatoid arthritis. *J Bone Joint Surg (Br) 1987; 69: 723-26.*

[13] MOLÉ D, ROCHE O, RIAND N, LEVIGNE C, WALCH G. Cemented glenoid component: results in osteoarthritis and rheumatoid arthritis. In: Walch G, Boileau P (eds): Shoulder arthroplasty, *Springer-Verlag, Berlin, 1999, 163-71.*

[14] NEYTON L, BOILEAU P, NOVÉ-JOSSERAND L, MD, EDWARDS TB, WALCH G. Glenoid bone grafting with a reverse design prosthesis. *J Shoulder Elbow Surg 2007;16: 71S-78S.*

[15] NEYTON L, SIRVEAUX F, ROCHE O, MOLÉ D, BOILEAU P, WALCH G. Results of revision surgery for glenoid loosening: a multicentric series of 37 shoulder prosthesis. *Rev Chir Orthop Reparatrice Appar Mot. 2004; 90(2): 111-21.*

[16] NEYTON L, WALCH G, NOVÉ-JOSSERAND L, MD, EDWARDS TB Glenoid corticocancellous bone grafting after glenoid component removal in the treatment of glenoid loosening. *J Shoulder Elbow Surg 2006;15: 173-9.*

[17] NORRIS TR, KELLY JD II, HUMPHREY CS Management of Glenoid Bone Defects in Revision Shoulder Arthroplasty: A New Application of the Reverse Total Shoulder Prosthesis. *Techniques in Shoulder and Elbow Surgery 2007;8(1): 37-46.*

[18] SIRVEAUX F, FAVARD L, OUDET D, HUGUET D, LAUTMAN S. Grammont inverted total shoulder arthroplasty in the treatment of glenohumeral osteoarthritis with massive and non-repairable cuff rupture. In: Walch G, Boileau P, Mole D, eds. 2000 Shoulder prostheses: two to ten year follow-up. *Montpellier: Sauramps Medical, 2001: 247-51.*

[19] SNEPPEN O, FRUENSGAARD S, JOHANNSEN HV, OLSEN BS, SOJBJERG JO, ANDERSEN NH. Total shoulder replacement in rheumatoid arthritis: proximal migration and loosening. *J Shoulder Elbow Surg 1996; 5:47-52.*

[20] SPERLING JW, COFIELD RH, O'DRISCOLL SW, TORCHIA ME, ROWLAND CM Radiographic assessment of ingrowth total shoulder arthroplasty. *J Shoulder Elbow Surg 2000; 9: 507-13.*

[21] TORCHIA ME, COFIELD RH, SETTERGREN CR. Total shoulder arthroplasty with the Neer prosthesis: long-term results. *J Shoulder Elbow Surg 1997; 6: 495-505.*

[22] WALL B, NOVÉ-JOSSERAND L, O'CONNOR DP, EDWARDS TB, WALCH G. Reverse Total Shoulder Arthroplasty: A Review of Results According to Etiology. *J Bone Joint Surg Am. 2007; 89: 1476-85.*

REVISION OF FAILED HEMI-ARTHRO-PLASTY TO REVERSE TOTAL SHOULDER ARTHROPLASTY THROUGH A TRANSHUMERAL APPROACH

F. GOHLKE, J. STEHLE, B. WERNER

The main indication for the reverse endoprosthesis (Grammont *et al.* 1987) is the painful and pseudoparalytic rotator cuff deficient shoulder in elderly patients of different aetiology. This disability can be the result of different entities: cuff tear arthropathy, proximal humerus fractures, rheumatoid arthritis and, recently revision shoulder arthroplasty. The value of reverse arthroplasty is predominantly proven for cuff arthropathy. For all other indications limited experience is available. The number of cases with revision reverse TSR published in literature is still small (DeWilde 2001, Levy *et al.* 2007, Flury *et al.* 2010).

The most frequent indication for reverse revision TSR is given in case of failed fracture hemi arthroplasty and, less frequently in instability and painful pseudoparalysis after total or hemiarthoplasty which was used in cases of cuff deficient shoulders. Numerous papers have shown that the results of primary and fracture arthroplasty are mostly inferior to osteoarthritis cases (Zyto *et al.* 1998, Boileau *et al.* 2001). According to Compito *et al.* (1994) and Boileau *et al.* (2002) the main reasons are tuberosity failure, stiffness, superior migration of the humeral head, loosening and nerve injuries. Especially in fracture sequelae type 3 or 4 (acc. to the classification of Boileau) hemiarthroplasty mostly yields only pain relief and limited functional improvement. Revision after unsatisfactory outcome in these patients using anatomic standard implants is rarely successful (Carroll *et al.* 2004).

MATERIAL

From 2000-2007 the senior author (F.G.) performed 103 revision arthroplasties as single stage procedure using reverse TSR. The majority were failed fracture hemiarthroplasties (n=60) and, in 7 cases implants of special design like bipolar or tumour prosthesis. In 13 cases reverse arthroplasty was used as a second stage procedure after removal of infected hemi fracture arthroplasty and temporary use of an antibiotics loaded spacer (results reported recently by Rolf *et al.* 2007).

Based on the experience with intra- and postoperative problems of our first cases we considered removal of well cemented stable stems or those with bony ingrowths as the main source of intraoperative complications. Therefore we looked for a new technique which provides faster and safer removal of the implant. A pectoralis major pediculated humeral window was preferred in order to avoid intraoperative fractures, preserve the blood supply of the humerus and to keep the stabilizing function of the pectoralis major muscle intact. We published our first series with this special surgical technique (transhumeral approach), which was prospectively evaluated, in 2007 (Gohlke and Rolf 2007). Posterior-lateral transfer of a fragment with the adherent Latissimus dorsi tendon was at this time only in 3 cases performed in order to improve external rotation. Long revision stems were used in all cases with humeral window in order to achieve sufficient anchorage length in the humeral shaft. Only for the first 2 cases short stems were available – one was revised to a long stem after 1.5 years, the second remained stable over 8 years (last follow-up).

The fragments and the humeral window of the proximal humerus were stabilized with 1-5 cerclage wires. In 4 cases further distal cerclage wires were used for the humeral diaphysis after splitting in order to remove the distal plug of bone cement. In 3 cases ultrasonography was used for removal of long distal cement plugs. All but two stems were cemented in a two stage procedure.

The material of our first series published by Rolf (2007) comprised of 34 revisions of failed fracture hemiarthroplasties (five men, 29 women). 25 patients were followed prospectively for up to 59 months postoperatively; an additional nine patients we re interviewed by telephone or writing using a validated Constant questionaire (n = 34, average age 68 years, 59-82 years). The average follow-up was 31.5 months (12-59 months).

Preoperatively, 24 patients were suffering from a significant loss of the anterior part of the deltoid muscle and/or partial denervation of the deltoid confirmed by EMG as a consequence of previous interventions.

In 28 patients, there was static anterosuperior migration of the humeral head or subluxation. Pseudoparalysis was diagnosed in all these patients as a consequence of rotator cuff insufficiency. In eight patients, intraoperative biopsies were positive without any apparent clinical signs of infection.

RESULTS

The preoperative age and gender related Constant Score improved from 17.5 to 63% postoperatively. Range of motion for active elevation and internal rotation was substantially improved (average elevation preoperatively 48°, postoperatively 125°). Pain was relieved in every patient. Function correlated to the extent of soft-tissue damage. 14 patients were very satisfied with the surgical outcome, 16 were satisfied and four dissatisfied. There were eight complications in total.

The gain of active mobility, especially active forward elevation, was mainly related to three parameters: Absence of complications, presence of teres minor and, the amount of deltoid muscle loss.

In none of the cases the bone of the proximal humeral window disappeared and a remodelling of the bone could be observed in 16 cases. Progressive resorption of the bone fragments as the result of devascularization due to complete stripping of the soft tissue attachments did not occur. This would be associated with the risk of early loosening and fatigue failure of the implant.

Inferior notching of the glenoid could surprisingly only observed in 4 patients (one grade II° and 3 grade I° acc. to Nerot). This finding was probably due to the short follow-up, inferior placement of the metaglène, use of a glenosphere with greater diameter in many cases or higher degree of tensioning comparing to normal reverse arthroplasty in order to avoid further dislocations.

Complications for the first series (published 2007): Three dislocations, one disconnection of the humeral metaphyseal component from the diaphysial stem after 15 months, and one case with heterotopic ossification. One periprosthetic fracture occured after adequate trauma (fall in the staircase after 11 months and postoperative radial nerve paresthesia with complete recovery).

One low grade infection recurred with gradually increasing swelling, moderate pain and CRP enhancement 3 months after surgery. This was successfully revised in a two stage procedure using an articulating Vancomycin and Gentamycin loaded spacer directed to the germ and second reverse TSR.

DISCUSSION

In literature little is known about the benefit of reverse arthroplasty as revision implant despite the fact that many centres are actually using this system in revision cases, preferably when the glenoid bone stock is well preserved (Jouve *et al.* 2005). The complication rate of this procedure seems to be considerably high (ranging from 11-37%). Our revision rate in 40 anatomical hemiarthroplasties which were revised to reverse TSR in a single stage procedure after more than 2 years follow-up were 20% (n=8, 5 dislocations, 1 impingement of heterotopic ossifications at the glenoid, 1 uncoupling of the stem, 1 late periporthestic fracture). At present reverse shoulder arthroplasty gets proven for revisions in failed hemiarthroplasties with cuff deficient shoulders. Caution is appropriate in case of:

- Active infections.
- Gross destruction of the glenoid or severe osteoporosis: Stable fixation of the metaglène may be impossible or includes the risk of early loosening. In those cases insertion of the reverse humeral component as a hemi solution combined with bone graft reconstruction and second stage conversion to a reverse TSR can be advocated. Especially in cases of a longstanding anterior-superior subluxation or complete dislocation the glenoid bone is weak and atrophic. Therefore the patients should be informed about the possible use of iliac bone grafting.
- Severe damage of deltoid muscle: The authors do not recommend this procedure in case of delta muscle palsy or destruction of more than 60% because the risk of dislocation is high and the benefit for the patient regarding gainof function poor.
- Asymetric scarring, severe stiffness and heterotopic ossification close to the plexus and the axillary nerve causing unbalanced soft tissues contractures. These cases required time consuming surgery which has a high risk of vascular or neurological complications.

- Destruction of the lower third of the humerus: In these cases even the longest revision stem which routinely is available may provide no stable reconstruction of the humerus. Bone grafting, bulk allografts and the use of special contoured fixation plates for the distal humerus or custom-made stems are required.
- Younger patients (less than 60 years): The first long-term results (Guery *et al.* 2006) point out that a sudden loss of function may occur after 6-7 years probably as a consequence of progressive inferior glenoid notching, or increasing polyethylene wear and particles disease.

The functional results of revision cases seem to be less favourable than those obtained in cuff tear arthropathy regarding both, active range of motion and muscle strength. De Wilde *et al.* (2001) first described in 5 cases (4 patients) an improvement of the Constant score from 14 to 62. We reported recently the clinical and X-ray results of the first 34 patients which were prospectively followed up over more than 1 year (mean 34 moonths). The function measured by the Constant score improved from 20 to 63% after year follow-up (Gohlke *et al.* 2007) and remained stable during a maximum of 8 years observed in some patients. Jouve *et al.* published the results of a prospective multicenter series of 45 patients suffering from different pathologies (38% fracture hemi arthroplasties) and a minimum follow-up of 2 years. In this series the Constant score improved from 18.7 to 55.6 with the greatest benefit obtained for pain and activities of daily living. 71% of their patients were satisfied with the procedure.

We found no signs of glenoid loosening or bone resorption of the humerus within the first 2 years.

We observed two late dislocations, one after 3 months and the second after 2 years with a breakage of the wires and displacement of the pediculated bone window which obviously did not heal. Both patients underwent latissimus dorsi transfer which probably was of adverse effect on bone healing. After refixation of the bone window with cerclage wires and reorientation of the force of the pectoralis major both remained stable without a humeral lengthener. The clinical results of the 6 patients treated with latissimus dorsi transfer revealed no significant difference in the active mobility or gain of function and score comparing to the rest.

After multiple revisions advanced damage of the soft tissue can be expected which contains loss of contractile elements of the deltoid muscle, significant scarring and asymmetric muscle atrophy. Therefore intra-operatively increased pretension by lengthening of the implant is mostly recommended in order to prevent instability. Excessive lengthening, however, has to be avoided because this includes the risk of overstretching of the brachial plexus and peripheral nerves (ulna and radial nerve), functional impairment and, reflex dystrophy. Moreover in the long run the soft tissues gradually elongate again which may lead to late instability. A well preserved pectoralis major can prevent this late complication even in case of loss of the anterior third of the delta muscle. Nevertheless significant lesions of the anterior delta muscle had an unfavourable influence on active anterior elevation in many patients. Two female patients suffered from secondary loss of active mobility and pain after fatigue fracture of the scapular spine after 5 and 17 months.

Therefore Chacon *et al.* (2009) recommended the use of composite bulk allograft in order to improve the ingrowths and long-term attachment of the soft tissues. They published lower rates of instability which may be influenced in part by the different design (greater lateral off-set of the glenosphere) of their glenoid component. However, this special design increases the shear forces on the baseplate and is therefore probably responsible for higher rates of early baseplate loosening in their series.

We feel that for the great majority composite bulk allografts do not provide significant advantages to revisions comparing to a surgical technique which preserves the body's own bone stock.

Recently we revised patients after resection of the proximal humerus and insertion of tumour prosthesis as salvage procedure causing chronic dislocations followed by very difficult conditions for further revisions. For such problems or advanced humeral bone loss according to grade 4 or 5 of our recently introduced classification (Gohlke and Werner 2009) allografts may offer a second line of defense.

CONCLUSION

Revision of hemiarthroplasty with reverse TSR is a technically demanding procedure with high complication rates between 15-45% but offers in most cases of failed arthroplasties with rotator cuff insufficiency a valuable option. Our first midterm results revealed no difference in the rate of early loosenings of the long revision stems or glenoid components comparing to standard procedures in cuff tear arthropathy.

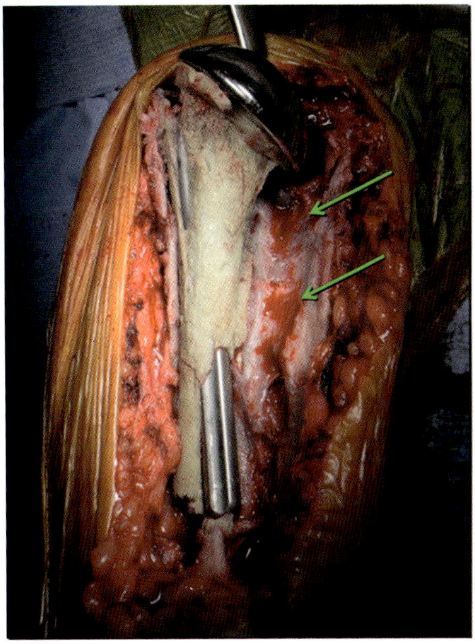

Fig. 1: ***Transhumeral approach with pectoralis pediculated humeral bone window. Note the bleeding of the bone due to preserved blood supply by the muscle attached to the fragment (arrows). Behind the bone window the ascending fibers of the Latissimus dorsi tendon are shown which can be used for tendon transfer.***

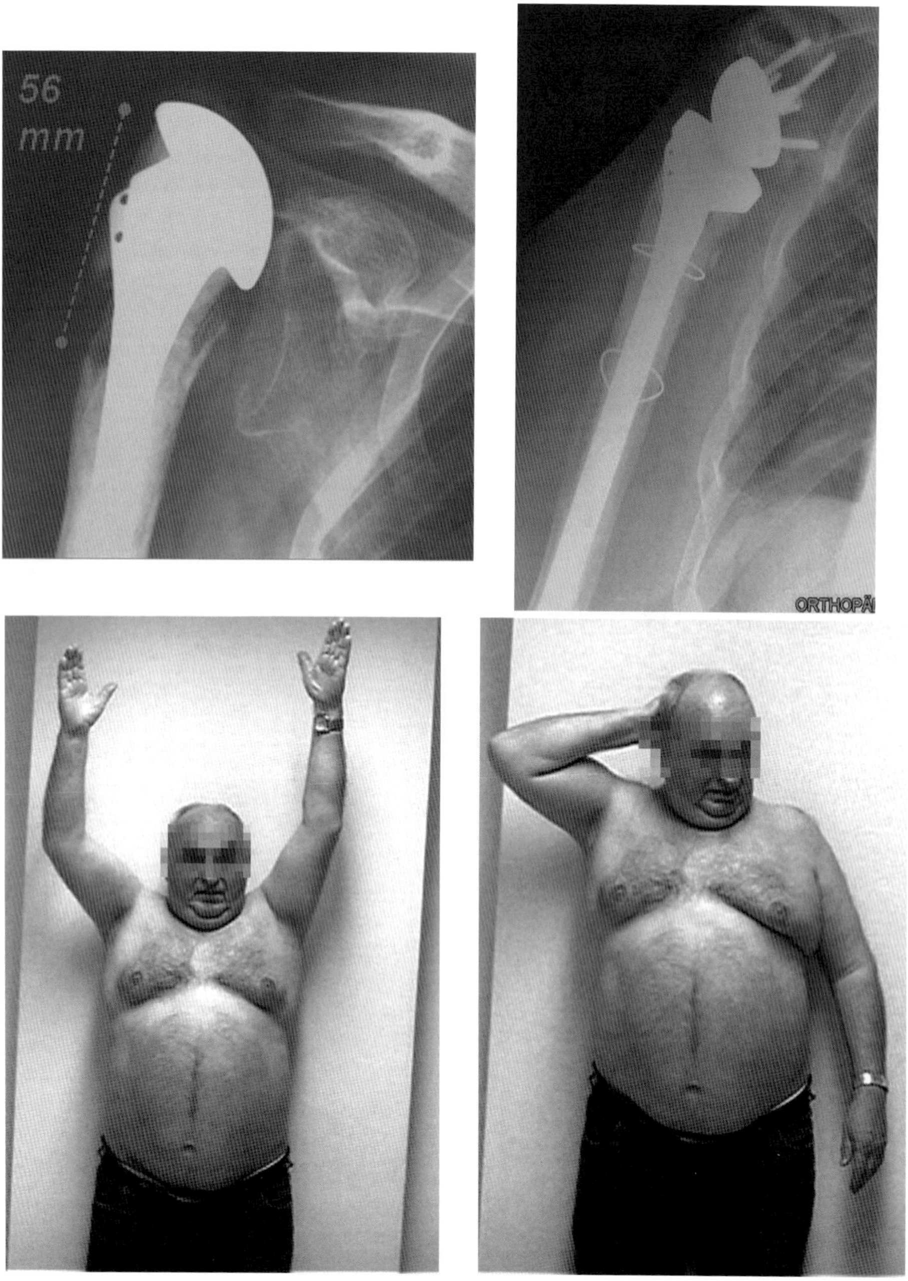

Fig. 2: 67 years old man with painful pseudoparalysis after fracture hemiarthroplasty with loss of tuberosities and metaphyseal bone of 5.8 cm, loss of the rotator cuff including teres minor. 2.5 years after revision reverse TSR he shows 165° active elevation and forward flexion due to an intensive education programme of the delta muscle.

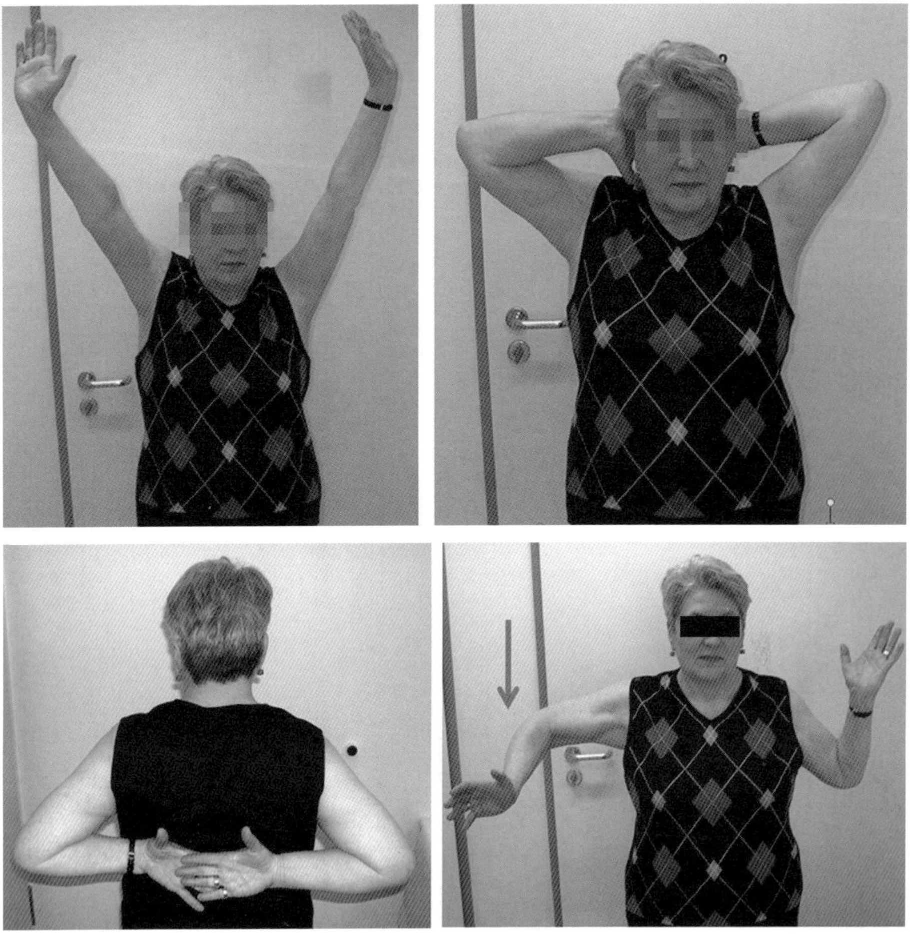

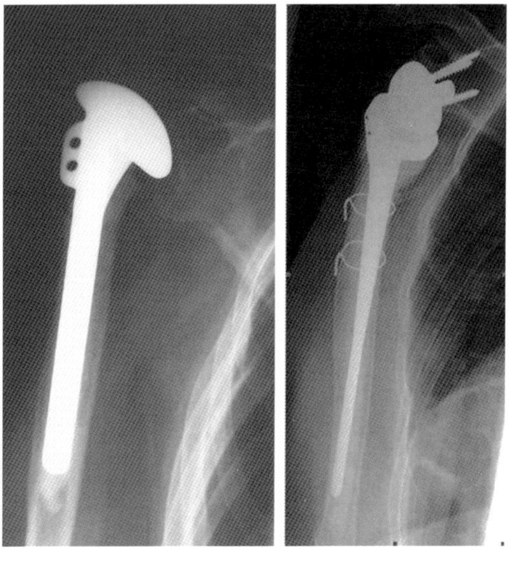

***Fig. 3:** Clinical result after revision of failed fracture arthroplasty 4 years after surgery in this 68 year old lady. Even looking perfect for active elevation and external rotation behind the head a closer examination reveals the weakness for external rotation with the arm in 90° of abduction.*

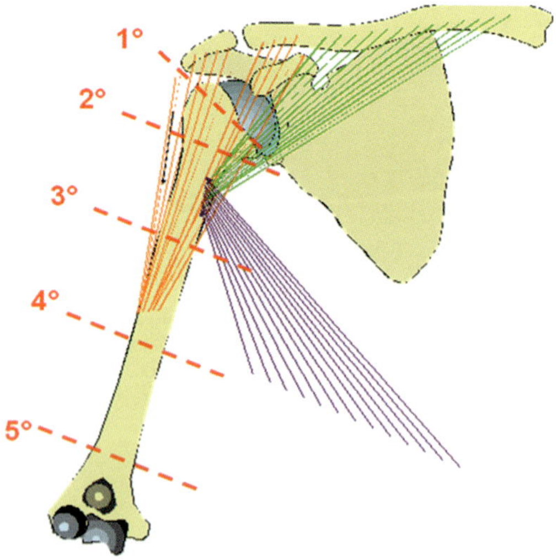

Fig. 4: Classifications of humeral bone loss (Gohlke and Werner 2009). Allografts, custom-made implants or tumour prosthesis may be required in advanced bone loss greater stage 3. Grade 1-3 can mostly be successfully treated by reverse TSR.

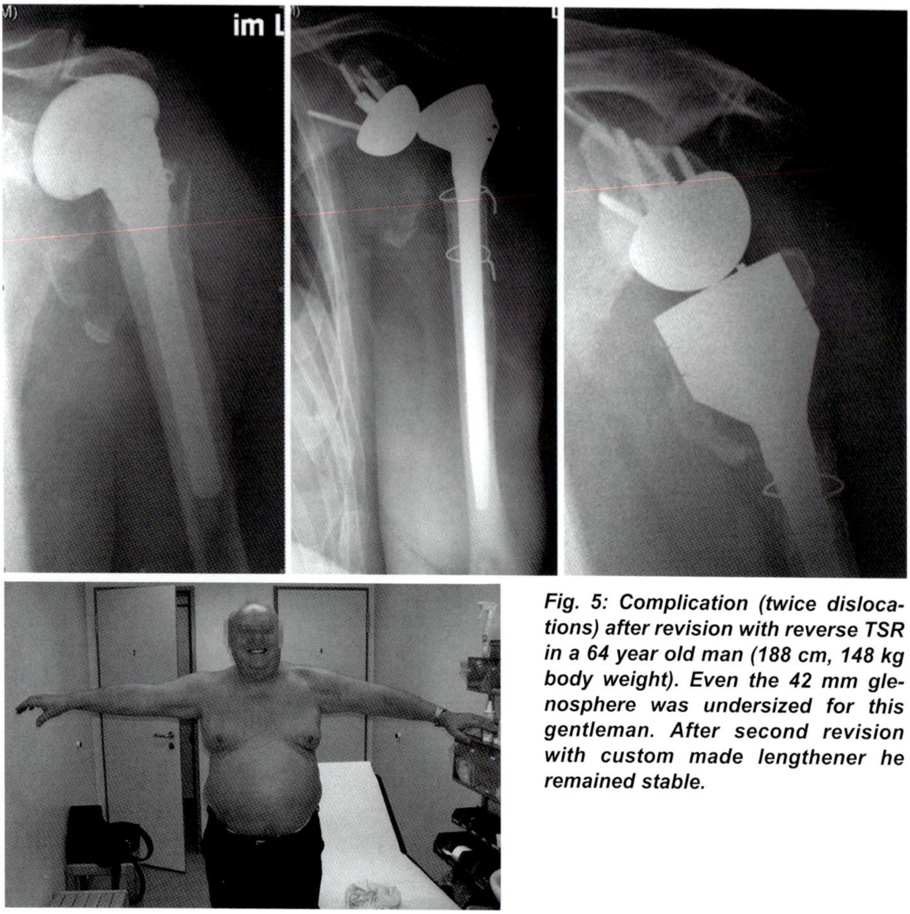

Fig. 5: Complication (twice dislocations) after revision with reverse TSR in a 64 year old man (188 cm, 148 kg body weight). Even the 42 mm glenosphere was undersized for this gentleman. After second revision with custom made lengthener he remained stable.

REFERENCES

[1] BOILEAU P, KRISHNAN SG, TINSI L, WALCH G, COSTE JS, MOLE D. Tuberosity malposition and migration: reasons for poor outcomes after hemiarthroplasty for displaced fractures of the proximal humerus. *J Shoulder Elbow Surg. 2002. 11: 401-12*

[2] BOILEAU P, TROJANI C, WALCH G, KRISHNAN SG, ROMEO A, SINNERTON R. Shoulder arthroplasty for the treatment of the sequelae of fractures of the proximal humerus. *J Shoulder Elbow Surg. 2001. 10: 299-308.*

[3] CARROLL RM, IZQUIERDO R, VAZQUEZ M Conversion of painful hemiarthroplasty to total shoulder arthroplasty: long-term results. *J Shoulder Elbow Surg 2004. 13: 599-603.*

[4] CHACON A, VIRANI N, SHANNON R, LEVY JC, PUPELLO D, FRANKLE M. Revision arthroplasty with use of a reverse shoulder prosthesis-allograft composite. *J Bone Joint Surg Am. 2009. 91: 119-27.*

[5] COMPITO CA, SELF EB, BIGLIANI LU Arthroplasty and acute shoulder trauma. Reasons for success and failure. *Clin Orthop 1994. 307: 27-36.*

[6] DE WILDE L, MOMBERT M, VAN PETEGEM P, VERDONK R Revision of shoulder replacement with a reversed shoulder prothesis (Delta III): report of five cases. *Acta Orthop Belg 2001. 47: 348-53.*

[7] FAVARD L, LAUTMANN S, SIRVEAUX F, OUDET D, KERJEAN Y, HUGUET D Hemiarthroplasty versus reverse arthroplasty in the treatment of osteoarthritis with massive cuff tear. In: Walch G, Boileau P, Molé: 2000 Shoulder prosthesis... two to ten year follow-up. *2001. 261-268, Sauramps Médical Montpellier.*

[8] FLURY MP, FREY P, GOLDHAHN J, SCHWYZER HK, SIMMEN BR Reverse shoulder arthroplasty as a salvage procedure for failed conventional shoulder replacement due to cuff failure-midterm results. *Int Orthop. 2010. (in print)*

[9] GOHLKE F, ROLF O Revision of failed fracture hemiarthroplasties to reverse total shoulder prosthesis through the transhumeral approach : method incorporating a pectoralis-major-pedicled bone window. *Operat Orthop Traumatol 2007. 19(2): 185-208.*

[10] GOHLK F, WERNER B Humeral bone defects in revision and primary shoulder arthroplasty. *Proc. SECEC 2009, Madrid*

[11] GUERY J, FAVARD L, SIRVEAUX F, OUDET D, MOLE D, WALCH G Reverse total shoulder arthroplasty. Survivorship analysis of eighty replacements followed for five to ten years. *J Bone Joint Surg Am. 2006 Aug; 88(8): 1742-7*

[12] LEVY JC, VIRANI N, PUPELLO D, FRANKLE M Use of the reverse shoulder prosthesis for the treatment of failed hemiarthroplasty in patients with glenohumeral arthritis and rotator cuff deficiency. *J Bone Joint Surg Br. 2007. 89(2): 189-195.*

[13] LEVY J, FRANKLE M, MIGHELL M, PUPELLO D The use of the reverse shoulder prosthesis for the treatment of failed hemiarthroplasty for proximal humeral fracture. *J Bone Joint Surg Am. 2007. 89(2): 292-300.*

[14] JOUVE F, WACH G, NOVÉ-JOSSERAND, NEYTON L, WALL B, LIOTARD JP Revision of shoulder arthroplasty with reverse prosthesis. Abstract Book of the 19th. *Congress of European Society for Surgery of the Shoulder and Elbow (SECEC), Rome 2005, P. 144.*

[15] ROLF O, STEHLE J, GOHLKE F Treatment of septic arthritis of the shoulder and periprosthetic shoulder infections. Special problems in rheumatoid arthritis. *Orthopade 2007. 36(8): 700-7.*

[16] VALENTI PH, BOUTENS D, NEROT C *et al.* Delta-3 reverse prothesis for osteoarthritis with massive cuff tear : long term results (> 5 years). In: Walch G, Boileau P, Molé: 2000 Shoulder prosthesis... two to ten year follow-up. 2001. *253-9, Sauramps Medical Montpellier.*

[17] WALL B, NOVÉ-JOSSERAND L, O'CONNOR DP, EDWARDS TB, WALCH G Reverse total shoulder arthroplasty: a review of results according to etiology. *J Bone Joint Surg Am 2007. 89(7): 1476-85.*

[18] WIRTH MA, ROCKWOOD CA Complications of shoulder arthroplasty. Clin Orthop 1994; 307: 47- 69.

[19] ZYTO K, WALLACE WA, FROSTICK SP, PRESTON BJ Outcome after hemiarthroplasty for three and four part fractures of the proximal humerus. *J Shoulder Elbow Surg 1998. 7: 85-9.*

REVERSE TOTAL SHOULDER ARTHROPLASTY AND GLENOID NOTCHING

B. JOST, C. GERBER

ABSTRACT

Introduction

Reverse total shoulder arthroplasty according to the concept of Grammont [1] can relieve pain and restore function in patients with cuff tear arthropathy or cuff deficient shoulders after trauma or prior fracture or prosthetic surgeries. The most frequently reported radiographic complication is inferior glenoid/scapular notching (fig. 1) with a reported incidence of up to 93% [2]. The clinical relevance of notching as well as the anatomic and radiographic parameters that predispose to its occurrence is not yet completely understood.

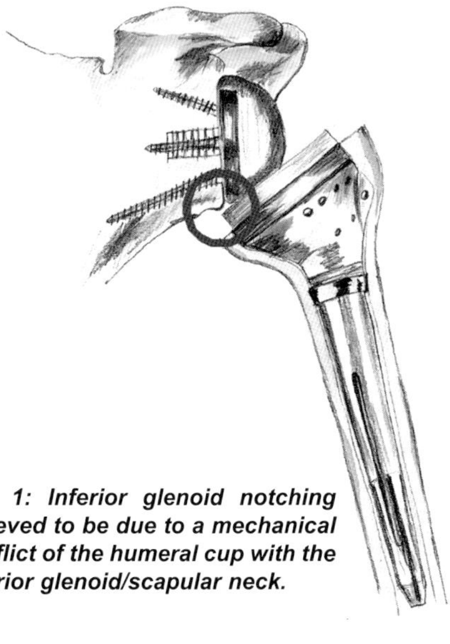

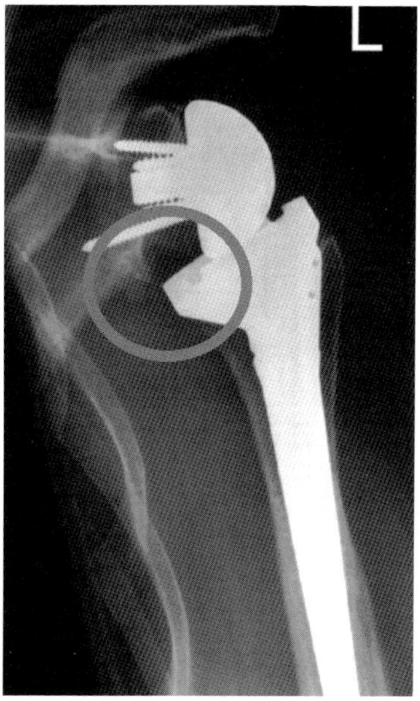

Fig. 1: Inferior glenoid notching believed to be due to a mechanical conflict of the humeral cup with the inferior glenoid/scapular neck.

Assessment and classification of inferior notching

Inferior glenoid notching is mainly and most reliably evaluated on true AP radiographs using fluoroscopic control to ensure the correct orientation of the hemispheric glenoid implant. The most widely used classification of Sirveaux [3] divides inferior scapular notching in 5 grades: *grade 0:* no bony defect/notching; *grade 1:* the defect concerns only the pillar; *grade 2:* the defect has contact with the lower screw of the baseplate; *grade 3:* the defect extends over the lower screw; *grade 4:* the defect extends under the baseplate.

Inferior glenoid notching should be distinguished from spur (or osteophyte) formation. A spur at the inferior scapula is frequently found after reverse shoulder arthroplasty and may be confused with scapular notching. The real or virtual line of the lateral margin of the scapula to the baseplate/glenosphere divides a spur (below the line) form notching (above the line).

Factors influencing inferior notching

Position of the glenosphere [4] : In an vitro study the effect of glenoid component positioning on glenohumeral range of motion was assessed in shoulder specimens. Of the four different positions of the glenosphere tested the position with the glenosphere extending beyond the inferior glenoid rim (configuration 3) had significantly improved adduction and abduction angles compared with all other test configurations (fig. 2).

Angle between glenosphere and scapular neck [5] : The angle between the glenosphere and the scapular neck is highly correlated with inferior notching. A notching index can be calculated with use of the height of implantation of the glenosphere and the postoperative prosthesis-scapular neck angle (fig. 3). This allows prediction of the occurrence of notching with a high sensitivity and specificity.

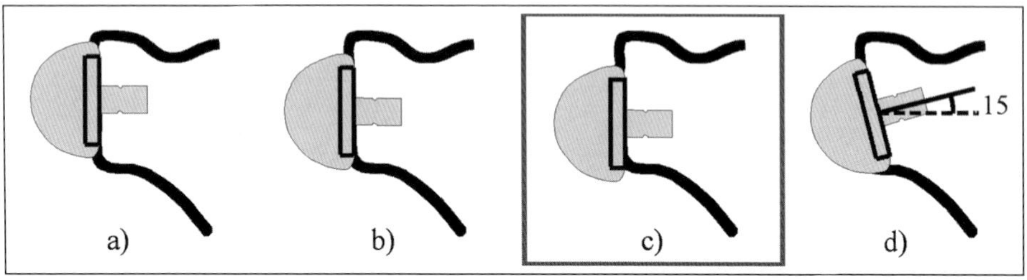

Fig. 2: Position 3 (red frame) with the baseplate flush with the inferior glenoid leading to an inferior overhang of the glenosphere is ideal.

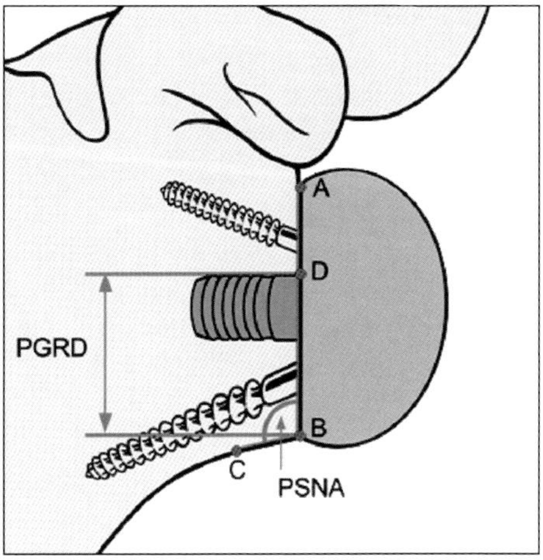

Fig. 3: The prosthesis scapular neck angle (PSNA) is the angle between the line A/B and B/C. The peg glenoid rim distance (PGRD) is the distance between D and B.

The height/position of implantation of the glenosphere has approximately an eight times greater influence on inferior notching than the prosthesis scapular neck angle (fig. 4).

Scapular notching and its impact on clinical outcome

The influence of inferior glenoid notching on the clinical outcome is not yet clear. In our own reported series [5] 77 consecutive shoulders with an irreparable rotator cuff defi-ciency managed with a reverse Delta III shoulder arthroplasty were reviewed after a minimum of 24 months. All shoulders that had development of inferior notching (34 shoulders or 44%) did so in the first fourteen months. The angle between the glenosphere and the

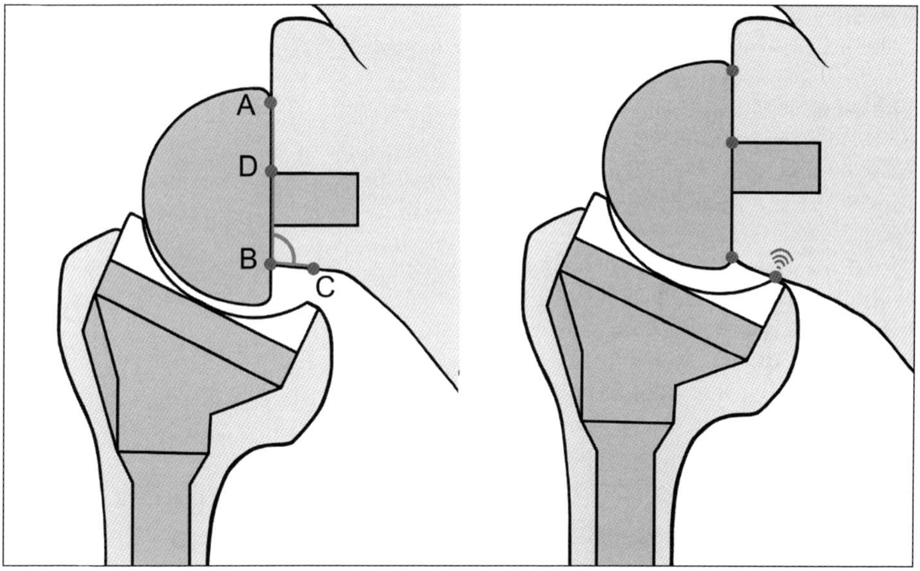

Fig. 4: A short PGRD and a small PSNA (left) has less risk for notching than a long PGRD and larger PSNA (right).

scapular neck (PSNA) ($r = 0.667$) as well as the craniocaudal position of the glenosphere (PGRD) ($r = 0.654$) were highly correlated with inferior notching ($p<0.001$) and inferior scapular notching was associated with a significantly poorer clinical outcome. Therefore it seems that inferior scapular notching after reverse total shoulder arthroplasty adversely affects the intermediate-term clinical outcome. It can be prevented by optimal positioning of the glenoid component.

In a multicentre study Sirveaux *et al.* [3] have also found a negative effect of scapular notching on clinical outcome with a significant negative influence of grades 3 and 4 on the Constant score. They reviewed 80 shoulders at a mean follow-up of 44 months after reversed shoulder prosthesis.

However, no effect on clinical outcome was noted on a midterm follow-up in a multicentre study reported by Lévigne *et al.* [6]. The causes and consequences of scapular notching after reverse shoulder arthroplasty were investigated in 337 consecutive shoulders. Scapular notching was a frequent finding, the first radiographic signs generally appeared within the first months and at last follow-up of 47 months 62% had scapular notching. Notching frequency and extension were correlated to the length of follow-up. Patients with high positioning of the baseplate and superior (upward) tilting of the glenosphere were more at risk for notching.

Summary and outlook

Inferior scapular notching is frequently found after reverse total shoulder arthroplasty and may ultimately lead to loosening of the glenoid component. However, inferior scapular notching does not seem to be ultimately correlated to clinical outcome and glenoid component failure. Although, inferior notching usually starts early after the operation it does not seem to progress uniformly and consistently over time and does necessarily compromise glenoid stability in all instances.

Several factors may reduce the incidence of inferior notching. In terms of prosthetic design a glenoid head which is at least hemispherical and a shallow socket/inlay should be more beneficial. Inferior positioning of the glenosphere seems to be ideal. Although, from a biomechanical point of view an inclinated glenosphere is better than an upward tilted glenosphere, excessive reaming of the inferior glenoid to increase inclination of the gleno-sphere should be avoided; the quality (subchondral bone) and quantity (diameter) of the inferior glenoid is of great importance for optimal component stability. Lateralisation of the centre of rotation with a bony increased offset (BIO-RSA) [7] may reduce notching.

However, even with optimal design and technique complete elimination of inferior notching is probably not realistic due to the specific biomechanical and design principles of a reversed prosthesis. Furthermore, other factors may contribute to the development of inferior notching such as individual or specific motion-sequences, especially in the scapulothoracic joint, independent of the prosthesis design and the implantation technique.

REFERENCES

[1] GRAMMONT PM, BAULOT E. Delta shoulder prosthesis for rotator cuff rupture. *Orthopedics 1993; 16: 65-8.*

[2] WERNER CM, STEINMANN PA, GILBART M, GERBER C. Treatment of painful pseudoparesis due to irreparable rotator cuff dysfunction with the Delta III reverse-ball-and-socket total shoulder prosthesis. *J Bone Joint Surg Am 2005;87: 1476-86.*

[3] SIRVEAUX F, FAVARD L, OUDET D, HUQUET D, WALCH G, MOLE D. Grammont inverted total shoulder arthroplasty in the treatment of glenohumeral osteoarthritis with massive rupture of the cuff. Results of a multicentre study of 80 shoulders. *J Bone Joint Surg Br 2004;86: 388-95.*

[4] NYFFELER RW, WERNER CM, GERBER C. Biomechanical relevance of glenoid component positioning in the reverse Delta III total shoulder prosthesis. *J Shoulder Elbow Surg 2005;14: 524-8.*

[5] SIMOVITCH RW, ZUMSTEIN MA, LOHRI E, HELMY N, GERBER C. Predictors of scapular notching in patients managed with the Delta III reverse total shoulder replacement. *J Bone Joint Surg Am 2007;89: 588-600.*

[6] LEVIGNE C, BOILEAU P, FAVARD L *et al.* Scapular notching in reverse shoulder arthro-plasty. *J Shoulder Elbow Surg 2008;17: 925-35 Epub 2008 Jun 16.*

[7] BOILEAU P, ROUSSANNE Y, BICKNELL R, BRASSART N, CHUINARD C. Bony increased-offset reverse shoulder arthroplasty (BIO-RSA). In: Boileau P, ed. Shoulder concepts 2008 Ar-throscopy & arthroplasty. *Montpellier: Sauramps médical; 2008.*

BIOMECHANICS OF REVERSE SHOULDER ARTHROPLASTY

M. WALKER, M. WILLIS, J. BROOKS, M. FRANKLE

ABSTRACT

The management of patients suffering from pain and decreased function as a result of rotator cuff dysfunction continues to evolve. Improvements in our diagnostic techniques have allowed us to describe a wide array of pathology related to rotator cuff disease and how it can produce a spectrum of symptomatology in our patients. More complete understanding of the biomechanics of the rotator cuff deficient shoulder has helped facilitate improved treatment options. Historically, hemiarthroplasty was the treatment of choice for rotator cuff deficient shoulders and for advanced rotator cuff arthropathy; however, results for this procedure have been unpredictable at best. Over the last three decades, reverse total shoulder arthroplasty has been introduced to help treat the cuff deficient shoulder, and has achieved reliable improvement in both pain and function. Initial designs were based mostly on theory, with little scientific evidence to support the design rationale. As such, several of these initial designs failed for various reasons. An improved understanding of the biomechanics of rotator cuff deficiency and reverse shoulder arthroplasty has facilitated the development of modern reverse arthroplasty designs. Based on sound biomechanical data, these improvements have helped overcome many of the mechanical failures of early designs. By advancing our understanding of the basic science and biomechanics of these implants, we aim to continue to improve in implant function and clinical results. This paper outlines the current understanding of the rotator cuff deficient shoulder and the reverse shoulder arthroplasty focusing both on scientific data and how the biomechanics of the shoulder relate to these topics.

HISTORICAL PERSPECTIVE

The term 'cuff tear arthropathy' (CTA) was first coined by Neer in 1983 to describe patients with massive rotator cuff tears in addition to various structural changes in the glenohumeral joint [50]. He observed joint changes such as superior displacement of the humerus, femoralization of the greater tuberosity, and acetabularization of the coracoacromial arch (fig. 1). Since his original description of CTA, it has been noted that rotator cuff dysfunction leads to a wide spectrum of glenohumeral joint disease (fig. 2). The basic pathology involves glenohumeral instability resulting from unbalanced dynamic forces across the joint; the spectrum of disease can involve severe glenoid and humeral sided wear, often in eccentric patterns. The initial surgical treatment advocated by Neer included hemiarthroplasty. However, subsequent published literature revealed that hemiarthroplasty for CTA had unpredictable and often poor results [11, 20, 50, 51, 56, 58, 66, 67].

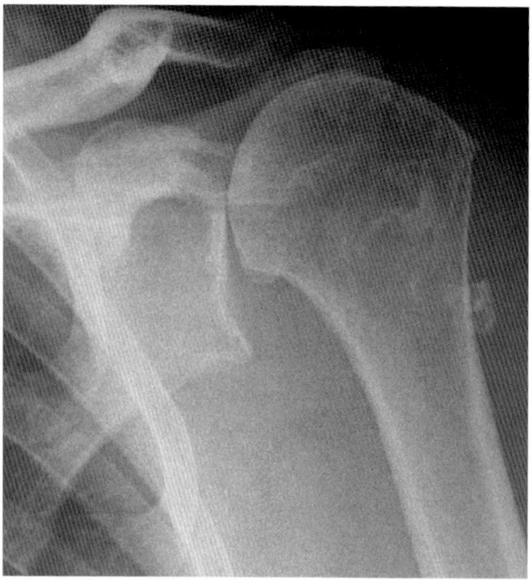

Fig. 1: True AP (Grashey View) of a shoulder with cuff tear arthropathy. The film demonstrates glenohumeral arthritis, superior glenoid wear, proximal humeral migration, and acetabularization of the acromion

Reverse design total shoulder arthroplasty was developed to address the need for a treatment with better clinical outcomes and more predictable functional results for the treatment of CTA. Initial designs (Fenlin, Gerard, Kessel, Kolbel, Liverpool, Neer, and Avery II) (fig. 3) utilized constrained devices that had high rates of clinical failure. These failures were likely related to their inability to withstand forces at the glenosphere-bone junction during attempted shoulder motion [2, 55]. These early failures lead to the development of a semi-constrained

Fig. 2: The spectrum of disease seen in rotator cuff tear arthropathy
Found in: LEVY JC. The spectrum of disease in the rotator cuff-deficient shoulder. In: Frankle MA, editor. Rotator cuff deficiency of the shoulder. *New York: Thieme Medical Publishers; 2008. p. 147-70.*

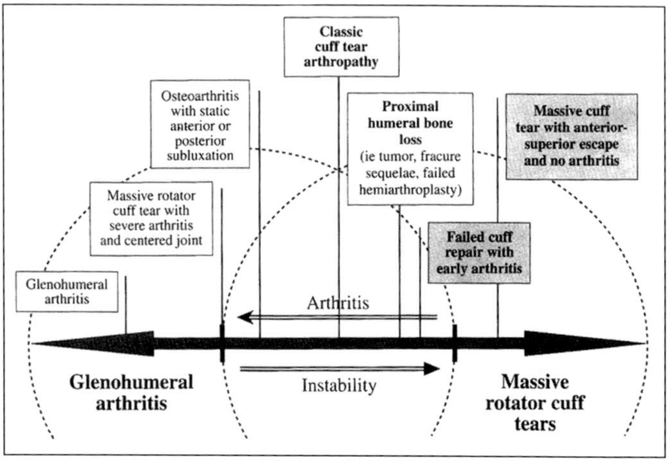

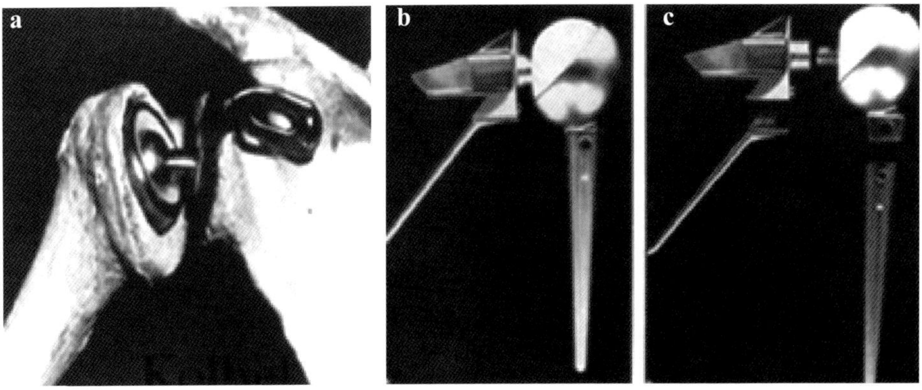

Fig. 3: Early reverse total shoulder arthroplasty designs include the Kolbel (a) and Fenlin (b,c).

reverse prosthesis by Paul Grammont in 1985 (fig. 4). The initial design employed a cemented humeral and glenoid component. Over time, this was subsequently modified and evolved in 1991 to the Delta III prosthesis, which used a large glenosphere (36 or 42mm) and a humeral component with a neck-shaft angle of 155 degrees (Fig. 4) (Depuy International Ltd., Warsaw, IN, USA) [30]. Initial clinical results of this prosthesis were very promising, with two year follow-up showing significant decreases in pain and improvement in clinical function in all 13 patients treated by Grammont [30]. These results were confirmed by Boulahia et al., who evaluated 16 patients and reported outcomes as good or excellent for all [8].

Biomechanically, the design of the Delta III was designed to transfer the center of rotation of the humerus medially and to lengthen the humerus. The theory was that by lengthening the humerus, the deltoid muscle would be placed on stretch, allowing for compression between the humerosocket and glenosphere and subsequently stabilizing the prosthetic articulation. Furthermore, medializing the glenoid center of rotation could allow for enhanced recruitment of deltoid muscle fibers; this in combination with humeral lengthening would allow for a more efficient deltoid lever arm [50]. Additionally, it was felt that a humeral center of rotation located as close as possible to the bone-glenosphere junction would decrease baseplate loosening and the failure seen in previous designs [7].

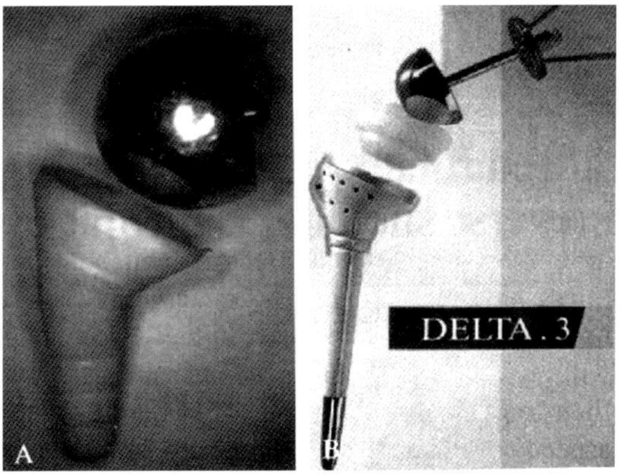

Fig. 4: A. Grammont's original reverse arthroplasty design. B. The Delta 3 reverse arthroplasty

Found in: KLEIN S, LEVY J, HOLCOMB J, PUPELLO D, FRANKLE M. Treatment of advanced rotator cuff dysfunction with reverse shoulder arthroplasty. *Minerva Ortop Traumatol 2009;60: 29-46.*

Despite the excellent clinical outcomes reported with the Delta III, several problems remain with this device. First, mechanical impingement between the medial aspect of the humeral component and the inferior scapula, or inferior scapular notching, is often observed. In fact, this is one of the most commonly reported problems with reverse shoulder arthroplasty and has been reported in several series ranging from 24.5 to 96% of cases [7, 65]. Second, the clinical results of the device revealed limitations in external rotation, prompting several authors to consider muscle transfers in an effort to restore external rotation [4, 5, 19, 28, 29, 64]. Finally, by medializing and moving the humerus distally, patients note a loss of the normal deltoid contour. This not only leads to cosmetic concerns, but may have the effect of decreasing the deltoid efficiency. This may also lead to a prosthetic design with less inherent stability [27]. Recognition of these problems lead to clinical and basic science studies aimed at improving the surgical technique and design of reverse shoulder arthroplasty.

In this paper, we review the basic biomechanical challenges associated with the rotator cuff deficient shoulder and the biomechanical rational for newer designs aimed at reducing complications related to reverse shoulder arthroplasty. We will review the current scientific evidence related to the function of reverse shoulder arthroplasty as well as factors which affect performance in patients undergoing reverse shoulder arthroplasty. Initially we will review basic shoulder biomechanics, then move to discussion of general aspects of total joint arthroplasty, and finally examine specific aspects of reverse shoulder arthroplasty including glenoid baseplate (metaglene) fixation, glenoid component position, glenohumeral stability, glenohumeral range of motion (ROM) and muscle function about the shoulder treated with a reverse prosthesis.

SHOULDER BIOMECHANICS: THE BASICS OF NORMAL AND CUFF DEFICIENT SHOULDERS

A normal shoulder works by balancing the proximal pull of the deltoid with the compressive force that the rotator cuff provides between the humeral head and the glenoid. This allows for a smooth range of motion of the shoulder and minimal translational movements of the glenohumeral joint. Matsen referred to this concept as concavity-compression [46]. In general terms, Matsen described this concept as a ball sitting in the concavity of a table [48]. The greater the depth of the concavity, the greater a displacing force must be to dislodge the ball for a given compressive load (fig. 5). In the normal shoulder, the rotator cuff muscles provide the compressive load to center the humeral head on the glenoid. These compressive forces are lost in the rotator cuff deficient shoulder, meaning that the primary problem of this pathology is one of inherent instability resulting from unbalanced muscle forces in the glenohumeral joint. With rotator cuff deficiency, the deltoid tends to pull the humerus proximally, leading to glenohumeral instability (fig. 6). In this case, the humeral head can migrate into the subacromial space. This can lead to changes in glenoid morphology, arthritis, and decreased motion from shortening of the deltoid and loss of the normal fulcrum for shoulder movement.

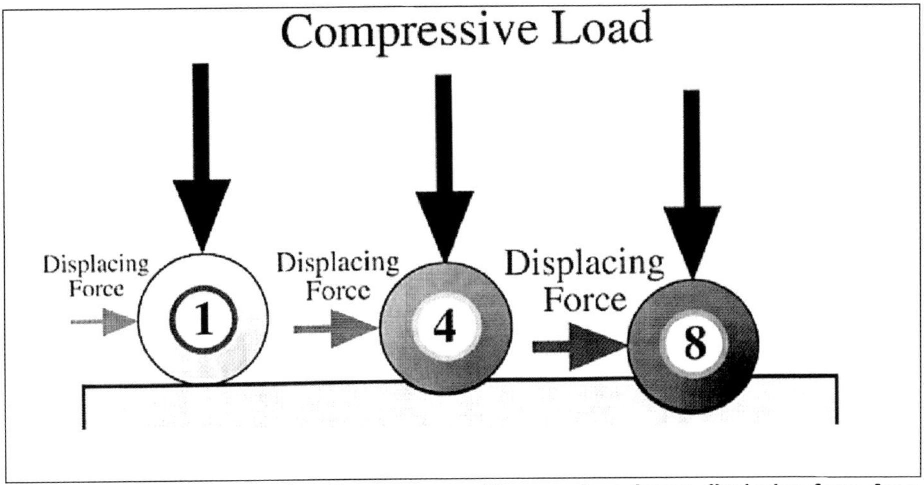

Fig. 5: Concavity-compression. Deeper concavities require a larger displacing force for a given compressive load.

Found in: MATSEN FA 3rd, LIPPITT SB. Principles of Glenohumeral stability. In: Matsen FA 3rd, Lippitt SB, DeBartolo SE. Shoulder surgery: principles and procedures. *Philadelphia: Saunders: 2004. p 83.*

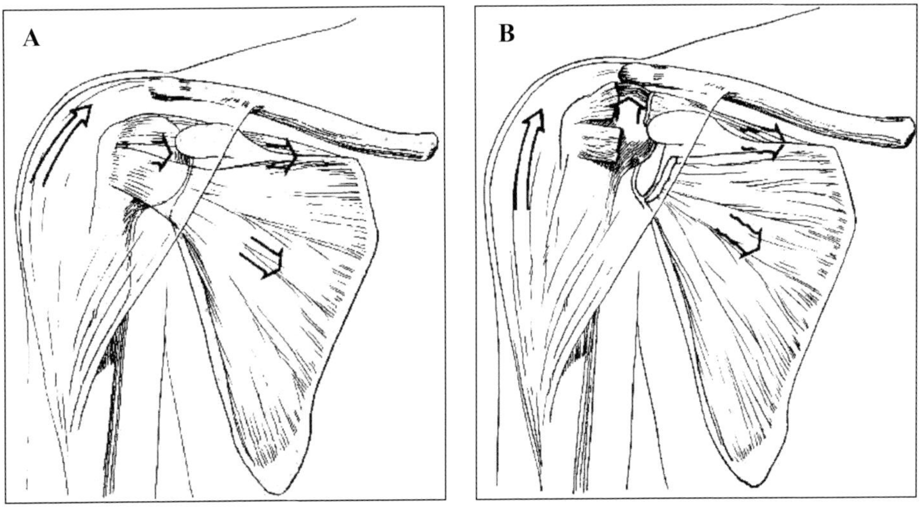

Fig. 6:
A) A normal shoulder showing the balance between the proximal pull of the deltoid and the compressive force provided by the rotator cuff muscles.
B) Loss of the rotator cuff musculature leads to instability in the shoulder joint from the unbalanced proximal pull of the deltoid.

Although treatment of patients with rotator cuff deficiency has focused on those patients with complete loss of the rotator cuff function, as with other disease processes, there exists a spectrum of pathological entities with various clinical presentations. Recognition of pathology beyond the deficient rotator cuff is thus essential in determining the proper treatment. One must evaluate the articular surface, ligamentous stability, soft-tissue compliancy, and peri-scapular musculature in conjunction with the degree of rotator cuff disease. Patients with capsular insufficiency, eccentric bone deficiency, and static or dynamic instability all may have varying degrees of rotator cuff deficiency. In these cases, selection of a conventional total shoulder arthroplasty is likely to have poor results.

Another biomechanical point proposed by Matsen is the concept of the glenoid center line [49]. In a normal glenoid, the center line represents a line perpendicular to the articular surface of the glenoid and directed, on average, approximately 10 degrees posterior (retroverted) to the plane of the scapula (fig. 7). The center line serves as the pillar under which the humeral head rests; glenohumeral and scapulothorasic motion are coupled to maintain the centerline beneath the humeral head throughout the shoulder's range of motion. In the rotator cuff deficient shoulder, unbalanced muscular forces disrupt this relationship of the humeral head to the glenoid center line, making this an important concept in reverse shoulder arthroplasty. The morphology of the glenoid can be highly variable in cuff deficient shoulders. Wear patterns on the glenoid can consist of no wear, superior, inferior, anterior, posterior, or global wear [25]. Abnormal wear patterns are likely due to the altered biomechanical and biochemical environment of the cuff deficient shoulder and often result in eccentric wear patterns on the glenoid [17, 50, 62]. The spectrum of disease can be quite varied; some patients have a loss of stability of such a degree, that the humerus is "disassociated" from the glenoid. Loss of the CA ligament can cause the humeral head to escape from the coracoacromial arch. In this situation there may be no articular cartilage loss because there is no longer contact between the humeral head and the glenoid. However, some patients can have less obvious loss of containment of the humeral head; the resulting instability can lead to articular erosion in eccentric positions. These patients tend to present with a greater degree of soft tissue contracture and asymmetric glenoid wear. Finally, a subset of patients have cuff deficiency that may result from an inflammatory disease, either crystalline arthropathy (Milwaukee shoulder) or rheumatoid disease. These patients often have central (or global) erosion of the glenoid with variable of amounts of stiffness or instability. These different wear patterns can make glenoid component placement difficult in reverse shoulder arthroplasty and recognizing them is critical. Identification of these patterns can assist in proper preoperative planning. Ideally, the glenoid

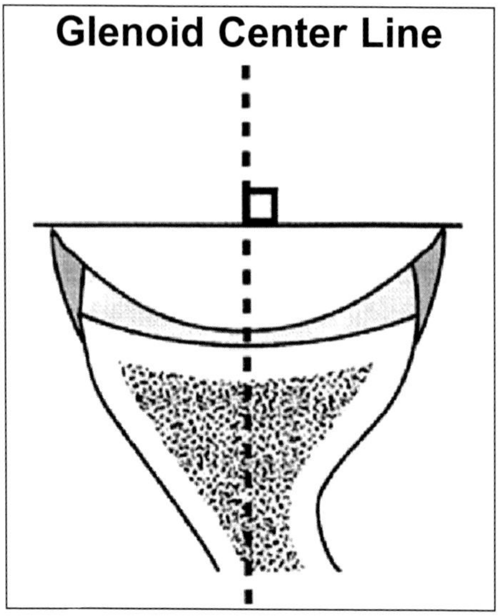

Fig. 7: The glenoid center line. This is a line perpendicular to the glenoid face.

Found in: MATSEN FA 3rd, LIPPITT SB. Principles of Glenohumeral stability. In: Matsen FA 3rd, Lippitt SB, DeBartolo SE. Shoulder surgery: principles and procedures. *Philadelphia: Saunders: 2004. p 89.*

component is placed along the glenoid centerline; this is the area that reproduces the normal version of the glenoid and allows for a stable and strong column of bone beneath the implant. Further, this is the vector through which a stable gleno-humeral relationship can be reproduced. However, in some cases, component placement in line with the glenoid center line is not possible due to glenoid bone deficiency. In cases of severe or eccentric glenoid wear, stable baseplate fixation can only be achieved by placing the component along the alternate glenoid center line (fig. 8) [25]. This alternate center line is defined as a line aiming at the dense bone where the scapular spine meets the body of the scapula, and is not necessarily perpendicular to the remaining glenoid face. The concept is to provide an ade-

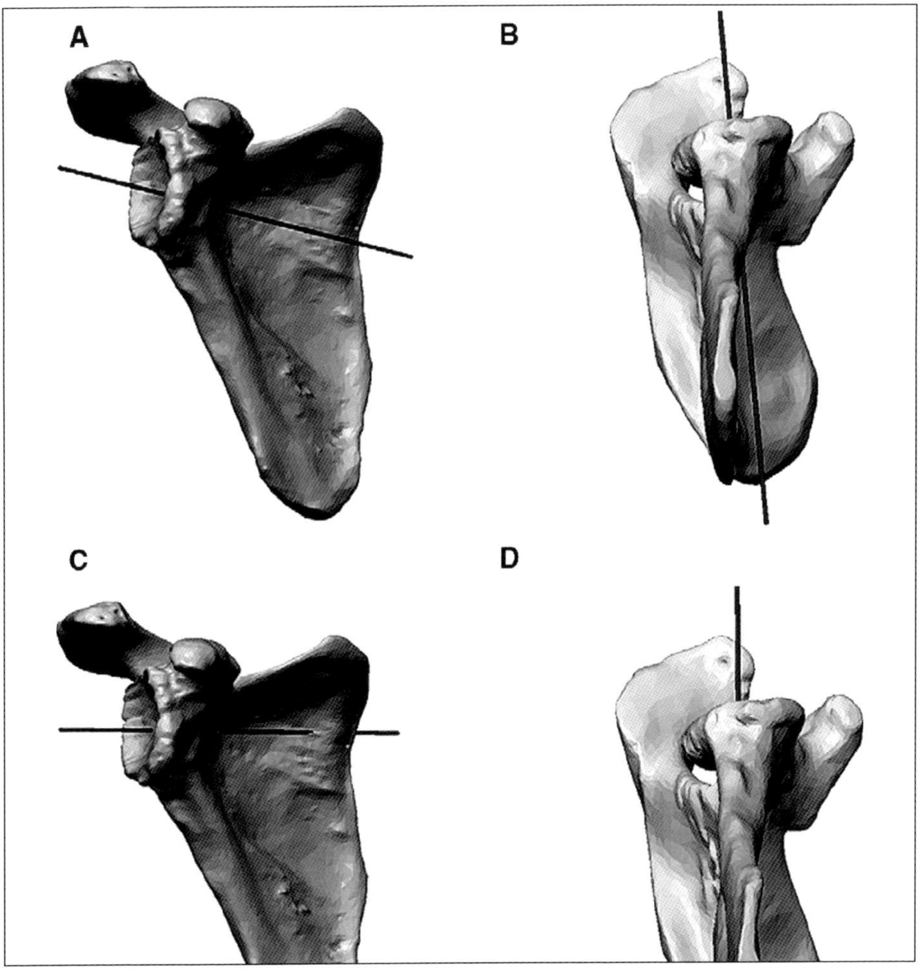

Fig. 8: A and B - Computer model demonstrating the glenoid center line.
C and D - Computer model demonstrating the alternate center line along the scapular spine

Found in: FRANKLE MA, TERAMOTO S, ZONG-PING LUO, LEVY J, PUPELLO D. Glenoid morphology in reverse shoulder arthroplasty: Classification and surgical implications. *J Shoulder Elbow Surg 2009 (18), 874-85.*

quate column of bone to achieve stability for baseplate fixation. Understanding the center line in the cuff deficient shoulder with little glenoid wear can provide excellent fixation for the glenoid baseplate in reverse arthroplasty; knowing what glenoid wear patterns make the centerline unusable allows surgeons to compensate for bone loss by achieving adequate fixation along the alternate centerline.

Another important alteration from normal shoulder mechanics seen in the cuff deficient shoulder involves the concept of impingement. This can occur between the greater tuberosity and the acromion and lead to acromial erosion or "acetabularization." In patients who have lost the dynamic stabilizers of the rotator cuff muscles, the humeral head migrates superiorly and leads to abutment underneath the acromion (fig. 1). Since instability is the main mechanical alteration in allowing impingement, methods to decompress the impingement (such as bony subacromial decompression) will ultimately be ineffective. In these cases, use of a fixed-fulcrum prosthesis such as a reverse can neutralize this dynamic instability.

TOTAL JOINT ARTHROPLASTY: THE BASICS

Basic principles of total joint arthroplasty, learned mostly from the total hip literature, can provide a conceptual framework to improve understanding of reverse shoulder arthroplasty. The key concepts relate to component fixation and prosthetic impingement.

Fixation in total joint arthroplasty has undergone considerable changes since Charnley introduced the total hip arthroplasty. Initial implants were fixed with cement, and this continues to be used with high frequency in certain situations. Cement provides initial stable prosthetic attachment by acting as a grout. However, long term failure of the cement-bone or cement-prosthetic interface is possible. As a result, the concept of osteointegration was introduced. In this case, coating the implants with certain materials or roughening the surface to allow the bone to ingrow or ongrow to the prosthesis could theoretically provide a longer lasting attachment and a decreased incidence of mechanical failure. Optimal bone ingrowth requires initial stable attachment of the prosthesis to the bone with micromotion at the bone-prosthetic interface of less then 150 microns and a surface with properties to allow osseous healing [41]. The optimal surface characteristics depend on the type of coating used, the porosity of the material (typically 65-80% for most orthopaedic applications), and optimal surface roughness of the coating [3].

Currently available reverse shoulder designs use a combination of cement for diaphyseal fixation of the humeral component, and a proximal coating for metaphyseal osseointegration. Individual implants vary on the extent of proximal porous coating. For example, the coating on the DJO, Zimmer Anatomical, Exactech Equinox, Affinis Inverse and the Universal Arrow System tends to be very light; the coating on the Lima SMR, Zimmer Trabecular and the Biomet Comprehensive is much heavier; all of these use cement distally. Other implants (DePuy and Tornier) rely solely on cement for fixation. It is important to note, though, that relatively little biomechanical or clinical data exists for humeral fixation in reverse shoulder arthroplasty. Previous work on humeral stem fixation in an anatomic stem suggested that both proximal and fully cemented humeral stems offer decreased micromotion and enhanced rotational stability when compared to a press fit technique [38]. Forces placed on the humeral component of the reverse shoulder arthroplasty may in fact be quite different.

Preliminary work on humeral component fixation using the reverse arthroplasty model suggested that proximal humeral bone loss could diminish humeral fixation in cemented humeral stems [35]. Additionally, modularity on the humeral side exacerbates the effect of humeral bone loss, as forces tend to be transmitted directly to the modular interface, resulting in an early failure point.

Glenoid fixation in reverse arthroplasty universally utilizes cementless techniques. Various fixation methods have been employed to achieve a stable attachment; in essence these involve either a press fit peg with peripheral screw fixation (Zimmer Anatomical, Exactech Equinox, Affinis Inverse, Universal Arrow System, Lima SMR, Zimmer Trabecular, DePuy Delta III, DePuy Delta Xtend, Tornier), or a central screw with peripheral screw fixation (DJO and Biomet Comprehensive). Most of these baseplate designs also have a coated backside with either a flat or concave surface for ingrowth or ongrowth as well as a variable configuration of peripheral screws for further stabilization. The goal on the glenoid side is to prevent micromotion and allow for bony ongrowth in order to decrease glenoid failure rates. Often, this is achieved by the basic AO principles of bone healing: compression and neutralization. Compression is achieved through either a central axis screw or peripheral unlocked screws. Once the baseplate is properly compressed to the glenoid bone, forces can be neutralized with locking screws, thereby minimizing micromotion [37].

Prosthetic impingement has been identified as an important method of failure in total hip arthroplasty. Impingement has been implicated in the production of prosthetic wear particles, a reduction in joint motion, and persistent pain and even prosthetic dislocation. This is often a result of improper component position or prosthetic selection. Positioning of the components in total joint arthroplasty is of utmost importance for several reasons. First, optimal positioning can avoid instability by providing patients with a functional range of motion within their native range [12]. Second, positioning can be optimized to avoid impingement. Impingement is a noted cause of polyethylene wear and component failure after total hip arthroplasty [47]. Impingement is also a noted clinical finding and complication in reverse shoulder arthroplasty that can be decreased by optimizing component positioning and prosthetic design. Impingement between the humerosocket and the inferior lateral scapular pillar results in the radiographic appearance of erosion of bone along the inferior scapular neck. This phenomenon, termed scapular notching, has been shown to result in inferior scapular wear, osteolysis, and polyethylene wear [55]. Impingement in reverse arthroplasty may also contribute to prosthetic instability, unexplained pain, and long term prosthetic loosening. Finally, component position is important to restore the function of the surrounding musculature of the joint. In total hip replacements this has been shown to be a reason for postoperative dislocation [16]; these concerns are also present in reverse shoulder arthroplasty.

GLENOID BASEPLATE (METAGLENE) FIXATION

In order to achieve secure fixation to the glenoid, it is important that the baseplate be well fixed to the highest quality bone available. Furthermore, the fixation must be stable enough to allow for osseous integration. Failure at the glenoid baseplate and has been attributed to the inability of the baseplate fixation to overcome the forces imparted to the interface prior to adequate bony ingrowth [23]. Chebli *et al.* emphasized the importance of glenoid fixation and peripheral screw placement into the highest quality glenoid bone stock [10]. This bone stock can be found in the three major columns of scapular bone, as described by Humphrey *et al.* They emphasize placing peripheral screws into either the base of the coracoid, the spine of the scapula, or the scapular pillar [40]. Both groups emphasize the importance of bone quality for optimal screw placement and suggest that screw purchase into good bone may reduce the incidence of failure at the bone-baseplate interface. However, due to the varied spectrum of disease seen in CTA, these optimal locations are not always readily available for prosthetic fixation. Pathologic changes in the glenoid often develop in the setting of rotator cuff deficiency.

Analysis of glenoid morphology in patients treated with reverse arthroplasty has helped to better understand these anatomical variations. Using a series of 216 glenoids which required reverse shoulder arthroplasty, Frankle *et al.* observed 62.5 percent of patients have a normal glenoid morphology [25]. In the setting of a normal glenoid, the anatomic center line can be used to provide glenoid baseplate fixation. Alternatively, 37.5 percent of glenoids had abnormal glenoid morphology, with eccentric bone loss either posteriorly (17.6%), superiorly (9.3%), anteriorly (4.2%), or globally (6.5%). In the setting of abnormal glenoid morphology, the anatomic center line could not provide optimal glenoid fixation and in this case the alternate center line was used.

Bone growth into or onto the prosthesis is the ultimate goal and can provide durable attachment of the component to the bone. To achieve bony ingrowth using a cementless prosthesis it is important to minimize micromotion to less than 150 micrometers (um) [41]. Hopkins *et al.* noted that micromotion between the baseplate and glenoid could be decreased by changing design factors of the prosthesis and altering the placement of peripheral screws. They showed that increasing the length, diameter, and inclination of the peripheral screws all decreased the micromotion in a reverse shoulder model [39]. Further, they showed that micromotion increases if the stiffness of the surrounding bone decreases, as in poor quality or osteoporotic bone [39].

It is possible to apply the basic principals of bone healing to enhance bony ingrowth to the baseplate. As advocated by the Association for the Study of Internal Fixation (ASIF), bone heals best in compression. All reverse designs advocate compression of the baseplate to the glenoid bone. This compression can be established by central axis or peripheral screws. For example, the DJO RSP utilizes a central lag screw to facilitate compression of the baseplate (fig. 9), while the Depuy Delta III establishes compression via a central post and peripheral

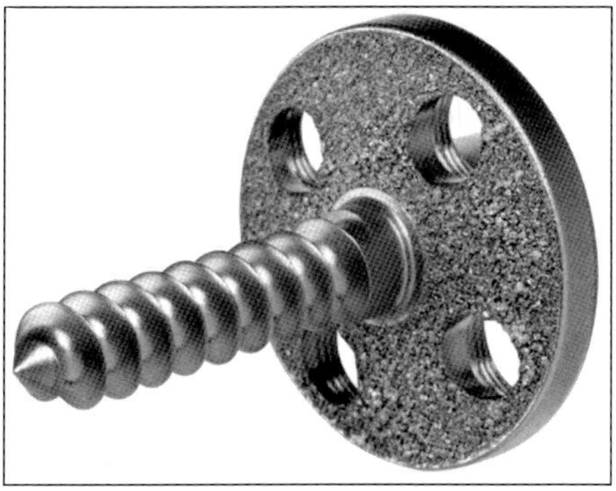

Fig. 9: Central 6.5 mm lag screw of the DJO RSP.

screws. These two designs were compared to evaluate the amount of compression achieved. A ten-fold difference was observed between the DJO RSP (2000N) and the Delta III (200N) [21].

Additionally, using a load-to-failure model, the central screw design was compared to the central post design. A 2.3 fold increase in load-to-failure was observed between the central screw (629 N) and the central post (269 N) [21].

While fixation with a central screw demonstrated promise in the lab, early clinical results using a central 6.5 mm lag screw in combination with 3.5 mm peripheral non-locked screws for glenoid fixation of a laterally offset glenosphere showed an initial high glenoid failure rate of approximately 10% [23]. Further analysis of these failures using Scanning Electron Microscopy (SEM) revealed a failure of bone ingrowth between the baseplate and the glenoid bone. These early clinical glenoid-sided failures prompted further analysis of glenoid component fixation. In a study of construct stiffness, Harmen et al evaluated different baseplate constructs using locked (5.0 mm) and unlocked screw (3.5 mm) combinations. Baseplates fixed with 5.0 mm locked screws were observed to have 29% less micromotion than those fixed with 3.5mm unlocked screws [37]. A subsequent clinical study using locked 5.0 mm peripheral screws showed that glenoid failure was reduced to 0.4% [13].

GLENOID POSITION

Optimal positioning of the glenoid component is currently an area of active research. Several different glenoid designs have been introduced and are currently available from different manufacturers. These range from glenoids with a glenohumeral center of rotation at the center of the glenoid baseplate (original Grammont design), to glenoids with eccentrically placed centers of rotation. Eccentric offset designs include lateral offset designs (DJO RSP), inferior offset designs (Depuy Xtend, Exactech), and variable offset designs (Biomet). Several basic science studies have been performed to determine the biomechanical forces on the glenoid with these different designs and to elucidate the optimal positioning of the glenoid component for these various designs. Studying optimal glenoid position has important consequences for maximizing the impingement free arc of motion.

Grammont believed that glenoid failure was related to the amount of shear stress across the glenoid component, and that simply medializing the center of rotation of the glenosphere to the glenoid face would dramatically reduce this stress. However, initially there was no information available to guide surgeons in optimal positioning of the baseplate on the glenoid in a way that could best minimize these shear stresses. Understanding of how component position can alter glenoid survival was not appreciated until 2006. While analyzing the initial failures of lateral offset reverse arthroplasties implanted with 3.5mm unlocked peripheral screws, it became apparent that they shared a common radiographic appearance of a superiorly tilted glenosphere [24]. This was not surprising, as patients initially treated with reverse shoulder arthroplasty often had superior glenoid wear, and baseplates were thus often implanted at the native glenoid inclination, superiorly tilting the component. Comparing different glenosphere implantation angles (15 degrees of superior tilt, 15 degrees of inferior tilt, and neutral tilt), Gutierrez *et al* demonstrated that inferior tilting the glenopshere 15 degrees, by preferentially reaming the inferior glenoid, resulted in the most uniform compressive forces and the least amount of tensile forces and micromotion [36]. Currently, the effect of baseplate position and distribution of forces across the baseplate-bone interface continues to be an area of active interest.

Gutierrez *et al.* investigated the forces at the baseplate-bone interface for three different glenosphere designs (concentric, lateral eccentric, and inferior eccentric) (fig. 10) placed in three different positions (superior tilt, neutral, and inferior tilt) (fig. 11). In this study a computer simulation was used, based on a previously validated biomechanical study, to evaluate the forces in the above mentioned conditions. The results showed a predictable pattern of forces at the baseplate-bone junction that

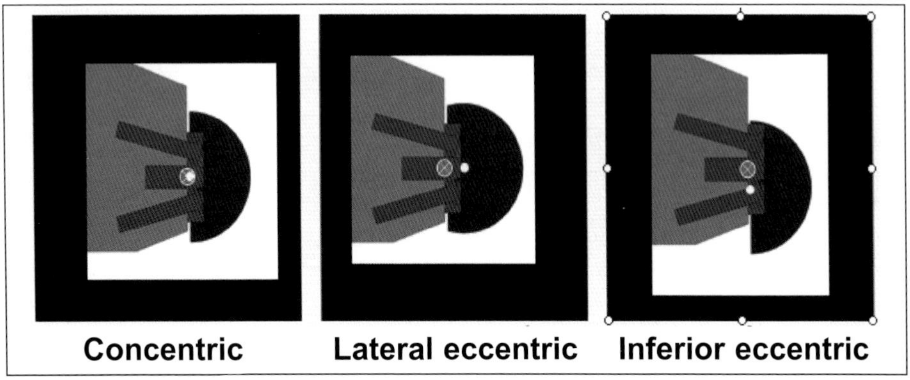

***Fig. 10:** Different glenosphere offsets. Concentric center of rotation: both the center of the baseplate and rotational center are in the same place. Lateral Eccentric center of rotation: The rotational center is lateral to the center of the baseplate. Inferior Eccentric: The rotational center is inferior to the center of the baseplate.*

corresponded with the type of offset used and the tilt in which the glenoid was placed (fig. 12). The most even distribution of forces was seen with a lateralized or concentric center of rotation placed in inferior tilt; the most uneven distribution of forces was seen with either a concentric or lateral center of rotation placed in superior tilt (fig. 13) [36]. Interestingly, those glenospheres with inferior offset demonstrated increasingly uneven forces in inferior tilt as opposed to neutral or even superior tilt.

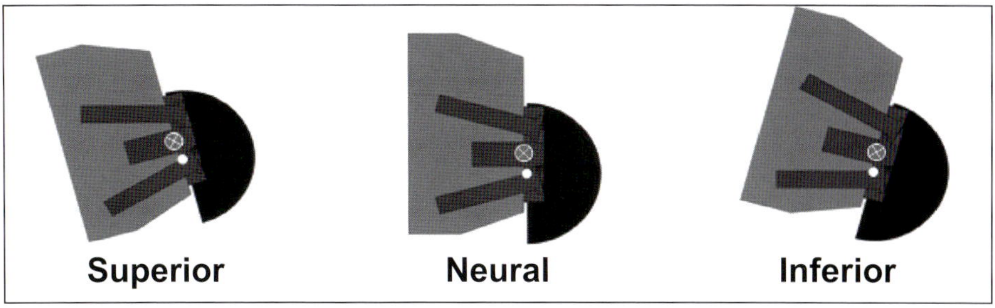

Fig. 11: Example of a glenosphere with an inferior eccentric center of rotation in different positions of glenosphere tilt.

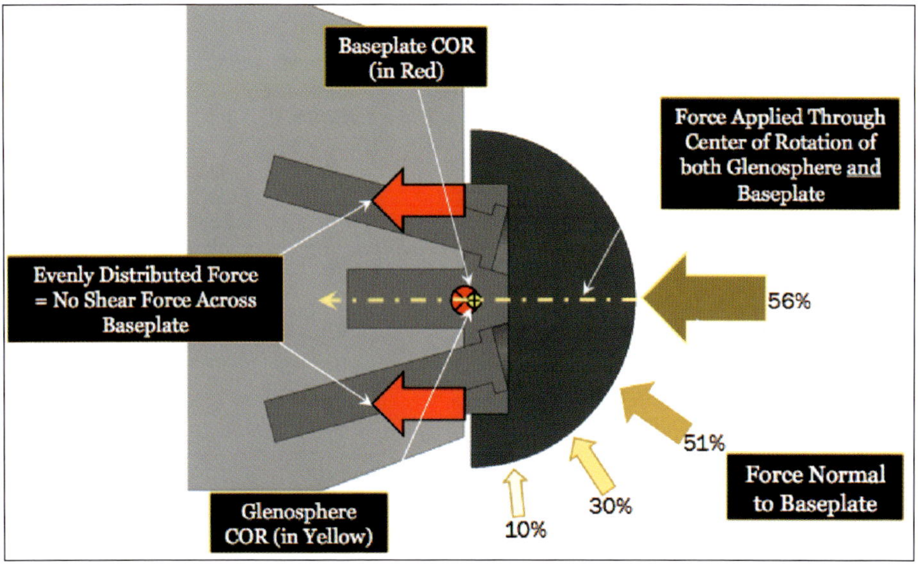

Fig. 12 A: Force distribution for glenospheres with centers of rotation at the glenoid surface (concentric).

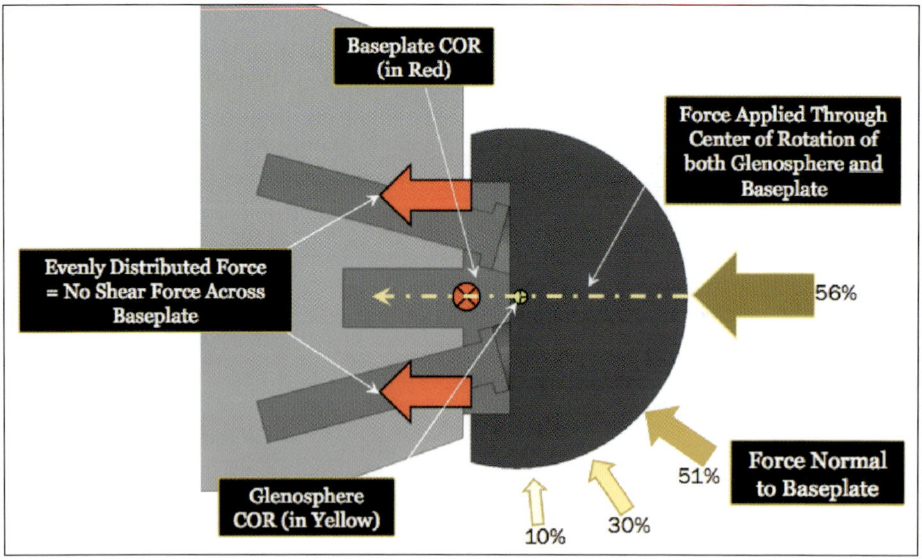

Fig. 12 B: Force distribution for glenospheres with laterally eccentric centers of rotation.

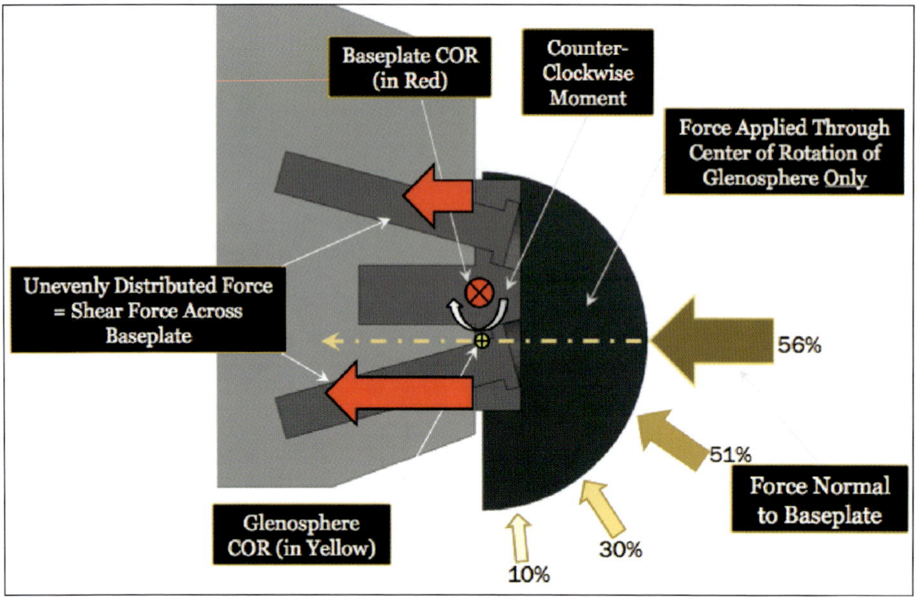

Fig. 12 C: Force distribution for glenospheres with inferiorly eccentric offset

	Glenosphere		Tilt
Most Even Distribution of Forces	Lateral	-	Inferior
↓	Concentric	-	Inferior
	Inferior	-	Neutral
	Inferior	-	Superior
	Concentric	-	Neutral
	Inferior	-	Inferior
	Lateral	-	Neutral
	Concentric	-	Superior
Most Uneven Distribution of Forces	Lateral	-	Superior

Fig. 13: Hierarchy of force distribution seen for different glenosphere eccentricities and tilts. The most even distribution of forces beneath the baseplate was seen with laterally eccentric glenospheres placed in inferior tilt.

STABILITY

If we consider the primary problem with cuff deficient shoulders to be one of a loss of stability of the glenohumeral joint due to the unbalanced pull of the deltoid, then we can understand how design changes can increase the stability of a reverse shoulder arthroplasty. Instability is common after reverse prosthesis, with rates of dislocation reported as high as 30% using the Grammont design [14, 53]. There are several factors that contribute to post-operative instability: soft tissue tension, glenosphere diameter, humeral-socket constraint, impingement, and axillary nerve/deltoid function.

Gutierrez *et al.* evaluated several factors of prosthetic design, including the compressive force on the prosthesis, the prosthetic socket depth, and the glenosphere size [32]. Using several different reverse prosthetic designs the authors evaluated the effect of changing the above variables and how that affected the stability of the prosthesis based on how much translational force (perpendicular to the prosthesis) was required to dislocate the prosthesis. They found a hierarchy of importance among these factors: the most important parameter for achieving stability was increasing the compressive forces on the prosthesis, followed by humerosocket depth. In contrast, glenosphere size was much less important in the stability of reverse shoulder arthroplasty. Further, they developed a mathematical model based on the mechanical data that was collected and validated that a critical determinant in translational stability was the relationship of the diameter of the socket to the diameter of the sphere. They called this the D/R ratio (diameter of the sphere/the radius of the humerosocket). Essentially, this showed that devices with an increased D/R ratio have more inherent stability; or, for the same size ball, a deeper socket would be more stable.

Ultimately, this is a matter of constraint; a deeper humerosocket concavity means a more constrained device that is harder to dislocate [1, 42]. The essence of the D/R ratio rests in the basis of Matsen's theory of concavity-compression [48]. In the native shoulder, Matsen discussed the balance stability angle; this is the maximum "angle that the net force on the humeral head forms with the glenoid centerline before dislocation occurs" [49]. He used this angle to calculate the stability ratio; the ratio of the translational force on the humerus to the compressive normal load on the humeral head (fig. 14). Problematic to prostheses with a deeper socket, however, is a decreased impingement free arc of motion.

Gutierrez *et al.* evaluated the effect of increasing constraint of the prosthesis (by increasing socket depth) on the range of motion of the glenohumeral joint [34]. Using a computer simulation, they found that in the majority of cases, increasing constraint decreased the impingement

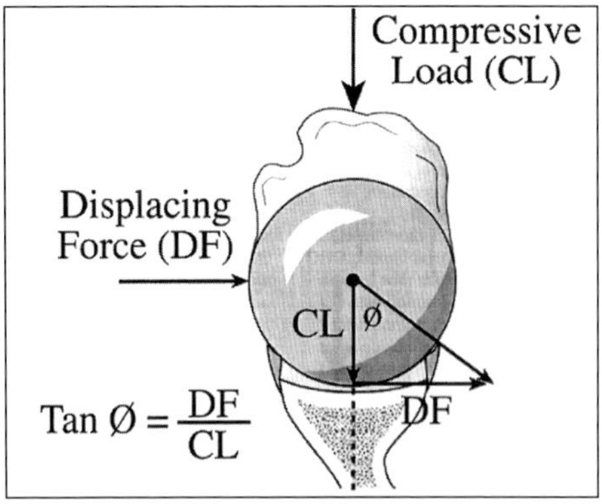

Fig. 14: The balance stability angle. This represents the maximum angle that the net force on the humeral head forms with the glenoid centerline prior to dislocation.

Found in: MATSEN FA 3rd, LIPPITT SB. Principles of Glenohumeral stability. In: Matsen FA 3rd, Lippitt SB, DeBartolo SE. Shoulder surgery: principles and procedures. *Philadelphia: Saunders: 2004. p 108.*

free arc of motion. More complex relationships between constraint and ROM were seen in a minority of the cases; the authors attributed the discrepancies to varying position of the glenosphere.

Clinical prosthetic instability in patients undergoing reverse shoulder arthroplasty is most common in clinical circumstances where there is glenoid or humeral sided bone loss. The loss of boney structures can create a loss of adequate displacement of the muscular envelope reducing compression on the prosthesis. In these cases, prosthetic selection is important and can compensate for these anatomical deficiencies. The restoration of anatomic position of the humerus in terms of the horizontal (lateral) offset of the tuberosity glenoid distance (east – west tension) as well as vertical offset acromial tuberosity distance (north-south tension) seems to provide a guide to restore anatomic soft tissue tension. This can be achieved through a variety of prosthetic design and surgical technique factors. The prosthetic factors include: use of varying glenosphere offset and size, different humeral neck-shaft angles (a varus or valgus humeral component), and varying the thickness of humeral inserts. Additionally, surgical techniques include: altering the level of the humeral osteotomy, offsetting placement of the humero-socket, and changing the placement of the glenosphere. Each of these design or surgical factors can help to re-tension the muscular envelope around the shoulder.

Boileau *et al.* noted that the remaining soft tissues can be tensioned with a Grammont-style device, but the vector of pull is no longer in an anatomic plane once the humerus is significantly elongated [7]. In fact, designs that medialize the center of rotation can place a distracting force on the humeral component in the case of glenoid bone loss, increasing the propensity of dislocation (fig. 15) [52].

An alternative method of establishing stability of the reverse shoulder arthroplasty is by increasing the acromial tuberosity distance (north – south shift) by lengthening the humerus. This can increase compression between the ball and socket and provide a stable reduction [7]. This can be achieved by several surgical and prosthetic adaptations. Placement of the glenosphere with inferior translation and inferior tilt effectively lengthens the humerus. Utilizing an inferiorly eccentric glenosphere, larger glenosphere with inferior overhang, a more valgus humeral neck shaft angle, and humeral augments can have a similar effect on lengthening the humerus. However, this is not without cost. Increasing humeral length carries the additional risk of acromion stress fracture, brachial plexopathy, deltoid over tensioning, and loss of motion.

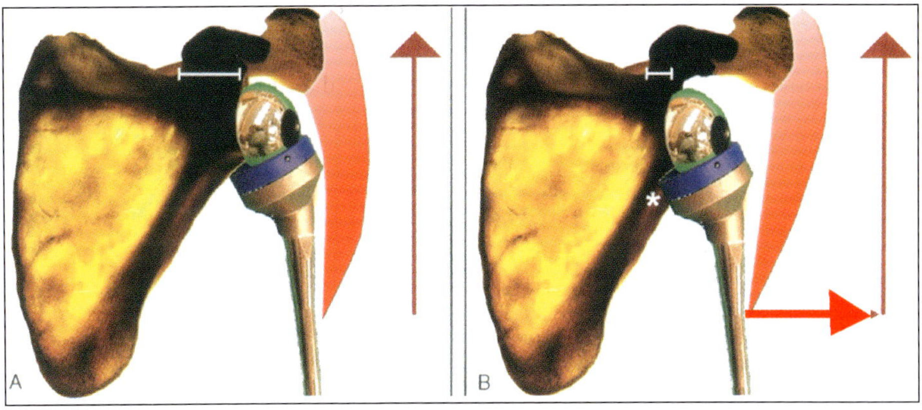

Fig. 15, A and B. A) Devices with lateralized centers of rotation allow the proximal pull of the deltoid to pull the humerus toward the glenosphere, thus increasing the compression and stability of the implant. B) Devices with medialized centers of rotation allow the deltoid to place a distraction moment on the prosthesis and increase the propensity for dislocation.

Found in: NORRIS, TOM R, KELLY, JAMES D. II, HUMPHREY, C. SCOTT. Management of Glenoid Bone Defects in Revision Shoulder Arthroplasty: A New Application of the Reverse Total Shoulder Prosthesis. *Techniques in Shoulder & Elbow Surgery. 8(1): 37-46, March 2007.*

Alternatively, an increase in compressive force across the glenohumeral joint can also be achieved by increasing the glenoid tuberosity distance (east – west shift). In this case, technique and design changes include: placement of a glenosphere with a greater lateral offset from the glenoid, using a more varus humeral component, and translating the humeral component so that the intramedullary stem is lateral to the socket. Potential problems with increasing the glenoid tuberosity distance may include greater component or boney impingement.

Freilich *et al.* evaluated the changes in capsular volume as well as vertical and horizontal shift of the humerus using several implant designs and several glenosphere and humerosocket sizes [26]. Their assumptions were that different reverse designs will be better suited to different clinical situations based on bone stock and soft tissue conditions. They found that the most important factor affecting intra-articular volume was the humeral neck-shaft angle; glenosphere diameter and offset had less of an effect. With regards to humeral displacement, the study showed that the most important factor in lateral displacement was the location of the glenosphere, followed by the humeral neck-shaft angle. Finally, deltoid length was affected most by the neck-shaft angle, with glenosphere location and humeral offset being less important.

It is important to remember, though, that stability is a complex issue with a multitude of implant and patient related factors that contribute to a stable arthroplasty. The amount of compression and the soft tissue tensioning are only two factors among many, with component position and impingement also playing an important role.

RANGE OF MOTION

Patient's shoulder function following reverse shoulder arthroplasty relates to the interaction of soft tissue tension, residual muscle function, and the potential motion provided by the prosthetic design used. The influence of prosthetic design on potential range of motion relates directly to impingement between the device and various locations about the shoulder such as the glenoid, acromion, and scapular neck. With many prosthetic designs, the medial aspect of the humeral socket impinges upon the inferior glenoid neck or scapular body; this often occurs in the resting position with the patient's arm at their side. A clear illustration of a limited range of motion occurs in adduction and results in scapular notching.

Several authors have suggested an adaptation of surgical technique as a method of avoiding the adduction deficit. This involves positioning the baseplate more inferiorly on the glenoid [43, 54]. Gerber *et al.* studied the effects of several different glenoid positions on impingement and range of motion after reverse shoulder arthroplasty. They found that inferior placement of the glenosphere with the inferior edge of the glenosphere 'hanging over' the inferior edge of the glenoid had a significant effect in improving adduction and abduction range of motion. Similar results were seen by Chou *et al.,* who showed that eccentric glenospheres with larger diameters can improve impingement free ROM [57]. Others have suggested that a combination of surgical technique adaptation and modification of prosthetic design can best limit the adduction deficit. Roche *et al.* showed that modification of the Grammont prosthesis by distalizing the glenoid and increasing the glenosphere thickness resulted in an improvement in impingement free ROM arc from 59 degrees to 109 degrees [57].
Other factors contributing to scapular notching were evaluated by Gutierrez *et al.* [33]. In order to best understand the hierarchal effects of both prosthetic design and adaptations of surgical technique, they used a virtual model with 243 simulated combinations to determine the hierarchy of factors necessary to avoid an adduction deficit. The factor which helped to best avoid an adduction deficit was a more varus humeral neck-shaft angle of 130 degrees, followed by an inferior glenosphere position on the glenoid, a 10-mm offset center of rotation lateral to the glenoid, inferior tilt of the glenosphere, and finally by a larger glenosphere size [34].

Furthermore, Gutierrez *et al.* used a computer simulation to assess different combinations of surgical and implant related factors when moving the humerus from 0 degrees of abduction to impingement [31]. This study showed that the most important factor for maximizing impingement free ROM was using a glenopshere with a center of rotation lateral to the glenoid. Next was inferior placement of the glenoid component, followed by inferior tilt of the glenoid component, the use of implants with a lower (more varus) neck-shaft angle, and finally using a larger glenosphere. Additionally, Gutierrez *et al.* characterized the ability of available reverse arthroplasty designs to maximize arc of motion [21]. They used an apparatus to simulate abduction of the humerus in the scapular plane and implanted six configurations of the RSP into a sawbones scapula and humerus. A linear correlation was found between abduction ROM and center of rotation offset relative to the glenoid: as center of rotation is lateralized, the ROM in abduction increased. Knowledge gained from these two studies can help maximize the potential ROM after reverse total shoulder arthroplasty. It is critical to appreciate that maximization of impingement free arc of motion is not only important in achieving ultimate range of motion, but it may play a critical role in the survivability of the implant. As noted in the hip arthroplasty experience, a major consequence of impingement is polyethylene wear, resulting in osteolysis and polyethylene disease. Impingement can be the cause of recurrent instability, loss of motion, and unexplained pain. In reverse shoulder arthroplasty, patients with scapular notching have been reported to have inferior clinical results and it may, in fact, lead to bone loss and catastrophic failure of the glenoid component [15, 60, 61]. Therefore, it would be helpful to minimize this complication and maximum effort should be made to optimize impingement free range of motion.

external rotation strength. Further, evidence suggests that those patients who do not have improvements in external rotation are less satisfied with their outcome [59].

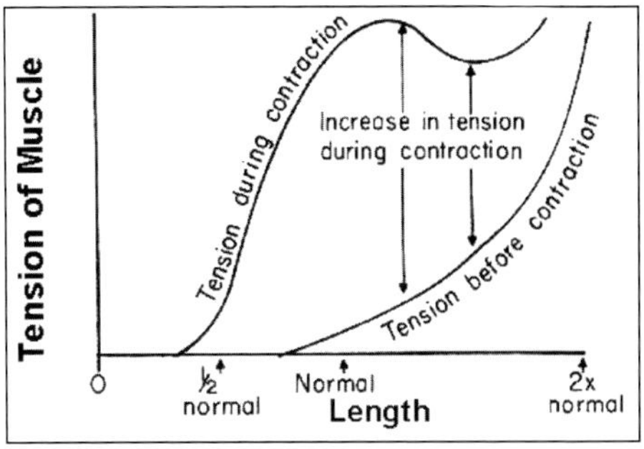

Fig. 16: The Blix Curve. Maximal muscle contraction is achieved at an optimal muscle length. Moving to lengths less than normal results in decreased tension during contraction.

MUSCLE FUNCTION: LOSS OF EXTERNAL ROTATION STRENGTH

Clinical results of reverse shoulder arthroplasty using the Grammont device repeatedly described improvements in pain relief and functional recovery, but a closer look revealed an unreliable improvement in external rotation. Some patients remain weak in external rotation, and some even show a loss in overall external rotation after surgery [6, 18, 59, 63, 65]. This is logical from a biomechanical standpoint if you consider the consequences of medializing the COR of the glenoid. By doing so, the length-tension relationship of the remaining muscles of the rotator cuff and shoulder are slackened (placed on a lower point on the Blix curve) (fig. 16). The vector of force is no longer in an anatomic plane with a distalized humerus. This altered anatomy decreases the efficiency of contraction and can explain the loss of

In contrast to the results seen using the Grammont device, return of external rotation using a prosthesis with a lateral center of rotation was observed more consistently. In order to help further understand this problem, Frankle *et al.* speculated that restoring the anatomical placement of the humerus would provide adequate tension of the remaining rotator cuff muscles, and hence provide for restoration of strength. This, theoretically, would allow for more normal function of those remaining muscles. In the setting of rotator cuff deficiency, the unstable, proximally migrated humerus prevented the remaining intact rotator cuff muscles from properly functioning. By restoring stability to the joint and tensioning the remaining muscles in a more anatomic fashion, external rotation could be restored. Additionally, utilizing a prosthetic design that maximized impingement-free arc of motion created the potential for functional recovery of external rotation. Clinical studies have confirmed that restoring the lateral offset of the humerus actually leads to an increase in external rotation postoperatively in a variety of pathological conditions [9, 13, 22, 44, 45]. Further, the authors felt that this would also help restore the stability of the glenohumeral joint by increasing the compression on the humerus, a factor that was compromised with medialization, and hence slackening of those rotator cuff muscles. Additionally, as mentioned above, restoring the maximal impingement free arc of motion is required to achieve at least passive rotational motion, a prerequisite for achieving active external rotation.

For patients with severe preoperative external rotational deficits, certain soft tissue procedures, such as latissimus dorsi and teres major transfers, have been shown to improve these deficits [4, 5, 19, 28, 29, 64]. Gerber speculated that the absence of the teres minor was predictive of external rotational weakness and advocated transferring motor units, specifically the latissimus dorsi, to help restore rotational weakness. Boileau also described a modification of the latissimus/teres minor tendon transfer to help improve rotational weakness. Finally, Grammont has speculated that the posterior deltoid could be recruited after reverse total shoulder arthroplasty to help improve rotational weakness, but there remains little biomechanical data to support this speculation.

CONCLUSIONS

The reverse shoulder arthroplasty design developed by Grammont was quite successful in decreasing pain and improving function in patients with rotator cuff deficiency. However, several problems were recognized with continued use of this implant. These problems lead to basic science and biomechanical studies aimed at improving the results of reverse shoulder arthroplasty. From these studies, increased attention has been given to glenosphere placement on the glenoid, glenosphere eccentricity, and the tilt in which the glenosphere is placed. Biomechanical studies have lead to modifications in surgical technique and advances in prosthetic design that have limited scapular notching and improved ROM and other functional outcomes for patients. Through continued research and improved understanding of the biomechanics of the rotator cuff deficient shoulder and the reverse shoulder arthroplasty, these clinical outcomes can continue to improve.

REFERENCES

[1] ANGLIN C, WYSS UP, PICHORA DR. Shoulder prosthesis subluxation: theory and experiment. *J Shoulder Elbow Surg. 2000;9: 104-14.*

[2] BAYLEY J, KESSEL L. The Kessel total shoulder replacement. In: Bayley J, Kessel L, eds. Shoulder Surgery. *New York: Springer-Verlag. 1982: 160-4.*

[3] BOBYN JD, TOH KK, HACKING SA, TANZER M, KRYGIER JJ. Tissue response to porous tantalum acetabular cups: a canine model. *J Arthroplasty. 1999;14: 347-54.*

[4] BOILEAU P, CHUINARD C, ROUSSANNE Y, BICKNELL RT, ROCHET N, TROJANI C. Reverse shoulder arthroplasty combined with a modified latissimus dorsi and teres major tendon transfer for shoulder pseudoparalysis associated with dropping arm. *Clin Orthop Relat Res. 2008; 466: 584-93.*

[5] BOILEAU P, CHUINARD C, ROUSSANNE Y, NEYTON L, TROJANI C. Modified latissimus dorsi and teres major transfer through a single delto-pectoral approach for external rotation deficit of the shoulder: as an isolated procedure or with a reverse arthroplasty. *J Shoulder Elbow Surg. 2007;16: 671-82.*

[6] BOILEAU P, WATKINSON D, HATZIDAKIS AM, HOVORKA I. Neer Award 2005: The Grammont reverse shoulder prosthesis: results in cuff tear arthritis, fracture sequelae, and revision arthroplasty. *J Shoulder Elbow Surg. 2006;15: 527-540.*

[7] BOILEAU P, WATKINSON DJ, HATZIDAKIS AM, BALG F. Grammont reverse prosthesis: design, rationale, and biomechanics. *J Shoulder Elbow Surg. 2005;14: 147S-161S.*

[8] BOULAHIA A, EDWARDS TB, WALCH G, BARATTA RV. Early results of a reverse design prosthesis in the treatment of arthritis of the shoulder in elderly patients with a large rotator cuff tear. *Orthopedics. 2002; 25: 129-33.*

[9] CHACON A, VIRANI N, SHANNON R, LEVY JC, PUPELLO D, FRANKLE M. Revision arthroplasty with use of a reverse shoulder prosthesis-allograft composite. *J Bone Joint Surg Am. 2009;91: 119-27.*

[10] CHEBLI C, HUBER P, WATLING J, BERTELSEN A, BICKNELL RT, MATSEN F, 3rd. Factors affecting fixation of the glenoid component of a reverse total shoulder prothesis. *J Shoulder Elbow Surg. 2008;17: 323-7.*

[11] COFIELD RH. Total shoulder arthroplasty with the Neer prosthesis. *J Bone Joint Surg Am. 1984;66: 899-906.*

[12] COVENTRY MB, BECKENBAUGH RD, NOLAN DR, ILSTRUP DM. 2,012 total hip arthroplasties. A study of postoperative course and early complications. *J Bone Joint Surg Am. 1974;56: 273-284.*

[13] CUFF D, PUPELLO D, VIRANI N, LEVY J, FRANKLE M. Reverse shoulder arthroplasty for the treatment of rotator cuff deficiency. *J Bone Joint Surg Am. 2008;90: 1244-51.*

[14] DE WILDE LF, VAN OVOST E, UYTTENDAELE D, VERDONK R. Results of an inverted shoulder prosthesis after resection for tumor of the proximal humerus. *Rev Chir Orthop Reparatrice Appar Mot. 2002; 88: 373-8.*

[15] DELLOYE C, JORIS D, COLETTE A, EUDIER A, DUBUC JE. Mechanical complications of total shoulder inverted prosthesis. *Rev Chir Orthop Reparatrice Appar Mot. 2002;88: 410-4.*

[16] DORR LD, WAN Z. Causes of and treatment protocol for instability of total hip replacement. *Clin Orthop Relat Res. 1998; 144-151.*

[17] ECKLUND KJ, LEE TQ, TIBONE J, GUPTA R. Rotator cuff tear arthropathy. *J Am Acad Orthop Surg. 2007;15: 340-9.*

[18] FAVARD L, LAUTMANN S, SIRVEAUX F, OUDET D, KERJEAN Y, HUGUET D. Hemi arthroplasty versus reverse arthroplasty in treatment of osteoarthritis with massive rotator cuff tear. In: Walch G, Boileau P, Mole D, eds. 2000 prothèses d'épaule recul de 2 à 10 ans. *Paris, France: Sauramps Medical. 2001: 261-268.*

[19] FAVRE P, LOEB MD, HELMY N, GERBER C. Latissimus dorsi transfer to restore external rotation with reverse shoulder arthroplasty: a biomechanical study. *J Shoulder Elbow Surg. 2008;17: 650-8.*

[20] FIELD LD, DINES DM, ZABINSKI SJ, WARREN RF. Hemiarthroplasty of the shoulder for rotator cuff arthropathy. *J Shoulder Elbow Surg. 1997;6: 18-23.*

[21] FRANKLE M. Rationale and Biomechanics of the Reverse Shoulder Prosthesis: The American Experience. In: Frankle M, eds. Rotator Cuff Deficiency of the Shoulder. *New York: Thieme. 2008: 76-104.*

[22] FRANKLE M, LEVY JC, PUPELLO D, SIEGAL S, SALEEM A, MIGHELL M, VASEY M. The reverse shoulder prosthesis for glenohumeral arthritis associated with severe rotator cuff deficiency. a minimum two-year follow-up study of sixty patients surgical technique. *J Bone Joint Surg Am. 2006;88 Suppl 1 Pt 2: 178-190.*

[23] FRANKLE M, SIEGAL S, PUPELLO D, SALEEM A, MIGHELL M, VASEY M. The Reverse Shoulder Prosthesis for glenohumeral arthritis associated with severe rotator cuff deficiency. A minimum two-year follow-up study of sixty patients. *J Bone Joint Surg Am. 2005; 87: 1697-1705.*

[24] FRANKLE MA, SIEGAL S, PUPELLO DR, GUTIERREZ S, GRIEWE M, MIGHELL MA. Coronal plane tilt angle affects risk of catastrophic failure in patients treated with a reverse shoulder prosthesis. *J Shoulder Elbow Surg. 2007; 16:e46.*

[25] FRANKLE MA, TERAMOTO A, LUO ZP, LEVY JC, PUPELLO D. Glenoid morphology in reverse shoulder arthroplasty: classification and surgical implications. *J Shoulder Elbow Surg. 2009;18: 874-85.*

[26] FREILICH R, GUTIERREZ S, PUPELLO D, LEE W, FRANKLE M. Analysis of joint volume, humeral displacement and deltoid length changes after reverse shoulder arthroplasty: hierarchy of surgical and implant-related factors. 56th annual meeting of the Orthopaedic Research Society, *New Orleans, LA, 6 March 2010.*

[27] GAGEY O, HUE E. Mechanics of the deltoid muscle. A new approach. *Clin Orthop Relat Res. 2000; 250-7.*

[28] GERBER C, MAQUIEIRA G, ESPINOSA N. Latissimus dorsi transfer for the treatment of irreparable rotator cuff tears. *J Bone Joint Surg Am. 2006;88: 113-120.*

[29] GERBER C, PENNINGTON SD, LINGENFELTER EJ, SUKTHANKAR A. Reverse Delta-III total shoulder replacement combined with latissimus dorsi transfer. A preliminary report. *J Bone Joint Surg Am. 2007;89: 940-7.*

[30] GRAMMONT PM, BAULOT E. Delta shoulder prosthesis for rotator cuff rupture. *Orthopedics. 1993;16: 65-8.*

[31] GUTIERREZ S, COMISKEY CA, LUO ZP, PUPELLO DR, FRANKLE MA. Range of impingement-free abduction and adduction deficit after reverse shoulder arthroplasty. Hierarchy of surgical and implant-design-related factors. *J Bone Joint Surg Am. 2008;90: 2606-15.*

[32] GUTIERREZ S, KELLER TS, LEVY JC, LEE WE, 3rd, LUO ZP. Hierarchy of stability factors in reverse shoulder arthroplasty. *Clin Orthop Relat Res. 2008;466: 670-6.*

[33] GUTIERREZ S, LEVY JC, LEE WE, 3rd, KELLER TS, MAITLAND ME. Center of rotation affects abduction range of motion of reverse shoulder arthroplasty. *Clin Orthop Relat Res. 2007;458: 78-82.*

[34] GUTIERREZ S, LUO ZP, LEVY J, FRANKLE MA. Arc of motion and socket depth in reverse shoulder implants. *Clin Biomech (Bristol, Avon). 2009;24: 473-9.*

[35] GUTIERREZ S, PUPELLO D, COMISKY C, FRANKLE M. Stability of reverse shoulder humeral implants in a proximal humeral bone loss model. 56th annual meeting of the Orthopaedic Research Society, *New Orleans, LA, 6 March 2010.*

[36] GUTIERREZ S, PUPELLO D, FRANKLE M. Effect of eccentric glenospheres and baseplate tilts on shear stress in reverse shoulder implants. 56th annual meeting of the Orthopaedic Research Society, *New Orleans, LA, 6 March 2010*

[37] HARMAN M, FRANKLE M, VASEY M, BANKS S. Initial glenoid component fixation in "reverse" total shoulder arthroplasty: a biomechanical evaluation. *J Shoulder Elbow Surg. 2005;14: 162S-167S.*

[38] HARRIS TE, JOBE CM, DAI QG. Fixation of proximal humeral prostheses and rotational micromotion. *J Shoulder Elbow Surg. 2000;9: 205-210.*

[39] HOPKINS AR, HANSEN UN, BULL AM, EMERY R, AMIS AA. Fixation of the reversed shoulder prosthesis. *J Shoulder Elbow Surg. 2008;17: 974-80.*

[40] HUMPHREY CS, KELLY JD, 2nd, NORRIS TR. Optimizing glenosphere position and fixation in reverse shoulder arthroplasty, Part Two: The three-column concept. *J Shoulder Elbow Surg. 2008;17: 595-601.*

[41] JASTY M, BRAGDON C, BURKE D, O'CONNOR D, LOWENSTEIN J, HARRIS WH. In vivo skeletal responses to porous-surfaced implants subjected to small induced motions. *J Bone Joint Surg Am. 1997;79: 707-14.*

[42] KARDUNA AR, WILLIAMS GR, WILLIAMS JL, IANNOTTI JP. Glenohumeral joint translations before and after total shoulder arthroplasty. A study in cadavera. *J Bone Joint Surg Am. 1997;79: 1166-74.*

[43] LEVIGNE C, BOILEAU P, FAVARD L, GARAUD P, MOLE D, SIRVEAUX F, WALCH G. Scapular notching in reverse shoulder arthroplasty. *J Shoulder Elbow Surg. 2008;17 :925-35.*

[44] LEVY J, FRANKLE M, MIGHELL M, PUPELLO D. The use of the reverse shoulder prosthesis for the treatment of failed hemiarthroplasty for proximal humeral fracture. *J Bone Joint Surg Am. 2007;89: 292-300.*

[45] LEVY JC, VIRANI N, PUPELLO D, FRANKLE M. Use of the reverse shoulder prosthesis for the treatment of failed hemiarthroplasty in patients with glenohumeral arthritis and rotator cuff deficiency. *J Bone Joint Surg Br. 2007;89: 189-95.*

[46] LIPPITT S, VANDERHOOFT JE, HARRIS SL, SIDLES JA, HARRYMAN DT, MATSEN FA. Glenohumeral stability from concavity-compression: A quantitative analysis. *J Shoulder Elbow Surg. 1993;2: 27-35.*

[47] MALIK A, MAHESHWARI A, DORR LD. Impingement with total hip replacement. *J Bone Joint Surg Am. 2007;89: 1832-42.*

[48] MATSEN F, LIPPITT S. Principles of glenohumeral stability. In: Matsen F, Lippitt S, DeBartolo S, eds. Shoulder Surgery: Principles and Procedures. *Philadelphia: Saunders. 2004: 83.*

[49] MATSEN F, LIPPITT S. Principles of glenoid concavity. In: Matsen F, Lippitt S, DeBartolo S, eds. Shoulder Surgery: Principles and Procedures. *Philadelphia: Saunders. 2004: 89.*

[50] NEER CS, 2nd, CRAIG EV, FUKUDA H. Cuff-tear arthropathy. *J Bone Joint Surg Am. 1983;65: 1232-44.*

[51] NEER CS, 2nd, WATSON KC, STANTON FJ. Recent experience in total shoulder replacement. *J Bone Joint Surg Am. 1982;64: 319-337.*

[52] NORRIS TR, KELLY JDI, HUMPHREY CS. Management of Glenoid Bone Defects in Revision Shoulder Arthroplasty: A New Application of the Reverse Total Shoulder Prosthesis. *Techniques in Shoulder & Elbow Surgery. 2007;8: 37-46.*

[53] NOVE-JOSSERAND L. Prosthetic instability: clinical presentation (early, late) type of reduction, unique or recurrent, causes etiologies, treatments, results. Poster presented at Nice Shoulder Course: *Arthroscopy and Arthroplasty Current Concepts, Palais de la Méditerranée, Nice, France, 2006.*

[54] NYFFELER RW, WERNER CM, GERBER C. Biomechanical relevance of glenoid component positioning in the reverse Delta III total shoulder prosthesis. *J Shoulder Elbow Surg. 2005;14: 524-28.*

[55] NYFFELER RW, WERNER CM, SIMMEN BR, GERBER C. Analysis of a retrieved delta III total shoulder prosthesis. *J Bone Joint Surg Br. 2004;86: 1187-91.*

[56] POLLOCK R, DELIZ E, MCILVEEN S, FLATOW E, BIGLIANI L. Prosthetic replacement in rotator cuff-deficient shoulders. *J Shoulder Elbow Surg. 1992;1: 173-86.*

[57] ROCHE C, FLURIN PH, WRIGHT T, CROSBY LA, MAULDIN M, ZUCKERMAN JD. An evaluation of the relationships between reverse shoulder design parameters and range of motion, impingement, and stability. *J Shoulder Elbow Surg. 2009;18: 734-41.*

[58] SANCHEZ-SOTELO J, COFIELD RH, ROWLAND CM. Shoulder hemiarthroplasty for glenohumeral arthritis associated with severe rotator cuff deficiency. *J Bone Joint Surg Am. 2001; 83-A: 1814-22.*

[59] SIMOVITCH RW, HELMY N, ZUMSTEIN MA, GERBER C. Impact of fatty infiltration of the teres minor muscle on the outcome of reverse total shoulder arthroplasty. *J Bone Joint Surg Am. 2007;89: 934-9.*

[60] SIMOVITCH RW, ZUMSTEIN MA, LOHRI E, HELMY N, GERBER C. Predictors of scapular notching in patients managed with the Delta III reverse total shoulder replacement. *J Bone Joint Surg Am. 2007;89: 588-600.*

[61] VAN SEYMORTIER P, STOFFELEN D, FORTEMS Y, REYNDERS P. The reverse shoulder prosthesis (Delta III) in acute shoulder fractures: technical considerations with respect to stability. *Acta Orthop Belg. 2006;72: 474-7.*

[62] VISOTSKY JL, BASAMANIA C, SEEBAUER L, ROCKWOOD CA, JENSEN KL. Cuff tear arthropathy: pathogenesis, classification, and algorithm for treatment. *J Bone Joint Surg Am. 2004;86-A Suppl 2: 35-40.*

[63] WALL B, NOVE-JOSSERAND L, O'CONNOR DP, EDWARDS TB, WALCH G. Reverse total shoulder arthroplasty: a review of results according to etiology. *J Bone Joint Surg Am. 2007;89: 1476-85.*

[64] WARNER JJ. Management of massive irreparable rotator cuff tears: the role of tendon transfer. *Instr Course Lect. 2001; 50: 63-71.*

[65] WERNER CM, STEINMANN PA, GILBART M, GERBER C. Treatment of painful pseudoparesis due to irreparable rotator cuff dysfunction with the Delta III reverse-ball-and-socket total shoulder prosthesis. *J Bone Joint Surg Am. 2005;87: 1476-86.*

[66] WILLIAMS GR, Jr, ROCKWOOD CA, Jr. Hemiarthroplasty in rotator cuff-deficient shoulders. *J Shoulder Elbow Surg. 1996;5: 362-7.*

[67] ZUCKERMAN JD, SCOTT AJ, GALLAGHER MA. Hemiarthroplasty for cuff tear arthropathy. *J Shoulder Elbow Surg. 2000;9: 169-172.*

LATERALIZATION IN THE DESIGN OF THE REVERSE SHOULDER ARTHROPLASTY IS IT DANGEROUS? IS IT USEFUL?

Ph. VALENTI, D. KATZ, Ph. SAUZIERES, A. KILINC

ABSTRACT

Background

Massive irreparable rotator cuff tear with a pseudoparalytic shoulder is the primary indication for total reverse shoulder arthroplasty (RSA). For this indication, previous studies have proved the success of this solution in restoring active anterior elevation. There are some drawbacks, however, such as the lack of internal and external rotation and the risk of glenoid notching due to humeral medialization. The aim of this study was to evaluate the clinical and radiographic results of a less medialized RSA integrated in the design of the prosthesis.

Method

Between October, 2003 and May, 2006, 76 less medialized RSAs (Arrow reverse prosthesis, Fournitures Hospitalières) were implanted in pseudoparalytic shoulders with rotator cuff deficiency. These patients were all retrospectively reviewed with a minimum follow-up of two years.

Results

The mean follow-up was 36 months. The absolute Constant score increased from 24 to 59, i.e. a gain of 35 points. Seventy-two patients were satisfied to very satisfied (94.8%) and 4 patients were dissatisfied (5.2%). The gain in active anterior elevation was 61° and the improvement in pain was 10 points. The gain in external rotation in adduction (ER1), was 15°, while that of external rotation in 90° of abduction (ER2) was 30°. Follow-up shows no inferior glenoid notching and two cases of glenoid loosening with this less medialized reverse prosthesis.

Conclusion

Less medialization of RSA improves both external and internal rotation, which are useful in the daily activities of older patients. The absence of glenoid notching is a positive factor for prosthesis survivorship, but longer follow-up and better analysis with CT scan are necessary to confirm these preliminary results.

INTRODUCTION

Reverse shoulder arthroplasty can yield satisfactory results in patients with pseudoparalysis of the shoulder due to glenohumeral osteoarthritis (OA) associated with an irreparable rotator cuff tear [5, 6, 23, 24, 26, 30]. Medializing and lowering the center of rotation improves the lever arm of the deltoid, particularly when the rotator cuff is deficient [1, 13, 14]. This design of the reverse prostheses, with a center of rotation (COR) at the level of the glenoid bone, decreases shearing forces at the glenoid component-bone interface and results in improved survivorship of the glenoid component compared with other constrained and semiconstrained designs [5, 20, 23, 24, 26, 30]. However, medialization of the COR and of the humeral stem encourages impingement of the humeral polyethylene (PE) insert on the scapular neck, resulting in inferior glenoid notching. The high reported rates of glenoid notching [15, 18, 22, 24, 25, 26, 27, 28, 30, 32] adversely affect the mid-term clinical outcome [25] and represent a potential risk of glenoid loosening in the long term [9].

As reported by Nyfeller *et al.* [21], mechanical failure of the base plate has been associated with PE wear, chronic inflammation of the joint capsule, and local osteolysis. Although good short- and mid-term clinical results were observed with the Delta III reverse prosthesis (DePuy, Warsaw, IN, USA), glenoid notching has been a frequent complication [15, 18, 22, 24, 25, 26, 27, 28, 30, 32].

Four therapeutic options have been reported to decrease the risk of glenoid notching and improve rotation:

- Lowering the position of the glenoid implant in its original form [25, 26] ;
- Improving the design of the prosthesis without modifying the COR by increasing the inferior overhang of the glenoid hemisphere ;
- A lateralization of the COR (6 to 8 mm) with a bone graft interposed between the native glenoid bone and the base plate has been described by Boileau *et al.* [3] as a bony increased offset reverse shoulder arthroplasty (BIO-RSA) ;
- A lateralization of the COR in the design of the prosthesis with its known risks of glenoid loosening [10, 28]. Frankle *et al.* [10] proposed a more lateralized COR to avoid glenoid notching, with better rotations compared to the results of Sirveaux *et al.* [26] but with a high complication rate (17%). Excessive lateralization of the COR results in increased torque and shear forces at the glenoid component-bone interface, as previously reported for constrained and semi-constrained designs [5, 24, 26, 30]. Improvement in the fixation of the base plate in semi-constrained prostheses can allow for moderate lateralization of the COR. In the Arrow reverse prosthesis (Fournitures Hospitalières, Mulhouse, France), the convex design of the base plate's medial surface, combined with press fit fixation (central keel and anterior extension) allows lateralization of the COR with good primary fixation.

The aim of this retrospective study is to describe the concept of a less medialized Arrow reverse prosthesis and report its clinical and radiographic results following implantation in patients presenting with a pseudoparalytic shoulder secondary to an irreparable rotator cuff tear.

MATERIALS AND METHODS

Patients

Between October, 2003 and May, 2006, 76 less medialized reverse prostheses (Arrow) were implanted consecutively by three surgeons (P.V., D.K., P.S.) for pseudoparalytic shoulders with massive rotator cuff tear. We excluded from this study reverse prostheses for post-traumatic OA, recent fracture-dislocation, chronic anterior locked dislocation, rheumatoid arthritis, and revisions of failed hemiarthroplasty or anatomic total shoulder arthroplasty. Contraindications to the surgery were deltoid paralysis, a history of chronic shoulder infection with a high-virulence organism, medial glenoid erosion extending as far as the coracoid process with an extensively-covering acromion, manual labor, and finally wheelchair- and crutch-dependent ambulation.

The mean patient age was 73 years (range, 52-90 years) with a female predominance (58 women versus 18 men). The dominant side was the most frequently impaired (56 dominant, 20 non-dominant). All the patients had previously received at least 6 months of physiotherapy, nevertheless active anterior elevation (AAE) remained less than 60°. The preoperative examination systematically includes standard radiographs and a CT-scan of the shoulder for the assessment of glenoid bone stock (the limiting factor to glenoid component implantation), muscular bulk of the deltoid and the remaining cuff muscles, and the degree of fatty infiltration of the remaining cuff muscles, using the classification of Goutallier *et al.* [12]. All the patients had a complete rupture of the supraspinatus and infraspinatus tendon, which were both retracted to the glenoid level. The mean fatty degeneration index (FDI) was 2.96 for supraspinatus and 2.91 for infraspinatus. The superior third of the subscapularis muscle was altered in 30% of cases with a FDI of 2.20. Teres minor was not analyzed in this series but no patient had a hornblower sign.

Operative Technique

All surgeries were begun with an antero-superior approach. The coracoacromial ligament was always cut and the acromion kept intact, particularly when the OA was already advanced. Wide resection of the capsule and degenerative fibrous tissue facilitated lowering of the humeral head in eccentric glenohumeral OA (stage IV or V, according to Hamada and Fukuda). Sectioning of the superior third of the subscapularis facilitated lowering the humeral head when the joint was stiff and the humeral head was fixed anteriorly in a subcutaneous position. The humeral bone cut was never done before the head was freed widely of the soft tissues. The inclination of the humeral bone cut was 135°, identical to the cut used for an anatomical prosthesis, given the universal character of the humeral stem. With the humeral cup inserted, the definitive inclination of the humeral component was 155°, which is identical to Delta and Tornier prostheses. Thus, more bone is cut in the metaphysis, but the cancellous metaphyseal bone is reused to provide a better press-fit for the stem. The retroversion angle chosen during the operation was around 20°.

To expose the glenoid via this antero-superior approach, particularly the inferior pole, a circumferential capsulectomy was absolutely essential. This allows the humeral head to be dislocated posteriorly and distally and the base plate to be positioned in a plane perpendicular to the glenoid. Proper glenoid exposure avoids malpositioning of the base plate, particularly with an upward orientation (superior tilt). Reaming the glenoid cavity was always performed sparingly, essentially removing the cartilage and conserving the subchondral bone. A superior or posterosuperior abrasion of the glenoid must be vigorously looked for preoperatively in order to prevent a superiorly-tilted glenoid base plate. The convex-backed, hydroxyapatite-covered base plate consists of a central keel and an anterior plate providing press-fit fixation to counter the shearing forces in the early degrees of abduction. Two divergent non-locking screws (5.5-mm diameter), reproducing the Grammont concept, provided definitive fixation for this base plate. The glenoid hemisphere was fitted on the base plate – rather than engulfing it – and fixed by both impaction and screwing. The prosthetic tension was assessed with a trial humeral insert: absence of scapular movement when the arm was raised to 80° was considered as suitable deltoid tension. A "+5" augment was used only 3 times to improve stability. An external rotation (ER) test with the elbow at the side rules out anterior decoaptation secondary to a posterior impingement of the humeral cup against the posterior aspect of the glenoid.

In very elderly patients with advanced osteopenia, the humeral stem was cemented. Indeed, the shape of the humeral stem – which is the same as that of the anatomical prosthesis (universal system) – and the maintenance of metaphyseal bone substance and inserting cancellous bone graft into the metaphysis, provided excellent primary stability. Passive physiotherapy was started immediately and patients living alone were transferred to a rehabilitation centre from the fifth postoperative day.

Clinical and Statistical Evaluation

All patients were examined by a single orthopaedic surgeon. The follow-up evaluation consisted of a physical examination, subjective satisfaction questionnaire, functional score (Constant-Murley) [7], and radiographs (anteroposterior [AP] and lateral outlet view).

Results were also assessed in light of previous surgical history as well as etiology using the classification of Hamada *et al.* [16]. Three groups were identified:

- **Group A** (17 cases) characterized by an eccentric humeral head without glenohumeral OA (Hamada stages I, II, and III).
- **Group B** (56 cases) characterized by an irreparable rotator cuff tear associated with an eccentric humeral head with glenohumeral OA (Hamada stages IV and V).
- **Group C** (3 cases) characterized by medialized, concentric OA and a non-functionnal, thin, atrophic rotator cuff, with an FDI greater than 3.

Presence or absence of glenoid notching on the radiographs and mechanical failure were also noted.

Statistical analysis was performed with InStat 3.0 software (GraphPad Inc, La Jolla, USA). Analysis consisted of a t-test (Student's test) with a $p<0.05$ for statistical significance between the preoperative and postoperative values.

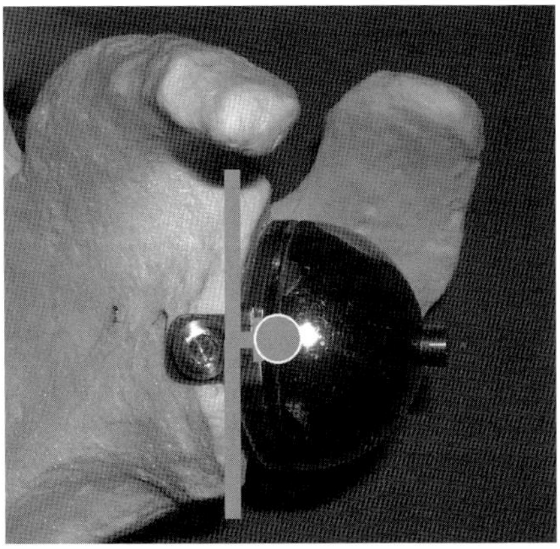

Fig. 1: The glenoid hemisphere is attached to the metal-base plate and not embedded in the glenoid. The center of rotation is thus not at level of glenoid bone but lateralized by 8.5 mm.

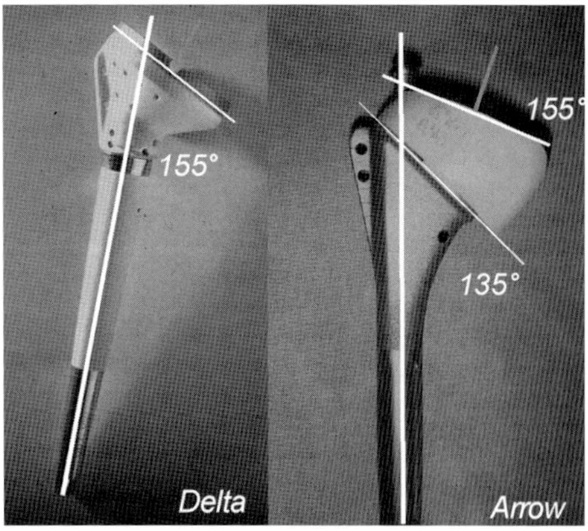

Fig. 2: The universal shape of the arrow humeral stem differs from the Delta Grammont prosthesis, which has a trumpet-shaped metaphysis that causes a medialization of the humerus.

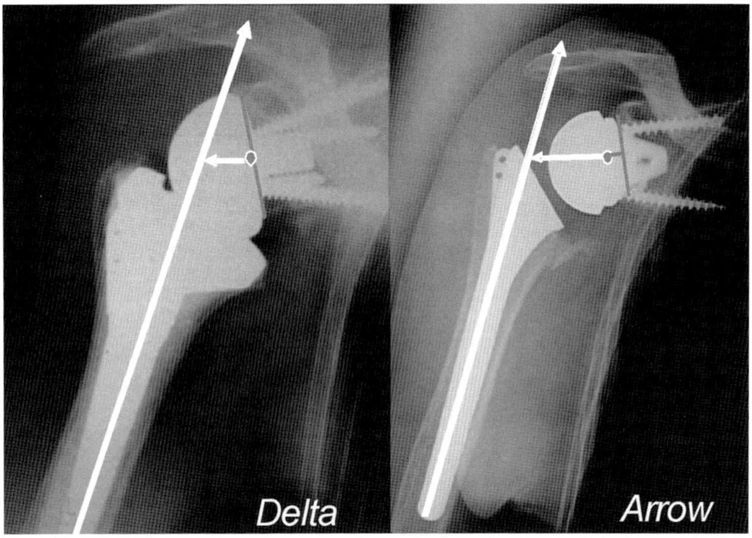

Fig. 3: The lateralization of the center of rotation associated with a lateralized humeral stem increases the stability of the RSA and restores the shoulder's contour.

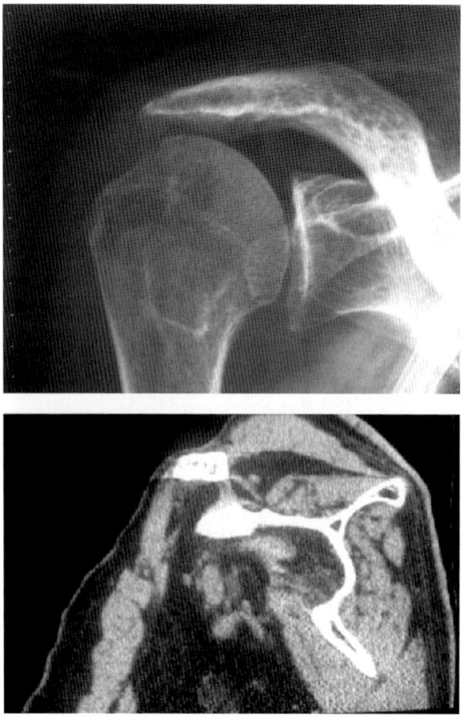

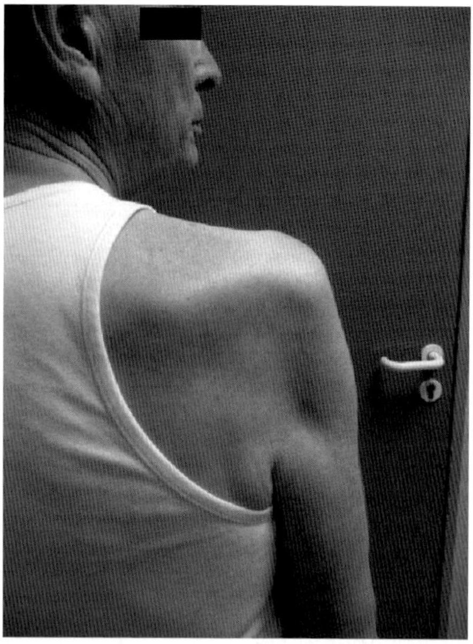

Fig. 4: A) Painful shoulder in a 74-year-old patient with limited anterior elevation, Hamada stage III; 4B) atrophic and irreparable rotator cuff tear.

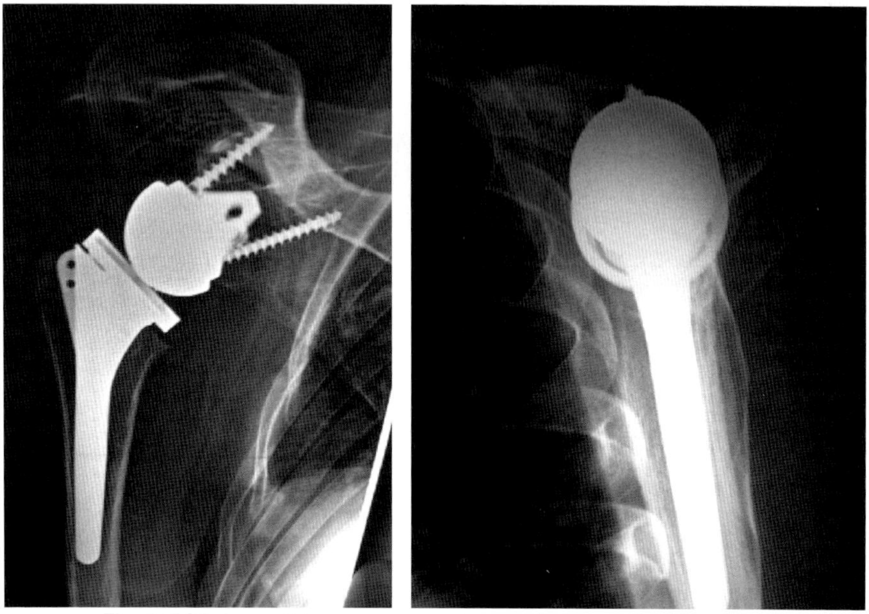

Fig. 5: RSA Arrow 2nd generation (anteroposterior and lateral views)

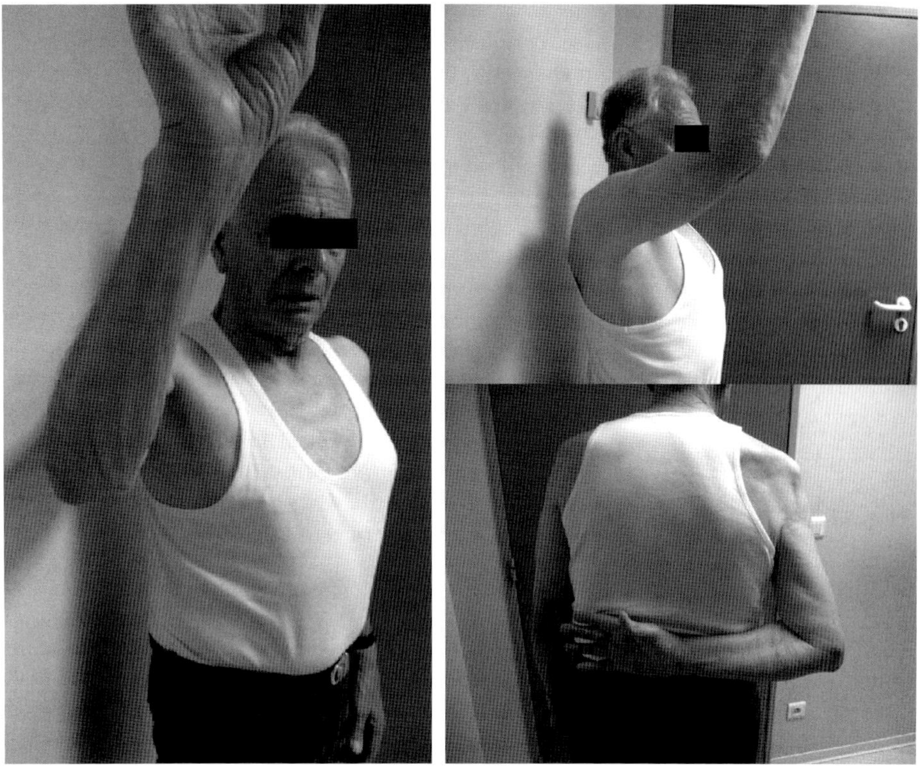

Fig. 6: Two-year follow-up – active anterior elevation of 120°, active external rotation in abduction of 70°, active internal rotation to L3 vertebral level.

Table 1: Preoperative and postoperative clinical results

	Preoperative	Postoperative	Gain
Constant Score (points)	24 (22-26)	59* (56-61)	35 (32-38)
Pain (points)	4 (3-5)	14* (13-14)	10 (9-11)
Active anterior elevation (°)	65 (58-72)	126* (121-132)	61 (52-70)
External rotation 1 (°)	15 (11-18)	30* (27-33)	15 (10-20)
External rotation 2 (°)	19 (14-24)	50* (45-55)	31 (24-38)
Internal rotation (points)	5,5 (5-6)	6,6* (6-7)	1 (1-2)
Strength (points)	1,6 (1-2,2)	6,3* (5,7-7)	4,8 (3,9-5,6)

RESULTS

All the patients were reviewed retrospectively. The mean follow-up was 36 months (24-48). The absolute Constant score improved from 24 to 59, representing a gain of 35 points. Twenty-nine patients were very satisfied and 43 were satisfied (together comprising 94.8%); 4 were dissatisfied (5.2%). According to the Constant score, the pain component was 13.88 representing a gain of around 10 points.

As summarized in Table 1, the gain in AAE was 61° (65° to 126°). The gain in ER with the arm adducted (ER1) was 15°, while it was 30° in ER with the arm at 90° of abduction (RE2) and of 1 point in internal rotation (IR).

Results according to the classification of Hamada *et al.* were:

In group B, the gain in AAE was only 54° compared with an 85° gain in group A. On the other hand, the gain in ER and IR in group A was 17°, which was higher than the gain of 9° in group B. This lesser result was related to more severe fatty degeneration of the rotator cuff muscles. However, there was no significant difference in the postoperative absolute Constant scores of the three groups.

No significant difference was found between the results of those who had or had not previously undergone surgery. (Seventeen of the 76 patients reviewed [22.3%] had undergone previous surgery.) The results were similar in the two groups, and among the patients who had undergone surgery the results did not vary with the type of previous surgery.

Radiographically, using AP and axillary views, at last follow-up, no patients had a notch in their scapular pillar with this less medialized reverse prosthesis. That said, one limitation was that we did not systematically obtain CT scans to analyze the glenoid bone, particularly in the posterior aspect of the pillar.

Complications

Fourteen patients suffered complications (16%), which can be divided into 2 groups:

- **Group 1** consists of 10 cases who experienced prosthetic dissociation related to a mechanical failure in the first-generation prosthesis implanted between April, 2003 and June, 2004. Six glenospheres separated from the base plate, and 4 impacted PE inserts detached from the humeral metaphyses they were impacted in. Those 10 patients underwent revision surgery. They received a second-generation prosthesis, with a final mean Constant score of 58.1 points, thus not significantly different from the uncomplicated cases.
  One patient was treated again and developed an infection. He is currently aseptic with a cement spacer awaiting reimplantation. Surgical revision was performed using a second-generation prosthesis, the glenoid hemisphere of which is impacted and screwed into the base plate. In the same way, the humeral insert is impacted and screwed into the humeral stem. Since starting to use this second-generation prosthesis (in the beginning of 2005), no mechanical failures have been recorded.
- **Group 2** consists of 4 patients (5%):
  One patient presented a late, aseptic glenoid loosening (in the 4th post-operative year) with a complete peripheral radiolucent line around the base plate and, clinically, with pain and a loss of AAE (70°). During the revision, no osseointegration was seen on the base plate. A

new base plate and hemisphere were implanted in combination with cancellous bone graft providing good-quality primary press-fit. Six months later, the shoulder was painless with an AAE of 130°. One patient presented a postoperative superior migration of the base plate caused by glenoid fracture during the initial implantation. The patient had limited AAE (80°) but no pain and refused revision. One patient had a stress fracture of the acromion which had been treated nonoperatively with a 20° loss of AAE. Finally, 1 patient had an axillary nerve palsy that was transitory and recovered partially.

DISCUSSION

Reverse shoulder arthroplasty following Grammont's principles has proved to be effective for restoring AAE. Yet, analysis of previously reported series has shown that the gain in ER and IR was very limited, and from the early postoperative months an inferior and posterior glenoid notch is found in a percentage varying from 40 to 70% [15, 18, 22, 24, 25, 26, 27, 28, 30, 32].

Authors have reported variable clinical repercussions from such glenoid notching: Sirveaux *et al.* [26] observed deterioration in the clinical result in type-3 and type-4 notches according to Nerot's classification [27]. Werner *et al.* [33] found after 44 months' follow-up that the glenoid notch had a negative influence on the Constant score. Delloye *et al.* [9] reported a fall in the Constant score if the notch reached the central keel, with the risk of glenoid loosening. On the other hand, Guéry *et al.* [15] seem to have shown with long-term follow-up that, however severe it is, the glenoid notch did not affect the Constant score. Thus patients with an inferior and posterior glenoid notch had, at short-term follow-up, a better ER1 due to reduced impingement [33].

Many recommendations have been made in the literature about preventing this glenoid notch from occurring:

De Wilde *et al.* [8] reported a series using a larger diameter glenosphere (42 mm). All authors [21, 25, 26, 32, 33] agree that the base plate should be placed as low as possible, flush with the inferior pole of the glenoid cavity. However, if the scapular pillar is very vertical, notching may still occur. According to Simovitch *et al.* [25], an inferior tilt of the metal back does not in theory prevent a notch from occurring.

Boileau *et al.* [3] proposed the BIO-RSA to lateralize the glenoid component of 7 to 10 mm. With this procedure, they reported only 3 cases of glenoid notching and 2 cases of partial osteolysis at the superior part of the graft in a series of 38 cases with a minimal follow-up of 12 months. The gain in elevation was a good 75° (61° preoperative to 136° postoperative), but the gain in active rotation (13° for ER and 4° for IR) was inferior to those obtained with the Arrow Reverse. The BIO-RSA procedure with a COR at the level of the new bone graft reproduces the concept of Grammont, but cannot definitively prevent glenoid notching. Thus, Boileau et al. still recommended implanting the base plate in a lower position.

In 1998, Frankle *et al.* [10] reported a less medialized reverse prosthesis with a more lateral COR close to the COR of a non-constrained anatomical prosthesis. The glenoid hemisphere consisted of 2/3 of a sphere and fitted into a flat-bottomed plate covered with hydroxyapatite fixed by a central stud and 3.5-mm peripheral screws. For 60 patients with a minimum follow-up of 2 years, the authors reported goods results in terms of ER (35.9°) with an AAE of 105° (lower than the results obtained with the Grammont prosthesis). On the other hand, 17% (i.e. 10 patients) had complications, including 7 cases of glenoid loosening, 2 cases of stress fracture of the base plate, and 1 case of infection. Of the 7 patients who underwent revision, 5 had a new RSA and 2 were transformed into hemiarthroplasties with a poor result as regards elevation. No notching was found with this much more lateralized prosthesis. Too much lateralization of the COR thus creates considerable shearing forces at the junction between the plate and the glenoid bone, which is not sufficiently compensated for by the fixation method. The authors reported that these cases of glenoid loosening occurred early before the second year and that no osseointegration was visible on the plate on revision. They therefore recommended improving the quality of fixation for the base plate, with a convex bottom, a 6.5-mm central compressive screw, and 5-mm peripheral screws locking into the plate. In addition, they proposed a more or less lateral COR depending on the quality of the glenoid bone. All these proposals ensued from in vitro work by Harman *et al.* [17].

In order to avoid the risk of glenoid notching and above all improve the gain in ER and IR, which is very useful in the everyday life of these elderly patients, we chose a reverse prosthesis with a less medialized design than Paul Grammont's original prosthesis. The COR is lateralized by 8.7 mm relative to the glenoid bone because the glenoid hemisphere is fitted to the plate. In addition, the shape of the metaphyseal part of the humeral stem creates more lateralization of the humerus than the trumpet-shaped Grammont prosthesis. This lateralization, admittedly less than that in the prosthesis designed by Frankle *et al.* [10], has led us to propose an improvement in the primary fixation of the glenoid implant: the base plate with a convex base, which is covered with hydroxyapatite and comes in 3 different sizes to provide optimal contact with the glenoid cavity's subchondral bone. A central keel and an anterior lug provide primary fixation that opposes torsional forces. This plate is also fixed by 2 superior and inferior divergent, non-locking screws to oppose shearing forces at the beginning of abduction. In our retrospective series of 76 cases with a minimum follow-up of 2 years, this lateralization produced a gain in ER (RE1 of 15° and RE2 of 32°) and IR (two vertebral levels), with a mean AAE of 126°. We did not detect any glenoid notches in standard radiographs (AP and axillary views) and only 2 cases of glenoid loosening occurred (1 early technical error and 1 late loosening).

CONCLUSION

Modification of the initial concept of Paul Grammont with a moderate lateralization of the prosthesis by around 10 to 12 mm provides goods functional results. There is a gain in active ER with considerable impact on the quality of life of the concerned elderly patients. The absence of glenoid notching at last follow-up is a good prognostic factor for the prosthesis' survivorship, but it is too early to make any assertions about the longevity of this "less medialized" reverse prosthesis. Longer follow-up is needed to confirm these good early results and support the proposal of this solution for the yet unsolved case of younger patients.

REFERENCES

[1] BAULOT E, CHABERNAUD D, GRAMMONT PM Results of Grammont's inverted prosthesis in omarthritis associated with major cuff destruction. A propos of 16 cases. *Acta Orthop Belg, 61 Suppl 1: 112-9, 1995.*

[2] BOHSALI KI, WIRTH MA, ROCKWOOD CA Jr Complications of total shoulder arthroplasty. *J Bone Joint Surg Am, 88(10): 2279-92, 2006.*

[3] BOILEAU P, CHUINARD C, BICKNELL R, PELEGRI C Bony increased offset reverse shoulder arthroplasty (BIO RSA); a biologic solution to scapular notching. *(Paper presented at : 10th International Congress of Shoulder and Elbow Surgery (Brazil)), 2007.*

[4] BOILEAU P, WATKINSON D, HATZIDAKIS AM, HOVORKA I Neer Award 2005: The Grammont reverse shoulder prosthesis: results in cuff tear arthritis, fracture sequelae, and revision arthroplasty. *J Shoulder Elbow Surg, 15(5): 527-40, 2006.*

[5] BOILEAU P, CHUINARD C, ROUSSANNE Y, NEYTON L, TROJANI C Modified latissimus dorsi and teres major transfer through a single delto-pectoral approach for external rotation deficit of the shoulder: as an isolated procedure or with a reverse arthroplasty. *J Shoulder Elbow Surg, 16(6): 671-82, 2007.*

[6] BOULAHIA A, EDWARDS TB, WALCH G, BARATTA RV Early results of a reverse design prosthesis in the treatment of arthritis of the shoulder in elderly patients with a large rotator cuff tear. *Orthopedics, 25(2): 129-33, 2002.*

[7] CONSTANT CR, MURLEY AH A clinical method of functional assessment of the shoulder. *Clin Orthop Relat Res, (214): 160-4, 1987.*

[8] DE WILDE LF, AUDENAERT EA, BERGHS BM Shoulder prostheses treating cuff tear arthropathy: a comparative biomechanical study. *J Orthop Res, 22(6): 1222-30, 2004.*

[9] DELLOYE C, JORIS D, COLETTE A, EUDIER A, DUBUC JE Mechanical complications of total shoulder inverted prosthesis. *Rev Chir Orthop Reparatrice Appar Mot, 88(4): 410-4, 2002.*

[10] FRANKLE M, LEVY JC, PUPELLO D, SIEGAL S, SALEEM A, MIGHELL M, VASEY M The reverse shoulder prosthesis for glenohumeral arthritis associated with severe rotator cuff deficiency. a minimum two-year follow-up study of sixty patients surgical technique. *J Bone Joint Surg Am, 88 Suppl 1 Pt 2: 178-90, 2006.*

[11] FRANKLIN JL, BARRETT WP, JACKINS SE, MATSEN FA 3rd Glenoid loosening in total shoulder arthroplasty. Association with rotator cuff deficiency. *J Arthroplasty, 3(1): 39-46, 1988.*

[12] GOUTALLIER D, POSTEL JM, BERNAGEAU J, LAVAU L, VOISIN MC Fatty muscle degeneration in cuff ruptures. Pre- and post-operative evaluation by CT scan. *Clin Orthop Relat Res, (304): 78-83, 1994.*

[13] GRAMMONT PM, BAULOT E Delta shoulder prosthesis for rotator cuff rupture. *Orthopedics, 16(1): 65-8, 1993.*

[14] GRAMMONT PMT, P LAFFAY, JP DERIES X Etude et réalisation d'une nouvelle prothèse d'épaule. *Rhumatologie, 39: 407-418, 1987.*

[15] GUERY J, FAVARD L, SIRVEAUX F, OUDET D, MOLE D, WALCH G Reverse total shoulder arthroplasty. Survivorship analysis of eighty replacements followed for five to ten years. *J Bone Joint Surg Am, 88(8): 1742-7, 2006.*

[16] HAMADA K, FUKUDA H, MIKASA M, KOBAYASHI Y Roentgenographic findings in massive rotator cuff tears. A long-term observation. *Clin Orthop Relat Res, (254): 92-6, 1990.*

[17] HARMAN M, FRANKLE M, VASEY M, BANKS S Initial glenoid component fixation in "reverse" total shoulder arthroplasty: a biomechanical evaluation. *J Shoulder Elbow Surg, 14(1 Suppl S): 162S-167S, 2005.*

[18] JACOBS R, DEBEER P, DE SMET L Treatment of rotator cuff arthropathy with a reversed Delta shoulder prosthesis. *Acta Orthop Belg, 67(4): 344-7, 2001.*

[19] NEER CS 2nd, CRAIG EV, FUKUDA H Cuff-tear arthropathy. *J Bone Joint Surg Am, 65(9): 1232-44, 1983.*

[20] NEER CS 2nd, WATSON KC, STANTON FJ Recent experience in total shoulder replacement. J Bone Joint Surg Am, 64(3): 319-37, 1982.

[21] NYFFELER RW, WERNER CM, SIMMEN BR, GERBER C Analysis of a retrieved delta III total shoulder prosthesis. *J Bone Joint Surg Br, 86(8): 1187-91, 2004.*

[22] RITTMEISTER M, KERSCHBAUMER F Grammont reverse total shoulder arthroplasty in patients with rheumatoid arthritis and nonreconstructible rotator cuff lesions. *J Shoulder Elbow Surg, 10(1): 17-22, 2001.*

[23] ROCKWOOD CA Jr The reverse total shoulder prosthesis. The new kid on the block. *J Bone Joint Surg Am, 89(2): 233-5, 2007.*

[24] SEEBAUER L, WALTER W, KEYL W Reverse total shoulder arthroplasty for the treatment of defect arthropathy. *Oper Orthop Traumatol, 17(1): 1-24, 2005.*

[25] SIMOVITCH RW, ZUMSTEIN MA, LOHRI E, HELMY N, GERBER C. Predictors of scapular notching in patients managed with the Delta III reverse total shoulder replacement. *J Bone Joint Surg Am, 89(3): 588-600, 2007.*

[26] SIRVEAUX F, FAVARD L, OUDET D, HUQUET D, WALCH G, MOLE D Grammont inverted total shoulder arthroplasty in the treatment of glenohumeral osteoarthritis with massive rupture of the cuff. Results of a multicentre study of 80 shoulders. *J Bone Joint Surg Br, 86(3): 388-95, 2004.*

[27] VALENTI PB, D NEROT C Delta 3 reversed prothesis for osteoarthritis with massive rotator cuff tear, long term results (>5 years). Shoulder prosthesis… two to ten years follow-up. *Sauramps Medical, Montpellier 253-259, 2001.*

[28] VALENTI PK, D SAUZIERES PH Is it useful to medialize a reverse shoulder arthroplasty? Clinical and radiological results of 51 delta and 51 Arrow prosthesis. *(Paper presented at: 10th International Congress of Shoulder and Elbow Surgery (Brazil)), 2007 Brazil.*

[29] VALENTI PK, D SAUZIERES PH What should we expect of the reverse shoulder arthroplasty in term of active anterior elevation? A review of 96 cases. *(Paper presented at EFORT), 2008 Nice.*

[30] VANHOVE B, BEUGNIES A Grammont's reverse shoulder prosthesis for rotator cuff arthropathy. A retrospective study of 32 cases. *Acta Orthop Belg, 70(3): 219-25, 2004.*

[31] VISOTSKY JL, BASAMANIA C, SEEBAUER L, ROCKWOOD CA, JENSEN KL Cuff tear arthropathy: pathogenesis, classification, and algorithm for treatment. *J Bone Joint Surg Am, 86-A Suppl 2: 35-40, 2004.*

[32] WALL B, NOVE-JOSSERAND L, O'CONNOR DP, EDWARDS TB, WALCH G Reverse total shoulder arthroplasty: a review of results according to etiology. *J Bone Joint Surg Am, 89(7): 1476-85, 2007.*

[33] WERNER CM, STEINMANN PA, GILBART M, GERBER C Treatment of painful pseudoparesis due to irreparable rotator cuff dysfunction with the Delta III reverse-ball-and-socket total shoulder prosthesis. *J Bone Joint Surg Am, 87(7): 1476-86, 2005.*

[34] WIRTH MA, ROCKWOOD CA Jr Complications of total shoulder-replacement arthroplasty. *J Bone Joint Surg Am, 78(4): 603-16, 1996.*

BIOMECHANICAL RATIONALE FOR BIO-RSA & METALLIC LATERALIZATION

A. TERRIER, A. FARRON

INTRODUCTION

Reversed Shoulder Arthroplasty with a Bony Increased Offset (BIO-RSA) has been proposed by Pascal Boileau to improve the mobility of the standard reversed shoulder arthroplasty (STD-RSA) by a lateralization of the center of rotation of the joint. Instead of using an eccentric glenosphere, this technique uses a bone graft taken from the humeral head to lateralize a standard glenosphere.

Impingement is indeed a problem with the non-anatomic design of reversed shoulder prostheses. Different solutions have been proposed, such as to lateralize the center of rotation of the joint. The improvement in mobility of this solution has been evaluated, in several anatomic planes, but not in activities of daily living, which may involve more complex kinematics [1].

Although lateralization of the rotation center improves mobility, there is still a worry that this could increase the torque between the glenoid component and the glenoid bone, weakening the fixation of the baseplate, and eventually leading to an increase in risk of failure. This has been evaluated for different lateralization values, by estimating the micromotion between the baseplate and the glenoid bone, using synthetic bone and numerical models [2-3]. This is, however, still not done for the BIO-RSA.

Therefore, the goal of this study was to test two hypotheses: 1) BIO-RSA improves the mobility by reducing impingement, as in metallic lateralization, 2) BIO-RSA does not weaken screw fixation. The two hypotheses were tested with a numerical musculoskeletal model of the shoulder. Mobility was evaluated by reproducing passive kinematics of 4 activities of daily living (ADL), and screw fixation was evaluated in an active movement of loaded abduction controlled by muscles. The standard RSA was compared to the BIO-RSA and to a metallic lateralization of the glenosphere.

METHODS

A numerical musculoskeletal model of the glenohumeral joint was used for this study [4-8]. This model is composed of the scapula, the humerus, the middle deltoid (MD), the anterior deltoid (AD) and the posterior deltoid (PD). The geometry of the scapula and humerus were obtained from CT images of a normal cadaveric shoulder. The local mechanical properties of the scapula were obtained from the same CT images, using the relationship between Hounsfield number and elastic modulus [9-11]. The contact between the muscles and the bones was considered, to replicate the deformation and wrapping of the muscles around the humeral head. The arm motion was actively controlled by the muscular activation. A feedback algorithm automatically predicted the muscular forces required to balance the arm weight and produce abduction in the scapular plane. This algorithm assumed fixed ratios of the muscular forces, derived from EMG and PCSA measurements, as proposed by Poppen and Walker [12].

The reversed Aequalis prosthesis (Tornier, Inc., Edina, MN) was used as a reference in this study. The glenosphere diameter was 36 mm and the humeral cup was perfectly congruent. The BIO-RSA had the same glenosphere, but a longer central peg (25 vs. 15 mm). The positioning of the 4 screws was different, the baseplate was inclined downward by 10°, and a bone graft of 10 mm was placed between the glenoid bone cut and the baseplate. The metallic lateralization (LAT-RSA) was based on the same configuration as the STD-RSA, but with a lateralization of 10 mm of the glenosphere. The geometric description of the STD-RSA and BIO-RSA was obtained from the manufacturer, but the LAT-RSA was created from the STD¬RSA. The prostheses were inserted into the musculoskeletal model according to manufacturer recommendations using a computer-aided design (CAD) software (www.solidworks.com). Each component positioning was performed by a senior orthopedic surgeon and assessed by the manufacturer. The compressive tightening force of the anterior and posterior screws was set to 100 N, according to a cadaveric study [13]. In the numerical analysis, metal parts were assumed rigid, while the polyethylene components were elastic ($E = 500$ MPa, $\nu = 0.4$).

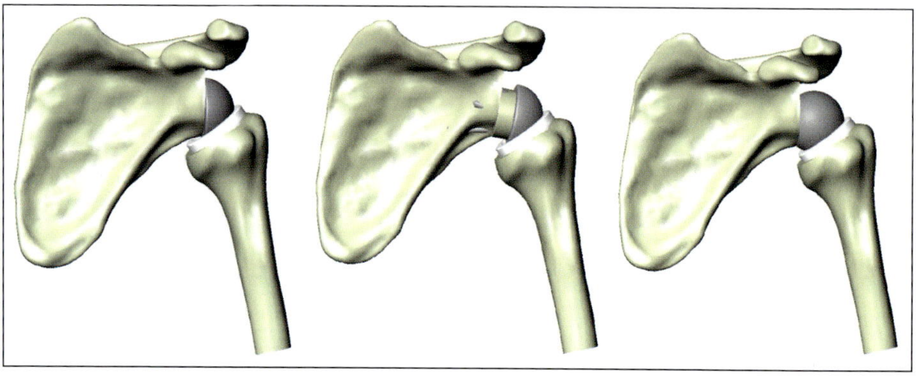

***Fig. 1:** The three configurations tested: the standard RSA (STD-RSA), the BIO-RSA, and the metallic lateralization (LAT-RSA).*

The mobility of the three prostheses was evaluated by testing all possible positions without impingement. We thus obtained a 3D map of impingement for the three angles of rotation of the glenohumeral joint, following the ISB recommendations [14]. With this map, any position of the humerus can be characterized as possible, or in mechanical conflict. This map was used to evaluate the percentage of possible movement compared to 4 different activities of daily living: **1)** hand to the contralateral shoulder, **2)** hand to mouth, **3)** combing hair, **4)** hand to back pocket [15]. The kinematics data, measured on healthy volunteers, were divided in three equal phases, for all 4 activities: the start, the middle, and the end of the movement. For each phase, the *in vivo* kinematic data were compared to the mobility map of the 3 prostheses, and the percentage of allowed movement, free of impingement, was evaluated.

The screw fixation of the three prostheses was evaluated during a simulated movement of loaded abduction in the scapular plane. Abduction was simulated from neutral elevation to 150 degrees of abduction, with the elbow in full extension. The arm weight was 37.5 N (5% of the body weight of a 75 kg person) and 10 N were added in the hand. The motion of the scapula was accounted for to provide the correct alignment of the muscle forces relative to the vertical direction of the arm weight force. A scapulo-humeral rhythm of 2:1 was assumed.

All numerical analyses were performed with the finite element solver Abaqus 6.7 (www.simulia.com). Linear hexahedral elements were used for the polyethylene component, and (modified) quadratic tetrahedral elements were used for the glenoid bone. All metallic parts, including screws, were assumed rigid. No friction was considered between the 2 articular surfaces. All interfaces were fully bonded.

For the three tested configurations, we evaluated the impingement positions, the muscle moment arms, the muscle forces, the joint reaction force, the screw force, and the bone strain around the screws. The screw force and bone (maximum principal) strain around screws corresponded only to the values between the screws and the glenoid bone, excluding the bone graft of the BIO-RSA.

RESULTS

The relative mobility of each prosthesis was improved by the BIO-RSA and the LAT-RSA, compared to the STD-RSA. This improvement was principally observed at the beginning of some movements, when the arm is in a resting position (elbow at the waist), and when the hand is at the low back (fig. 2). When the hand is on the contralateral shoulder, we observed an impingement at the end of the movement with the BIO-RSA and LAT-RSA, which was greater than for the STD-RSA.

Regarding the moment arms, forces, and bone strain around screws, similar trends were observed during the entire abduction movement. We therefore limited the results presentation to the values at 60 degrees of abduction, which were the most critical. The moment arms of the three deltoid heads decreased by about 10% with the BIO-RSA and STD-RSA, compared to the STD-RSA. This induced an increase of the muscular force of about 10% in each deltoid head. The joint reaction force also increased by about 10% in the BIO-RSA and LAT-RSA. The force between each screw and the glenoid bone

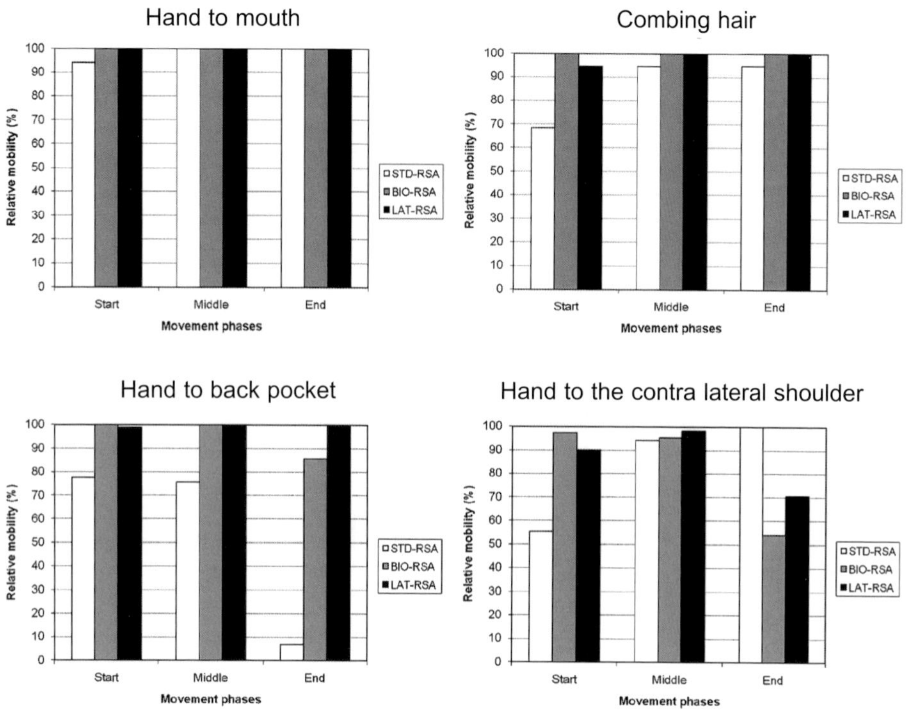

Fig. 2: The relative mobility of each prosthesis, for the 4 movements considered, in the 3 phases of the movement.

was rather similar for each prosthesis. Overall, the screw force was approximately 2 times higher in the superior screw (≈ 240 N) than in the other screws (≈ 110 N). There was however a higher force in the inferior screw of the BIO-RSA (≈ 190 N) compared to the STD-RSA (≈ 80 N) and LAT-RSA (≈ 90 N), but it was partly balanced by a lower force (≈ 230 N) in the superior screw of the BIO-RSA compared to the LAT-RSA (≈ 270 N). Finally, these changes in screw forces between each prosthesis, were slightly transferred into bone strain around the screws. Overall, there were indeed only small differences between each screw, and each prosthesis (Fig. 3). On average, the bone strain was near its physiologic value (≈ 0.1%), and below the damaging value (≈ 1%).

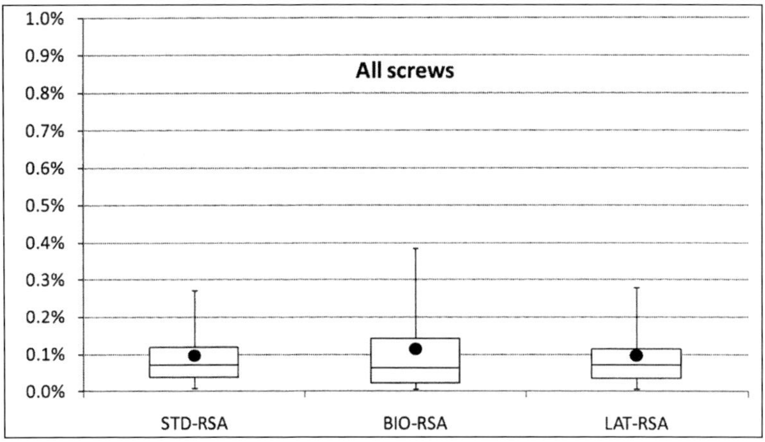

***Fig. 3:* Bone glenoid (maximum principal) strain around all screws, for each prosthesis. The complex distribution of the strain around the 4 screws is summarized in boxplots by the lower quartile, the median, the upper quartile, the 10th and 90th percentile. The black dot represents the average.**

DISCUSSION

Reverse shoulder arthroplasty is a relatively new technique to treat glenohumeral arthritis coupled with rotator cuff deficiency. Although results are rather good, there are still some concerns, mainly with the impingement caused by the non-anatomic reverse prosthesis. Metallic lateralization of the joint center has been proposed to limit the impingement and increase mobility. Recently, Pascal Boileau has presented a new technique using a bone graft taken from the humeral head to achieve the lateralization. This technique, using a specific baseplate, was compared to a classic reversed prosthesis and to a metallic lateralized prosthesis, using a numerical musculoskeletal model of the shoulder.

The mobility analysis confirmed the improvement of the BIO-RSA, which was similar to the mobility of the LAT-RSA. The fixation quality of the screws was evaluated by estimation the glenoid bone strain around each screws. Overall, the strains were similar for each prosthesis and below the damage value of 1%. The results of mobility were consistent with previous studies [1] as the results of screw fixation, which can be compared to stability analysis of the baseplate [2-3].

The strength of the present study was to compare the three prostheses within the same numerical framework, which has however some limitations. The most important one is certainly with associated the simulated movement. Although mobility was evaluated in 4 activities of daily living, the screw fixation was only tested for a loaded abduction in the scapular plane. We might indeed observe a different behavior, and have different conclusions for other movements. We, however, assume that this movement can be associate with the most frequent loaded activities supported by the glenohumeral joint.

To conclude, BIO-RSA and the equivalent metallic lateralization improve mobility, without increasing the risk of glenoid component failure.

ACKNOWLEDGEMENTS

This study was financially supported by Tornier (Tornier Inc, Edina, MN). The authors also thank Yves-Alain Ratron (Research director, Tornier) and Prof. Pascal Boileau for their help.

REFERENCES

[1] GUTIERREZ S, LEVY JC, LEE WE, 3rd, KELLER TS, MAITLAND ME. Center of Rotation Affects Abduction Range of Motion of Reverse Shoulder Arthroplasty. *Clin Orthop Relat Res 2007.*

[2] HARMAN M, FRANKLE M, VASEY M, BANKS S. Initial glenoid component fixation in "reverse" total shoulder arthroplasty: a biomechanical evaluation. *J Shoulder Elbow Surg 2005;14: 162S-7S.*

[3] HOPKINS AR, HANSEN UN, BULL AM, EMERY R, AMIS AA. Fixation of the reversed shoulder prosthesis. *J Shoulder Elbow Surg 2008; 17: 974-80.*

[4] TERRIER A, MERLINI F, PIOLETTI DP, FARRON A. Total shoulder arthroplasty: Downward inclination of the glenoid component to balance supraspinatus deficiency. *J Shoulder Elbow Surg 2009.*

[5] TERRIER A, REIST A, MERLINI F, FARRON A. Simulated joint and muscle forces in reversed and anatomic shoulder prostheses. *J Bone Joint Surg Br 2008; 90: 751-6.*

[6] TERRIER A, MERLINI F, PIOLETTI DP, FARRON A. Comparison of polyethylene wear in anatomical and reversed shoulder prostheses. *J Bone Joint Surg Br 2009; 91: 977-82.*

[7] TERRIER A, REIST A, VOGEL A, FARRON A. Effect of supraspinatus deficiency on humerus translation and glenohumeral contact force during abduction. *Clin Biomech 2007; 22: 645-51.*

[8] TERRIER A, VOGEL A, CAPEZZALI M, FARRON A. An algorithm to allow humerus translation in the indeterminate problem of shoulder abduction. *Med Eng Phys 2008; 30: 710-6.*

[9] CARTER DR, HAYES WC. The compressive behavior of bone as a two-phase porous structure. *J Bone Joint Surg Am 1977; 59: 954-62.*

[10] MANSAT P, BAREA C, HOBATHO MC, DARMANA R, MANSAT M. Anatomic variation of the mechanical properties of the glenoid. *J Shoulder Elbow Surg 1998;7: 109-15.*

[11] RHO JY, HOBATHO MC, ASHMAN RB. Relations of mechanical properties to density and CT numbers in human bone. *Med Eng Phys 1995; 17: 347-55.*

[12] POPPEN NK, WALKER PS. Forces at the glenohumeral joint in abduction. *Clin Orthop 1978: 165-70.*

[13] TERRIER A, KOCHBECK S, MERLINI F, GORTCHACOW M, PIOLETTI DP, FARRON A. Tightening Force and Torque of Nonlocking Screws in a Reverse Shoulder Prosthesis. *Clinical Biomechanics Accepted for publication.*

[14] WU G, VAN DER HELM FC, VEEGER HE, *et al.* ISB recommendation on definitions of joint coordinate systems of various joints for the reporting of human joint motion-Part II: shoulder, elbow, wrist and hand. *J Biomech 2005; 38: 981-92.*

[15] VAN ANDEL CJ, WOLTERBEEK N, DOORENBOSCH CA, VEEGER DH, HARLAAR J. Complete 3D kinematics of upper extremity functional tasks. *Gait Posture 2008; 27:120-7.*

BONY INCREASED-OFFSET REVERSED SHOULDER ARTHROPLASTY (BIO-RSA): THE BENEFITS OF BONY LATERALIZATION

P. BOILEAU, G. MOINEAU, Y. ROUSSANNE, K. O'SHEA

ABSTRACT

Background

Scapular notching, prosthetic instability, limited shoulder rotation, and loss of shoulder contour are problems associated with the current medialized design reverse shoulder arthroplasty (RSA). We hypothesized that the addition of cancellous bone graft, harvested from the humerus, and placed beneath the baseplate of the RSA would heal, effectively creating a scapula with a long neck. We further hypothesized that such bony lateralization would prevent the above-mentioned problems, and protect the glenoid component from loosening.

Material and Methods

A bony increased-offset RSA (BIO-RSA) was implanted into 45 consecutive patients (mean age, 72 years) with a rotator cuff-deficient shoulder. An autogenous bone graft harvested from the humeral head was placed between the baseplate and the reamed glenoid surface, secured in place using a lengthened central peg (+25 mm) and 4 screws. Patients with severe glenoid bone loss or humeral head necrosis were not included. All patients underwent prospective clinical, plain radiographic and CT-scan assessment except 3 patients who died before two-year follow-up. The mean follow-up was 28 months (24 to 40 months).

Results

The bone graft healed completely to the native glenoid in 41 cases and partially in one case. No graft resorption under the baseplate and no glenoid loosening was observed at latest follow-up. Scapular notching (inferior and/or posterior) was identified in 9 patients. Mean active anterior elevation improved from 86° to 146° (+61°), external rotation from 13° to 23° (+10°), and internal rotation from 4.4 to 5.6 points (+1.2). The absolute Constant Score improved from 31 to 67 points ($p<0.0001$). The adjusted Constant improved from 44 to 93% ($p<0.0001$). The Subjective Shoulder Value (SSV) increased from 33% to 75% ($p<0.0001$). No postoperative instability was observed and the shoulder contour was maintained.

Conclusions

Despite the advanced age of the patients, bone grafts harvested from the humeral head and placed under the glenoid baseplate of an RSA healed in all cases. Biomechanically, keeping the center of rotation at the bone-glenoid interface avoids increasing the torque on the glenoid component. The clinical advantages of the BIO-RSA are decreased scapular notching, enhanced prosthetic stability, maintenance of shoulder contour; all while preserving active mobility. With regard to the prevention of glenoid loosening, while respecting the principles of Grammont, bony lateralization is, in our opinion, more appropriate than prosthetic lateralization.

Level of evidence

Therapeutic study, Level IV (case series - no, or historical control group)

INTRODUCTION

In patients with pseudo-paralysis related to rotator cuff deficiency, the Grammont reverse shoulder arthoplasty (RSA) represents a major advance in the restoration of shoulder function [8, 11, 13, 17, 18, 33, 35, 36]. The two basic biomechanical principles of the Grammont prosthesis are: ***1)*** medialization of the gleno-humeral center of rotation and, ***2)*** lowering of the humerus [7]. The resultant effect of these principles is to reduce torque on the glenoid component and increase the deltoid lever arm, overcoming the weak or absent rotator cuff musculature [7, 37]. To date, the reported rate of glenoid component loosening in the Grammont RSA has been relatively low, ranging from 2-5% [7, 8, 35, 38]. A number of problems and complications specific to this prosthesis have been reported in the literature; however, all of them can be attributed to its medialized design. The first of these, scapular notching, has been observed in 50 to 96% of postoperative radiographs [7, 8, 30, 32, 33, 38, 44]. Infero-medial impingement of the humeral insert against the pillar of the scapula during adduction and rotation of the arm is associated with polyethylene wear, potentially resulting in osteolysis from the generated particulate wear debris [7, 30, 35]. Large scapular notches, encroaching upon the inferior-most screw are associated with decreased functional results and glenoid loosening [34, 35]. *Limited post operative shoulder rotation*, although depending in part on the state of the remaining rotator cuff muscles, is also related to the limited excursion of the cup around the medialized glenosphere [6]. With the arm held by the side, impingement of the cup against the glenoid neck may be a limiting factor in achieving gleno-humeral rotation. Anterior scapular impingement may restrict internal rotation while posterior impingement restricts external rotation. *Prosthetic instability* occurs in 3 to 6% of Grammont RSA's [4, 15, 29]. In addition to the potential for instability arising from impingement of the cup on the glenoid neck, humeral medialization reduces the tension on the peri-articular soft tissues. Both early dislocation, as a result of direct impingement and late, as a result of wear of the polyethylene cup, have been observed. Finally, humeral medialization raises a cosmetic concern as some patients dislike the loss of their normal shoulder contour [6].

In an attempt to address these problems, recent authors have proposed a change in the design of Grammont's prosthesis, promoting an *increased-offset* RSA [14, 39]. Such *prosthetic lateralization*, achieved by increasing the offset of the glenosphere or baseplate, potentially decreases the risk of scapular notching while improving shoulder stability and rotation. The disadvantage of prosthetic lateralization is the increased torque or shear force applied to the glenoid component. In a biomechanical study, Harman et al demonstrated a four-fold increase in displacement of the glenoid component during eccentric loading, when comparing a + 7mm increased-offset baseplate prosthesis to the medialized design of the Grammont prosthesis [22]. Not surprisingly, in clinical practice, *increased-offset RSA* led to increased rates of glenoid loosening and screw breakage. Frankel et al reported the clinical and radiological results of 60 patients operated with a lateralized RSA (RSP, Encore Medical). At a mean follow-up of 21 months, while no scapular notching was observed, eight baseplate failures in seven patients required revision, equivalent to a 12% rate of glenoid loosening [14]. In comparison, Guéry et al, in a series of 80 patients with cuff tear arthritis (CTA) treated with the Grammont prosthesis, reported a 4% rate of glenoid loosening at 10 to 15 years follow up [19].

In an attempt to address the problematic issues encountered with RSA, we adopted a novel approach. Our hypothesis was that *bony lateralization* of RSA would be preferable to metallic prosthetic lateralization. Rather than changing Grammont's RSA, a design proven successful over 20 years, we have sought to solve some of the problems related to humeral medialization by improving the surgical technique and implant. In 2006, we started to bone graft the reamed glenoid surface with a disc of cancellous bone graft, harvested from the humeral head, during implantation of RSA. Our goal was to obtain a bony lateralization of the prosthesis that would keep the center of rotation at the glenoid bone-prosthesis interface (fig. 1). The autogenous bone graft is secured in place using a modified baseplate, which has a lengthened central peg (+25 mm) and accepts 4 screws. Once the bone graft has healed to the native glenoid, the torque on the glenoid component should be minimized, protecting from glenoid loosening, while the problems related to medialization (notching, instability, limited rotation, loss of shoulder contour) should be prevented. This original procedure is called '*bony increased-offset reversed shoulder arthroplasty*' or 'BIO RSA'.

The aim of the present prospective study is to report the clinical and radiological results of the BIO-RSA with a minimum two-year follow-up. We hypothesized that: ***1)*** a bone graft to the native glenoid using a disc of cancellous bone harvested from the humeral head during RSA would heal, not resorbing under the baseplate despite the advanced age of the patients; ***2)*** bony lateralization of the RSA would offer the advantage of being faithful to Grammont's principle, keeping the center of rotation at the glenoid bone-prosthesis interface, thus avoiding glenoid loosening; ***3)*** bony lateralization of the RSA would not compromise the deltoid lever arm and would still allow restoration of active elevation despite the deficiency of the rotator cuff; and ***4)*** glenoid bone grafting during RSA would be beneficial for the patient by decreasing the rate of scapular notching, improving stability, and preserving shoulder rotation and shoulder contour.

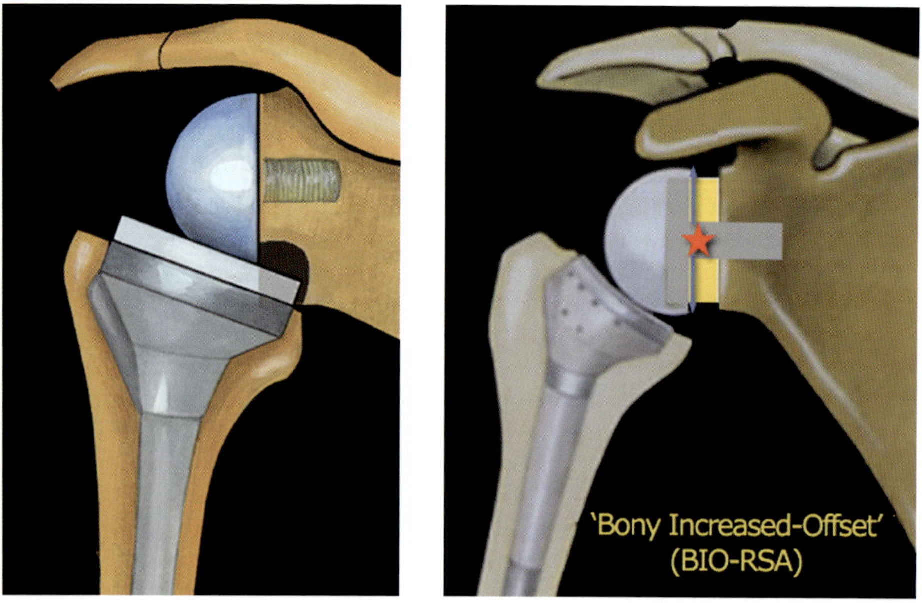

Fig. 1: The medialized design of the Grammont (inferior scapular impingement) and the concept of the BIO-RSA (Bony-increased offset Reversed Shoulder Arthroplasty), which gives more clearance for the cup around the sphere while still keeping the center of rotation within the scapula.

MATERIAL AND METHODS

Patient Selection

The BIO-RSA was offered as a treatment to patients presenting with a painful and pseudo-paralytic shoulder related to cuff tear arthritis (CTA), failed rotator cuff surgery or the sequelae of a proximal humeral fracture. The study protocol required the implantation of the same reverse geometry prosthesis in all patients, incorporating a glenoid bone graft harvested from the humeral head, fixed with a specific baseplate with a lengthened central peg and four screws. The postoperative protocol consisted of clinical, plain radiographic and CT scan follow-up at a minimum of two years following prosthetic implantation.

We excluded from the present investigation: ***1)*** patients with severe glenoid bone deficiency either in the vertical plane (Favard stage E3) or in the horizontal plane (Walch type B2 and C) [13,42] as it was felt that their inclusion would not have permitted evaluation of the benefits of the bony lateralization; ***2)*** cases where it would not have been possible to harvest a humeral bone graft such as: patients with severe humeral deficiency as occurs in end-stage CTA with humeral head necrosis and/or collapse i.e. Hamada and Fukuda stage 5 [21], some cases of rheumatoid arthritis, proximal humeral tumors or patients with failed previous arthroplasty; ***3)*** patients who underwent the procedure using a bone graft other than autologous humeral head, such as iliac crest bone graft or allograft.

The risks and benefits of the procedure were explained to the patients. All patients gave written, informed consent and local institutional review board approval was obtained.

Operative Technique

All operations were performed by the senior author (PB) or under his direction. The procedure was carried out under general anesthesia with interscalene block in the 'beach-chair' position. Although feasible through an anterosuperior deltoid splitting approach, a delto-pectoral approach was used in all cases.

The implant used was the Aequalis™ Reversed (Tornier Inc., Houston) which is a reverse ball and socket prosthesis designed according to Grammont's principles [17, 18]. The conventional baseplate has a 15 mm long central peg. In order to accommodate the bone graft and facilitate stable fixation in the native glenoid, a specific metaglene with a lengthened central peg (25 mm) was designed and implanted in all cases. The circular baseplate is 29 mm in diameter, has a rough surface, and is hydroxyapatite coated (fig. 2).

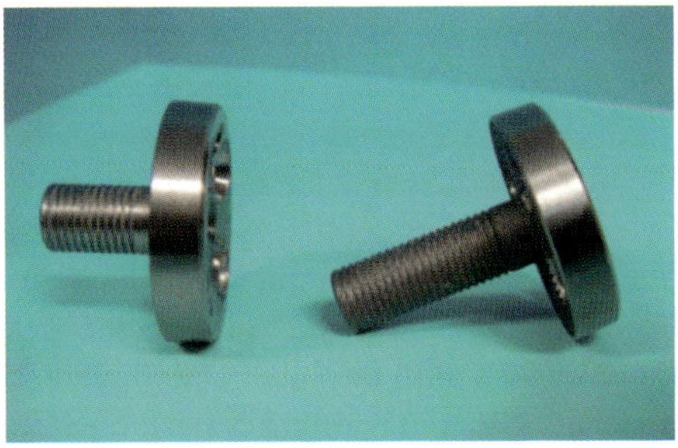

Fig. 2: Standard baseplate with a 15mm long central peg and BIO-RSA baseplate with lengthened peg (25 mm) used for primary fixation in the native glenoid vault.

The surgical technique comprises ***three principal operative steps.***

Humeral Bone Graft Harvesting and Humeral Osteotomy (fig. 3)

Any remaining subscapularis tendon is detached from the lesser tuberosity. In all cases, the postero-superior cuff (supra- and infra-spinatus) was absent. If still present, the long head of the biceps tendon is tenodesed. Following anterior dislocation of the head, humeral preparation is performed. A 155° inclined humeral guide is placed at the summit of the head and set parallel to the forearm axis (0 to 30° according to the transepicondylar axis). No attempt is made to modify the native humeral retroversion. The ring of the humeral guide is placed in contact with the humeral head. A 2.5 mm threaded guide-wire is inserted in the axis of the humeral head until it catches the opposite humeral cortex. A ***bell-saw*** is used to create a cylinder of cancellous bone, 29 mm in diameter, corresponding to the dimensions of the baseplate. The humeral head cartilage is then reamed until the underlying cancellous bone is exposed. A cannulated drill is used to drill a central hole, 8mm in diameter, and the guide wire is removed. A ***cutting-guide*** is then inserted to harvest the desired thickness of bone graft (10 mm or 7 mm) with the aid of an oscillating saw. The disc of cancellous bone graft, harvested from the humerus is inserted along the lengthened central peg until it reaches the posterior surface of the baseplate. This disc may be either symmetrical or asymmetrical to compensate for cases where a degree of superior or posterior glenoid wear is encountered. In cases of asymmetrical grafting, the cylinder of graft is marked with a sterile pencil to assist in orientation according to the baseplate and the location of glenoid wear.

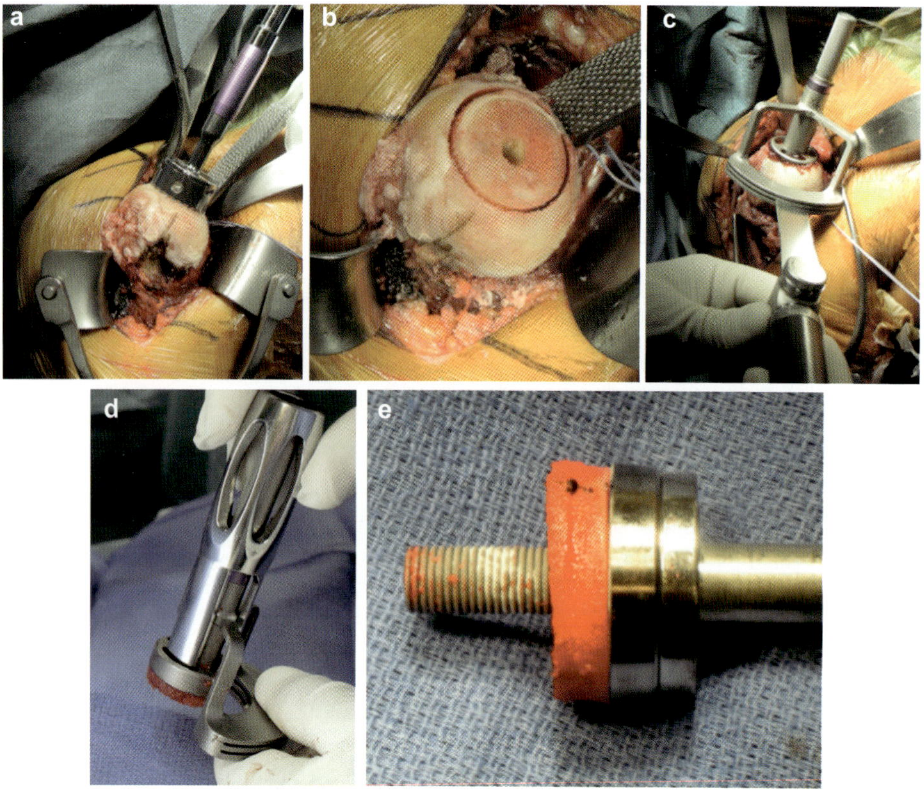

Fig. 3 (a-e): The pure cancellous bone graft, harvested from the humerus is inserted along the lengthened central peg until it reaches the posterior surface of the baseplate.

Glenoid Step

Achieving adequate glenoid exposure is the key technical point of this procedure. An anteroinferior capsulotomy and circumferential labral excision are performed. After partial detachment of the triceps origin, a specific retractor with two twisted ears (Playboy™ retractor, Tornier Inc.) is inserted to enable exposure of the inferior part of the glenoid surface. The vertical (meridian) and horizontal (equator) axes of the glenoid are marked with electro-cautery. The glenoid guide (29 mm in diameter) is placed flush with the inferior border of the glenoid and, the previously used 2.5 mm threaded wire is inserted into the glenoid with either 0° or 10° of inferior tilt in case of superior glenoid wear. A glenoid reamer is advanced on this wire. The reamer should be started while not yet in continuity with the glenoid surface so as to avoid iatrogenic fracture. The reamer is used to flatten the glenoid surface until the subchondral plate is reached. Glenoid reaming is performed to a depth of approximately 5 mm. The goal of the glenoid reaming is: ***1)*** to reach the cancellous bleeding bone, while ***2)*** avoiding superior tilt of the baseplate which has been shown to be associated with glenoid component loosening. It is crucial that the reamed glenoid surface be cancellous and/or bleeding to optimize the probability of bone graft healing. Although easily obtained at the inferior part of the glenoid, it is more difficult to achieve at the superior part of the glenoid where the bone is dense and cortical. Consequently, in addition to glenoid reaming, small drill holes (2.5 mm) are made at the periphery of the glenoid in order to obtain a complete bleeding bone surface (fig. 4). The central hole is then over drilled to 8 mm, using a "self-stop" drill bit. The baseplate, together with the harvested bone graft, is impacted into the central drilled hole. In a manner equivalent to plate osteosynthesis, fixation is obtained with two 4.5 mm AO compressive (anterior and posterior) and two 4.5 mm locking screws (inferior and superior). The anterior and posterior AO screws are placed first for compression of the bone graft against the prepared bleeding glenoid surface and are inserted in a convergent direction. The superior and inferior locked screws are inserted divergently: the aim is to place one screw into the base of the coracoid and one into the inferior scapular pillar in order to achieve the maximum possible purchase. The glenosphere is then fixed to the metaglene via a morse taper and countersunk set screw. The glenosphere diameter chosen depends on the size of humerus i.e. the size of the patient. The 36 mm diameter glenosphere is usually used in frail elderly women while the 42 mm is preferred in men. The thickness of the disc of cancellous bone graft is adjusted according to the size of the sphere. A 10mm graft is used for a 36 mm sphere and a 7 mm graft for a 42 mm sphere as the 42 mm sphere is already more lateralized than the 36 mm.

Humeral Step

This is performed preferentially following the glenoid step in order to avoid fragilization of the humerus and scratching of the glenosphere with the humeral component during the dislocation maneuver. The metaphyseal "cheese grater" reamer (32 or 42 mm) is used to remove the remaining cancellous bone from the proximal humeral epiphysis, allowing placement of the neck component. Diaphyseal reaming is performed sequentially with broaches of 6, 9, 12, and 15 mm; the diameter of

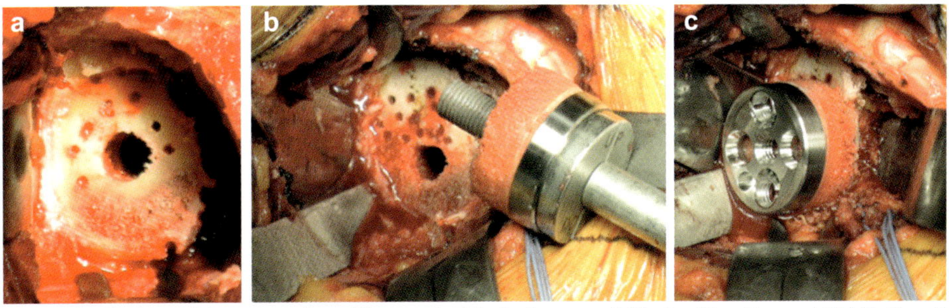

Fig. 4 (a-c): Glenoid preparation: The central hole is over-drilled with a 8mm drill bit. Small drill holes (2.5mm) are made at the periphery of the glenoid face in order to obtain a complete bleeding bone surface. The baseplate, with the cancellous bone graft inserted along the lengthened central peg, is impacted until it reaches the cancellous glenoid surface and then fixed with four screws.

stem chosen corresponding to the broach which comes into contact with the diaphyseal cortical bone. The humeral trial component is then inserted in the medullary canal and a standard +6mm polyethylene (PE) cup is inserted. The prosthesis is reduced and prosthetic stability and tension is assessed. Usually, in primary cases a polyethylene of greater thickness than 6mm is not required as the prosthetic lateralization results in enhanced stability and soft-tissue tension. The trial is removed and the definitive humeral implant is cemented into the medullary canal in the planned degree of retroversion. A definitive standard PE humeral insert is impacted into the humeral neck. The humeral component is then reduced by gentle traction applied to the arm in slight abduction while simultaneously applying direct pressure on the humeral neck. A "shoehorn" is often used to assist in the reduction maneuver. After the shoulder has been reduced with final implants in position, the shoulder is put through a full passive range of motion to check for any evidence of instability or impingement. The subscapularis tendon is reattached to the lesser tuberosity using three to four transosseous sutures that are placed before humeral cementation and prosthesis implantation. The deltopectoral interval is closed and a drain on closed suction is left in place for 24 hours.

Postoperative Management

Patients are discharged from the hospital one or two days after surgery. A sling is worn during the first four weeks. The rehabilitation protocol used for the BIO-RSA is not different to that used for a standard RSA. Self-directed rehabilitation with pendular exercises are started immediately (5 times a day, 5 minutes each session). The patient is encouraged to use his/her hand immediately for activities of daily living such as eating, drinking, holding a newspaper or a book to read, typewriting, dressing, etc. After four weeks, formal rehabilitation with a physiotherapist is started. Aquatherapy in a swimming pool is recommended. No heavy lifting is allowed until after 12 weeks so as to ensure that solid bony union of the graft has been obtained. Return to all types of activities, including gardening or leisure sports (swimming, golfing) is permitted at 3 to 6 months postoperatively.

Clinical Evaluation

All patients were prospectively evaluated at 3, 6, 12 months by the surgeon (PB), and yearly thereafter by two independent observers (GM and YR). The Constant and Murley functional score was measured preoperatively and at each review [10, 12, 31]. The clinical results were graded according to the Constant score: a Constant score adjusted for age and gender of $\geq$100% was considered excellent, between 85-99% good, between 65-84% fair and inferior to 65% poor. The range of motion measured consisted of forward elevation in the scapular plane, external rotation (in adduction & in abduction) and internal rotation. Strength was measured using a hand-held dynamometer with the arm elevated 90° in the scapular plane. Any episode of instability (i.e., prosthetic subluxation or dislocation) during the follow-up period was recorded. Patients were asked to rate their satisfaction with the outcome. They were also asked to estimate the value of their shoulder as a percentage of an entirely normal shoulder (the SSV- Subjective Shoulder Value), preoperatively and at the last review [16].

Radiological Evaluation

All shoulders had postoperative plain radiographic assessment using fluoroscopy and magnification control according to the recommendations of Lévigne [25]. Radiographs were analyzed for evidence of bone graft healing, presence of radiolucent lines around the components, uncoupling or loosening of glenoid components, scapular notching and inferior osteophytes or spurs. Inferior scapular notching was carefully evaluated and graded according to the Nérot classification system [7].

CT-Scan Evaluation

Post-operative computed tomography was performed in all cases. Two independent examiners (GM and YR) analyzed all CT scans using OsiriX® software. Intra-observer and inter-observer reliability testing confirmed the reproducibility of the radiological and CT-scan evaluation. Parameters examined included bone graft healing, graft resorption or lysis, presence of radiolucent lines or glenoid loosening and the presence of scapular notching.

Two zones were divised, one above and one below the central peg on the true antero-posterior view in order to evaluate bone graft healing. ***Bone graft healing*** was considered as complete if no radiolucent line was observed in either of the two zones, partial if a radiolucent line was observed in one of the two zones, and absent if a radiolucent line was observed in the two zones. The same two zones were analyzed for evidence of Bone graft resorption or lysis. Images were carefully evaluated for inferior, posterior and anterior scapular notching. ***Inferior scapular notching*** was evaluated on the coronal slice passing directly through the middle of the glenoid peg. The distance between the middle of the lengthened glenoid peg and the inferior border of the graft is 14mm. Inferior notching was considered present if this distance measured less than 14mm. In a similar manner, axial slices were examined for the presence of ***anterior or posterior notching***.

Statistical Analysis

The d'Agostino-Pearson test was used to analyze data distribution. Pre- and post-operative data was analyzed for statistically significant differences between means; paired values were compared using the paired t-test and unpaired results were compared with the Mann-Whitney test (MWT). The Chi-squared test (Chi2) and Fisher's exact test (FET) for small numbers were used to compare categorical data. The significance level was set at $p<0.05$.

RESULTS

Patient Population

Between March 2006 and March 2008, 45 consecutive patients with cuff-deficient shoulders who underwent RSA combined with glenoid bone grafting were prospectively followed. No patient was lost to follow-up, but three patients died from unrelated conditions before two years post-operatively, leaving 42 patients available for complete functional, radiological and CT assessment. The average duration of follow-up was 28 months (range, 24 to 40 months). Forty-two shoulders in 42 patients constituted the study group. There were 28 women and 14 men; in 32 cases, the dominant side was affected. The average age of the patients at the time of surgery was 72 years (range 52 to 86 years). Before undergoing surgery, all patients had exhausted conservative treatment which consisted of physical therapy for a minimum of six months and/or intra-articular corticosteroid injections. In 27 cases, the pre-operative diagnosis was cuff tear arthritis (CTA); 12 patients had failed previous rotator cuff surgery: 8 had failed rotator cuff repair (6 open and 2 arthroscopically) and 4 had failed biceps tenodesis (with acromioplasty in 2 cases); 3 patients had sequelae of proximal humeral fractures. All patients had complete tears of the supraspinatus and infraspinatus with variable involvement of the subscapularis and teres minor.

Complications

No cases of glenoid loosening, prosthetic dislocation or subluxation were observed. No patient had to be revised or reoperated during the period of follow up. One patient had a temporary post-surgical brachial plexus palsy with complete recovery at 6 months post-operatively.

Clinical results

The functional results, according to the Constant score, the mobility and the subjective results according to the subjective Shoulder Value (SSV) are summarized in Table I.

Table 1: Functional Results

	Preoperative	Postoperative	Gain	P Value (tests)
Active Mobility				
AAE (°)	86 ± 35 (20 to 160)	146 ± 21 (80 to 170)	+60 (-20 to 130)	<0.0001 (MWT)
AER (°)	12.8 ± 21.4 (-40 to 50)	22.9 ± 16.4 (-10 to 70)	+10 (-20 to 60)	<0.01 (t-test)
AIR (level)	4.4 ± 2.2 (0 to 10)	5.7 ± 2.5 (0 to 10)	+1.3 (-10 to 10)	<0.031 (MWT)
Constant Score				
Pain / 15 points	5.5 ± 3.4 (0 to 15)	12.7 ± 2.8 (5 to 15)	+7 (-10 to 15)	<0.0001 (MWT)
Activities / 20 points	7 ± 3.3 (5 to 12)	16.5 ± 2.9 (10 to 20)	+9.5 (-2 to 18)	<0.0001 (t-test)
Range of motion / 40 points	17 ± 9.6 (4 to 38)	30.4 ± 5.8 (14 to 40)	+13 (-8 to 30)	<0.0001 (MWT)
Strength / 25 points	1.8 ± 4.9 (0 to 10)	7 ± 3.8 (0 to 18)	+5 (-3 to 18)	<0.0001 (MWT)
Absolute Constant Score /100 points	**31 ± 13** **(8 to 60)**	**66.6 ± 11** **(31 to 88)**	**+35** **(-15 to 64)**	<0.0001 (MWT)
Adjusted Constant Score (%)	**44 ± 18.4** (13 to 87)	**93.4 ± 15.6** (48 to 136)	**49** (-22 to 100)	<0.0001 (MWT)
Subjective Shoulder Value (SSV) (/100%)	**34 % ± 16** (10 to 80)	**75 % ± 14** (30 to 95)	**+41 %** (-15 % - 70 %)	p<0.0001 (MWT)

AAE = Active Anterior Elevation; **AER** = Active External Rotation; **AIR** = Active Internal Rotation. Each parameter has been reported as a mean value, with standard deviation and range.

Thirty-nine patients (93%) were satisfied or very satisfied with their functional result. According to the adjusted Constant score, the clinical results were excellent or good in 32 patients (76%), fair in 8 patients and poor in 2 patients.

The gain in active mobility was respectively +60° for anterior active elevation, +10° for active external rotation and +1.3 points for internal rotation. Only one patient had negative external rotation with the arm at side. Mean active external rotation in abduction was 53° (range 10°-90°). Thirty-six patients (86%) were able to internally rotate at least to the sacrum.

Radiological Results

Radiographic images were available for analysis in all 42 patients. Bone graft healing was complete in the upper zone in 41 cases and doubtful in 1 case. Healing was complete in the lower zone in all 42 cases (fig. 5). There were no cases of glenoid component loosening at latest follow-up. No lucent lines around the peg or around the screws were observed in any case. There was no evidence of any humeral-side component loosening or failure. Inferior scapular notching was observed in 8 cases (19%). According to the Nérot classification, it was classified as grade 1 in 5 cases, as grade 2 in two cases and as grade 3 in one case. An inferior osteophyte (spur) along the scapula was observed in 17 cases at the level of the pillar.

CT Scan Results

Computed tomographic analysis at a minimum of 2 years following surgery was available for all 42 patients. Bone graft healing was considered to be complete in 41 cases. One bone graft was considered to have healed partially because of a persistent radiolucent line observed at the interface between the graft and the native glenoid above the central peg. No radiolucent line was observed at the

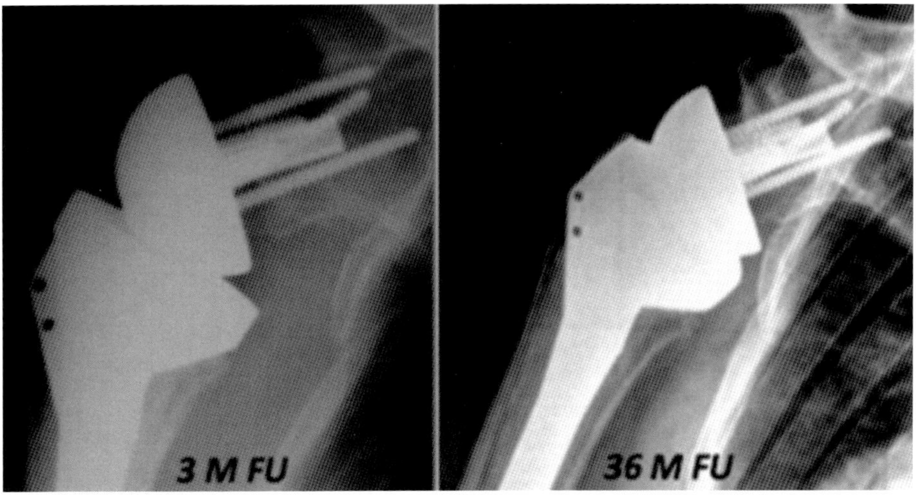

Fig. 5: Radiological results: A/P views showing bone graft evolution (3 months and 36 months follow-up) with complete healing and no scapular notching at latest follow-up. Note the low and inferiorly tilted positioning of the glenoid implant in addition to its lateralization.

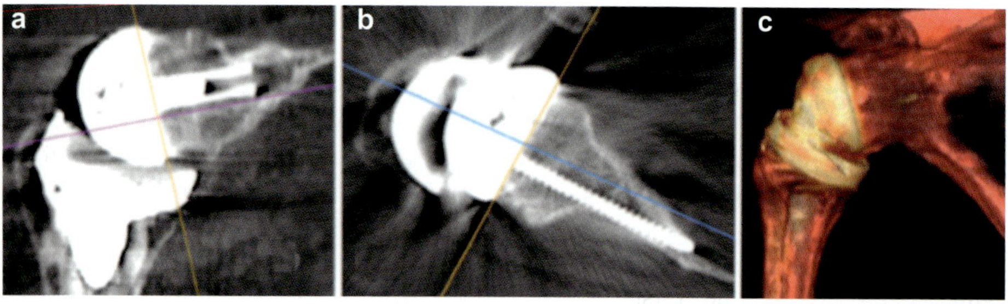

Fig. 6: CT scan at 36 months follow-up showing bone graft healing in the frontal plane (A), axial plane below the peg (B) and 3D reconstruction demonstrating the lengthened scapular neck (C).

inferior part of this graft (fig. 6). No graft resorption was observed except partial lysis of the inferior part of the graft corresponding to the observed cases of inferior scapular notching. The same 8 cases of inferior scapular notching observed on the plain radiographs were confirmed on CT imaging. A posterior notch was observed in 3 cases, isolated in two cases and associated with an inferior notch in one patient. No cases of anterior scapular notching were encountered.

DISCUSSION

Two separate prosthetic designs of RSA (*Grammont-medialized* and *metallic-lateralized*) are currently available for implantation, each with distinct advantages and drawbacks. On one hand, the medialized design RSA of Grammont practically eliminates the problem of glenoid loosening, while being at the same time responsible for some other problems and complications as reported in the literature [8, 11, 13, 17, 18, 33, 35, 36]. Scapular notching, prosthetic instability, limited mobility in rotation, and cosmetic concerns are the main disadvantages related to the medialized design of the Grammont prosthesis. To avoid or minimize these potential shortcomings, other authors have recently proposed lateralized-offset RSA [14, 39]. Such implants have the potential to generate greater torque at the bone-implant interface, with the net effect of increasing the rate of glenoid loosening [22]. This *metallic lateralization* takes place at the baseplate level or at the sphere level or both. Consequently, the prosthetic center of rotation is not located in the scapula but inside the prosthesis itself. In many ways, this prosthetic (metallic) lateralization represents a 'return to the past', leading to repeat the same mistakes as the previous generation when early designs of RSA failed due to glenoid loosening [3, 6, 9, 12].

The question therefore arises: is it be possible to retain some of the advantages of Grammont's medialized concept, keeping the center of rotation within the scapula, while in addition benefiting from a lateralized design RSA which reduces the problems of scapular notching, prosthetic instability, limited rotation and loss of shoulder contour? In an attempt to answer this question, we have proposed a procedure aimed at achieving bony lateralization of the RSA (instead of a *metallic lateralization*) (fig. 1). The concept is to graft the glenoid with a cancellous bone graft, harvested from the humeral head, securely fixing it in situ with the help of a lengthened baseplate peg and screws (fig. 3, 4).

This original procedure with a modified implant is called 'bony increased-offset reversed shoulder arthroplasty' or 'BIO-RSA'. While the principle of the BIO-RSA was simple and apparently sound from a biomechanical perspective, it needed to be verified in clinical practice. There were a number of potential concerns with this novel technique. Firstly, as the RSA is a semi-constrained prosthesis, performed predominantly in elderly patients with decreased healing potential, there is a theoretical risk of nonunion and/or resorption of the bone graft, the consequence of which would be glenoid loosening. Secondly, the functional effect of bony lateralization on shoulder motion was unclear: while shoulder rotation could theoretically be improved, in the setting of rotator cuff deficiency it was unknown whether lateralization would allow the deltoid to function sufficiently to permit active elevation above the horizontal level.

The present study confirms our *first hypothesis*: despite the advanced age of the operated patients in our series (72 years), the bone graft healed completely to the native glenoid in 41 cases and partially in one case. We did not observe any instance of bone graft resorption or lysis under the baseplate at a mean follow-up of 28 months. Bone graft healing was followed closely with sequential radiographs (at 3, 6, 12 months) and with CT-scans in all patients (fig. 5 and 6). We believe that a number of factors are responsible for the satisfying healing rates between the bone graft and the native glenoid: ***1)*** autograft, not allograft was used; ***2)*** the bone graft was applied to a bleeding cancellous surface on the native glenoid; ***3)*** the specially designed baseplate incorporated a longer central peg enabling strong primary fixation in the native glenoid; ***4)*** Four additional screws (2 locking and 2 compressive) provided strong supplementary fixation of the bone graft; ***5)*** after 30° of abduction, the forces applied to the glenoid component of a reversed prosthesis are mainly compressive and therefore, promote bone graft healing [7, 11, 17]. By reaming the glenoid surface with a 10° inferior inclination, compressive forces were further favored. Our radiological results clearly exceed the disappointing results reported after glenoid bone grafting in non constrained shoulder prostheses, where a detrimental shear force is generated during abduction [2, 24, 28].

In relation to our *second hypothesis*, no radiographic evidence of glenoid component loosening or screw breakage was identified at a mean follow-up of 28 months. As a result of the bone graft healing to the native glenoid, the bony lateralization maintains the centre of rotation at the glenoid-bone interface, thereby minimizing torque on the glenoid component. In doing so, Grammont's main biomechanical principal has been adhered to [3, 7, 11, 17]. From a technical standpoint, it is desirable to place the baseplate and bone graft flush to the inferior glenoid rim for at least two reasons (fig. 4): ***1)*** a *biological reason:* the lower part of the glenoid is proven to be well vascularized while the superior is almost avascular [1, 41]; ***2)*** *a mechanical reason:* the lower part of the glenoid is larger, offering a more stable platform for the bone graft. Nyffeler has recommended such inferior placement in order to improve motion and avoid scapular notching [30, 34].

The present clinical study confirms our *third hypothesis*: *bony lateralization* during RSA does *not* compromise the deltoid lever arm and enables active elevation above the horizontal level in patients with a cuff-deficient shoulder. The mean active elevation at review was 146° in our patients, representing a significant gain of 60° (Table 1). These results are equivalent to those reported for patients with CTA treated using a standard medialized Grammont RSA [4, 8, 14, 15, 23, 36, 40, 43]. The fact that the lateral displacement of the centre of the sphere does *not* decrease the deltoid moment arm is an important finding. As mentioned previously, the Grammont RSA is based on two biomechanical principles: lowering of the humerus and medialization of the center of rotation [6, 15, 17, 26]. According to our results, in a cuff-deficient shoulder, lowering the humerus (i.e., lengthening and tensioning the deltoid fibers) appears to be the more important biomechanical factor in restoring active elevation and allowing the deltoid to overcome the weak or absent rotator cuff muscles.

With regard to our *fourth hypothesis*, we have demonstrated that bony lateralization of the RSA provides clear advantages in terms of scapular impingement in all directions, prosthetic stability and shoulder contour. Bony lateralization facilitates the optimal positioning of the glenoid component, keeping the humeral cup away from the pillar of the scapula and decreasing the rate of inferior notching. Only 8 patients (19%) had inferior scapular notching in this series and only one patient had a grade 3 notch. The decreased rate of inferior scapular notching found with the BIO-RSA is a significant finding since in a number of studies, inferior notching has been shown to adversely affect mid-term clinical outcomes [15, 17, 34]. We feel that the low rate of inferior scapular notching is the result of both the low and lateral placement of the baseplate, as low placement alone has not been proven to solve the problem of inferior notching [27, 43].

Most studies reporting results of the Grammont/Delta RSA have found a significant gain in active elevation but almost no gain in active rotation. Indeed, some patients lose active internal rotation following RSA, not succeeding in putting their arm behind their back [8, 14, 23, 36, 40, 43]. Our results showed significant improvement in both external rotation (from 13° to 23°) and internal rotation (from sacral level to L3) (fig. 7). We feel that the improved rotation can be explained by the increased lateral offset, created by the glenoid bone grafting, providing more clearance for the humeral cup around the glenosphere during rotation with the arm at side. A further positive point brought by the BIO-RSA is the gain in shoulder stability provided by the bony lateralization. In a recent multicenter study of 450 patients operated with a RSA, prosthetic instability was encountered in 6% of the cases [29]. In our study, no case of subluxation or dislocation has been recorded at the current follow-up. In addition to the improved mobility and stability, bony lateralization preserves shoulder contour, approximating the appearance of the normal contralateral side (fig. 7).

The present study has some limitations: there is no control group, the number of patients is small and the follow-up is short. However, since bone graft healing has been observed in all patients with a minimum two-year follow-up, there is no reason to believe that the results will deteriorate over time. Although further clinical and radiological assessment is mandatory, these early results encourage us to continue performing this procedure. We acknowledge that the technique of bony lateralization itself has some limitations: the procedure cannot be performed in cases of humeral bone loss or deficiency (humeral head necrosis, previous failed

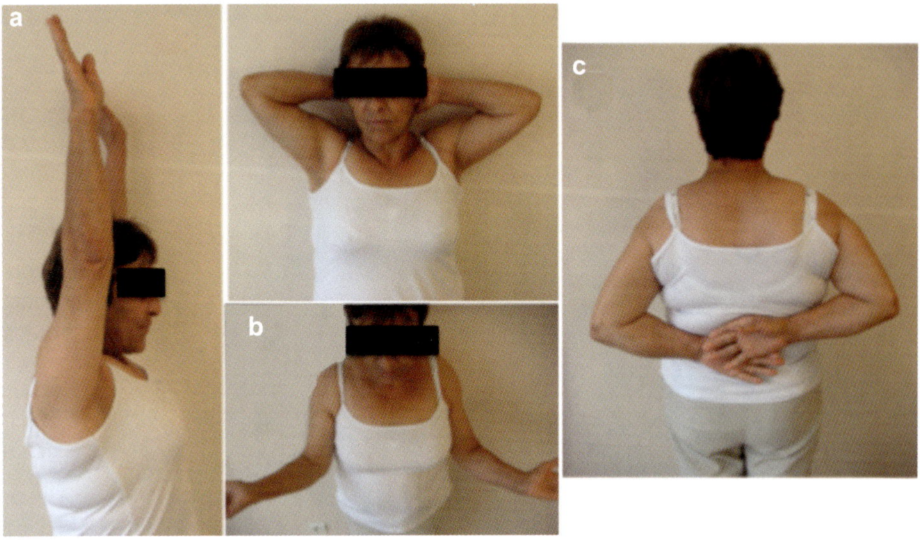

Fig. 7: Clinical results in a 70 years old patient at 29 months follow-up after BIO-RSA. From left: active anterior elevation is 170° (a), external rotation 45° (b), internal rotation to L1 (c); The Constant Score is 79 pts and the shoulder contour compares favorably to the contralateral side.

prostheses). However, if the surgeon wants to keep the benefits of bony lateralization in cases of humeral deficiency, an iliac crest bone graft is a reasonable substitute. Finally, it should be mentioned that the BIO-RSA does not lengthen or increase the complexity of the surgical procedure in comparison to a standard RSA. The exposure and reaming of the glenoid is facilitated by the fact that only one single small (29 mm) reamer is used to abrade the glenoid surface. Since there is no need to introduce large (36 and 42 mm) reamers inside the joint, glenoid exposure and preparation is easier.

In summary, the present study demonstrates that glenoid bone grafting during RSA, with a cancellous bone graft harvested from the humeral head, is a safe procedure. Bone graft healing is reliably obtained and no glenoid loosening has been observed with a minimum two-year follow-up. The bony lateralization of the RSA obtained with this procedure (bony increased-offset reversed shoulder arthroplasty or BIO-RSA) provides the major advantage of maintaining the prosthetic center of rotation at the prosthesis-glenoid interface. The adherence to one of the Paul Grammont's basic biomechanical principles has the net effect of reducing torque on the glenoid component. By providing more clearance for the humeral cup around the glenoid sphere, the BIO-RSA minimizes scapular impingement in all directions: inferiorly (decreased rate of scapular notching), (anteriorly (preserved internal rotation), posteriorly (preserved external rotation), and even superiorly. In addition, as a result of enhanced soft tissue tensioning, the BIO-RSA provides for a more stable articulation and a better preservation of shoulder contour, all while preserving active elevation.

REFERENCES

[1] ABRASSART S, STERN R, HOFFMEYER P. Arterial supply of the glenoid: an anatomic study. *J Shoulder Elbow Surg 2006;15(2): 232-8.*

[2] ANTUNA S, SPERLING JW, COFIELD RH. Reimplantation of a glenoid component after component removal and allograft bone grafting: a report of 3 cases. *J Shoulder Elbow Surg 2002;11(6): 637-41.*

[3] BAULOT E, CHABERNAUD D, GRAMMONT PM. Results of Grammont's inverted prosthesis in omarthritis associated with major cuff destruction. Apropos of 16 cases. *Acta Orthop Belg 1995;61 Suppl 1: 112-9.*

[4] BAULOT E, VALENTI P, GARAUD P, BOILEAU P, NEYTON L, SIRVEAUX F, NAVEZ G, ROCHE O, MOLÉ D, FAVARD L, GUERY J, LE DU C, GERBER C, WALCH G, NOVÉ-JOSSERAND L. Résultats des prothèses inversées. *Rev Chir Orthop Reparatrice Appar Mot 2007;93: 63-92.*

[5] BAYLEY JL, KESSEL L. The Kessel total shoulder replacement. In: Shoulder surgery. *New York: Springer Berlin Heidelberg; 1982.*

[6] BOILEAU P, WATKINSON DJ, HATZIDAKIS AM, BALG F. Grammont reverse prosthesis: design, rationale, and biomechanics. *J Shoulder Elbow Surg 2005;14(1 Suppl S): 147S-61S.*

[7] BOILEAU P, WATKINSON D, HATZIDAKIS AM, HOVORKA I. Neer Award 2005: The Grammont reverse shoulder prosthesis: results in cuff tear arthritis, fracture sequelae, and revision arthroplasty. *J Shoulder Elbow Surg 2006; 15(5): 527-40.*

[8] BOULAHIA A, EDWARDS TB, WALCH G, BARATTA RV. Early results of a reverse design prosthesis in the treatment of arthritis of the shoulder in elderly patients with a large rotator cuff tear. *Orthopedics 2002; 25(2): 129-33.*

[9] BROSTROM LA, WALLENSTEN R, OLSSON E, ANDERSON D. The Kessel prosthesis in total shoulder arthroplasty. A five-year experience. *Clin Orthop Relat Res 1992(277): 155-60.*

[10] CONSTANT CR, MURLEY AHG A clinical method for functional assessment of the shoulder. *Clin Orthop Relat Res 1987; 214: 160-4.*

[11] DE WILDE LF, MIDDERNACHT B, DE ROO PJ, VAN MAELE G, DE WILDE LF. Consequences of scapular anatomy for reversed total shoulder arthroplasty. *CORR 2008.*

[12] ELLMAN H, HANKER G, BAYER M. Repair of the rotator cuff. End-result study of factors influencing reconstruction. *J Bone Joint Surg Am 1986; 68(8): 1136-44.*

[13] FAVARD L, LAUTMANN S, SIRVEAUX F. Hemi arthroplasty versus reverse arthroplasty in the treatment of osteoarthritis with massive rotator cuff tear. In: Walch G BP, Mole D, editors., ed. 2000 Shoulder prosthesis two to ten year follow-up. *Montpellier: Sauramps Medical; 2001: 261-8.*

[14] FRANKLE M, LEVY JC, PUPELLO D, *et al.* The reverse shoulder prosthesis for glenohumeral arthritis associated with severe rotator cuff deficiency. a minimum two-year follow-up study of sixty patients surgical technique. *J Bone Joint Surg Am 2006; 88 Suppl 1 Pt 2: 178-90.*

[15] GERBER C, PENNINGTON SD, NYFFELER RW. Reverse Total Shoulder Arthroplasty. *J Am Acad Orthop Surg 2009; 17: 285-95.*

[16] GILBART MK, GERBER C. Comparison of the subjective shoulder value and the Constant score. *J Shoulder Elbow Surg 2007; 16(6): 717-21.*

[17] GRAMMONT PM, BAULOT E. Delta shoulder prosthesis for rotator cuff rupture. *Orthopedics 1993; 16(1): 65-8.*

[18] GUÉRY J, FAVARD L, SIRVEAUX F, OUDET D, MOLE D, WALCH G. Reverse total shoulder arthroplasty. Survivorship analysis of eighty replacements followed for five to ten years. *J Bone Joint Surg Am 2006; 88(8): 1742-7.*

[19] GUTIÉRREZ S, LEVY JC, FRANKLE MA, CUFF D, KELLER TS. Evaluation of abduction range of motion and avoidance of inferior scapular impingement in a reverse shoulder model. *J. Should. Elbow Surg. 17, 608-15.*

[20] GUTIÉRREZ S, ZONG-PING L, LEVY JONATHAN, FRANKLE MA. Arc of motion and socket depth in reverse shoulder implants. *Clin Biomech (Bristol, Avon). 2009; 24(6): 473-9.*

[21] HAMADA K, FUKUDA H, MIKASA M, KOBAYASHI Y. Roentgenographic findings in massive rotator cuff tears. A long-term observation. *Clin Orthop Relat Res 1990(254): 92-6.*

[22] HARMAN M, FRANKLE M, VASEY M, BANKS S. Initial glenoid component fixation in "reverse" total shoulder arthroplasty: a biomechanical evaluation. *J Shoulder Elbow Surg 2005;14(1 Suppl S): 162S-7S.*

[23] HATZIDAKIS AM, NORRIS TM, BOILEAU P. Reverse shoulder arthroplasty: indications, techniques, and results. *Techn Shoulder Elbow Surg 2005(6): 135-49.*

[24] HILL JM, NORRIS TR. Long-term results of total shoulder arthroplasty following bone-grafting of the glenoid. *J Bone Joint Surg Am 2001; 83-A(6): 877-83.*

[25] LÉVIGNE C, BOILEAU P, FAVARD L, *et al.* Scapular notching in reverse shoulder arthroplasty. In: Medical S, ed. Nice Shoulder Course Reverse Shoulder Arthroplasty. *Montpellier 2006: 353-72.*

[26] MATSEN III FA, BOILEAU P, WALCH G, GERBER C, BICKNELL RT. The reverse total shoulder arthroplasty. *Instr Course Lect 2008; 57: 167-74.*

[27] MOLÉ D, FAVARD L. Cuff Tear Arthritis. SOFCOT Symposium (in French) under the direction of Molé D. & Favard L. *Rev. Chir. Orthop. 2007, 93, suppl. au n° 6, 3S37-3S94.*

[28] NEYTON L, BOILEAU P, NOVE-JOSSERAND L, EDWARDS TB, WALCH G. Glenoid bone grafting with a reverse design prosthesis. *J Shoulder Elbow Surg 2007; 16(3 Suppl): S71-8.*

[29] NOVÉ-JOSSERAND L, WALCH G. Instability after RSA. In: Médical S, ed. Nice Shoulder Course Reverse Shoulder Arthroplasty. *Montpellier; 2006.*

[30] NYFFELER RW, WERNER CM, GERBER C. Biomechanical relevance of glenoid component positioning in the reverse Delta III total shoulder prosthesis. *J Shoulder Elbow Surg 2005; 14(5): 524-8.*

[31] RICHARDS RR, AN KN, BIGLIANI LU, *et al.* A standardized method for the assessment of shoulder function. *J Shoulder Elbow Surg 1994; 3(347352).*

[32] SEEBAUER L. Total reverse shoulder arthroplasty: European lessons and future trends. *Am J Orthop 2007; 36(12 Suppl 1): 22-8.*

[33] SEEBAUER L, WALTER W, KEYL W. Reverse total shoulder arthroplasty for the treatment of defect arthropathy. *Oper Orthop Traumatol 2005; 17(1): 1-24.*

[34] SIMOVITCH RW, ZUMSTEIN MA, LOHRI E, HELMY N, GERBER C. Predictors of scapular notching in patients managed with the Delta III reverse total shoulder replacement. *J Bone Joint Surg Am 2007; 89(3): 588-600.*

[35] SIRVEAUX F, FAVARD L, OUDET D. Grammont inverted total shoulder arthroplasty in the treatment of glenohumeral osteoarthritiswith massive cuff rupture of the cuff. Results of a multicenter study of 80 shoulders. *J Bone Joint Surg Br 2004; 86: 388-95.*

[36] SIRVEAUX F, FAVARD L, OUDET D, HUGUET D, LAUTMAN S. Grammont inverted total shoulder arthroplasty in the treatment of glenohumeral osteoarthritis with massive and non repairable cuff rupture. In: Walch G BP, Mole D, editors., ed. 2000 Shoulder prosthesis two to ten year follow-up *Montpellier: Sauramps Medical; 2001:247-52.*

[37] TERRIER A, REIST A, MERLINI F, FARRON A. Simulated joint and muscle forces in reversed and anatomic shoulder prostheses. *J Bone Joint Surg Br 2008; 90: 751-6.*

[38] VALENTI PH, BOUTENS D, NEROT C. Delta 3 reversed prosthesis for osteoarthritis with massive rotator cuff tear: long term results (>5 years). *Shoulder Prosthesis 2000: 253-9.*

[39] VALENTI P, SAUZIERES P, COGSWELL L, O'TOOLE G, KATZ D. The reverse shoulder prosthesis-surgical technique. *Tech Hand Up Extrem Surg 2008; 12(1): 46-55.*

[40] VANHOVE B, BEUGNIES A. Grammont's reverse shoulder prosthesis for rotator cuff arthropathy. A retrospective study of 32 cases. *Acta Orthop Belg 2004; 70(3): 219-25.*

[41] VON SCHROEDER HP, KUIPER SD, BOTTE MJ. Osseous anatomy of the scapula. *Clin Orthop Relat Res 2001(383): 131-9.*

[42] WALCH G, BADET R, BOULAHIA A, KHOURY A. Morphologic study of the glenoid in primary glenohumeral osteoarthritis. *J Arthroplasty 1999; 14(6): 756-60.*

[43] WALL B, NOVE-JOSSERAND L, O'CONNOR DP, EDWARDS TB, WALCH G. Reverse total shoulder arthroplasty: a review of results according to etiology. *J Bone Joint Surg Am 2007; 89(7): 1476-85.*

[44] WERNER CM, STEINMANN PA, GILBART M, GERBER C. Treatment of painful pseudoparesis due to irreparable rotator cuff dysfunction with the Delta III reverse-ball-and-socket total shoulder prosthesis. *J Bone Joint Surg Am 2005; 87(7): 1476-86.*

POLYETHYLENE WEAR IN ANATOMIC AND REVERSED SHOULDER PROSTHESES

A. FARRON, A. TERRIER

INTRODUCTION

Polyethylene wear is a recurrent problem in joint arthroplasty. In addition to permanent deformation or complete destruction of the component, small debris particles are also associated with inflammatory reactions of the surrounding bone, eventually leading to the failure of the bone between the implant and the host bone, and implant loosening.

In anatomic total shoulder arthroplasty, failure of the glenoid polyethylene component is the main cause of complication, often related to periprosthetic osteolysis and aseptic loosening [1]. Polyethylene wear of anatomic prostheses has been clinically observed on retrieved glenoid components. For reversed shoulder prostheses, polyethylene wear is usually related to scapular notching. However, the surface wear of the humeral cup is still unexplained. In reversed prostheses, the glenohumeral force is lower and the contact area is higher than in anatomic prostheses [2]. Consequently, the contact pressure should thus be much lower, but the volumetric wear might be as abondant in reversed prostheses as in anatomic prostheses.

The goal of this study was thus to estimate the volume of polyethylene wear of a reversed prosthesis, and compare it to an anatomic prosthesis, during one year of activities of daily living (ADL).

METHODS

A numerical musculoskeletal model of the glenohumeral joint was used for this comparative study [2]. The model included the scapula, the humerus and 6 scapulo-humeral muscles: middle, anterior, and posterior deltoid, supraspinatus, subscapularis and infraspinatus combined with teres minor. Arm motion and joint stability was achieved by muscles, allowing for natural translation of the humeral head. The muscle activation patterns were derived from EMG data and controlled by a synchronization algorithm. Arm weight was 37.5 N (5% bodyweight). The reversed (RP) and anatomic (AP) Aequalis prostheses were positioned in the numerical model according to manufacturer recommendations. For the RP, the rotator cuff muscles were deactivated since this prosthesis is used when these muscles are partly or completely deficient. Linear wear was defined by H = k.p.s, where *k* is the wear factor, *p* the contact pressure and *s* the sliding distance. Pressure and sliding were provided by the musculoskeletal model. The wear factor was pressure dependent, based on experimental relationships [3]. Eight levels of abduction were considered. Their daily frequency was estimated from in-vivo recorded data on healthy volunteers during activities of daily living (Table 1) [4]. One year of use was simulated to predict the linear and volumetric wear. The volumetric wear was the difference of volume between the original and worn component.

RESULTS

With the AP, the contact pattern on the glenoid surface moved rapidly from the inferior to the superior side during the first 30 degrees of abduction, and then went back to the inferior side. It reached 20 MPa at 90° of abduction. With the RP, the contact pattern on the humeral cup surface remained at the inferior side. Overall, contact pressure was 20 times lower with the RP than with the AP (fig. 1).

One year of use produced a maximum linear wear of 0.2 mm with the AP, and 0.13 mm with the RP (Fig. 2). The volumetric wear was 8.4 mm^3 with the AP, but reached 44.6 mm^3 with the RP.

Abd. level	10°	30°	50°	70°	90°	110°	130°	150°
Daily freq.	13021	6790	5557	2678	633	153	34	37

Table 1. Daily frequency associated to each abduction level

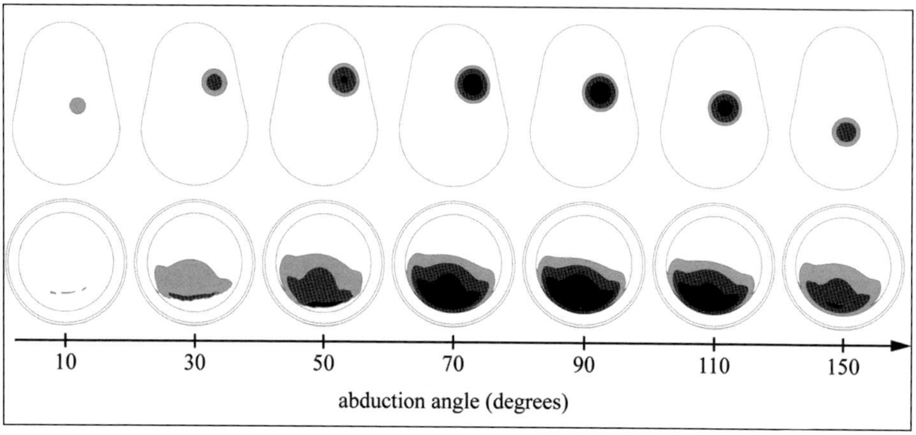

Fig. 1: Contact pattern with the AP (top) and RP (bottom)

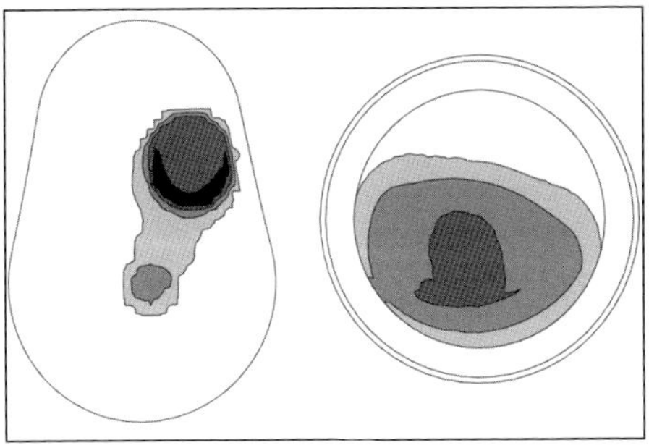

Fig. 2: Linear wear on the polyethylene glenoid component of the AP (left) and the humeral cup of the RP (right) after one year of use.

DISCUSSION

Polyethylene wear particles were found around humeral and glenoid components of AP removed after aseptic loosening associated osteolysis [5, 6]. This loosening process might occur in the same way with RP if the amount of wear is comparable. Since this potential problem has not been reported yet, this study aimed to estimate and compare the polyethylene associated to an AP and a RP. Using a numerical musculoskeletal shoulder model, one year of simulated activities of daily living produced 5 times more volumetric wear with the RP than with the AP, which confirms a potential polyethylene wear problem with RP.

Within the limitations of numerical analyses, the musculoskeletal model provided a comparative analysis of the two prostheses in the same conditions. The motor and stabilizing function achieved by muscles allowed for the natural translation of the humeral head of the AP and the increased muscle moment arm of the RP. A variable wear factor was essential because of the large range of contact pressure involved. Although activities of daily living were only characterized by abduction cycles in the scapular plane, the in-vivo recorded shoulder kinematics provided a realistic estimate of the shoulder use. Since kinematics was measured on healthy volunteers, the patient activity was probably overestimated. The wear mechanism complexity was not fully reproduced here. Cold flow deformation and cross-shear was not accounted for, but would have little effect on the simulated movements.

Polyethylene particles are a matter of concern with AP. Infiltration of these particles within the bone-implant interface can induce a progressive implant loosening. According to the present results, this problem should not be underestimated with RP. It might indeed be associated to the higher level of humeral stem loosening reported with RP. The long term survival of RP might be improved by using a highly cross-linked polyethylene, which has better abrasion resistance but lower plastic resistance.

ACKNOWLEDGEMENT:

This study was partly supported by Tornier Inc., Edina, MN.

REFERENCES

[1] MATSEN *et al. J Bone Joint Surg Am, 2008; 90(4): p. 885-96.*

[2] TERRIER *et al. J Bone Joint Surg Br, 2008; 90(6): p. 751-6.*

[3] SAIKKO. *Proc Inst Mech Eng [H], 2006; 220(7): p. 723-31.*

[4] COLEY *et al.* 2008. *Gait & Posture.*

[5] WIRTH *et al. J Bone Joint Surg Am, 1999; 81(1): p. 29-37.*

[6] KLIMKIEWICZ *et al. J Shoulder Elbow Surg, 1998; 7(4): p. 422-6*

INFLUENCE OF SPHERE DIAMETER ON RADIOGRAPHIC AND CLINICAL RESULTS OF RSA

L. DE WILDE

ABSTRACT

Background

The reverse total shoulder arthroplasty is an effective treatment for cuff tear arthropathy. Glenosphere size seems to be a matter of debate because some surgeons advocate the biggest possible size while others advise a small one.

Hypothesis

The purpose of this study is to determine the clinical and radiographic differences of a 38 mm glenosphere versus a 42 mm one.

Material and Methods

We compared the clinical and radiographic results of 14 patients with a 42 mm glenosphere and 4 with a 38 mm glenoshere of which all the variable parameters that might have influenced these results, were eliminated as much as possible.

Results

We found for the glenosphere 42 mm a better deltoid muscle power, a better passive adducted external rotation, a better passive abducted external rotation, a slightly better active external rotation, and a smaller active and passive internal rotation than for the 38mm version.

Radiographically a greater lengthening and prosthetic overhang to the glenoid was seen for the 42 mm glenosphere.

Discussion and Conclusion

This is the first study trying to evaluate the clinical and radiographic effects after changing one prosthetic design parameter. It does not show a statistically significant difference between the two analyzed glenosphere sizes, suggesting the original design of the initial "Grammont" prosthesis was nearly optimal. If the rotator cuff remnants are spared to prevent dislocation it seems advisable to balance the benefits of a greater glenosphere, more soft-tissue tension, and greater prosthetic overhang to the inferior glenoid against the risk of overstretching and dysfunction of the remaining cuff.

INTRODUCTION

Reverse total shoulder arthroplasty is proven to be a successful treatment of cuff tear arthropathy. This type of treatment restores the lost stable glenohumeral fulcrum, in a more favorable biomechanical configuration, which enables the shoulder joint to be abducted by the deltoid muscle solely.

Despite the good clinical results of this treatment, proven by many orthopedic centers, many questions remain to optimize this type of treatment.

One of these questions is about the size of the glenosphere. Some surgeons advocate the biggest possible size [1, 9] and others advise a small one [2].

Because there are arguments to defend both options this study is designed to determine whether the orthopedic surgeon should concentrate on the size of the glenosphere in reverse total shoulder arthroplasty.

THEORETICAL BACKGROUND

The size of the glenosphere of the reverse total shoulder arthroplasty influences on the total length of the total prosthesis in the scapular [3] and axial [10] planes of the body. The use of a bigger glenosphere makes the surgical procedure technically more challenging because the increased prosthetic bulkiness reduces the intraoperative visibility of the baseplate [4] and stretches the soft tissues more.

The length of the musculotendinous unit

The remaining length of the musculotendinous unit depends not only on the total length of the prosthesis but also on the position of this prosthesis on the bone. This influence can be situated at the glenoid side and at the humeral side.

Nowadays the method of choice is to implant the glenosphere as distally as possible on the glenoid to create a prosthetic overhang to the bone [7, 8]. If the base plate is not placed as distally as possible, the lengthening of the musculotendinous unit will be altered.

The size of the glenosphere will also influence this length but the net gain will be limited [9] (see figure 1).

The thickness of the polyethylene inlay will also influence the total length of the musculotendinous unit but the net gain of an extra 3mm lengthening will have a limited effect on the power of the deltoid, similarly to the size of the glenosphere.

Finally the height of the implanted humeral component will affect this prosthetic length as well. This height is the result of the osseous humeral cut and depends on the height of the humeral fixation in reference to this cut.

The lengthening of the musculotendinous unit in the scapular and axial plane of the body has its impact on the strength of the remaining rotator cuff [6].

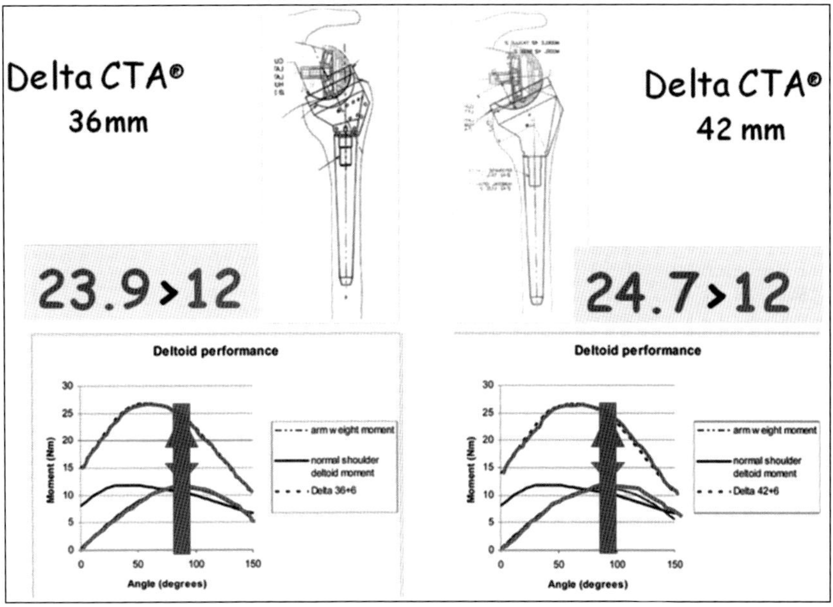

Fig. 1: Biomechanical comparison of the influence of the radius of the glenosphere on the power of the glenoid in a computerized model. The net gain on the power due to the larger glenosphere is limited.

The amount of stretching is determined by the size of the glenosphere but also by the relationship between the humeral and glenoid components [10]. The main biomechanical reason is the change in rotational movement of an anatomic prosthesis versus a reversed one: a spinning versus a hinging rotation [4]. This implies that a difference in position of the glenohumeral relationship in the axial plane of the body of 10 degrees will have a change of approximately 5 mm in the length of the remaining rotator cuff [11].

The orthopedic surgeon needs to bear in mind that the excursion of the rotator cuff remnants will increase with by 20% to 25% in reverse settings.

With the rotator cuff muscles having an average length of 17.5 cm (infraspinatus and subscapularis), and for the teres minor 8cm, it is obvious that a 36- or 38-mm configuration, which stretches the musculotendinous unit up to 2 or 3 cm respectively, will be more important for the teres minor than for the subscapular remnant.

The stability of the prosthetic unit

According to the literature a smaller radius of the glenosphere guarantees a greater stability of the reverse total shoulder prosthesis [2]. This is only applicable if absolute values are taken into account and the comparison of the smaller glenosphere to the larger one is done with the same cup depth or radius and not with a depth or a radius of the same relation to the size. Taking a similar prosthetic relationship into account, the size of the glenosphere nor the depth of the cup interferes with the stability (parallelism between both curves). Therefore it seems more appropriate to concentrate on the optimal stability ratio (contact area versus prosthetic stability) than on the size of the glenosphere. Moreover stability is not only dependent on the size of the glenosphere or prosthetic contact area, it also depends on the periprosthetic room around the glenosphere [10, 11] and on the periprosthetic tension [12]. The latter will mainly be higher for a larger glenosphere configuration than for a small one.

The difficulty of the surgical procedure

In the original Delta CTA reverse total shoulder prosthesis – as is the case for many commercially available designs – the glenosphere was still hemispheric. This implies that the radius determines the maximum prosthetic bulkiness [4]. Every surgeon will agree that it is more difficult to assemble a larger glenosphere to a baseplate fixed with screws on the glenoid than a smaller one. Reduction of the prosthetic bulkiness by implanting a hemispheric glenosphere makes this type of surgery easier without interfering with the radius of the glenosphere (fig. 2).

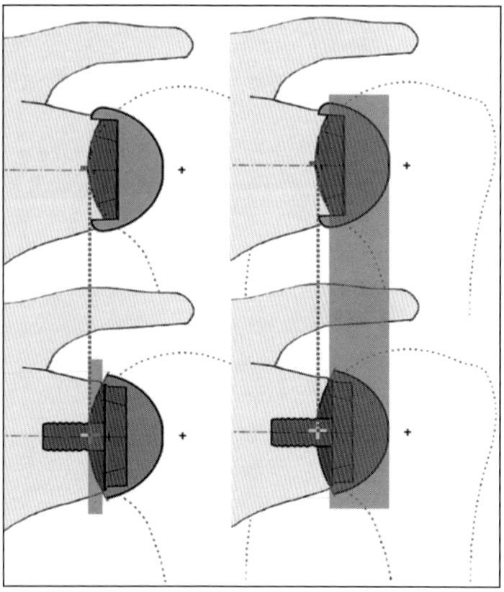

Fig. 2: Schematical comparison of the influence of the effect of a curved base plate versus a flat beseplate. If the center of rotation is identical, it has its consequences on the removal of glenoid bone by reaming (less for the curved baseplate) and for the bulkiness of the glenosphere (less than half a sphere for the curved baseplate with an identical radius).

CLINICAL CONSEQUENCES

In order to overcome the problem of comparing apples and oranges, these theoretical consequences need to be taken into account in a clinical study. To study clinically the difference in outcome between a large-sized and a small-sized glenosphere, we tried, as much as possible to minimize the number of the above-mentioned influencing parameters.

MATERIALS AND METHODS

We limited our study to a population with a proven irreparable cuff tear of the postero-superior rotator cuff with or without osteoartritis.

Inclusion criteria: fatty degeneration of the supraspinatus and infraspinatus of more than grade 3 according to the criteria of Goutallier; no fatty degeneration of the subscapularis; rupture of less than one cm of the proximal subscapular tendon; the long head of the biceps tendon is present, tenodezed, tenotomized or absent; a stiff shoulder with a loss of less than 25% of the passive mobility compared to the opposite side if not explained by osteonecrosis or severe osteoarthritis deformans; absence of any preoperative and postoperative complications.

Clinically all patients were preoperatively and postoperatively (at 1 year follow-up) evaluated by the Constant-Murley score [18]. The passive mobility in the prone position and the active external rotation were measured.

The same surgeon operated on all the patients while convinced that the larger glenosphere would benefit his patients most.

All patients were operated with the same approach (supero-posterior, McKenzie approach with a resection of the distal clavicle). They were all treated with a DeltaXtend reverse total shoulder prosthesis (DePuy Ltd, Leeds, UK). The base plate was always positioned flush with the inferior border of the glenoid. This needed a section of the triceps tendon from its origin for all patients. All base plates were fixed with two angular stable screws to the scapular bone. The relation of the humeral and glenoid prostheses in the axial plane of the body was always with an opening wedge of 30° according to the technique of Karelse *et al.* [10]. The intraoperative tension of the prosthesis was adapted so that no opening wedge occurred at the extremes of articular motion between both prosthetic components. No conflict was allowed intraoperatively in testing the prosthesis between the humeral tuberosities or shaft and the acromion and/or coracoid process.

In all cases a high-mobility polyethylene layer was used which has an identical proportional contact area for the 38 mm and 42 mm configurations.

All prosthesis were implanted uncemented according to the guidelines of the surgical technique.

A radiographic examination was done preoperatively and postoperatively (at one year follow-up). The severity of the cuff tear arthropathy was graded according to Hamada [19] and Favard [20]. The lengthening of the upper arm was measured as the increase in Acromio-Humeral distance on an AP-view of the adducted arm according to De Wilde *et al.* [3]. The prosthetic overhang to the glenoid was quantified in millimeters. A greading of a scapular notching according to Nérot [21] was done.

A statistical comparison between the 38 mm and 42 mm glenospheres was done.

The difficulty of the surgical procedure was rated by the surgeon as easy, moderate, or difficult, taking into account the bony dissection/preparation, the implantation of the prosthetic components and the assembling of the prosthesis.

RESULTS

All patients were female with a mean age of 72 years (61-84). Eighteen patients were included in this study. Fourteen were treated with a 42 mm glenosphere but only four with a 38 mm glenosphere. The follow-up was always at 12 months. A high-mobility polyethylene insert of 3 mm and 6 mm was placed in 6 patients, and a 9 mm lengthener was used twice for the the 42 mm glenosphere. A high mobility insert of 3 mm and 6mm was placed twice for the 38 glenosphere.

The preoperative and postoperative Constant-Murley score is presented in

Table 1. The preoperative scores are comparable for both groups.

The internal rotation (hand in back) was peroperatively at a mean of L4 (S1-D7) for 38 mm and a mean of D12 (SIJ-D4) for 42 mm and postoperative it changed to a mean of D12 (SIJ-D7) for 38 mm and to a mean of L4 (Trochanter-D7) for 42 mm postoperative.

The external rotation is evaluated passively and actively with the elbow at the side (ER1 = adducted external rotation) and with the elbow ninety degrees abducted (ER2 = abducted external rotation) and the results are found in Table 2.

The active internal rotation was evaluated with the belly-press and Gerber test. All (38 mm and 42 mm) had a positive preoperative belly-press test as well as a positive Gerber test. For the 42 mm configuration a belly-press test was powerful for 11/14 and a Gerber test for 9/14. For the 38 mm configuration the belly-press test and Gerber test was powerful for all (4/4).

We classified 1 patient as Hamada 1, 4 patients Hamada 2, 3 and 4B, 5 patients as Hamada 4A. According to Favard's classification we had four E0, eight E1, two E3, four E2 and no E4.

The radiographic evaluation is summarized in Table 3.

The difficulty ratio of the procedure for 2 in the 42 mm group and 1 in the 38 mm group were graded as moderately difficult, and all the others were graded as easy.

Table 1: Clinical evaluation with the Constant-Murley score in absolute values: evaluation of pain, activities of daily living (ADL), mobility, and power.

	38 mm preop CS	42 mm preop CS	38 mm 1y po CS	42 mm 1y po CS
Pain	8(4.5 -14)	8(0 - 3)	14(14.5 -15)	13(10.5 - 15)
ADL	8(1 - 13)	6(3 - 18)	17(9 - 20)	18(10 - 20)
Mobility	19(0 - 30)	15(2 - 32)	33(36 - 40)	34(14 - 40)
Power	3(0 - 8)	3(0 - 10)	2(3 - 10.5)	3(0.5 - 10.5)
Total	38(5.5 - 63)	32(7- 67.5)	66(64 - 83.6)	68(38.5 - 80.5)

Table 2: Active and passive external rotation evaluation for the 38 mm and 42 mm configuration preoperatively and postoperatively.

	38 mm preop		42 mm preop		38 mm postop		42 mm postop	
	ER1	ER2	ER1	ER2	ER1	ER2	ER1	ER2
Passive	47°(20-80)	47°(30-70)	29°(0-80)	66°(60-90)	15°(10-40)	37°(20-80)	28°(10-30)	51°(30-90)
Active	17°(10-40)	20°(10-60)	7°(-10-40)	17°(0-70)	3°(-10-80)	28°(20-60)	20°(10-90)	40°(10-80)

Table 3: Radiological evaluation: scapular notching according to Nérot, acromiohumeral distance, and prosthetic overhang.

	38 mm preop CS	42 mm preop CS	38 mm 1y po CS	42 mm 1y po CS
Notching according to Nérot (mm)	Not applicable	Not applicable	Stage 0: 4	Stage 0: 12 Stage 1: 2
Acromiohumeral distance	2.2 mm (0-5.5)	1.7 mm (0-4)	35.1 mm (20-45.5)	40 mm (26-55)
Acromiohumeral distance difference (mm)	Not applicable	Not applicable	32.9 mm (14.5-42.5)	38.3 mm (22.2-55)
Prosthetic overhang (mm)	Not applicable	Not applicable	6.4 mm (5.5-7)	9.1 mm (6-12)

DISCUSSION

This study tries to evaluate the clinical and radiographic impact of a difference in glenoid size for a reverse total shoulder arthroplasty. As known from the literature, there is a discrepancy between the clinical results favoring the use of a smaller glenosphere [17] and the theoretical considerations that are in favor of the use of a larger glenosphere [1, 9].

In an effort to limit all the interfering parameters of this type of surgery this study applied a strict inclusion protocol leading to a rather limited study-population. Of course this is the major weakness of this study, but due to the strict application of the inclusion criteria, we believe this is the first study that can clinically and radiographically evaluate the short-term effect of the size of the glenosphere in reverse total shoulder arthroplasty.

The results of this study showing that for a posterosuperior cuff tear arthropathy this type of treatment is effective at the short term agree with the literature [6, 7, 20, 21]. It is not possible to make a statistically significant difference between both groups using the Constant-Murley score. The postoperative evaluation of the external rotation reveals a decrease in the passive adducted external rotation. This effect is greater for the smaller glenosphere. The gain in passive range of motion of the abducted external rotation is more important for the bigger glenosphere. This study reveals an improvement in active external rotation for both sizes. This gain is more important for the larger glenosphere and in abduction. This is in contrast with the literature, which states that the external rotation is reduced or at most maintained in the presence of a teres minor, as was the case in all of our patients [6, 7]. Placing our base plate as distally as possible to create a prosthetic overhang to the glenoid might be a possible explanation.

Unfortunately, this study found a slight decrease in internal rotation, both active and passive, with this type of treatment despite the high-mobility polyethylene insert and the caution to position as accurately as possible the prosthesis in the axial plane of the body. Fortunately this decrease remained limited and is more in favor of the smaller configuration. This can be explained by the fact that the subscapularis tendon was not or only partially ruptured, which might lead to more muscular scarring, loss of propriorecep-tion [14,] or dysfunction due to overstretching in the larger configuration.

Creating a firm prosthetic overhang to the bone had a positive effect on the scapular notching which was only seen in 2 cases at stage 1 according to Nérot [21]. This effect is not related to the size of the glenosphere. The use of a bigger glenosphere guarantees a greater prosthetic overhang to the glenoid bone but the use of a smaller glenosphere always permits the creation of an overhang of at least 5 mm. Because this overhang is not only present in the scapular plane of the body but also in the axial plane, this might explain the more pronounced dysfunction of the subscapularis tendon due to more stretch and excursion in the larger configuration.

Although all the surgical interventions were done with the use of a cutting guide this study shows that the lengthening of the upper arm seems to be variable up to 25 mm independent of the size of the glenosphere. Nevertheless this lengthening is more pronounced for the larger configuration than for the smaller configuration. The reason for this inconsistent lengthening cannot only be explained by the thickness of the polyethylene inlay which was limited within 6 mm for both configurations. Another reason might be the disappearance of the greater tuberosity due to stress shielding postoperatively (Wolff's law). The more pronounced lengthening in the 42 mm configuration might explain the slightly more powerful abduction. On the other hand, the surgeon must be cautions not to "overstretch" the joint as it might endanger the neurovascular bundle [15]. To the best of our knowledge no studies are available yet to quantify the optimal lengthening of the deltoid and or rotator cuff remnants in experimental or in clinical settings.

The possible esthetic improvement due to reduced dimpling of the deltoid region using a greater radius was not addressed in this study. We believe it is difficult to measure this objectively as it is too dependent on the absolute morphologic/biometric values.

Although this study could not reveal strong statistical clinical or radiographic arguments to use a glenosphere 42 mm, one might argue against using this configuration in the treatment of cuff tear arthropathy because it only makes the surgery more difficult due to the prosthetic bulkiness. Nevertheless this study supports the tendency that a bigger glenosphere creates more range of motion actively and passively. This is a reason amongst others the design team of the DeltaXtend opted for a slightly bigger glenosphere (38 mm instead of 36 mm) and reduced its morphology to less than a hemisphere. In this design the largest diameter of this sphere is still slightly less bulky than the 36 mm of the hemispheric configuration (Fig. 2). The only adverse effect of this reduction of the prosthetic bulkiness is the decrease in contact area making this design theoretically more vulnerable to increased polyethylene wear.

CONCLUSION

This study is the first to evaluate the clinical and radiographic effect of changing one prosthetic design parameter. Because it does not show a clear difference between the glenosphere sizes, one can only conclude that the original design of the initial "Grammont" prosthesis was nearly optimal.

We believe caution is needed not to extrapolate the conclusion of this study to revision, posttraumatic or tumor indications where there may exist a need for detachment and/or resection of the rotator cuff complex or the impossibility of reattachement. Sparing as much as possible of the remaining rotator cuff seems to be advisable, as the subscapularis insufficiency seems to be important in explaining a higher dislocation rate [16]. If the rotator cuff remnants are spared to prevent dislocation it seems to be advisable to balance the benefits of a greater glenosphere, more soft-tissue tension, and greater prosthetic overhang to the inferior glenoid against the risk of overstretching and dysfunction of the remaining cuff.

REFERENCES

[1] CHOU J, MALAK SF, ANDERSON IA, ASTLEY T, POON PP. Biomechanical evaluation of different designs of glenospheres in the SMR reverse total shoulder prosthesis: Range of motion and risk of scapular notching. *J Shoulder Elbow Surg. 2009; 18: 354-9.*

[2] GERBER C, PENNINGTON SD, NYFFELER RW. Reverse total shoulder arthroplasty. *J Am Acad Orthop Surg. 2009 May; 17(5): 284-95.*

[3] DE WILDE LF, PLASSCHAERT FS, AUDENAERT EA, VERDONK RC. Functional recovery after a reverse prosthesis for reconstruction of the proximal humerus in tumor surgery. *Clin Orthop Relat Res. 2005 Jan;(430): 156-62.*

[4] MIDDERNACHT B, DE ROO PJ, VAN MAELE G, DE WILDE LF. Consequences of scapular anatomy for reversed total shoulder arthroplasty. *Clin Orthop Relat Res. 2008 Jun; 466(6): 1410-8.*

[5] DE WILDE L, AUDENAERT E, BARBAIX E, AUDENAERT A, SOUDAN K. Consequences of deltoid muscle elongation on deltoid muscle performance: a computerised study. *Clin Biomech. 2002 Aug; 17(7): 499-505.*

[6] BOILEAU P, WATKINSON DJ, HATZIDAKIS AM, HOVORKA I. Neer Award 2005: The Grammont reverse shoulder prosthesis: Results in cuff tear arthritis, fracture sequelae, and revision arthroplasty. *J Shoulder Elbow Surg 2006; 15: 527-40.*

[7] WERNER CM, STEINMANN PA, GILBART M, GERBER C. Treatment of painful pseudoparesis due to irreparable rotator cuff dysfunction with the Delta III reverse-ball-and-socket total shoulder prosthesis. *J Bone Joint Surg Am 2005; 87: 1476-86.*

[8] NYFFELER RW, WERNER CML, GERBER C. Glenoid component positioning in the reversed delta III total shoulder prosthesis. *J Shoulder Elbow Surg 2005; 14: 524-8.*

[9] DE WILDE LF, AUDENAERT EA, BERGHS BM. Shoulder prostheses treating cuff tear arthropathy: a comparative biomechanical study. *J Orthop Res, 2004, 22 (6): 1222-30.*

[10] KARELSE AT, BHATIA DN, DE WILDE LF. Prosthetic component relationship of the reverse Delta III total shoulder prosthesis in the transverse plane of the body. *J Shoulder Elbow Surg. 2008 Jul-Aug; 17(4): 602-7.*

[11] NYFFELER RW, SHEIKH R, ATKINSON TS, JACOB HA, FAVRE P, GERBER C. Effects of glenoid component version on humeral head displacement and joint reaction forces: an experimental study. *J Shoulder Elbow Surg. 2006 Sep-Oct; 15(5): 625-9.*

[12] KREKEL PR, DE BRUIN PW, VALSTAR ER, POST FH, ROZING PM, BOTHA CP. Evaluation of bone impingement prediction in pre-operative planning for shoulder arthroplasty. *Proc Inst Mech Eng H. 2009 Oct; 223(7): 813-22.*

[13] VAN SEYMORTIER P, STOFFELEN D, FORTEMS Y, REYNDERS P. The reverse shoulder prosthesis (Delta III) in acute shoulder fractures: technical considerations with respect to stability. *Acta Orthop Belg. 2006 Aug; 72(4): 474-7.*

[14] KASTEN P, MAIER M, RETTIG O, RAISS P, WOLF S, LOEW M. Proprioception in total, hemi- and reverse shoulder arthroplasty in 3D motion analyses: a prospective study. *Int Orthop. 2009 Dec; 33(6): 1641-7.*

[15] VAN HOOF T, GOMES GT, AUDENAERT E, VERSTRAETE K, KERCKAERT I, D'HERDE K. 3D computerized model for measuring strain and displacement of the brachial plexus following placement of reverse shoulder prosthesis. *Anat Rec (Hoboken). 2008 Sep; 291(9): 1173-85.*

[16] EDWARDS TB, WILLIAMS MD, LABRIOLA JE, ELKOUSY HA, GARTSMAN GM, O'CONNOR DP. Subscapularis insufficiency and the risk of shoulder dislocation after reverse shoulder arthroplasty. *J Shoulder Elbow Surg. 2009 Nov-Dec; 18(6): 892-6.*

[17] FAVARD L, GERBER C, BERHOUET J, BACLE G, NÉROT C, GARAUD P, MIDDERNACHT B, KARELSE A, DE WILDE L. The shoulder with eccentric omarthrosis. *Rev Chir Orthop Reparatrice Appar Mot. 2007 Oct; 93(6 Suppl): 40-50. [Article in French]*

[18] CONSTANT C, MURLEY A. A clinical method of functional assessment of the shoulder. *Clin Orthop Relat Res, 1987; 214: 160-4.*

[19] HAMADA K, FUKUDA H, MIKASA M, KOBAYASHI Y. Roentgenographic findings in massive rotator cuff tears. *Clin Orthop Relat Res,1990; 254: 92-6.*

[20] SIRVEAUX F, FAVARD L, OUDET D, HUQUET D, WALCH G, MOLE D. Grammont inverted total shoulder arthroplasty in the treatment of glenohumeral osteoarthritis with massive rupture of the cuff. Results of a multicentre study of 80 shoulders. *J Bone Joint Surg Br. 2004 Apr; 86(3): 388-95.*

[21] VALENTI PH, BOUTENS D, NEROT C. Delta 3 reversed prosthesis for arthritis with massive rotator cuff tears : long term results (> 5 years). In: G. Walch (ed). Schouders 2000 Protheses. Two to ten years follow-up, *Sauramps Medical, Montpellier, 2001, pp 252-9.*

RESULTS OF GLENOID BONE GRAFT IN PRIMARY REVERSE SHOULDER ARTHROPLASTY

C. LÉVIGNE, J. GARRET, S. GROSCLAUDE

In the setting of total shoulder arthroplasty, glenoid defects present significant technical challenges. The results of non-constrained anatomic prostheses – cemented or uncemented – combined with glenoid reconstruction are highly variable [1-3]. Reverse shoulder arthroplasty with bone graft is known to achieve acceptable functional results in arthropathy associated with cuff insufficiency and severe superior glenoid wear [4]. The reverse prosthesis has been suggested as a treatment for anteroposterior defects also, accepting the anatomy in the case of a small defect, or combined with glenoid reconstruction if the defect is more significant.

Compared to allograft or bone substitutes, structural bone autograft is the most reliable material, and is usually sculpted from a portion of the resected humeral head or from the iliac crest.

The aim of the study is to analyse the results of reverse shoulder arthroplasty combined with structural autograft for arthropathy associated with glenoid defects.

MATERIAL AND METHODS

This is a retrospective multicenter study of 34 cases of reverse arthroplasty implanted between 1998 and 2007 for five different aetiologies: cuff tear arthropathy (CTA) with superior defects in 18 cases, osteonecrosis and cuff deficiency with an inferior defect in 2 cases, rheumatoid arthritis with a superior defect in 5 cases and an anterior defect in one case, osteoarthritis with static posterior instability and a posterior defect (type B2 of Walch classification [5]) in 4 cases, and post-surgical static anterior instability with an anterior defect in 4 cases.

Preoperative mean Constant score was 22 pts (range, 3-46 pts). Active anterior elevation averaged 63° (range, 20-130°). Mean active external rotation with arm at the side was 10° (range, -60-90°).

Three grades of defect were defined according to the distance between a vertical line drawn flush to the most medial point of the defect and a vertical line drawn flush to the most medial point of the spinoglenoid notch, a radiographic landmark that we found to be the most reproducible regardless of beam orientation (fig. 1): Grade1 (minor) - if glenoid wear extends less than 1/3 of the distance between the original joint line and the vertical line at the spinoglenoid notch; grade 2 (moderate) - if glenoid wear extends between 1/3 and 2/3 of this distance; grade 3 (severe) if it reaches beyond 2/3 of this distance. Using this classification, the glenoid defect was defined as grade 1 in 3 cases, grade 2 in 12 cases and grade 3 in 19 cases.

A structural corticocancellous autograft was used in all cases, harvested from the iliac crest in 10 cases, from the resected humeral head in 23 cases and from both in 1 cases. The graft was secured using baseplate screws in 22 cases and by independent metallic screws in 12 cases. The reversed prosthesis was implanted simultaneously in 32 cases and as a second stage in two cases, 9 and 10 months later. The prosthesis implanted was a Grammont-type reverse prosthesis in all cases consisting of 3 Delta™ (Depuy) and 31 Aequalis Reversed™ (Tornier) prostheses.

RESULTS

Two patients experienced complications unrelated to the graft: one patient had a postoperative persistent incomplete brachial plexus palsy and one patient had a diaphyseal humeral fracture distal to the stem at 14 months postoperatively which required plate osteosynthesis. They were excluded for the clinical results but radiographic analysis of the graft and glenoid was reliableat the last follow-up and we kept these two patients in radiographic result.

Two patients were revised, 8 and 9 months after the index procedure, for migration of the baseplate: one was converted to a hemiarthroplasty. In the other case, a reverse shoulder arthroplasty was re-implanted. The status of these two cases before revision was included in the results as some baseplate migrations had not been reoperated upon and because we considered these cases to represent graft-related complications. All other patients were reviewed with a minimum of two years follow-up. The mean follow-up was 40 months (range, 8-86mths).

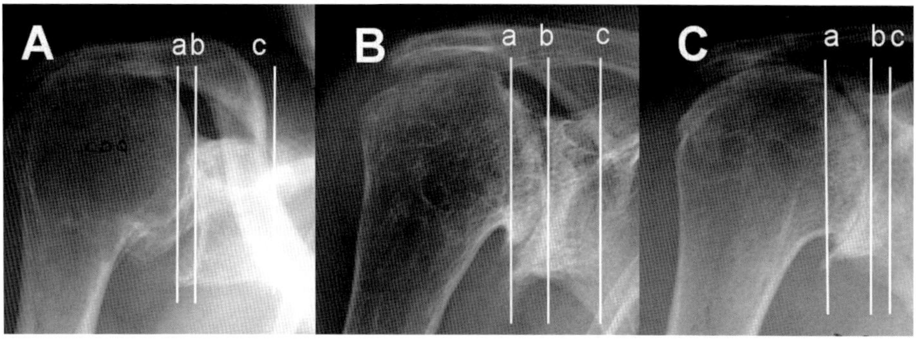

Fig. 1: Classification of the 3 grades of glenoid defect on AP view: (a) if the vertical line figuring the original joint line, (b) is the vertical line is flush with the most medial point of the defect and (c) is the vertical line is flush with the most medial point of the spinoglenoid notch. A- Grade1: ab < 1/3 ac, B- grade 2 : ab= 1/3-2/3 ac, C- grade 3 : ab > 2/3.

At last follow-up, the mean Constant score was 59 points (range, 19-98pts). The functional result was excellent in 10 cases (score >70pts), good in 14 cases (score 50-70pts), fair in 4 cases (score 30-50pts) and poor in 4 cases (score <30pts). Active anterior elevation reached an average of 133° (range, 50-170°) while active external rotation with arm at the side was 17° on average (range, -20-50°).

Radiographic evaluation was possible in 34 cases. 6 cases of baseplate migration associated with graft failure (18%) were observed. Graft healing was observed in 27 cases and could not be assessed in one case. We noted partial graft resorption in 5 cases, with resorption under the baseplate in 2 of these and extending beyond the bearing surface in 3 cases. Scapular notching was observed in 13 cases (46%). The results according to grade of defect demonstrated a significant association between grade 3 defects and both the likelihood of a poorer clinical results (worse constant score, active elevation and external rotation) and the probability of glenoid failure (table 1).

In relation to the defect location, anterior defects were significantly associated with a lower postoperative Constant score, active elevation and increased probability of glenoid failure (Table 2).

DISCUSSION

The radiographic evaluation of the grade of glenoid defect may be difficult on the AP view due to the lack of reproducible landmarks. In this study, we attempted to quantify the defect using a classification that we have used previously for rheumatoid arthritis [6], whereby glenoid wear is measured relative to the projection of the base of the coracoid process. This appeared to be an imprecise method, possibly due to the variability of both the defect location and the orientation of the radiologic beam. We observed that the projection of the spinoglenoid notch was clearer, more accurate and reproducible regardless of the defect location or beam orientation. While this new classification requires validation, it proved to be helpful and relevant in this study (fig. 1).

Table 1

	N	Constant score (pts)	AAE(°)	AER(°)	XR migration (nb)
Grade 1	3	62	147	26	0
Grade 2	12	69	153	21	0
Grade 3	17	53	108	15	6 (35%)

Table 2

	N	Constant score (pts)	AAE (°)	AER (°)	XR migration (nb)
Superior	20	63	133	16	4 (20%)
Inferior	3	64	143	23	0
Posterior	4	70	153	18	0
Anterior	5	41	108	20	2 (40%)

Glenoid migration is frequently encountered with autograft treatment of severe glenoid defects (35%). Of the 6 cases of migration observed, the central peg of the baseplate either did not reach the native glenoid (n=4) (fig. 2) or reached the native glenoid but, as reported in the operative report, without achieving primary stability (n=2) (fig. 3). We hypothesize that it is critical to obtain primary stability in the native bone with the central peg. A longer central peg may be required (25 mm instead of 15 mm) if the native bone is noted to be weak or of poor quality. We recommend using a long pegged glenoid in all cases of grade 2 or 3 defects. If a longer peg is not available or insufficient to achieve good stability, separate screw fixation of the graft is required and may be the key to achieving graft healing (fig. 4). Recently, two ingenious techniques have been described which benefit from first placing the graft on the baseplate around the central peg before securing both to the native glenoid. Norris described this technique using iliac crest, Boileau using resected humeral head [7, 8]. It is also advisable to stimulate healing by drilling the native sclerotic bone in advance of securing the baseplate.

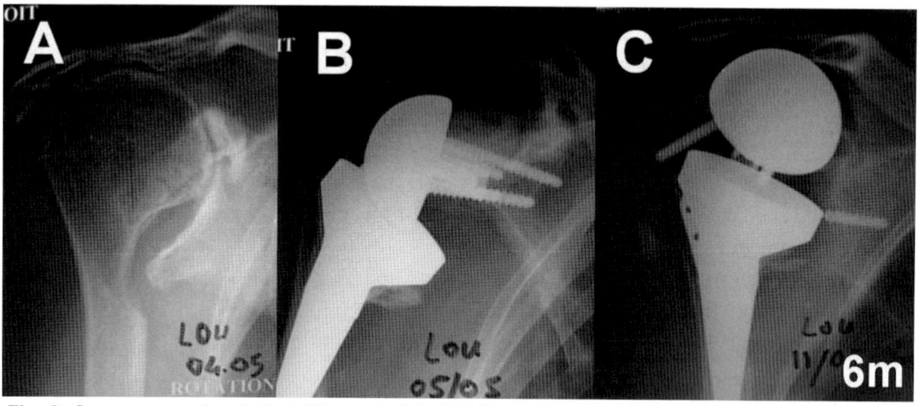

Fig. 2: Severe superior defect (A) treated by RSA combined with graft. Standard central peg not reaching the native glenoid (B). Migration of the baseplate after 6 months (C).

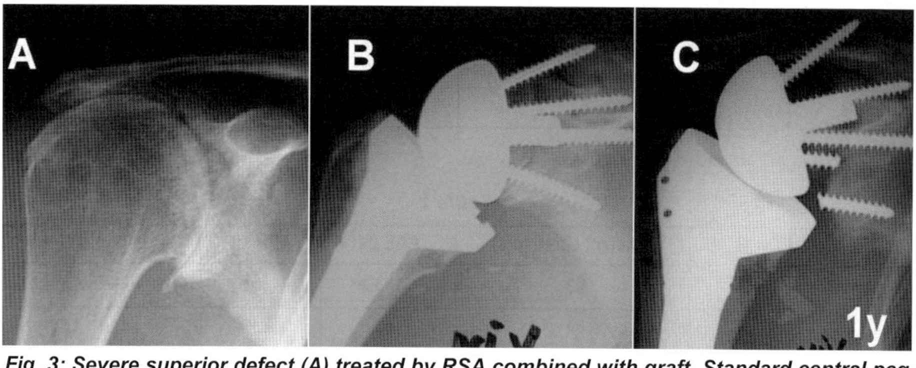

Fig. 3: Severe superior defect (A) treated by RSA combined with graft. Standard central peg reaching the native glenoid, reported as having poor bone quality (B). Migration of the baseplate after 12 months (C).

If the glenoid prosthesis cannot be stably implanted into the graft and glenoid, we suggest a minimal interval of 6 months before considering a second stage implantation of a reverse prosthesis. The 2 cases where a two-stage strategy had been adopted achieved graft healing and good functional results (fig. 5).

Partial resorption of the graft was observed in only 5 cases. If located under the baseplate it may progress and therefore requires surveillance. If located out the baseplate compression area, it likely represents a lack of mechanical constraint.

Scapular notching was frequent in the series (46%). Of the 13 cases, 11 prostheses were positioned too superiorly on the glenoid, an essential factor in the genesis of scapular notching [9-11] (fig. 6). A predisposing factor, that should be considered when preparing the glenoid, is the fact that the defect is frequently located at the superior part of the glenoid (10 cases out of 13). Ideally, the baseplate/graft should be flush with the inferior border of the glenoid and inferiorly tilted (fig. 7).

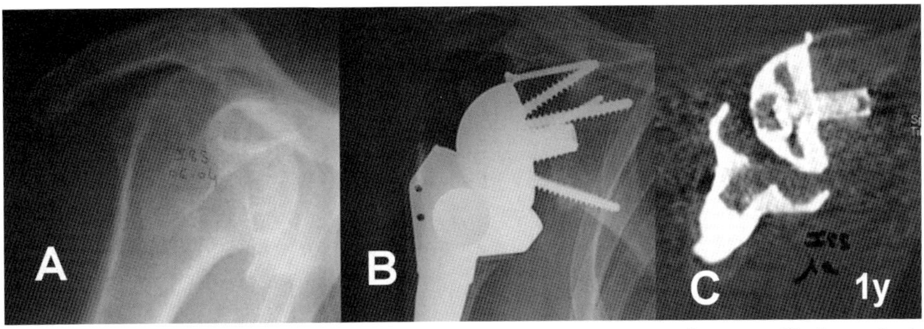

Fig. 4: Severe superior defect (A) treated by RSA combined with graft secured independently using screw fixation. Standard central peg not reaching the native glenoid (B). No migration of the baseplate after 12 months and healing of the graft (C).

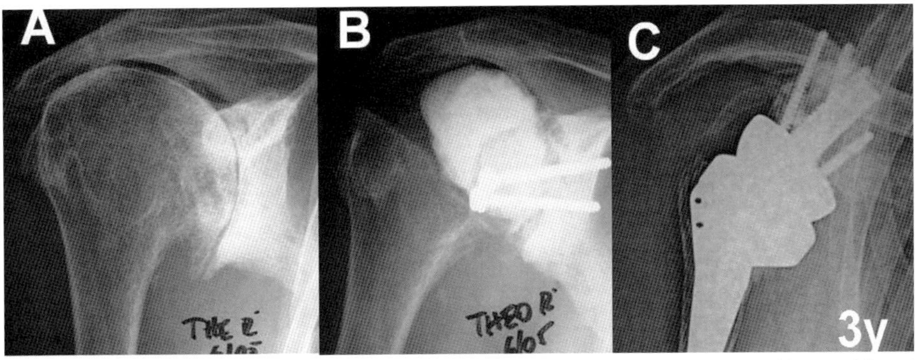

Fig. 5: Severe superior defect (A) treated by two staged procedure: screwed iliac and head graft at the first stage with cement spacer (B) and 8 months later second stage RSA with the result after 3 years (C).

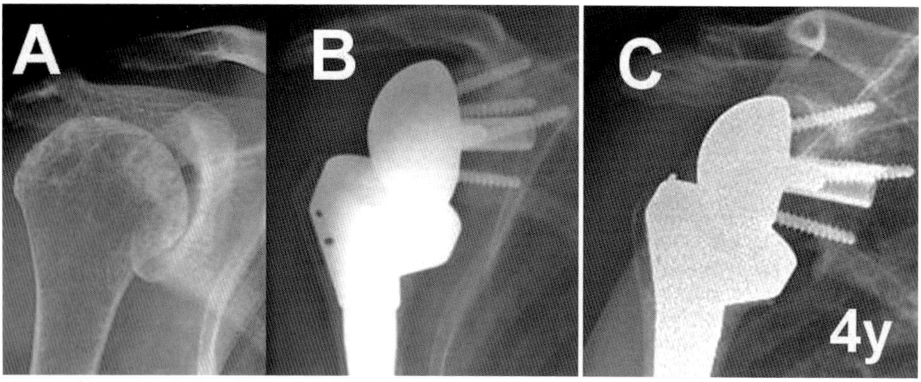

Fig. 6: Superior defect (A) treated by RSA combined with graft. The lower point of the sphere is not lower than the scapular neck (B). Scapular notching (C).

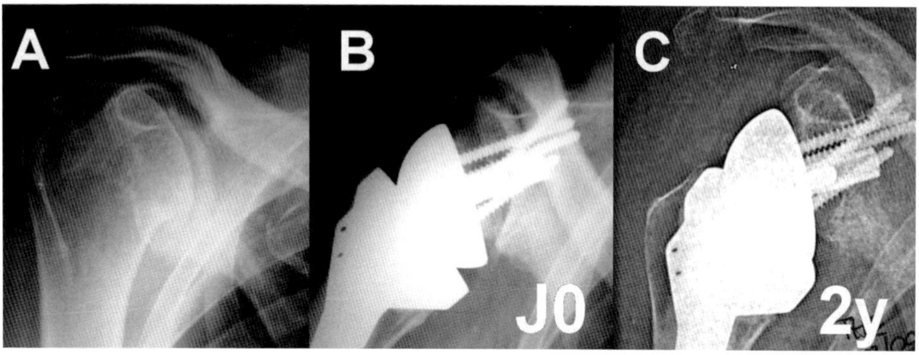

Fig. 7: Severe superior defect (A) treated by RSA combined with graft (B). Note the long peg in native glenoid. The sphere is in an ideal low position and is inferiorly tilted. 2 years follow-up (C).

In conclusion, reverse shoulder arthroplasty combined with structural glenoid bone graft is associated with a high risk of baseplate migration. Severe defects and anterior defects are particular risk factors. Analysing the causes of failure suggests that primary stability of the baseplate is the key factor in achieving graft healing and a good functional result.

REFERENCES

[1] NEER CS, MORRISON DS Glenoid Bone-Grafting in Total Shoulder Arthroplasty. *J Bone Joint Surg 1988; 70(8): 1154-62*

[2] STEINMANN SP, COFIELD RH Bone grafting for glenoid deficiency in total shoulder replacement. *J Shoulder Elbow Surg 2000; 9(5): 361-7.*

[3] HILL JM, NORRIS TR Long-Term Results of Total Shoulder Arthroplasty Following Bone-Grafting of the Glenoid. *J Bone Joint Surg 2001; 83(6): 877-83.*

[4] NEYTON L, BOILEAU P, NOVÉ-JOSSERANT L, EDWARDS TB, WALCH G Glenoid bone grafting with a reverse design prosthesis. *J Shoulder Elbow Surg 2007; 16(3S): 71-8*

[5] WALCH G, BADET R, BOULAHIA A, KHOURY A. Morphologic study of the glenoid in primary glenohumeral osteoarthritis. *J Arthroplasty 1999; 14: 756-60.*

[6] LÉVIGNE C, FRANCESCHI JP. Rheumatoid arthritis of the shoulder. Radiologic presentation and results of arthroplasty. In: G Walch and P Boileau, *Editors, Shoulder Arthroplasty, Springer, Berlin 1999: 221-32.*

[7] RICE RS, SPERLING JW, MILETTI J, SCHLECK C, COFIELD RH Augmented Glenoid Component for Bone Deficiency in Shoulder Arthroplasty. *Clin Orthop Relat Res 2008; 466; 579-83.*

[8] BOILEAU P, MOINEAU G, ROUSSANNE Y, O'SHEA K. Bony Increased-Offset Reversed Shoulder Arthroplasty (BIO-RSA). The Benefits of Bony Lateralization *Clin Orthop Rel Res. 2010 (in press).*

[9] SIRVEAUX F, FAVARD L, OUDET D, HUQUET D, WALCH G, MOLE D. Grammont inverted total shoulder arthroplasty in the treatment of glenohumeral osteoarthritis with massive rupture of the cuff. Results of a multicentre study of 80 shoulders. *J Bone Joint Surg Br 2004; 86(3): 388-95.*

[10] NYFFELER RW, WERNER CM, GERBER C. Biomechanical relevance of glenoid component positioning in the reverse Delta III total shoulder prosthesis, *J Shoulder Elbow Surg. 2005; 14(5): 524-8.*

[11] LÉVIGNE C, BOILEAU P, FAVARD L, GARAUD P, MOLÉ D, SIRVEAUX F, WALCH G. Scapular notching in reverse shoulder arthroplasty. *J Shoulder Elbow Surg. 2008; 17(6): 925-35.*

REVISION OF GLENOID COMPONENT IN REVERSE SHOULDER ARTHROPLASTY

D. MOLÉ, C. DEZALY, F. SIRVEAUX

INTRODUCTION

Three main stages presided over the development of reverse shoulder prosthesis: its description and inception by Paul Grammont at the end of the 1980s, its acceptance by major shoulder surgeons owing to the results it produced in cuff tear arthropathy during the 1990s, and finally its significant growth between 2000 and 2010, when it was more significantly used in situations of salvage surgery where it yielded results that an anatomic prosthesis could not achieve. During each of these three stages, the main objection raised regarding reverse prostheses was that they were considered to be a final surgical procedure beyond which, in the event of a problem, no solution was available. From this perspective, Paul Grammont described, from the outset, a shoulder cup which may cap the humeral part of the prosthesis if the glenoid implant needed to be removed. It is also with this eventuality in mind that we are all committed to reserving reverse prostheses for elderly patients in order to limit the impact of its failures.

Is it now time to reconsider these ideas? Is a reverse prosthesis truly the ultimate shoulder surgery? Is it possible, with modern graft techniques, to replace a failed reverse prosthesis and, in particular, its glenoid component? In setting out to answer these questions, we conducted a multicentered study, in which we focused on cases of replacement of the glenoid component of a reverse prosthesis, aiming to analyze the remedial actions and their outcomes.

PATIENTS AND METHODS

This retrospective study considered patients who were reoperated on for full or partial replacement of the glenoid part of a reverse prosthesis before December 31, 2008. 8 centers fully participated in this study. Patients were examined with more than one year follow-up; the analysis focused on the postoperative complications and revisions, the functional Constant score, the degree of active elevation and subjective results. The implants in place were monitored with control X-rays.

Among 73 patients who underwent a revision, 62 (85%) met the criteria of this study. Of those patients, 38 were women and 24 were men, their mean age being 67 years (29-81) when the reverse prosthesis was implanted for various etiologies (Table 1).

Thirty-one patients (50%) had had previous surgery, 31 patients had never been operated on. Only 4 patients (10%) had medical conditions which could potentially compromise the outcome of their arthroplasty (Parkinson's disease, paraplegia and two radiotherapy sequelae). In 39 cases, preoperative X-rays were available; the glenoid was normal or slightly worn (E0 or E1 type in the Favard classification) in 65% of cases. The surgical approach used for implanting of the prosthesis was delto-pectoral in 37 cases (60%), antero-superior in 25 cases (40%). In 6 cases (10%), the glenoid had been grafted (3 humeral heads, 3 iliac crests) at the time the reverse prosthesis was implanted. The reoperation for removal or replacement of the glenoid part took place, on average, 44 months (2-159) after implantation of the prosthesis. 34 patients (55%) had been reoperated on before the end of the third postoperative year. The etiology that led to revision (Table 2) was predominantly glenoid loosening (33 cases - 53%) and postoperative infection (23 cases - 37%). Re-intervention resulted in implanting a new reverse prosthesis in 33 patients (53%), to conversion into hemi-arthroplasty in 16 cases (26%) and to the removal of the implants in 13 cases (21%).

RESULTS

In only 2 cases (3.2%), intraoperative complications occurred: a glenoid fracture, treated by a coracoid transfer facing an hemi-arthroplasty, and a tuberosity fracture treated by osteosuture. None had future repercussions. However, a postoperative complication occures in 12 cases (19%) ; in 9 of these (19%) an attempt of RSA reimplantation was concerned. They were:
- *Instability:* 3 cases. Orthopedic reduction and a recurrent dislocation requiring open reduction and change of insert treated two early and isolated episodes.
- *Iterative glenoid loosening:* 2 cases. These were two cases of early aseptic loosening (3 and 9 months), one of which was reoperated on for a new reverse gle-

Table 1: Etiology of initial reverse prosthesis

Fracture	Fracture sequelae	CTA	Massive cuff tear	Primary OA	RA	HA revision	TSA revision
4 cases	14 cases	19 cases	9 cases	2 cases	6 cases	3 cases	5 cases
(6.4%)	(22.6%)	(30.6%)	(14.5%)	(3.2%)	(9.7%)	(4.8%)	(8.1%)

Table 2: Etiology of revision

Infection	Glenoid loosening	Instability	Disassembly
23 cases (37.1%)	33 cases (53.2%)	4 cases (6.4%)	2 cases (3.2%)

noid with a long peg baseplate and iliac crest bone graft.
- *Residual infection:* 7 cases. This concerned the resetting of 4 reverse prostheses and 3 hemi-arthroplasties (no resection-arthroplasty). 4 of these 7 patients were already infected before surgery. 3 were reoperated on for debridement. In the 4 others, the infection was uncertain and was treated with antibiotics.

A reoperation was necessary in 5 cases (8%) for chronic instability (1 case) for early loosening of the glenoid (1 case) and for infection (3 cases). In 3 cases, the reoperation involved a patient whose intervention had consisted in implanting a new reverse prosthesis.

With a mean follow-up of 48 months (12-175), the overall results were quite poor, which confirms the serious shortcomings of reverse prostheses failure. The Constant score increased by 15 points (21.8 → 36, 4); the effect on pain was good (5.1/15 → 10.7/15), the effect on active anterior elevation was poor (59.4° → 78.3°). The results differ depending on the type of intervention (Table 3).

The implanting of a new reverse prosthesis (Constant: 46.2 - pain: 11.7 - active anterior elevation: 103°) provides a significantly better functional outcome than conversion into hemi-arthroplasty (Constant 31.8 - pain: 11.1 - active anterior elevation 65.9°) and resection of the implants (Constant: 19.1 - pain: 8.1 - active anterior elevation: 35.7°). The results should be interpreted by taking into consideration the longer follow-up for hemi-arthroplasty and resection arthroplasties. It should be noted that resection-arthroplasty resulted in a loss of functional results with drop of 7 points in the Constant score between the state prior to the replacement and the score obtained at latest follow-up.

The implanting of a new reverse prosthesis (N = 32) (Table 4) was performed for glenoid loosening in 23 cases, and chronic infection in 9 cases. In 15 cases, the intervention was exclusively related to the glenoid, the humeral stem being left untouched, in 17 cases (9 infections with two-stage procedure, 8 glenoid loosenings with suspected bipolar loosening), the humeral stem was also changed. The results do not differ in these two subpopulations except a better active elevation when the humeral stem was left in place (110,6° vs 96,5°). When both components (glenoid and humeral part) of the prosthesis were changed (N = 17), this change

Table 3: Results of revision surgery

	Preoperative			Last Follow-up				
	Pain	Active Flexion	Constant Score	Pain	Active Flexion	Constant Score	Subjective (% satisfied)	F.U. (months)
Global series (n=62)	5.1	59.4	21.8	10.7	78.3	36.4	64%	48.3
RSA (n=32)	5.3	63.9	23.2	11.7	103	46.2	91%	34.2
HA (n=16)	3.5	47.3	15.2	11.1	65.9	31.8	56%	63.7
Resection Arthroplasty (n=14)	6.6	62.1	26.1	8.1	35.7	19.1	15%	63

Table 4: Results of revision for RSA

		Constant score (last F.U.)	Pain (last F.U.)	Active Flexion (last F.U.)
Isolated glenoid replacement (n=15)		48.1	11.5	110.6
Glenoid + stem replacement	1 stage (n=6)	41.3	12.5	88.3
	2 stage (n=11)	43.1	11.3	93.9
	Total (n=17)	44.5	11.9	96,5

was effected in one stage in 6 cases, in 2 separate stages in 11 cases (with or without the use of a spacer). There is no significant difference in outcome between these two subpopulations.

Hemi-arthroplasty (n = 16) was performed in 11 cases using the Grammont artifice (cup on the humeral implant left in place) and in 5 cases with replacing of the stem and use of an anatomic humeral prosthesis.

The results, both objective and subjective, were significantly better when the humeral stem was replaced (Table 5).

Subjectively, finally, 40 patients (64%) were satisfied or very satisfied with their re-intervention, while 22 (36%) were disappointed or dissatisfied. The satisfaction rate was 91% when a new reverse prosthesis was implanted, 56% when using a hemi-arthroplasty and 15% in case of resection-arthroplasty.

GLENOID LOOSENING

Thirty-three patients in this series were reoperated on for glenoid loosening of a reversed prosthesis. It is the most common etiology of these cases of surgical revision. The average age was 67.5 years at the time of the reverse prosthesis. 4 patients (12%) had a medical condition that could potentially interfere with the subsequent evolution of their prosthesis (1 Parkinson's disease, a paraplegic, two radiotherapy sequelae). The etiology of the reversed prosthesis was in 17 cases only (51%) a cuff tear arthropathy or massive rotator cuff tear, 7 patients (21%) were operated on for fracture sequelae, 5 (15%) for rheumatoid arthritis and 3 (9%) for TSA loosening. The average delay between the reverse prosthesis and the glenoid component revision is 51 months; 15 patients (45%) were operated on before the end of the second year. Loosening was coupled with a disassembling of the glenoid in 2 cases with prosthetic instabi-

Table 5: Conversion to HA

	Pain (last F.U.)	Constant score (last F.U.)	Active Flexion (last F.U.)	Subjective (% satisfied)
Conversion HA/No stem removal (n=11)	10.7	30.4	69.5	45.4%
Conversion HA/stem removal (n=5)	12	35	58	80%

lity in 1 case and with bipolar loosening in 3 cases. The septic loosenings were excluded from this analysis.

The reoperation consisted in 20 cases (61%) in the re-implanting of a new reverse glenoid (implanted in one stage in 17 cases and in 2 stages in 3 cases). In 12 cases (33%) the loosening of the glenoid was treated by conversion into hemi-arthroplasty, and finally, in 1 case, all the prosthetic components were removed for resection-arthroplasty. In 15 out of 20 cases (75%), the glenoid required a further bone graft (13 iliac crests, 1 allograft, 1 bone substitute).

A postoperative complication after reoperation occurred in 5 cases (8%): it was a postoperative infection in 3 cases (1 reoperation for resection-arthroplasty, 2 medical treatments), chronic instability in 1 case (reoperated on for open reduction and insert replacement) and early glenoid loosening in 1 case (reoperation for further change in reversed glenoid). Therefore 3 patients were reoperated on, bringing the rate of a second revision to 1%.

With a mean follow-up of 39 months, the results (Table 6) show a significant improvement in terms of pain, active elevation and Constant score: 24 patients (73%) were satisfied with the outcome.

The analysis of the results depending on the type of implant put in place is very much in favor of the reverse prosthesis. 19 patients (56%) have a reverse prosthesis, 18 (95%) are satisfied with an average Constant score of 48.7, a pain score of 12 and an active anterior elevation of 110°. 12 patients (36%) underwent hemi-arthroplasty, 5 (42%) are satisfied with an average Constant score of 31, a pain score of 10.5 and an active anterior elevation of 70°. 2 patients had undergone a resection-arthroplasty (one originally intended, one after postoperative infection). None is satisfied with a Constant score of 14.5, a pain score of 5 and an active anterior elevation of 25°. It is worth noting that for these two patients, revision for glenoid loosening has led to functional loss (Constant score and active anterior elevation) and an increase in pain. Among patients with a reverse prosthesis in place, the fact that a transplant had been used in the re-location glenoid made no difference, regardless of whether the surgery had been performed in 1 or 2 stages.

Table 6: Results of revision surgery for glenoid loosening

	Preoperative			Last Follow-up			
	Pain	Active Flexion	Constant score	Pain	Active Flexion	Constant score	Subjective (% satisfied)
Global series (n=33)	3.9	53	16.8	11.1	89.8	40.2	72.7%
RSA (n=19)	4.1	58.2	19.1	12.1	109.5	48.7	94.7%
HA (n=12)	3.1	52	13.6	10.5	70.4	31	41.7%
Resection arthroplasty (n=2)	7.5	35	18	5	25	14.5	0%

INFECTION

Infection is, in order of frequency, the second leading cause of revision of the glenoid component in our series. 23 patients (37%), with an average age of 66 years were affected by this problem. The etiology leading to the implanting of a reversed prosthesis was, in 9 cases only (39%). Cuff tear arthropathy or massive cuff rupture. It was, in 5 cases (22%), fracture sequelae and in 5 cases (22%) revision surgery after hemi-arthroplasty or total shoulder prosthesis. The average time between the introduction of the reverse prosthesis and glenoid adjustment for infection is 38 months. 13 patients (57%) were reoperated on within 3 years. 5 (22%) were reoperated on beyond the fifth year, most likely for a hematogenous infection. The infection was associated in 5 cases (22%) with chronic instability.

The re-operation consisted in 9 cases (39%) in the implanting, in 2 stages of a new reverse prosthesis, in 3 cases (13%) in a conversion into hemi-arthroplasty (always performed in 2 stages) and in 11 cases (43%) a resection-arthroplasty. No postoperative complications occurred following this revision surgery. No reoperation was necessary.

The infection was overcome in 19 cases (83%). In 4 cases (17%) infection was still present or highly doubtful; of these 2 cases of replacement of reversed glenoid in 2 stages and 2 cases of resection-arthroplasty. The results (Table 7) of the glenoid revision surgery of a reverse prosthesis for infection were disappointing.

The Constant score barely increased (from 31.1 before surgery to 31.6); loss of active anterior elevation (63° against 75° preoperatively) is offset by the relief of pain (10.6 against 7.2 preoperatively). However, 11 patients (48%) are satisfied with the results. The results are, once again, correlated with the implants in place with a clearly better result for reverse prostheses (Constant score of 42.8 - pain score of 11.3 - active anterior elevation 84°) compared with hemi-arthroplasties and resection - arthroplasties. Once again, the latter result in loss of functional efficiency.

Table 7: Results of revision surgery for infection

	Preoperative			Last Follow-up			
	Pain	Active Flexion	Constant score	Pain	Active Flexion	Constant score	Subjective (% satisfied)
Global series (n=23)	7.2	75.2	31.1	10.6	63.4	31.6	52.2%
RSA (n=9)	8.2	84.4	34.8	11.3	95	42.8	77.7%
HA (n=3)	7	65	25.6	14	56.6	38.3	100%
Resection arthroplasty (n=11)	6.8	73.6	29.5	9	39.1	20.6	18%

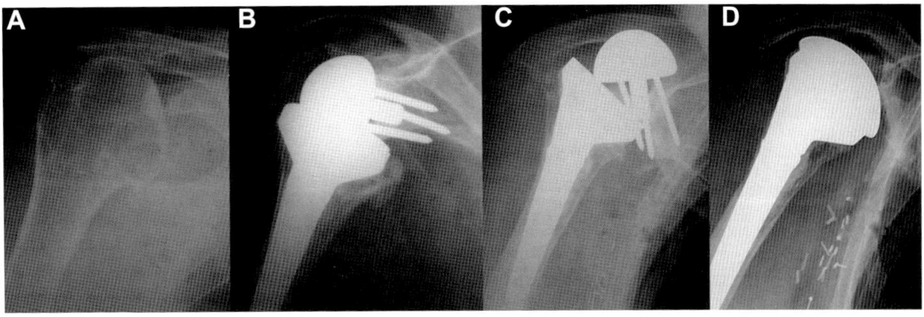

***Fig. 1: Conversion to HA without stem replacement - A and B: RSA for CTA** (Feb. 1996); **C: Glenoid loosening** (May 1999); **D: Conversion to HA** (May 1999)*

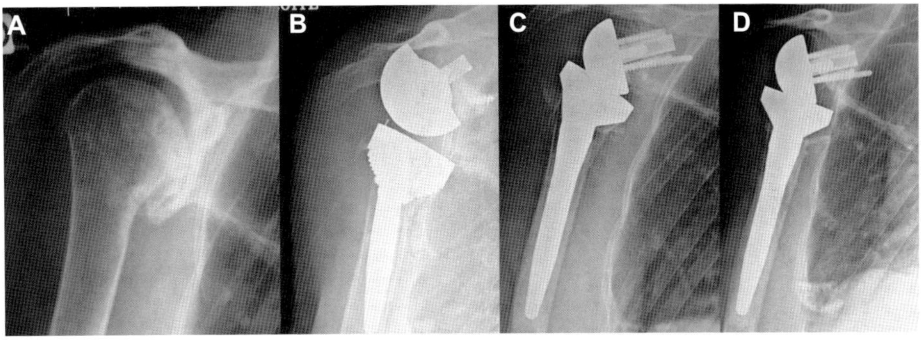

***Fig. 2 : One stage RSA exchange - A and B: RSA for CTA** (Feb. 2007); **B: Glenoid loosening** (Aug. 2008); **C: One stage RSA exchange with glenoid graft** (Aug. 2008); **D: Last follow-up** (Sept. 2009)*

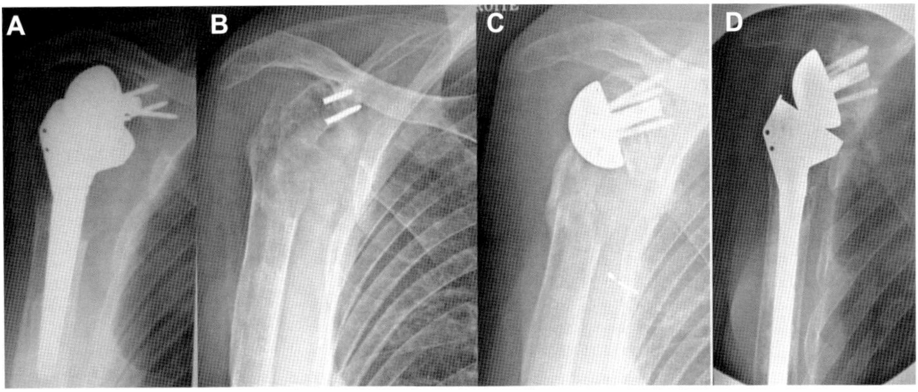

***Fig. 3: 2 stages RSA exchange for glenoid loosening - A: RSA for CTA / Glenoid loosening** (Janv. 2008); **B: Résection arthroplasty** (Feb. 2008); **C: First stage : Glenoid revision with iliac crest** (Apr. 2008); **D: Second stage : Humeral revision** (Jun. 2008)*

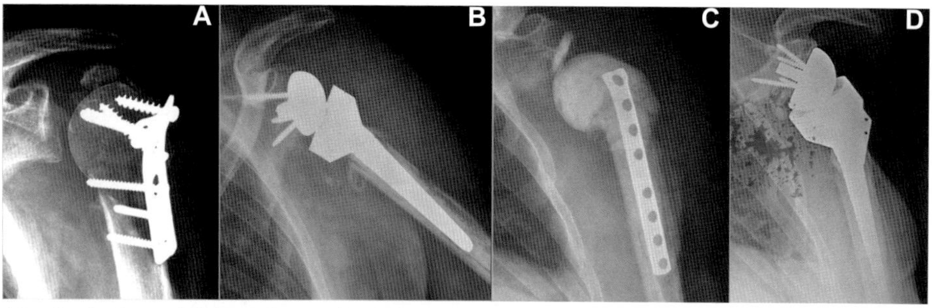

***Fig. 4 : 2 stages RSA exchange for infection - A: Upward humerus fracture** (Jan. 2002); **B: RSA for fracture sequelae** (Nov. 2002)**: sepsis; C: First stage : RSA removal / spacer** (Jul. 2003)**; D: Second stage: RSA** (Nov. 2003)*

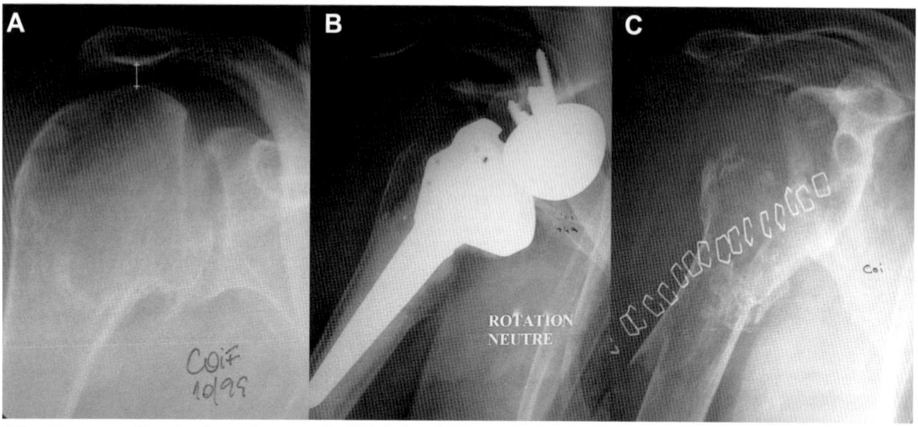

***Fig. 5 : resection/arthroplasty - A: RSA for CTA** (Oct. 1999)**; B: Infection and glenoid loosening** (Jan. 2004)**; C: Resection arthroplasty** (Jui. 2004)*

DISCUSSION - CONCLUSION

The first finding concerning this series is the low number of cases that were reported. Only 73 patients underwent reoperation for failure of the glenoid component of a reverse prosthesis in 8 centers specializied in shoulder surgery which extensively use this implant. This confirms, indirectly, the efficiency and stability of reverse prostheses, which undermines the claim that they were associated with a high risk of glenoid loosening.

Although of a rare occurrence, revision surgery is however most often linked to glenoid loosening (53% of cases); in order of frequency, postoperative infection is the second dominant etiology. The prosthesis in question had been implanted in patients who were relatively young (mean age 67 years) for different etiologies. The revision is premature in most cases (55% before the end of the third post-operative). The rate of postoperative complications (19%) and reoperation (8%) is analogous to those of originally implanted reverse prostheses.

This study validates the hypothesis that the implanting of a new reversed glenoid prosthesis (32 cases - 52%) is feasible, regardless of whether its re-implanting is performed with or without bone grafting, in one or two stages. With a average follow-up of 48 months, only 2 glenoids (6%) had loosened. It delivers results in every way superior to the conversion into hemi-arthroplasty and resection-arthroplasty. It should therefore be favored.

This study also shows that any decision involving a resection-arthroplasty should be taken with caution. With 14 cases of this series, this intervention results in lower functional efficiency, both in terms of the Constant score and active elevation.

Lastly, mechanical complications (glenoid loosening) can be corrected more effectively than infectious complications.

LONG-TERM OUTCOMES WITH THE REVERSE SHOULDER PROSTHESIS: 10 TO 15 YEARS OF FOLLOW-UP

L. FAVARD, G. ALAMI, A. YOUNG, C. DEZALY, V. FALAISE

INTRODUCTION

Since Neer's early work [15], shoulder arthroplasty has gradually become a reliable and widely used solution for the treatment of glenohumeral arthropathy. However, unlike the knee or hip, the shoulder owes most of its stability to the rotator cuff, the integrity of which is a prerequisite for the success of a traditional shoulder arthroplasty. In fact, the outcomes of arthroplasty are generally disappointing when a major compromise exists in the rotator cuff [2], as is the case with massive cuff tears with pseudoparalysis (MCT), cuff tear arthropathy (CTA), some cases of rheumatoid arthritis (RA), certain failed arthroplasties requiring revision, and fracture sequelae involving tuberosity malunion.

In the above situations, the absence of the rotator cuff causes the humeral head to ride proximally, which after total shoulder arthroplasty (TSA) increases the risk of rapid glenoid loosening through the rocking-horse effect [9]. To avoid this risk, it is possible to leave the glenoid as it is and perform a hemiarthroplasty (HA) or a bipolar arthroplasty; but the outcomes in these situations are often somewhat disappointing with limited improvement [1, 6, 16, 22]. Moreover, the progressive upward displacement of the humeral head causes wear of the coracoacromial arch, putting the patient at risk of a progressively deteriorating functional result [18]. Another possibility is using a constrained prosthesis with a fixed center of rotation, but various series have shown high complication rates – loosening in particular – gradually causing the abandonment of such implants [12, 13, 17].

Lastly, a Grammont-type [10] reverse shoulder arthroplasty (RSA) can be used. Some studies of this solution [3, 19] have reported satisfactory outcomes, possibly because of its medialized center of rotation and increased deltoid lever arm. But those studies have only reported short- or mid-term outcomes, so wear and loosening cannot be properly assessed.

We therefore carried out this study with two goals:

- to evaluate the outcomes of RSA after more than 10 years of follow-up with functional results and cumulative survival curves to prosthetic revision, and
- to analyze the effects of preoperative etiology on those outcomes.

MATERIALS AND METHODS

Between 1992 and 1999, 145 Delta (DePuy) RSAs were implanted in 138 patients. There were 110 women and 28 men – a sex ratio of 4:1 respectively. Mean age at the time of surgery was 72.4 years (range, 44 to 87). The dominant shoulder was involved in 117 cases. In 7 cases both shoulders were treated. The procedures were performed in 5 centers by senior surgeons specialized in shoulder surgery.

The patients had various initial etiologies, which we divided into the following 3 groups: **group A** – CTA, osteoarthritis (OA) with at least 2 involved cuff tendons, and massive cuff tear with pseudoparalysis (MCT); **group B** – failed HA, failed TSA, and fracture sequelae (FS); and **group C** – RA, fractures, tumor, and instability. Accordingly, 92 prostheses fell in group A, 39 in group B, and 14 in group C. Twenty shoulders had undergone previous surgery: 7 acromioplasty, 5 cuff repair, 7 long-head-of-biceps tenotomy, and 1 deltoid rotation flap.

The approach used was anterosuperior in 50 cases and deltopectoral in 95. All glenoid implants were uncemented, and humeral implants were cemented in 118 cases and uncemented in 27.

Clinical evaluation was carried out using the rating system of Constant and Murley [5] as well as documentation of active shoulder range of motion (ROM). Preoperative radiographs included an axillary view and antero-posterior, double-oblique views in neutral, internal, and external rotation. Radiographs at review included the same views, taken with the help of fluoroscopy whenever possible.

Survival curves were established with the Kaplan-Meier technique and with 95% confidence intervals according to Rothman. **Two end-points** were retained:
- implant revision, defined by glenoid or humeral replacement or removal, or conversion to HA; and
- a poor clinical outcome with an absolute Constant score of less than 30.

Survival curves were both cumulative and segmented according to etiology. Moreover, comparisons of instantaneous survivorship were carried out with the homogeneity test.

RESULTS

At the time of review, 45 patients had died with their prosthesis in place and 2 had died without their prosthesis. Of the 98 living patients, 51 were seen again, 7 were interviewed by phone, and 30 were lost to follow-up. For deceased patients, information on the prosthesis was obtained either from medical records or by telephone from the patient's family. Mean follow-up was 94.5 months (range, 2 to 203), and mean age at review was 79.4 years (range, 67 to 92).

The following **complications** were documented:
- 12 infections, treated with prosthetic removal (6), lavage and retention (4), or no surgery (2).

- 6 dislocations, reduced under general anaesthesia, then treated with a metal augment (2), conversion to HA (1), or no surgery (3).
- 4 glenoid dissociations (by unscrewing), treated with retightening without revision (2), component revision (1), or no surgery (1). Both the latter two cases involved glenoid loosening.
- 6 cases of glenoid loosening. Two occurred early in association with component malposition and were converted to HA, 1 had a reoperation for a glenoid revision 10 years postoperatively, 1 became infected and had a resection, and 2 were not reoperated on because of age or poor medical condition.
- 2 cases of humeral loosening, 1 of which was revised and the other patient died without reoperation.

The survival curve to prosthetic removal showed an **overall survivorship of 92% at 10 years and 84% at 15 years** (Fig. 1). At 10 years, segmentation according to etiology showed a 97% survivorship for group A and 88% for group B (Fig. 2). This difference was not significant (p=0.06).

Twelve prostheses required revision: 5 in group A, 5 in group B, and 2 in group C. Six prostheses were removed for septic loosening, one for early loosening following malpositioning, one for glenoid loosening associated with unscrewing, 2 for glenoid loosening 3 years postoperatively, 1 for humeral loosening, and 1 for pain and notching without loosening (although the glenoid component was revised at 10 years).

The survival curve to a Constant score of less than 30 showed an overall survivorship of 90% at 10 years and 77% at 15 years (Fig. 3). Segmentation according to etiology showed a significant difference at 10 years in favor of group A compared to group B (Fig. 4). There were no significant differences between those two groups otherwise – their main characteristics are summarized in Table I.

The number of patients with a minimum follow-up of 10 years was 58. Mean follow-up for this sub-population was

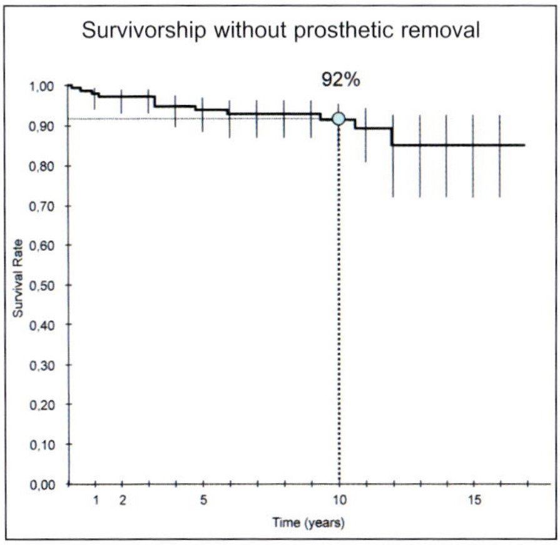

Fig. 1: Overall survivorship of RSA to revision (Kaplan-Meier method, Rothman's 95% confidence intervals).

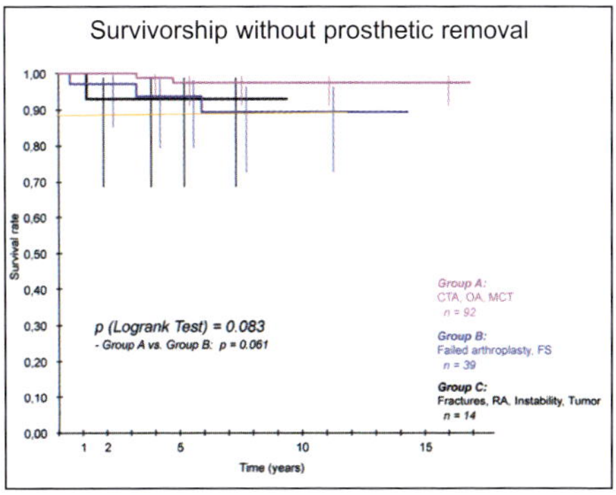

Fig. 2: Survivorship of RSA to revision, segmented according to etiology (Kaplan-Meier method, Rothman's 95% confidence intervals).

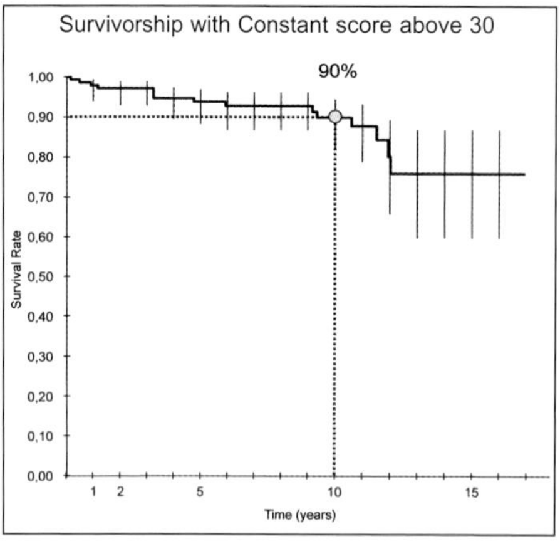

Fig. 3: Overall survivorship of RSA to low Constant score (<30) (Kaplan-Meier method, Rothman's 95% confidence intervals).

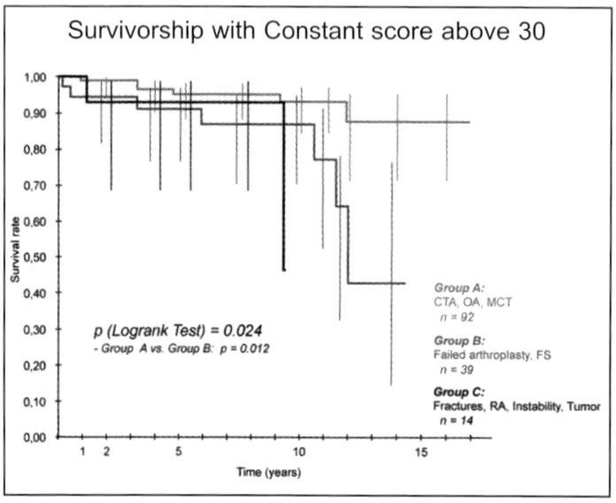

Fig. 4: Survivorship of RSA to low Constant score (<30), segmented according to etiology (Kaplan-Meier method, Rothman's 95% confidence intervals).

142 months (range, 120 to 203). We were able to establish a Constant score at more than 10 years for 51 patients. Among these patients, at the time of this review, 36 were in group A, 15 in group B, and none in group C. At the last follow-up, all parameters of the Constant score had significantly improved. Active ROM significantly improved in anterior elevation (121° ± 30°), but there was no improvement in external rotation with the elbow at the side (2° ± 15°).

DISCUSSION

This study is unique because of its long-term follow-up of more than 10 years. Our results show that the overall survivorship of the reverse shoulder prosthesis to removal is good even 10 years after implantation, in particular if it had been implanted for **CTA, OA**, or **MCT**. However, functional results did deteriorate progressively after 9 years. Group C represented a small and inhomogeneous group that was difficult to compare with the other groups with any useful conclusions. Nevertheless, in comparing groups A and B this study shows an advantage in using this prosthesis in CTA, OA, and MCT.

Table I: Main characteristics of groups A and B. Group A: osteoarthritis, cuff tear arthropathy, massive cuff tear; Group B: revision of hemiarthroplasty or revision of total shoulder arthroplasty, or fracture sequelae. (AAE, active anterior elevation.)

	Follow-up (mo.)	Age	Postoperative Constant score	AAE
Group A	145 ± 23	72 ± 5	57.2 ± 17	125 ± 28
Group B	135 ± 14	70 ± 7	50 ± 17	109 ± 31

The landmark study [14] reporting the results of RSA in the specific context of CTA found similar results, with 89% survivorship at 10 years. Yet, the mean follow-up in that study was only 51 months. In a very similar study, Guery [11] concentrated on the appearance of the survival curve, which showed a break **between 1 and 3 years** representing prosthetic revision and affecting more specifically a group of etiologies other than CTA. In fact, most of the prosthetic revisions occurred during that early period because of either **infection** or **rapid loosening**. Our study agrees with those findings, and the frequency of infection complicating RSA has been reported in other series too [4, 8, 20, 21].

The onset of glenoid problems during the early postoperative years is often the result of either a "technologic" problem, such as glenoid unscrewing, or a technical error, where the glenoid prosthesis was placed in a mechanically suboptimal position. The now-resolved problem of glenoid unscrewing was clearly an important contributor to past failures. It is important to remember that the cases at hand were often the earliest RSAs to be performed by the involved surgeons. The above problems aside, the glenoid-component fixation seems strong and durable, with minimal or no glenoid problems once the initial 3- to 4-year period has passed.

In the Guery study [11], the survival curve showed a second break after the 6th year. This break corresponded to a progressive decline in functional results. We found a similar **break at around 9 years**, also with declining **functional results**. Possible causes for this deterioration are the delayed consequences of radiographic abnormalities [14] and posterior extension of cuff tears into teres minor (with loss of active external rotation in abduction).

As for using this prosthesis in cases of revision of HA or TSA, it appears that caution is required, as this group had the highest revision rate. Pertinent to this problem is the important role played by native bone stock in implant fixation. The survival study presented during the "Nice Shoulder Course 2006" [7] and the study by Wall [20], despite being retrospective and with fairly short follow-up, provide additional information on the relatively high complication risk in cases of RSA for HA and TSA revision. This risk is also significant in RSA for fracture sequelae.

In **conclusion**, our study with a minimum follow-up of 10 years leads to the following recommendations:

- RSA should be reserved primarily for CTA, OA, or MCT.
- Extreme care must be taken to prevent infection and initial malpositioning of the glenoid component to minimize the need for early revision.
- The progressive deterioration of functional results after 9 years highlights the need for selecting the appropriate indications for RSA, especially in younger patients.

REFERENCES

[1] ARNTZ CT, S JACKINS, FA MATSEN 3rd. Prosthetic replacement of the shoulder for the treatment of defects in the rotator cuff and the surface of the glenohumeral joint. *J Bone Joint Surg Am. 1993;75: 485-91.*

[2] BARRETT WP, JL FRANKLIN, SE JACKINS, CR WYSS, FA MATSEN 3rd. Total shoulder arthroplasty. *J Bone Joint Surg Am. 1987;69: 865-72.*

[3] BAULOT E, D CHABERNAUD, PM GRAMMONT. [Results of Grammont's inverted prosthesis in omarthritis associated with major cuff destruction. Apropos of 16 cases]. *Acta Orthop Belg. 1995;61 Suppl 1: 112-9.*

[4] BOILEAU P, D WATKINSON, AM HATZIDAKIS, I HOVORKA. Neer Award 2005: The Grammont reverse shoulder prosthesis: results in cuff tear arthritis, fracture sequelae, and revision arthroplasty. *J Shoulder Elbow Surg. 2006;15: 527-40.*

[5] CONSTANT CR, AH MURLEY. A clinical method of functional assessment of the shoulder. *Clin Orthop Relat Res. 1987, 160-4.*

[6] DURANTHON LD, B AUGEREAU, H THOMAZEAU, E VANDENBUSSCHE, S GUILLO, F LANGLAIS. Bipolar arthroplasty in rotator cuff arthropathy: 13 cases. *Rev Chir Orthop Reparatrice Appar Mot. 2002;88: 28-34.*

[7] FAVARD L, J GUERY, R BICKNELL, P GARAUD, F SIRVEAUX, P BOILEAU. Survivorship of the reverse prosthesis. Reverse Shoulder Arthroplasty. N. C. Shoulder. *Montpellier, Sauramps Medical. 2006: 373-380.*

[8] FRANKLE M, S SIEGAL, D PUPELLO, A SALEEM, M MIGHELL, M VASEY. The Reverse Shoulder Prosthesis for glenohumeral arthritis associated with severe rotator cuff deficiency. A minimum two-year follow-up study of sixty patients. *J Bone Joint Surg Am. 2005;87: 1697-705.*

[9] FRANKLIN JL, WP BARRETT, SE JACKINS, FA MATSEN 3rd. Glenoid loosening in total shoulder arthroplasty. Association with rotator cuff deficiency. *J Arthroplasty. 1988;3: 39-46.*

[10] GRAMMONT P, P TROUILLOUD, J LAFFAY, X DERIES. Etude et realisation d'une nouvelle prothèse d'épaule. *Rhumatologie. 1987; 39: 407-418.*

[11] GUERY J, L FAVARD, F SIRVEAUX, D OUDET, D MOLE, G WALCH. Reverse total shoulder arthroplasty. Survivorship analysis of eighty replacements followed for five to ten years. *J Bone Joint Surg Am. 2006;88: 1742-7.*

[12] LAURENCE M. Replacement arthroplasty of the rotator cuff deficient shoulder. *J Bone Joint Surg Br. 1991;73: 916-9.*

[13] LETTIN AW, SA COPELAND, JT SCALES. The Stanmore total shoulder replacement. *J Bone Joint Surg Br. 1982;64: 47-51.*

[14] MOLE D, L FAVARD Excentered scapulohumeral osteoarthritis. *Rev Chir Orthop Reparatrice Appar Mot. 2007;93: 37-94.*

[15] NEER CS 2nd, KC WATSON, FJ STANTON. Recent experience in total shoulder replacement. *J Bone Joint Surg Am. 1982;64: 319-37.*

[16] PETROFF E, H MESTDAGH, C MAYNOU, JM DELOBELLE. Arthroplasty with a mobile cup for shoulder arthrosis with irreparable rotator cuff rupture: preliminary results and cineradiographic study. *Rev Chir Orthop Reparatrice Appar Mot. 1999;85: 245-56.*

[17] POST M. Constrained arthroplasty of the shoulder. *Orthop Clin North Am. 1987;18: 455-62.*

[18] SANCHEZ-SOTELO J, RH COFIELD, CM ROWLAND. Shoulder hemiarthroplasty for glenohumeral arthritis associated with severe rotator cuff deficiency. *J Bone Joint Surg Am. 2001;83-A: 1814-22.*

[19] SIRVEAUX F, L FAVARD, D OUDET, D HUQUET, G WALCH, D MOLE. Grammont inverted total shoulder arthroplasty in the treatment of glenohumeral osteoarthritis with massive rupture of the cuff. Results of a multicentre study of 80 shoulders. *J Bone Joint Surg Br. 2004;86: 388-95.*

[20] WALL B, L NOVE-JOSSERAND, DP O'CONNOR, TB EDWARDS, G WALCH. Reverse total shoulder arthroplasty: a review of results according to etiology. *J Bone Joint Surg Am. 2007;89: 1476-85.*

[21] WERNER CM, PA STEINMANN, M GILBART, C GERBER. Treatment of painful pseudoparesis due to irreparable rotator cuff dysfunction with the Delta III reverse-ball-and-socket total shoulder prosthesis. *J Bone Joint Surg Am. 2005;87: 1476-86.*

[22] WORLAND RL, DE JESSUP, J ARREDONDO, KJ WARBURTON. Bipolar shoulder arthroplasty for rotator cuff arthropathy. *J Shoulder Elbow Surg. 1997;6: 512-5.*

PATTERN OF LOOSENING OF POLYETHYLENE KEELED GLENOID COMPONENTS IN PRIMARY OSTEO-ARTHRITIS

A MULTICENTER STUDY WITH FOLLOW-UP > 5 YEARS

G. WALCH, A. YOUNG, P. BOILEAU

ABSTRACT

Introduction

Radiolucent lines adjacent to cemented glenoid components are frequently observed following total shoulder arthroplasty. Previous studies have demonstrated that these radiolucencies influence the clinical outcome and are progressive in nature, leading to glenoid loosening. While micromotion at the junction of the bone and cement is thought to be responsible, an accurate analysis of the causes and forces responsible is lacking. The aim of this study was to analyze the long-term radiological glenoid changes following TSA in order to better understand the mechanisms responsible for loosening.

Materials and Methods

Between 1991 and 2003, in 10 European centers, 611 shoulder arthroplasties were performed for primary osteoarthritis using a third generation anatomic prosthesis with a cemented all-polyethylene keeled glenoid component. Full radiographic and clinical follow-up greater than 5 years was available for 518 shoulders. Kaplan-Meier survivorship analysis was performed with glenoid revision for loosening and radiological glenoid loosening as end points. Clinical outcome was assessed with the Constant score, adjusted Constant score, patient satisfaction score, subjective shoulder value and range of movement.

Results

After a mean follow-up of 103.6 months (61-209 months), the Constant score improved significantly ($p<0.0001$) from 30.1 points pre-operatively to 65.2 points at latest follow-up, with all subscores also improving significantly ($p<0.0001$). The active anterior elevation increased from 91.5 to 138.1 degrees ($p<0.0001$), and active external rotation increased from 7.9 to 33.2 degrees ($p<0.0001$). 90.3% of patients were either very satisfied or satisfied with their outcome and the average SSV was 77.1%.

Radiological loosening was found in 166 cases (32%). Glenoid loosening was limited to a complete lucency in 30 cases and there were 136 cases with migration of the component. Three patterns of glenoid component migration were mainly observed: a superior tilt was observed in 52 cases (10%); a posterior tilt was observed in 33 cases (6.3%); and a subsidence of the glenoid component was observed in 41 cases (7.9%). Superior tilting of the glenoid was statistically associated with the following risk factors ($p<0.05$): low positioning of the glenoid component; type of glenoid preparation for the keel (i.e. curettage versus compaction); and proximal migration of the humeral head. Subsidence of the glenoid component was statistically associated with excessive reaming of the glenoid ($p <0.001$) for the convex back prostheses. Posterior tilting of the glenoid component was statistically associated with posterior instability of the humeral head ($p <0.01$) and excessive reaming to correct posterior glenoid erosion. Survivorship with the end-point being glenoid revision for loosening was 99.8% at 5 years, 95.9% at 10 years and 77.5% at 15 years. Survivorship with the end-point being radiological loosening (RLL>12) was 99% at 5 years, 70.1% at 10 years, and 25.8% at 15 years.

Discussion-Conclusion

The three patterns of migration observed in this study underscore the importance of the supporting bone beneath the glenoid component. Anchorage with a keel, or even pegs, may provide rotational stability but cannot resist the compressive or eccentric posterosuperior forces exerted on the glenoid in TSA. It seems essential to maximize the support under the glenoid implant, and therefore we recommend consideration of the following:

- Optimization of the design and size of the implant;
- Limit the amount of reaming so as to not sacrifice the subchondral or sclerotic glenoid bone;
- Reduce the destruction of bone needed for anchorage, i.e. keel preparation by compaction rather than curettage technique;
- Reduce the size of the keel, or the number of pegs, that undermines and diminishes the supporting bone and also increases the surface area available for micromotion and osteolysis.

INTRODUCTION

The radiological results of cemented polyethylene keeled glenoid components are typically analyzed by the presence or absence of lucencies at the junction of the bone and cement. The percentage of radiolucent lines has been reported to range from 0 to 90% depending on the duration of follow-up, the etiology and type of prosthesis [1-5]. These lucencies reflect micromotion at the junction of the bone and cement, but due to the variability in the rates reported, short follow-up less than 5 years and limited series, an accurate analysis of the causes and forces responsible cannot be made. The clinical impact of radiolucent lines has been debated, with some authors believing that they were most often asymptomatic, while others instead found deterioration in clinical outcome [6-8]. Even if the radiolucent lines are not always clinically relevant, their evolutive nature is however accepted by most authors, and they can progress to a complete radiological loosening (continuous lucent line greater than 2 mm) and a migration of the glenoid component (tilt and or subsidence) [2, 9-13].

The aim of our study was to examine specifically the migration of the glenoid component in a large number of cases with the same etiology, primary osteoarthritis, and with a follow-up of more than 5 years. Our hypothesis was that by analyzing the rates and patterns of migration, and considering the influence of different techniques used by different surgeons, we would better understand the mechanisms responsible for glenoid loosening.

MATERIALS AND METHODS

Between 1991 and 2003, in 10 European centers, 611 shoulder arthroplasties were performed for primary glenohumeral osteoarthritis as described by Neer [14] using a cemented all-polyethylene keeled glenoid component with either a flat or convex back In all cases the same unconstrained, cemented, third generation anatomic implant (Aequalis: Tornier Inc, Minneapolis) was used. Cases operated on with a metal-back glenoid component were excluded for this series, as well as cases with bone grafting of the glenoid.

In an effort to obtain a pure series of primary osteoarthritis, shoulders with an inflammatory arthropathy, post infectious arthropathy, neurological problem, osteonecrosis (post traumatic, idiopathic) or post-traumatic arthritis were excluded. Additional exclusion criteria included any shoulder with a history of shoulder trauma (fracture or soft tissue injury), instability (surgically or non surgically treated), rotator cuff tear involving the infraspinatus, or prior shoulder surgery.

Of the 611 prostheses implanted for primary glenohumeral OA, 36 patients died before 5 years follow-up, 37 were lost to follow-up, 20 sent a questionnaire and refused to perform radiographs, leaving 518 TSA in 437 patients (71 bilateral), which forms the basis of this study. The average age at surgery was 67.7 years (range 35-90), there were 68% women and 61.1% were implanted in the dominant side.

CLINICAL ANALYSIS

All patients in this series were evaluated preoperatively with a Constant score consisting of four individual scores for pain 15 points, activity 20 points, active mobility 40 points, and strength 25 points [15]. The absolute Constant score was subsequently adjusted for age and sex. In addition, active preoperative mobility for forward flexion in the plane of the scapula and external rotation at the side was recorded (Table I).

The postoperative evaluation was performed on all shoulders at the time of the latest follow-up or immediately before revision and consisted of a Constant score, mobility evaluation and a subjective patient assessment graded by asking the patients to rate their outcome as very satisfied, satisfied, uncertain or disappointed. Additionally, a subjective shoulder value (SSV) was determined by asking the patient to score their shoulder as a percentage of a normal shoulder [16].

Table I : Preoperative and Postoperative clinical data

	Preop + std dev	Postop + std dev	"p"
Pain (0-15 pts)	3.7 ± 2.4	11.9 ± 3.5	.0001
Act. Daily living (0-20 pts)	7.2 ± 2.9	16.3 ± 4.3	.0001
Mobility (0-40 pts)	15 ± 6.9	29.9 ± 8.3	.0001
Strength (0-15 pts)	4.2 ± 4.8	7 ± 4	.0001
Constant Score 100 pts	30.1 + 12.3	65.2 ± 16.8	.0001
Adj.Constant Sc	40.1 ± 16.5	93.8% ± 25.3	.0001
Act.Forw. Elevation	91.5° ± 28	138.1° ± 33.1	.0001
Act.Ext. Rot. at side	7.9° ± 15.7	33.2° ± 20	.0001
Subjective results		VS= 65.7% S= 24.6% D= 7.9% - UH= 1.5%	
SSV (%)		77.1% ± 21%	

OPERATIVE TECHNIQUE

All TSA were performed via the deltopectoral approach. The subscapularis was tenotomized at the level of the anatomical neck in 434 cases, it was detached from the lesser tuberosity in 80 cases, and an osteotomy of the lesser tuberosity was performed in 4 cases. There were 12 cases with associated repair of the supraspinatus and 381 cases with tenotomy or tenodesis of the biceps tendon.

Resection of the humeral head was performed at the level of the anatomical neck after removal of osteophytes under direct vision. The goal was to respect the original inclination and retroversion of each individual.

Regarding glenoid preparation, there were different techniques used in different centers. Two different techniques of glenoid keel preparation were used according to surgeon preference, the curettage technique as described by Neer [4] and the compaction technique as described by Gazielly [17]. Some centers performed no reaming of the glenoid surface, whereas others reamed generously in an attempt to achieve optimal seating of the glenoid component and a normal version of the glenoid component. The reaming technique was known to be more aggressive in one center, but it was not possible to objectively quantify this except that the percentage of small glenoids used was more frequent and perforation of the anterior cortex with leak of cement was almost systematic (fig. 1). Excessive reaming decreases the amount of available glenoid bone surface area for support and also decreases the depth of bone for the keel slot.

A flat-back glenoid component was used in 217 cases whereas a convex-back component was used in 301 cases.

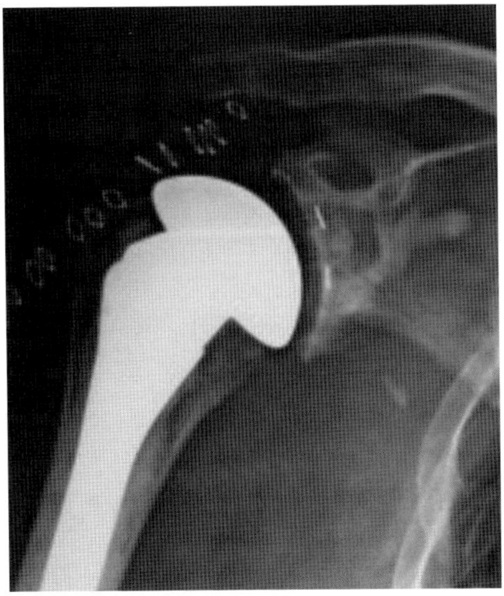

Fig. 1 : Perforation of the anterior cortex with leak of cement. Excessive reaming decreases the depth of bone for the keel slot.

The postoperative immobilization was slightly different from one center to another, but generally consisted of 30 days in a sling, immediate early passive rehabilitation while protecting the subscapularis repair, and active rehabilitation after 45 days. Muscle strengthening exercises were never recommended.

RADIOGRAPHIC ANALYSIS

The preoperative, initial postoperative and most recent radiographs were evaluated. Anteroposterior views in neutral, internal and external rotation, and an axillary view were systematically performed under fluoroscopic control. Radiographs at the latest follow-up were assessed by three authors, two of them being involved in the operations, and one independent observer. The radiographs were evaluated to determine the presence of glenohumeral subluxation, a periprosthetic lucent line and a shift in the position of the components. Glenohumeral subluxation was evaluated according to Torchia & Cofield [6] on the AP view in neutral rotation. The presence of periprosthetic radiolucent lines around the glenoid component was scored according to Molé [18] (0 point for no radiolucency to 18 points for radiolucencies exceeding 2 mm in 6 zones). A score of 0 to 6 points is considered to indicate no loosening, 7 to 12 points is possible loosening, and 13 to 18 points is definite loosening. Any migration or shift of the component received by convention a score of 18 points and was also considered as definite radiological loosening. The type of migration was defined as superior tilt, posterior tilt, or subsidence in the case of medial migration; two of the three examiners had to agree regarding the existence and type of migration.

A preoperative Arthro-CT was available in 369 cases and MRI or Arthro-MRI in 69 cases allowing for analysis of the glenoid shape in the horizontal plan and the state of the rotator cuff tendons and muscle. A partial articular side tear of the supraspinatus was present either on the preoperative imaging or intraoperatively in 9.6% of the cases (42 cases) and a complete full thickness tear in 7.5% (33 cases). The state of the muscles was assessed according to the fatty infiltration method described by Goutallier [19] (Table II).

Glenoid shape in the horizontal plane was classified according to the Walch classification [20]: Type A_1 was present in 115 cases (23%), type A_2 in 116 cases (23.2%), type B_1 in 82 cases (16.4%), type B_2 in 105 cases (21%) type C in 5 cases (1.0%) and was impossible to classify in one case (0.2%).

Table II : Preoperative Fatty Infiltration of the Rotator cuff muscles

Infraspinatus muscle	
Stage 0	
Stage 1	155 (31%)
Stage 2	29 (5.8%)
Stage 3	3 (0.6%)
Stage 4	0
Supraspinatus muscle	
Stage 0	
Stage 1	158 (31.6%)
Stage 2	35 (7.05%)
Stage 3	1 (0.2%)
Stage 4	1 (0.2%)
Subscapularis muscle	
Stage 0	
Stage 1	134 (26.8%)
Stage 2	40 (8%)
Stage 3	8 (1.6%)
Stage 4	0

STATISTICAL ANALYSIS

The differences among subgroups were tested by ANOVA for the quantitative variables, followed by post-hoc Bonferroni tests or Kruskal-Wallis tests (quantitative variables not normally distributed) or by Chi-square tests for Fisher exact test (qualitative variables). The correlations between quantitative variables were analyzed by the Spearman correlation coefficient. Survivorship analyses were performed according to the method of Kaplan-Meier [21]. A statistical regression was performed to analyze the effects of glenoid preparation (curettage or compaction), reaming of the glenoid surface, the design of the implant (flat or convex), age at operation, sex and the operated side.

RESULTS

Five-hundred-eighteen TSA with complete radiographic and clinical follow-up were reviewed at a mean of 103.6 months (range 60 to 219 months). Three-hundred-eighty-three cases (74%) had a follow-up between 5 and 10 years, 109 cases (21%) had a follow-up between 11 and 15 years, and 21 cases (5%) had a follow-up of greater than 15 years.

COMPLICATIONS AND REVISIONS

The most frequent complication was secondary rotator cuff tear but the main cause for revision was glenoid loosening (Table III). Among the 46 revisions (8%) performed at an average of 10 years, 26 (4.5%) were done for glenoid loosening. With end-point being glenoid revision, and with a confidence interval of 95%, the survivorship of the glenoid component was 99.8% [95% CI: 0.994 ; 1] at 5 years, 95.9% [0.937; 0.982] at 10 years and 77.5% [0.675; 0.876] at 15 years (fig. 2).

Table III : Complications & Revisions

	Complications	Revisions
Humeral Fracture distal to the stem	4	2
Humeral stem migration	3	3
Sepsis	4	4
Cuff tear	29	1
Subscapularis rupture	13	2
Anterior dislocation	1	1
Posterior Dislocation	3	2
Neurologic Complication	3	
Stiffness	5	5
Glenoid loosening	26	26
TOTAL	**91 (15.8%)**	**46 (8%)**

The survivorship of the flat back component with end-point being glenoid revision was significantly less than the convex-back (fig. 3).

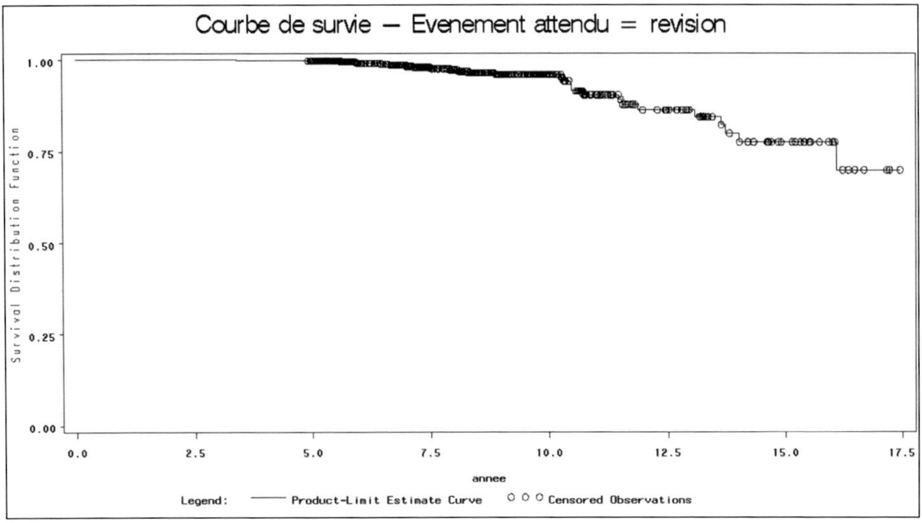

Fig. 2 : Survivorship of keeled PE glenoid component in Primary OA with end-point being glenoid revision.

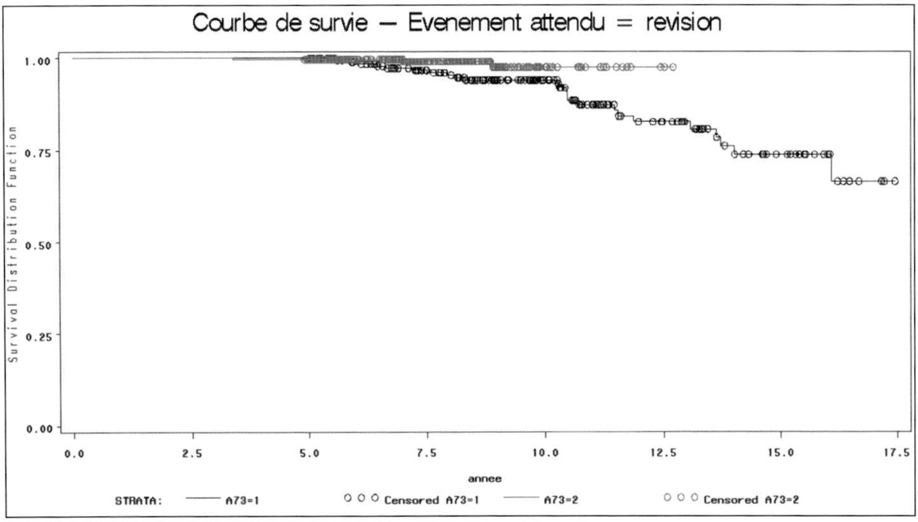

Fig. 3 : Survivorship of flat-back (black curve) and convex-back (grey curve) glenoid with end-point being glenoid revision.

CLINICAL RESULTS

The Constant score improved significantly ($p<0.0001$) from 30.1 points pre-operatively to 65.2 points at latest follow-up, with all subscores also improving significantly ($p<0.0001$) (Table 1). The active anterior elevation increased from 91.5 to 138.1 degrees ($p<0.0001$), and active external rotation increased from 7.9 to 33.2 degrees ($p<0.0001$). At latest follow-up, 90.3% of patients were either very satisfied or satisfied with their outcome. The average Subjective Shoulder Value was 77.1%.

RADIOLOGICAL RESULTS

An anterior subluxation was seen on the axillary view in 18 cases (3.5%), and a posterior subluxation in 25 cases (4.8%). Superior subluxation of the humeral head with regard to the center of the glenoid was observed to be mild in 69 cases (13.3%), moderate in 52 cases (10%), and severe in 37 cases (7.1%).

The average RLL score was 7.97 ± 6.5. There was no radiological loosening (score 0 to 6) in 272 cases (52.5%), possible loosening (score 7 to 12) in 80 cases (15.4%), and definite radiological loosening in 166 cases (32%).

The glenoid RLL score was correlated with the duration of postoperative follow-up ($p<0.0001$) (fig. 4). Glenoid preparation with the compaction technique gave a smaller RLL score than with the curettage technique ($p<0.001$). The type of component (flat versus convex) also had a statistical influence with better results for RLL observed with the convex-back ($p<0.01$). The preoperative shape of the glenoid also had a statistical influence ($p<0.01$), with better results for RLL with glenoid type A_1 and A_2 than B_1 and B_2. The RLL and the loosening rate were also statistically greater if the prosthesis was implanted in the dominant side than in the non-dominant side ($p=0.0008$). The presence of severe subluxation of the humeral head on the latest radiographs was correlated with a higher RLL score (<0.0001). All of the postoperative clinical parameters were strongly correlated ($p<0.0001$) with the RLL score: pain; activity; mobility; strength; Constant score; adjusted Constant score; active forward elevation; active external rotation; subjective results; and SSV.

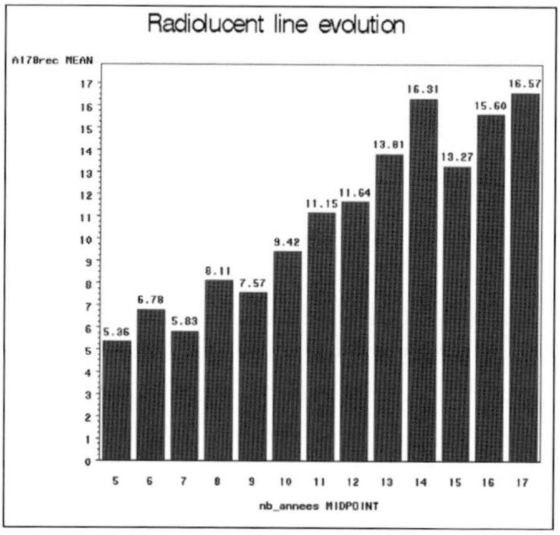

Fig. 4 : Relationships between follow-up and Radiolucent line score.

We did not find any correlation between RLL and any of the following: sex; age at operation; preoperative rupture of the supraspinatus; preoperative fatty infiltration of the infraspinatus muscle or subscapularis; humeral head size; glenoid size; vertical position of the glenoid; and tilt of the glenoid in the coronal plane.

Survivorship with end-point being radiological loosening (RLL>12), and with a confidence interval of 95%, was 99% [95% CI: 0.99; 1] at 5 years, 70.1% [0.65; 0.76] at 10 years, and 25.8% [0.17; 0.34] at 15 years (fig. 5). The survivorship of the convex component was significantly less than the flat-back (fig. 6).

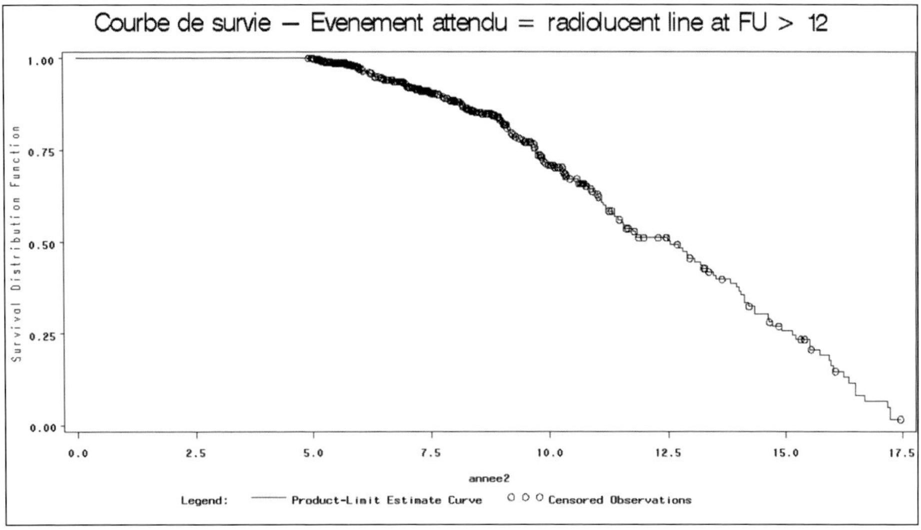

Fig. 5 : Survivorship of keeled glenoid component in primary OA with end-point being Radiological loosening (Radiolucent line >12).

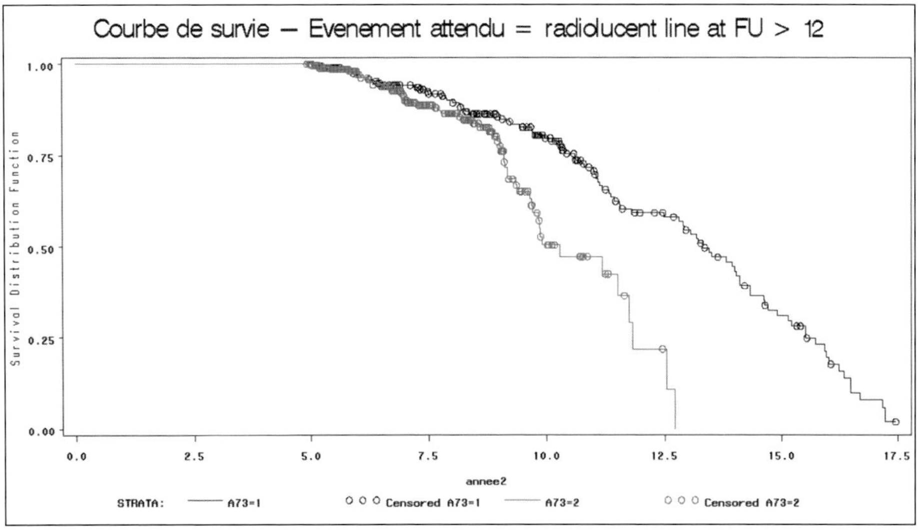

Fig. 6 : Survivorship of flat-back (in black) and convex-back (in grey) glenoid with end-point being Radiological loosening (Radiolucent line >12).

MIGRATION OF THE GLENOID COMPONENT

There were 166 glenoids that had a RLL score of greater than 12 or had migrated. The loosening was limited to a complete lucency greater than 1 mm in 30 cases and there were 136 migrated components.

The migration of the glenoid component was corrrelated with: younger age at operation ($p=0.0076$); increased duration of follow-up ($p<0.0001$); dominant side ($p=0.0019$), preoperative glenoid type B_1 and B_2 versus type A_1 and A_2 ($p<0.0001$); flat back glenoid versus convex back ($p<0.0001$); curettage technique versus compaction technique ($p<0.0001$).

A superior tilt was observed in 52 cases (10%) and was correlated with: duration of follow-up ($p<0.0001$); lower position of the glenoid component on the immediate postoperative radiographs ($p=0.0015$) (fig. 7); superior tilt in the coronal plane on the immediate postoperative radiographs ($p=0.0052$); and superior subluxation of the humeral head ($p<0.0001$).

Subsidence of the glenoid component was observed in 41 cases (7.9%) and was strongly correlated with the convex-back glenoid and the surgical center, i.e. subsidence was exclusively seen in the centers that performed motorized reaming (fig. 8, 9, 10) ($p<0.0001$).

A posterior tilt was observed in 33 cases (6.3%) and was correlated with the preoperative glenoid shape types B1 and B2 ($p<0.001$) (fig. 11, 12).

In 10 cases (1.9%) we observed either dislocated glenoid components (4 cases), anterior tilt (3 cases), or combined complex displacements (3 cases).

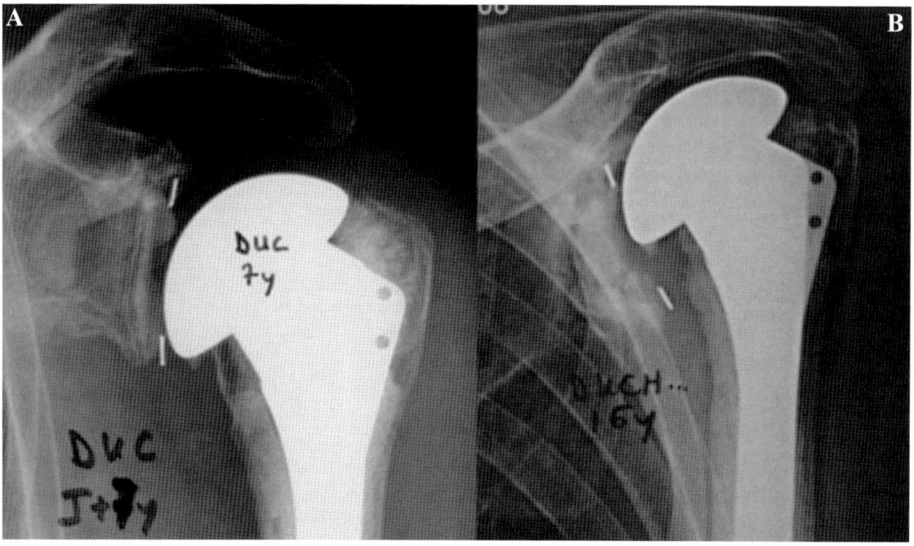

Fig. 7 : initial lower position of the glenoid component (7A) was correlated with secondary superior tilt (7B).

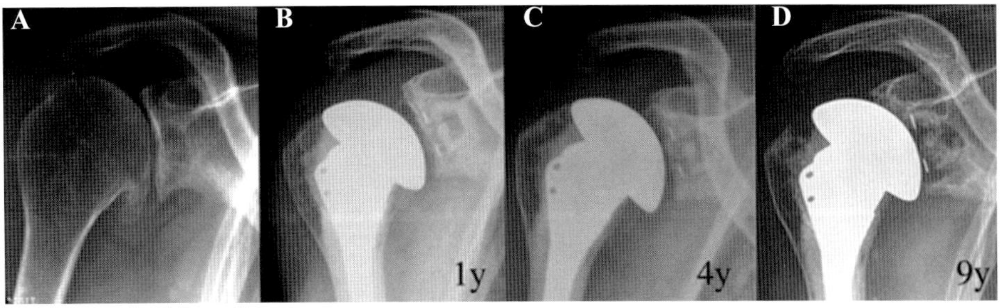

Fig. 8 : Primary OA (8A) operated on with TSA. Initial good radiological result at 1 year (8B) and 4 years (8C) with secondary subsidence of the glenoid component after 9 years(8D).

SINKING IN

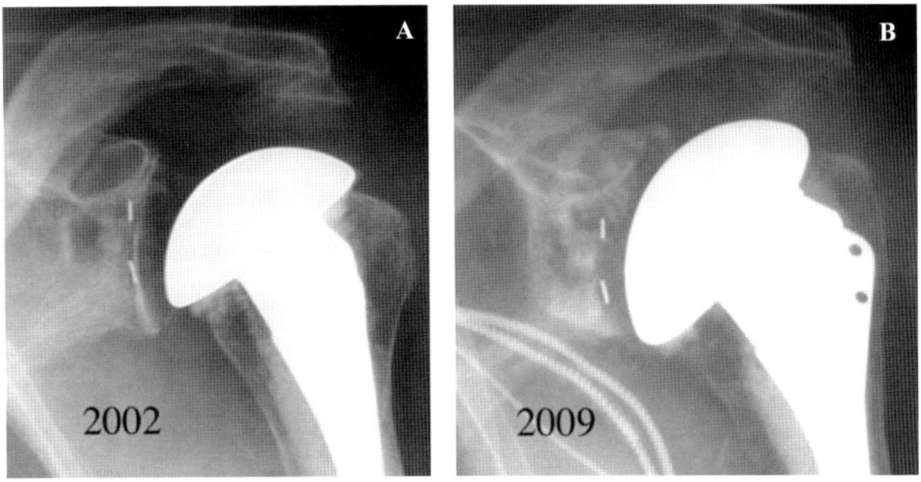

Fig. 9 : Initial correct radiological result (9A) with secondary subsidence of the glenoid component at seven years follow-up (9B).

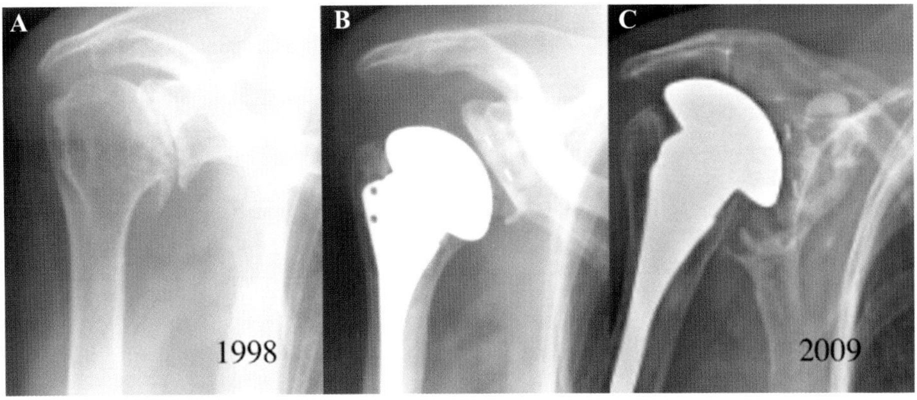

Fig. 10 : Primary OA (10A) treated by TSA with flat-back keeled glenoid component (10B). Excessive reaming lead to secondary subsidence of the glenoid component (10C).

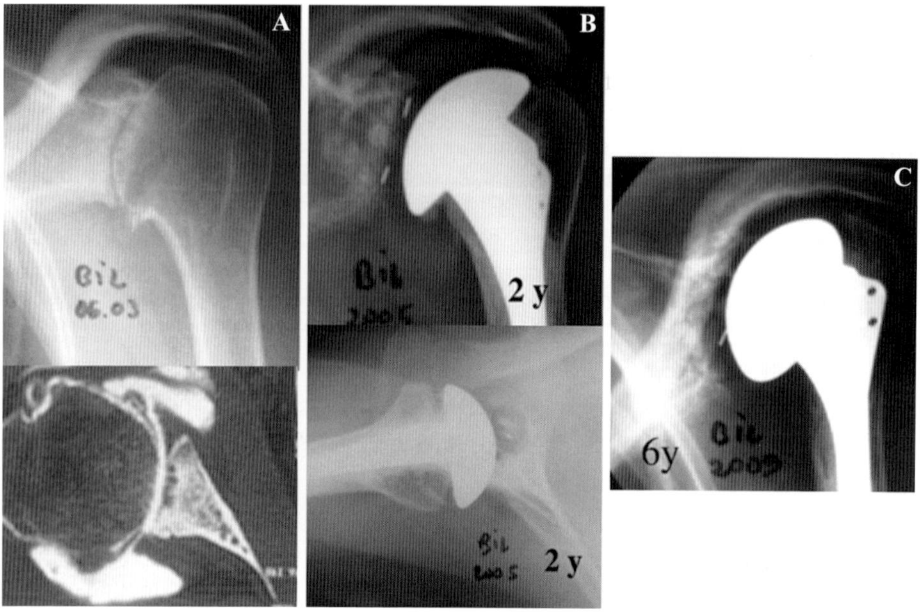

Fig. 11 : Primary OA with B2 glenoid (11A), X-rays at 2 y postop show recurrence of posterior instability of the HH (11B) and radiological loosening at 6 years.

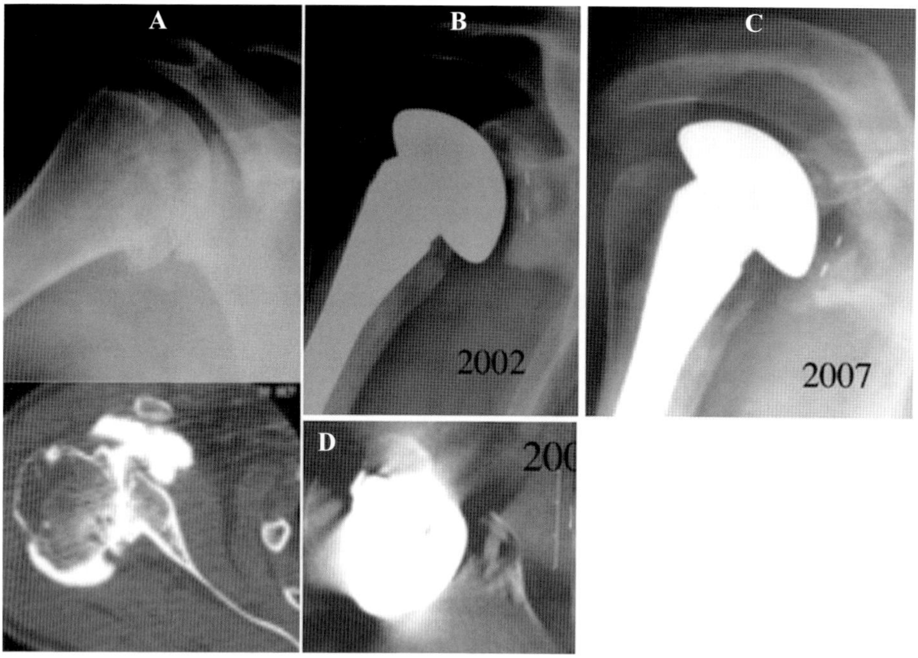

Fig. 12 : Primary OA with B2 glenoid (12A) postop X-rays (12B), and 5 y follow-up (12C) showing a posterior tilt (12D) of the glenoid component.

DISCUSSION

We have reported a series of 518 keeled polyethylene glenoid components implanted for primary osteoarthritis of the shoulder with a minimum follow-up of 5 years. The survivorship without revision for glenoid loosening of 99.8% at 5 years, 96% at 10 years, and 77.5% at 15 years in our study compares favorably with that reported by the Mayo Clinic series for an all-polyethylene keeled component [6, 22]. Survivorship with end-point being radiological loosening in our series was 99% at 5 years, 70.1% at 10 years, and 25.8% at 15 years. The rate of radiological loosening is difficult to compare with the literature as there is no consensus regarding the definition and no survivorship analyses have been published with end-point being radiological loosening. In a report of the long-term follow-up of TSA with the Neer prosthesis, Torchia et al reported definite (19 out of 34 cases) or probable (3 out of 34 cases) radiological loosening in 65% of cases with a diagnosis of primary osteoarthritis at an average radiographic follow-up of 9.6 years [6]. Regarding a series of 64 pegged and keeled glenoid prostheses implanted for osteoarthritis and followed up for an average of 5.1 years, Haines *et al.* [23] reported a Kaplan-Meier survival curve of 78% at 7 years and 46% at 10 years for glenoid components with end point being "at risk" (i.e. lucency of at least 2 mm in all zones or component migration) or revised; the authors found a correlation between radiological loosening and preoperative erosion of the glenoid.

Several factors significantly associated with the development of glenoid radiological loosening have been identified in this series: duration of follow-up; dominant arm; method of glenoid preparation; preoperative type of glenoid; and the design of the component back side, i.e. flat versus convex. However, gender, age at operation, and mismatch did not have a statistical influence. The influence of follow-up confirms that radiolucent lines at the bone cement interface are evolutive in nature. We also confirmed that, although not all of the radiologically loose glenoids were revised, there was a clear statistical association between radiological loosening and the clinical outcome, with all objective and subjective criteria highly influenced by the RLL score.

With a mean follow-up of 103.6 months, 136 glenoid components (26.2%) were observed to have migrated. Torchia and Cofield reported a shift in the glenoid component in 38% of cases in their long-term follow-up of TSA with the Neer prosthesis [6]. Three major patterns of migration of the glenoid component were observed in our series and suggested the underlying mechanisms responsible for loosening:

- *Superior* tilting was seen in 10% of cases, caused by superior translation of the humeral head and the gradual sinking of the implant into the bone. This pattern was favored by pathological ascension of the humeral head as a result of secondary rotator cuff rupture and implanting the glenoid component in a low position. This pattern of loosening has been previously described as the "rocking horse" phenomenon in association with massive rotator cuff tears [24]. We found this complication in a series of patients with primary glenohumeral osteoarthritis without serious rupture of the rotator cuff at the time of surgery. Greater eccentric loading of the humeral head on the glenoid caused by the superior translation of the humeral head required at the beginning of arm elevation explains the biomechanical forces responsible for this pattern [25]. We therefore recommend maximum preservation of the sclerotic subchondral bone in the upper part of the glenoid and use of a glenoid component with a more oval shape rather than pear-shaped to increase the superior bone support and better resist eccentric loading. We now recognize that many of our prostheses that were implanted in the early 1990s had multiple problems: sacrifice of important bone in the glenoid preparation by curettage, low position of the glenoid and pear shaped component.

- *Subsidence* was observed in 7.9% of cases, however it was found exclusively in the centers that used motorized reaming during glenoid preparation for the convex glenoid component. In osteoarthritic glenoids, many patients have lost their normal concavity in favor of a more flattened shape and convex reamers in these cases tend to sacrifice the subchondral or hard sclerotic bone. The preservation of subchondral bone and a solid osseous support appears to be important for resistance against compressive forces. Cement and polyethylene play no long-term role in the resistance to subsidence, only the bone can withstand these stresses over time.
- *Posterior* tilt was observed in 6.3% of cases and was statistically correlated with posterior instability of the humeral head, frequently observed in primary OA associated with glenoid types B_1 and B_2. The eccentric loading caused by the automatic posterior translation [25] of the humeral head also increases the posterior constraints. The reaming that is sometimes necessary in biconcave glenoids to correct the posterior wear and allow glenoid components to be implanted in neutral retroversion adds to bone fragility and likely plays a role in the development of posterior tilt. It now seems preferable to accept a slight retroversion, perhaps up to 15 degrees, rather than to ream and excessively sacrifice the support offered by the subchondral or sclerotic bone. The limit beyond which consideration should be given to using a reverse prosthesis in association with bone grafting of the posterior defect, since the baseplate in RSA transmits compressive loads and not shear forces as experienced in TSA to better stabilize any underlying bone graft, remains to be defined.

These important underlying mechanisms responsible for loosening, identified by studying the migration patterns of the glenoid component in primary osteoarthritis, stress the importance of bone support. The anchorage keel (or pegs) provides rotational stability but this does not resist either compressive forces or posterosuperior eccentric loading. It therefore appears important to maximize bone support during insertion of the glenoid component in TSA, particularly in the upper and posterior parts of the glenoid where the greatest stresses are experienced in raising the arm.

Our specific recommendations regarding the glenoid component of TSA based on the results of this multicenter study are as follows:

1) Optimization of the glenoid component design (greater width of the upper part) and increased size to take advantage of all of the available support offered by arthritic glenoids.
2) Limit the amount of reaming performed so as to not sacrifice the strong subchondral or sclerotic bone.
3) Minimize the amount of bone sacrificed for insertion of the glenoid anchor by reducing the size of the keel and preparation of the slot by compaction

rather than by curettage. For pegged glenoids, decrease the number of pegs that are not essential and unnecessarily weaken the supporting bone and also increase the bone cement surface area exposed to micromotion and therefore osteolysis.

In conclusion, we have reported a 32% rate of radiological loosening and 4.5% rate of revision for loosening of the glenoid component at a mean of 104 months in a series of 518 total shoulder prostheses implanted for primary glenohumeral osteoarthritis. Tilting or subsidence of the glenoid component was observed in 136 cases and has highlighted the importance of preservation of glenoid bone stock, and in particular the sclerotic subchondral bone appears to be the only factor that can resist in the long-term the stresses imposed by the humeral head.

REFERENCES

[1] AMSTUTZ HC, THOMAS BJ, KABO JM, JINNAH RH, DOREY FJ. The Dana total shoulder arthroplasty. *J Bone Joint Surg Am. Sep 1988; 70(8): 1174-82.*

[2] COFIELD RH. Total shoulder arthroplasty with the Neer prosthesis. *J Bone Joint Surg Am. Jul 1984; 66(6): 899-906.*

[3] FIGGIE MP, INGLIS AE, FIGGIE HE, 3rd, SOBEL M, BURSTEIN AH, KRAAY MJ. Custom total shoulder arthroplasty in inflammatory arthritis. Preliminary results. *J Arthroplasty. Mar 1992; 7(1):1-6.*

[4] NEER CS 2nd, WATSON KC, STANTON FJ. Recent experience in total shoulder replacement. *J Bone Joint Surg Am. Mar 1982; 64(3): 319-37.*

[5] RAISS P, ALDINGER PR, KASTEN P, RICKERT M, LOEW M. Total shoulder replacement in young and middle-aged patients with glenohumeral osteoarthritis. *J Bone Joint Surg Br. Jun 2008; 90(6): 764-69.*

[6] TORCHIA ME, COFIELD RH, SETTERGREN CR. Total shoulder arthroplasty with the Neer prosthesis: long-term results. *J Shoulder Elbow Surg. Nov-Dec 1997; 6(6): 495-505.*

[7] SOJBJERG JO, FRICH LH, JOHANNSEN HV, SNEPPEN O. Late results of total shoulder replacement in patients with rheumatoid arthritis. *Clin Orthop Relat Res. Sep 1999(366): 39-45.*

[8] STEWART MP, KELLY IG. Total shoulder replacement in rheumatoid disease: 7- to 13-year follow-up of 37 joints. *J Bone Joint Surg Br. Jan 1997; 79(1): 68-72.*

[9] THROCKMORTON TW, ZARKADAS PC, SPERLING JW, COFIELD RH. Pegged versus keeled glenoid components in total shoulder arthroplasty. *J Shoulder Elbow Surg. Feb 9.*

[10] SZABO I, BUSCAYRET F, EDWARDS TB, NEMOZ C, BOILEAU P, WALCH G. Radiographic comparison of flat-back and convex-back glenoid components in total shoulder arthroplasty. *J Shoulder Elbow Surg. Nov-Dec 2005; 14(6): 636-42.*

[11] WIRTH MA, ROCKWOOD CA, Jr Complications of total shoulder-replacement arthroplasty. *J Bone Joint Surg Am. Apr 1996; 78(4): 603-16.*

[12] YIAN EH, WERNER CM, NYFFELER RW *et al.* Radiographic and computed tomography analysis of cemented pegged polyethylene glenoid components in total shoulder replacement. *J Bone Joint Surg Am. Sep 2005; 87(9): 1928-36.*

[13] BOYD AD Jr, THOMAS WH, SCOTT RD, SLEDGE CB, THORNHILL TS. Total shoulder arthroplasty versus hemiarthroplasty. Indications for glenoid resurfacing. *J Arthroplasty. Dec 1990; 5(4): 329-36.*

[14] NEER CS 2nd Replacement arthroplasty for glenohumeral osteoarthritis. *J Bone Joint Surg Am. Jan 1974; 56(1): 1-13.*

[15] CONSTANT CR, MURLEY AH. A clinical method of functional assessment of the shoulder. *Clin Orthop Relat Res. Jan 1987(214): 160-64.*

[16] GILBART MK, GERBER C. Comparison of the subjective shoulder value and the Constant score. *J Shoulder Elbow Surg. Nov-Dec 2007; 16(6): 717-21.*

[17] GAZIELLY DF. Comment je scelle un implant glénoïdien en polyéthylène convexe à quille avec ma technique de compaction d'os spongieux. *Maîtrise Orthopédique 2007; 162(Mar) : 6-11.*

[18] MOLÉ D, ROCHE O, RIAND N, LÉVIGNE C, WALCH G. Cemented glenoid components: results in osteoarthritis and rheumatoid arthritis. In: Walch G, Boileau P, *eds. Shoulder Arthroplasty. Berlin: Springer; 1999: 163-171.*

[19] GOUTALLIER D, POSTEL JM, BERNAGEAU J, LAVAU L, VOISIN MC. Fatty muscle degeneration in cuff ruptures. Pre- and post-operative evaluation by CT scan. *Clin Orthop Relat Res. Jul 1994(304): 78-83.*

[20] WALCH G, BADET R, BOULAHIA A, KHOURY A. Morphologic study of the glenoid in primary glenohumeral osteoarthritis. *J Arthroplasty. Sep 1999; 14(6): 756-60.*

[21] KAPLAN EL, MEIER P. Nonparametric estimation from incomplete observations. *J Amer Statist Assn. 1958; 53: 457-81.*

[22] FOX TJ, CIL A, SPERLING JW, SANCHEZ-SOTELO J, SCHLECK CD, COFIELD RH. Survival of the glenoid component in shoulder arthroplasty. *J Shoulder Elbow Surg. Nov-Dec 2009; 18(6): 859-63.*

[23] HAINES JF, TRAIL IA, NUTTALL D, BIRCH A, BARROW A. The results of arthroplasty in osteoarthritis of the shoulder. *J Bone Joint Surg Br. Apr 2006; 88(4): 496-501.*

[24] FRANKLIN JL, BARRETT WP, JACKINS SE, MATSEN FA, 3rd Glenoid loosening in total shoulder arthroplasty. Association with rotator cuff deficiency. *J Arthroplasty. 1988;3(1): 39-46.*

[25] KARDUNA AR, WILLIAMS GR, WILLIAMS JL, IANNOTTI JP. Kinematics of the glenohumeral joint: influences of muscle forces, ligamentous constraints, and articular geometry. *J Orthop Res. Nov 1996; 14(6): 986-93.*